Acquired Aphasia

Acquired Aphasia

SECOND EDITION

Edited by

MARTHA TAYLOR SARNO

Department of Rehabilitation Medicine
New York University School of Medicine
New York, New York

ACADEMIC PRESS, INC.
Harcourt Brace Jovanovich, Publishers
San Diego   New York   Boston
London   Sydney   Tokyo   Toronto

Copyright © 1991, 1981 by Academic Press, Inc.
All Rights Reserved.
No part of this publication may be reproduced or transmitted in any
form or by any means, electronic or mechanical, including photocopy,
recording, or any information storage and retrieval system, without
permission in writing from the publisher.

Academic Press, Inc.
San Diego, California 92101

United Kingdom Edition published by
Academic Press Limited
24–28 Oval Road, London NW1 7DX

Library of Congress Cataloging-in-Publication Data

Acquired aphasia / edited by Martha Taylor Sarno. -- 2nd ed.
        p.   cm.
    Includes bibliographical references.
    Includes indexes.
    ISBN   0-12-619321-5   (alk. paper)
    1. Aphasia.   I. Sarno, Martha Taylor.
    [DNLM: 1. Aphasia.   WL 340.5 A186]
    RC425.A26   1991
    616.85'52--dc20
    DNLM/DLC
    for Library of Congress   90-1008
                                                                   CIP

Printed in the United States of America
91   92   93   94   9   8   7   6   5   4   3   2   1

Contents

13
Acquired Aphasia in Children   425
DOROTHY M. ARAM

14
Aphasia after Head Injury   455
HARVEY S. LEVIN

15
The Psychological and Social Sequelae of Aphasia   499
JOHN E. SARNO

16
Recovery and Rehabilitation in Aphasia   521
MARTHA TAYLOR SARNO

Contributors

Numbers in parentheses indicate the pages on which the authors' contributions begin.

MARTIN L. ALBERT (405), Aphasia Research Center, Boston University School of Medicine, Veterans Administration Medical Center, Boston, Massachusetts 02130

DOROTHY M. ARAM (425), Department of Pediatrics, Case Western Reserve University School of Medicine, and Rainbow Babies and Children's Hospital, Cleveland, Ohio 44106

RHODA AU (405), Clinical Neurology, Veterans Administration Medical Center, Boston, Massachusetts 02130

ARTHUR BENTON (1), Departments of Neurology and Psychology, University of Iowa, Iowa City, Iowa 52242

RITA SLOAN BERNDT (223), Department of Neurology, University of Maryland Medical School, Baltimore, Maryland 21201

SHEILA BLUMSTEIN (151), Department of Linguistics, Brown University, Providence, Rhode Island 02912, and Boston Aphasia Research Center, Veterans Administration Medical Center, Boston, Massachusetts 02130

HUGH W. BUCKINGHAM, JR. (271), Program in Linguistics and Department of Speech, Louisiana State University, Baton Rouge, Louisiana 70803

ALFONSO CARAMAZZA (181), Cognitive Science Center, The Johns Hopkins University, Baltimore, Maryland 21218

ANTONIO DAMASIO (27), Division of Behavioral Neurology, University of Iowa College of Medicine, Iowa City, Iowa 52242

HANNA DAMASIO (45), Division of Behavioral Neurology, University of Iowa College of Medicine, Iowa City, Iowa 52242

HOWARD GARDNER (373), Psychology Department, Boston University School of Medicine, and Veterans Administration Medical Center, Boston, Massachusetts 02130

KERRY HAMSHER (339), Section of Neurology, University of Wisconsin Medical School, Milwaukee, Wisconsin 53201

EDITH KAPLAN (313), Departments of Neurology and Psychiatry, Boston University School of Medicine, Boston, Massachusetts 02130

HARVEY S. LEVIN (455), Division of Neurosurgery, University of Texas Medical Branch, Galveston, Texas 77550

LORAINE K. OBLER (405), Department of Neurology, Boston University School of Medicine, and Aphasia Research Center, Veterans Administration Medical Center, Boston, Massachusetts 02130

BRENDA C. RAPP (181), Cognitive Science Center, Johns Hopkins University, Baltimore, Maryland 21201

ALEXANDRA REHAK (373), Department of Psychology, Boston University School of Medicine, and Veterans Administration Medical Center, Boston, Massachusetts 02130

ANTHONY RISSER (73), Neuropsychology Department, Faxton-Children's Hospital, Utica, New York 13502

JOHN SARNO (499), Department of Rehabilitation Medicine, New York University School of Medicine, Howard A. Rusk Institute of Rehabilitation Medicine, New York, New York 10016

MARTHA TAYLOR SARNO (521), Department of Rehabilitation Medicine, New York University School of Medicine, Howard A. Rusk Institute of Rehabilitation Medicine, New York, New York 10016

OTFRIED SPREEN (73), Department of Psychology, University of Victoria, Victoria, British Columbia, V8W 2Y2 Canada

ELLEN WINNER (373), Department of Psychology, Boston College, Boston, Massachusetts 02167

Preface to the Second Edition

In preparation for the second edition of *Acquired Aphasia* each author was challenged to keep the original historical context while updating and adding new concepts and research results developed in the past decade. In some instances this was not possible. A case in point are the chapters by Rita Sloan Berndt and Alfonso Caramazza, who coauthored a chapter on lexical-semantic aspects of aphasia in the first edition but who have written separate chapters in this edition on sentence processing and lexical deficits respectively, reflecting the extraordinary amount of new work that has emerged in these areas.

Several authors have been added. Rhoda Au, along with Loraine Obler and Martin Albert, revised the chapter on language in the elderly aphasic. Alexandra Rehak joined Howard Gardner and Ellen Winner on artistry in aphasia, and Brenda Rapp collaborated with Alfonso Caramazza on the lexical deficits chapter. An entirely new chapter on acquired aphasia in children was contributed by Dorothy Aram. Regrettably, Harold Goodglass did not participate in the revision of his original chapter with Edith Kaplan. The chapter on auditory comprehension is not included in this edition since it was not possible for the author, Karen Riedel, to do a complete revision at this time.

I am indebted to Antonia Buonaguro and John Sarno for their assistance and support in reviewing the revised volume and to Laureen VanOudenrode for her secretarial help.

Preface to the First Edition

During the past two decades, aphasia has been a subject of increasing interest to a variety of disciplines beyond those of speech pathology, medicine, and psychology. Once the exclusive province of the neurologist, to whom we owe a great debt for pioneer work, aphasia is now studied as well by speech and language pathologists, linguists, cognitive psychologists, neuropsychologists, and others. The burgeoning of clinical and academic activity is the primary impetus for this volume, whose purpose it is to provide an authoritative text and reference book for graduate students, clinicians, and research workers in the many fields now concerned with aphasia.

The contents and roster of contributors reflect the view that no single discipline or author can be expert in all of the areas that contribute to our knowledge of aphasia. It is the editor's intent, therefore, to provide to the student of aphasia a comprehensive, almost exhaustive text by bringing together the writing of some of the most prolific and knowledgeable workers in the field of aphasia. Many of the contributors are pioneers in the areas of their special interest. The result is that all aspects of aphasia are treated in depth; indeed, each chapter is a review of the subject under discussion. The fact that the authors come from a diversity of disciplines adds to the richness and authority of the text.

The breadth of the book may also be judged by the fact that there are chapters on artistry and aphasia, aphasia in children, in closed-head injury, and in the elderly, as well as the emotional aspects of aphasia. Topics relevant to a comprehensive understanding of the disorder are included. "Trendy" subjects have been avoided. A textbook cannot be all things to all people, but the experience and sophistication of the authors of this volume have resulted in a work of broad applicability.

Issues and problems, diversity and controversy are liberally represented.

Though the physiology of communication in health and disease remains an enigma at the most basic level, there is a large body of information on the subject reflecting a century of hard work and creative energy. It is another purpose of this volume to provide the student a distillation of that great effort and a thorough review of our knowledge to date.

The volume is logically organized for courses in aphasia. Chapters on the history, anatomy, and nature of aphasia set the stage for reviews of other dimensions of the disorder (e.g., phonology, auditory comprehension, etc.). The "special" chapters alluded to above add to the completeness and uniqueness of the work and reflect the fact that certain populations require different insights and management.

It should be noted that the scope of this volume does not permit a review of the techniques and practice of aphasia therapy. Broad principles have been outlined, but to cover that subject in detail would require another textbook equal to this in length. Aphasia therapy cannot be conducted by formula; it is a process that grows out of the specific needs of the patient and the knowledge and imagination of the therapist.

I am deeply grateful to the authors whose chapters comprise this book. My special thanks to Hanna Damasio for the anatomical illustrations which she created for her chapter, to the patients and staff of the Speech Pathology Service of the Institute of Rehabilitation and Medicine, to Karen Riedel, Eric Levita, and Margaret Naeser for their invaluable help, and to Rae Dorin and Esther Toledo for typing assistance. I am indebted to my father, Abril Lamarque, for his guidance in the overall graphic design, and to Antonia Buonaguro for her dedicated help with all stages of the project. I am especially grateful to my husband, John, for pointing up the need for such a text and for his support, encouragement, and incisive criticism.

NEW YORK
1981

1

Aphasia: Historical Perspectives

ARTHUR BENTON

The origins of aphasic disorder no doubt go back to the distant past. The association between disturbed speech and traumatic head injury must have been quite familiar to all primitive people who enjoyed the gift of speech. In any case, references to speechlessness as a sign or form of disease can be found in the earliest medical writings, for example, the Edwin Smith Surgical Papyrus, an Egyptian manuscript that dates back to 1700 B.C. and that is believed to be a copy of a still older manuscript (Breasted, 1930).

Early Contributions

Aphasia in Greek Medicine

The Hippocratic writings (ca. 400 B.C.) include many descriptions of speech disturbances, usually within the setting of protracted and often fatal illness. However, it is not clear exactly what was meant by such terms as *aphōnos* and *anaudos;* translators have given them various meanings depending upon their context. Thus, whether distinctions were made between aphasia, dysarthria, muteness, and aphonia is not known. A passage in the Coan Prognosis (No. 353 in the translation of Chadwick & Mann, 1950) associates speechlessness following convulsions "with paralysis of the tongue, or of the arm and right side of the body" (p. 248). Another passage in the Coan Prognosis (No. 488 in the Chadwick–Mann translation) states that "an incised wound in one temple produces a spasm in the opposite side of the body" (p. 263). Taken in

ACQUIRED APHASIA, SECOND EDITION

combination, the two observations provide a basis for relating speech disorder to injury of the left hemisphere. There is no evidence that the correlation was made.

Aphasia in Roman Medicine

Some developments during the Roman period deserve mention. The Latin author and commentator, Valerius Maximus (ca. A.D. 30), described the first case of traumatic alexia (Benton & Joynt, 1960). Soranus of Ephesus and other medical writers of the period differentiated loss of speech due to paralysis of the tongue from that resulting from other causes (Creutz, 1934). However, the other causes were not specified, and whether these physicians had in mind a distinction between an articulatory and an amnesic type of aphasia is uncertain. Also during this period physicians and philosophers localized specific cognitive functions in different regions of the brain, more often in the cerebral ventricles than in the substance of the brain itself (Benton, 1976; Pagel, 1958). Perception was assigned to the lateral ventricles, reasoning to the third ventricle, and memory to the fourth ventricle. The ventricles and their connections were conceived as forming the structural basis for a dynamic process in which sensory information is received and integrated in the lateral ventricles, reflected upon in the third ventricle, and placed into a memory store in the fourth ventricle.

Aphasia in the Renaissance

One development during the Renaissance was the application of this schema of ventricular localization to specific problems of diagnosis and treatment. Antonio Guainerio, a fifteenth-century physician, mentioned two aphasic patients; one could say only a few words and the other showed paraphasic misnaming. Reasoning deductively, he ascribed their condition to an excessive accumulation of phlegm in the fourth ventricle with consequent impairment of "the organ of memory" (Benton & Joynt, 1960). Direct surgical intervention to alleviate traumatic aphasia was another feature of Renaissance medicine. Reports describing cases of depressed skull fracture in which removal of bone fragments in the brain led to restoration of speech in the patient were published by Nicol Massa and Francisco Arceo (Benton & Joynt, 1960; Soury, 1899).

The following statement by Johann Schenck von Grafenberg (1530–1598) indicates that at least some physicians of the time understood that brain disease could cause a nonparalytic type of speech disorder:

I have observed in many cases of apoplexy, lethargy and similar major diseases of the brain that, although the tongue was not paralyzed, the patient could not speak because, the faculty of memory being abolished, the words were not produced. (Benton & Joynt, 1960, p. 209)

Later writers made the same point. For example, in 1742 Gerard Van Swieten wrote that he had seen "many patients whose cerebral functions were quite sound after recovery from apoplexy, except for this one deficit—in designating objects, they could not find the correct names for them" (Benton & Joynt, 1960, p. 211). These observations formed the basis for the classification of motoric and amnesic types of aphasic disorder that was made in the early nineteenth century.

Credit for the first explicit, albeit very brief, description of the syndrome of alexia without agraphia goes to Gerolamo Mercuriale (1530–1606). In the course of discussing cerebral localization of function, he cited the case of a printer who had lost the ability to read after sustaining an epileptic seizure. He could still write but could not read what he had written. Mercuriale regarded the deficit as symptomatic of a partial loss of memory (Meunier, 1924).

Seventeenth-Century Contributions

Relatively detailed descriptions of cases that leave no doubt that the patient was truly aphasic are first encountered in the seventeenth century. Two of these case reports are of particular interest. One, published in 1676 by Johann Schmidt, is entitled "Loss of Reading Ability Following Apoplexy with Preservation of Writing." In it Schmidt described a patient who suffered from a paraphasic expressive speech disorder after a stroke. Eventually he recovered oral speech but was still completely alexic. He could write to dictation but "could not read what he had written even though it was in his own hand. . . . No teaching or guidance was successful in inculcating recognition of letters in him" (cited in Benton & Joynt, 1960, p. 209).

The second case report, entitled "On a Rare Aphonia," described a patient with a nonfluent expressive speech disorder and an equally severe incapacity for repetition. She was unable to repeat even short phrases, such as "God will help." Within this context of grossly defective conversational and repetitive speech, however, she showed remarkably preserved capacity for serial speech. Once she was started off, she could recite the Lord's Prayer, Biblical verses, and the like. It was this dissociation that led Peter Rommel, the author of the paper published in 1683, to designate his case as an instance of a "rare aphonia" (see Benton

& Joynt, 1960, for translations of the Latin texts of Schmidt and Rommel).

Eighteenth-Century Descriptions

Many allusions to different forms of aphasic disorder appeared during the eighteenth century. Among them was the first description, in 1745 by Olaf Dalin, of preservation of the capacity to sing in a patient with a severe expressive speech disorder (see Benton & Joynt, 1960, for a translation of the Swedish text).

The 1770 monograph of Johann Gesner entitled "Speech Amnesia" was the first major study of the disorder (see Benton, 1965). It was a landmark contribution on a number of counts. From a clinical standpoint, the six case reports in it provided a wealth of information about such diverse features of aphasia as jargonaphasia and jargonagraphia, inability to read aloud with preserved ability to read silently for understanding, greater impairment in reading one language than another, and preservation of the ability to recite familiar prayers within the setting of defective conversational speech. Moreover, in contrast to most earlier authors, Gesner emphasized that word-finding difficulties and paraphasic speech reflect not a loss of memory in general but a specific type of memory loss, namely, speech amnesia. Finally, and perhaps most importantly, Gesner was the first to advance a theory of the nature of aphasic disorders in terms of "speech amnesia." In discussing jargonaphasia, he insisted that it did not signify a dementia but only a specific type of forgetting. He pointed out that ideation and the memory for words must be distinguished from each other. Ideation is evoked by the perception of physical objects and the action of the sensory nerves. The evocation of words follows ideation, and hence additional neural energy or action is required for it to take place. Therefore, it is understandable that brain disease could impair the memory for words but leave ideation intact so that a patient might be able to recognize an object and know its significance, yet misname it or not be able to name it at all. The physical basis for such a disturbance in verbal memory was a sluggishness (Trägheit) in the relationships among the different parts of the brain.

Thus, in a rather vague way, Gesner advanced an associationist theory of aphasia, which stated that the disorder consisted of a failure to connect a perception or idea with its appropriate linguistic sign. He called the disorder SPEECH AMNESIA, as had his predecessors, but he went a step further by ascribing to what today we would call ASSOCIATIVE PROCESSES. Some 25 years later, Alexander Crichton (1798)

TABLE 1.1

Knowledge of Aphasia in 1800

Clinical Descriptions
  Nonfluent aphasia: Speechlessness
  Fluent aphasia: Anomia, paraphasia, jargonaphasia (Van Swieten, 1742; Gesner, 1770)
  Agraphia (Gesner, 1770; Linné, 1745)
  Alexia without agraphia (Mercuriale, ca. 1580; Schmidt, 1676)
  Preserved capacity for serial speech (Rommel, 1683)
  Preserved capacity for singing (Dalin, 1745)
  Dissociation in reading different languages (Gesner, 1770)
  Unawareness of defect (Van Goens, 1789; Crichton, 1798)
  Lack of emphasis on comprehension defects (Morgagni, 1762)

Theory
  Defective "organ of memory" (Guiainerio, 1481; Schenck von Grafenberg, 1583)
  Defective associational processes (Gesner, 1770; Crichton, 1798)

Neuropathologic Concepts
  Ventricular localization: Fourth ventricle (Guainerio, 1481)
  Disease of the brain

---

expressed the idea with greater clarity. Writing about paraphasic speech, he suggested that this

> very singular defect of memory . . . ought rather to be considered a defect of that principle, by which ideas, and their expressions, are associated, than of memory; for it consists in this, that the person, although he has a distinct notion of what he means to say, cannot pronounce the words which ought to characterize his thoughts. (Crichton, 1798, p. 371)

Table 1.1 presents a summary of the knowledge of aphasia that had been gained by 1800. It is evident that a substantial amount of information about the disorder was available to the well-informed physician or layman. For the most part, this knowledge was of a clinical nature. Little had been written about the basic nature of the aphasic disorders, although brief statements of an associationist theory had been made by Gesner and Crichton. The neurological bases of aphasia remained quite obscure since the primitive state of eighteenth century neuroanatomy and neurophysiology precluded the possibility of establishing meaningful correlations.

Aphasia: 1800–1860

During the first decades of the nineteenth century, further advances were made along all lines: clinical knowledge, theoretical formulation, and neuropathology. A number of clinical studies contributed to knowledge of the phenomenology of aphasia. Osborne (1833) described a highly educated patient with severe jargonaphasia who nevertheless was able to understand oral speech and to read. He could even read foreign languages, and, in contrast to his grossly defective speech, his writing was only mildly affected. Lordat (1843) reported what appears to be the first case of dissociation of language loss in a polyglot. The patient could hardly say a word in French but could speak fluently in his native Languedoc. Bouillaud (1825a) described involuntary echolalia in aphasic patients and called attention to the extreme verbosity of some patients. Marcé (1856) wrote a paper on agraphia in which he showed that the severity of the impairment in writing could vary independently of that in oral speech. He therefore postulated the existence of a cerebral center for writing that was distinct from the center for oral speech. A decade later, Ogle (1867) confirmed the independence of the two forms of expressive language disability and employed the term AGRAPHIA to designate impairment in writing.

More sophisticated theoretical formulations of the nature of aphasia were also advanced. The most important was that made by Jean-Baptiste Bouillaud (1796–1881), who classified aphasic disorders into two basic types, one being articulatory and the other amnesic in nature. Bouillaud (1825a) insisted that it was necessary to "distinguish two different phenomena in the act of speech, namely the power of creating words as signs of our ideas and that of articulating these same words. There is, so to speak, an internal speech and an external speech" (p. 43, translation by author). He then pointed out that "it is not uncommon to observe suspension of speech sometimes solely because the tongue and its congenerous organs refuse the pronunciation of words and sometimes because the memory of these words escapes us" (p. 43). Thus, one must distinguish between "two causes which can lead to loss of speech, each in its own way; one by destroying the organ of memory of words, the other by an impairment in the nervous principle which directs the movements of speech" (Bouillaud, 1825b, pp. 285–286).

The validity of Bouillaud's division of aphasic disorders into an articulatory, apraxic, aphemic category and an amnesic category is still generally accepted under the rubric of "nonfluent" and "fluent" types of aphasia. Lordat (1843) proposed essentially the same classification when he distinguished between "verbal asynergy," or loss of the ability to pronounce words, and "verbal amnesia," or loss of memory for words. His concept of verbal asynergy was based on his observation of cases of aphasia "in which the patient has a clear idea of the words he should utter and in which the muscles of speech are completely free from paralysis" (cited in Benton, 1964, p. 323). Lordat also discussed the relationship between intelligence and language and concluded that they were essentially independent; aphasia was neither a sign nor a cause of dementia.

The problem of the neuropathological basis of the aphasic disorders was first brought into prominence by the anatomist and phrenologist Franz Joseph Gall (1758–1828). His theory held that the human brain was an assemblage of organs, each of which formed the material substrate of a specific cognitive ability or character trait. Among the approximately 30 traits localized in his system were two cerebral "organs" of language, one for speech articulation and the other for word memory, which he placed in the orbital region of the frontal lobes.

Gall's hypothesis that the brain is not a unitary equipotential organ, but instead consists of an aggregate of functionally specialized areas, attracted both loyal supporters and vigorous opponents. No issue was more hotly debated than his localization of speech and language in the frontal lobes, and there was no more ardent champion of the concept than Jean-Baptiste Bouillaud, who marshaled clinical as well as pathological evidence to support the contention. However, Bouillaud's evidence was not altogether convincing, and, in any case, empirical testing of the hypothesis by others did not support it. For example, the clinical pathologist Gabriel Andral (1797–1876) reported on the clinical status during life of 37 patients in whom he had found lesions of the frontal lobes on autopsy. Speech disturbances had been present in 21 patients, whereas 16 had shown no signs of speech disorder. Moreover, Andral had seen 14 cases of aphasia with lesions confined to postrolandic areas and not involving the frontal lobes. He therefore concluded that "loss of speech is not a necessary result of lesions in the anterior lobes and furthermore it can occur in cases in which anatomical investigation shows no changes in these lobes" (Andral, 1840, p. 368; translation by author).

Aphasia: 1861–1900

Paul Broca

The protracted controversy over the validity of Gall's placement of language centers in the frontal lobes was no nearer resolution in 1860 than in 1830, but it did serve a most important function. It provided the impetus for the surgeon and physical anthropologist Paul Broca (1824–

1880) to examine the brains of two aphasic patients who had been under his care during the last months of their lives. The autopsy findings showed that the lesion that was ostensibly responsible for the nonfluent aphasic disorder shown by these patients during life was situated in both cases in the posterior part of the left frontal lobe. At the time, Broca interpreted his findings as supporting the Gall–Bouillaud thesis that the seat of language was in the frontal lobes, and he made no particular reference to the fact that the lesions were left sided. As he collected additional cases, however, his attention was drawn to the unilateral nature of the lesion causing the nonfluent impairment of speech to which he gave the name APHEMIA. Reporting in 1863 on the autopsy findings in eight aphasic patients (Broca, 1863), he noted that all had lesions on the left frontal lobe. He rather cautiously added, "I do not dare to draw a conclusion and I await new findings." The "new findings" were soon forthcoming, and in 1865 Broca enunciated his famous dictum, "We speak with the left hemisphere."

The validity of Broca's generalization was readily confirmed, and the doctrine of hemispheric cerebral dominance for language was born. At practically the same time, a number of clinicians added the qualification that left hemisphere dominance for speech held only for right-handed persons; in left handers the right hemisphere appeared to be dominant for language function.

Broca's discovery led to a major revolution in medical and physiological thinking. From a medical standpoint, aphasia was transformed from a minor curiosity to an important symptom of focal brain disease. From a physiological standpoint, the reality of cerebral localization was established, and this led to a period of intense investigation of functional localization in both animal and human subjects (Benton, 1977; Young, 1970).

The place of Marc Dax (1771–1837) in this history deserves mention. In the 1860s his son, Gustav Dax (1815–1893), asserted that in 1836 Marc Dax had written a paper in which he assembled a mass of evidence to show that aphasia was related to disease of the left hemisphere. This unpublished paper, entitled "Lesions of the Left Hemisphere Coinciding with Forgetfulness of the Signs of Thought," was then published by Gustav Dax in 1865. There followed a minor controversy over whether Dax or Broca should be accorded priority for the discovery of left hemisphere dominance for speech (see Critchley, 1964). Analysis of the question indicates that, although Marc Dax did write the remarkable paper that his son published three decades later, there is no evidence that he presented it at a regional medical meeting in Montpellier, as was claimed (Joynt & Benton, 1964). Apparently the paper remained a private document. Thus, it seems that Dax did discover the special relationship between left hemisphere disease and aphasia about 25 years before Broca's first observation (Benton, 1984). However, he did not make his discovery known to the medical world other than through the distribution of copies of his paper to two or three friends.

The Contribution of Carl Wernicke

When Broca made his localization, he emphasized that he did not mean to imply that all forms of aphasia were related to left frontal lobe disease but only the motoric type, which he called aphemia and which was essentially the same as the articulatory and asynergic types of the disorder described by Bouillaud and Lordat. It remained for a German neuropsychiatrist, Carl Wernicke (1848–1905), to demonstrate that the occurrence of the other major type of aphasic disorder, that is, the amnesic type, was related to disease of the left temporal lobe. In a monograph published in 1874 (when he was 26 years old), Wernicke described the major features of what he called SENSORY APHASIA, now called WERNICKE'S APHASIA. These features were fluent but disordered speech, analogous disturbances in writing, impaired understanding of oral speech, and impairment in both oral and silent reading. The crucial, or at least most frequently occurring, lesion associated with this aphasic syndrome was situated in the hinder part of the first temporal gyrus of the left hemisphere, the region now known as WERNICKE'S AREA.

Wernicke's contribution was by no means limited to this discovery, important as that was (Geschwind, 1967). He pointed out the danger of mistaking sensory aphasia, characterized by disordered speech and impaired understanding, with a confusional or even a psychotic state. He also emphasized the necessity for distinguishing between an aphasic impairment in naming objects from an agnosic (or asymbolic) failure to recognize objects, a point made by Freud (1891) some 15 years later. Moreover, as will be seen, he not only accounted for known aphasic syndromes from the rather simple neural model that he developed, but also correctly predicted the existence of syndromes that had not been described at the time.

The Associationist School

Broca and Wernicke were not only localizationists but also associationists. Like Gesner and Crichton, they thought of aphasic disorders as disturbances in attaching appropriate verbal labels to ideas, objects, or events, with basic intellectual capacity remaining essentially intact. In addition, their discoveries provided a basis for classifications of aphasic disorders as well as schematic models to explain their nature. For the most part, these models depicted the anatomic structures and neural mechanisms that were presumed to underlie language performances. The typical formulation was in terms of interconnected cortical centers that served as depositories for the auditory and visual memories of words and of the movement patterns of speech and writing. Models of this type were proposed by most of the leading aphasiologists of the late nineteenth century, such as Wernicke, Lichtheim, Charcot, and Bastian.

The schema of Lichtheim (1885), an elaboration of a simpler model proposed by Wernicke, postulated the existence of five interconnected cortical centers, four of which serve different aspects of language: a center of the memory-images of the movement patterns of oral speech (M); a center of the memory-images of word sounds (A); a center of the memory-images of the movement patterns of writing (W); and a center of the memory-images of written words (V). A fifth cortical area (C) was designated as a center in which concepts or ideas to be expressed were formulated. Lichtheim was not alone in postulating such a center, but most of the "diagram makers," to use Head's (1926) derisive term, regarded intellectual activity as a function of large areas of the cerebral cortex outside the region bounded by the language centers. The five centers were connected not only with each other but with other cortical and subcortical areas. For example, the auditoverbal and visuoverbal centers were intimately associated with the corresponding cortical receiving areas for audition and vision. Arrows in his diagram indicated the direction of flow of information from one center to another.

Reasoning deductively from his models, Lichtheim predicted the existence of seven major aphasic syndromes. Some of them were familiar to clinicians; others were still of a hypothetical nature. He reasoned that a lesion of Center M would produce the clinical picture of Broca's aphasia as then conceived: pervasive impairment in oral speech expression with preservation of the ability to understand oral speech and to read silently. Writing to dictation and spontaneous writing would be impaired because, according to the diagram, the underlying neural mechanisms involve Center M, these performances being typically mediated by "speaking to oneself." On the other hand, writing from copy, a purely visuographic performance not involving "speaking to oneself," would be preserved.

The already familiar syndrome of Wernicke's sensory aphasia was, of course, produced by a lesion in Center A. In addition to defective understanding of oral speech and defective silent reading, the patient would also show inability to repeat and to read aloud, since the neural mechanisms underlying these performances involve transmission of information from the primary auditory and visual cortical receiving centers to Wernicke's area, in which Center A is located. Oral speech expression would be paraphasic, because the lesion of Center A prevented appropriate transmission of sound-images to the center for speech utterance.

Both Broca's aphasia and Wernicke's aphasia could be classified as "central" aphasic disorders in the sense that they were produced by lesions in the cortical centers in which memory-images or representations were stored. In his original formulation, Wernicke (1874) considered what would be the outcome of a lesion interrupting the connection between Centers A and M (i.e., impairing the conduction of information from Wernicke's area to Broca's area). Because Center A was intact, the patient's understanding of oral speech as well as his or her silent reading would be preserved. Moreover, the patient's oral speech expression would be fluent, because Center M was also intact. Nevertheless, oral speech expression would be disordered, that is, paraphasic, because the break in the connection between Centers A and M prevented effective translation of sound-images into spoken sounds. Wernicke called this aphasic syndrome, which had not been described clinically up to that time and was therefore of a hypothetical character, CONDUCTION APHASIA to distinguish it from syndromes due to lesions in the cortical centers. Lichtheim agreed with this formulation and added an important defining feature to the syndrome, namely, the inability to repeat spoken utterances. Subsequent clinical observation has confirmed the existence of the syndrome of conduction aphasia that Wernicke had deduced from his model (Benson, 1979; Benson & Geschwind, 1971; Benson et al., 1973; H. Damasio & Damasio, 1980).

Another syndrome postulated by Lichtheim concerned the consequences of a break in the connection between the concept center (C) and the expressive speech center (M). He predicted that spontaneous speech would be impoverished since ideas could not reach verbal expression. On the other hand, because the basic mechanisms of speech are intact, strictly linguistic performance such as repetitive speech and reading aloud would be preserved. The understanding of speech would also be spared, since both Center A and its connection with Center C remain intact. The real existence of this syndrome, designated by Wernicke (1886) as TRANSCORTICAL MOTOR APHASIA, has also been confirmed by subsequent clinical observation (Benson, 1979; Benson & Geschwind, 1971; Rubens, 1976).

These were (in rather oversimplified terms) some of the aphasic syndromes deduced by Wernicke, Lichtheim, and other diagram makers from their models of the neural mechanisms underlying normal and pathological language performances. Their approach was notably successful in some respects, and it possessed the merit of linking aphasic disorders with brain function. However, there was general agreement that it was only partially successful in accounting for the diverse phenomena of aphasia and the curious combinations of symptoms often encountered in aphasic patients. Moreover, serious objections to this associationist–anatomical approach were advanced by clinicians who viewed aphasia as being more than a linguistic disorder in the narrow sense and considered that it was as much a defect in thinking as in speech (Goodglass, 1988).

The Cognitive School

The influential French clinician Armand Trousseau (1801–1867) was the first major figure to challenge the assumption that thinking per se is not impaired in uncomplicated aphasic disorder. Attacking Broca's concept of aphemia, he cited cases from the literature and his own practice to show that aphasic patients, whose disability appeared on superficial examination to be of a purely linguistic nature, in fact showed numerous intellectual defects. He concluded categorically that "intelligence is always lamed" in aphasia (Trousseau, 1865).

This theme was then developed in greater depth by the English neurologist John Hughlings Jackson (1835–1911), who may be considered to be the founder of the "cognitive school" in the field of aphasia. Following an earlier brief formulation by the French physician Jules Baillarger (1809–1890), he distinguished between two levels of speech: emotional (or automatic) and intellectual. It is the intellectual level of utterance, involving the statement of "propositions," that is impaired in the aphasic patient, who may show considerable preservation of automatic language in the form of interjections, oaths, clichés, and recurring utterances. Jackson (1878) then pointed out that the basic unit of language is not the word but the meaningful proposition.

> To speak is not simply to utter words, it is to propositionise. A proposition is such a relation of words that it makes one new meaning; not by a mere addition of what we call the separate meanings of the several words; the terms of the proposition are modified by each other. Single words are meaningless, and so is any unrelated succession of words. The unit of speech is the proposition. A single word is, or is in effect, a proposition, if other words in relation are implied. (p. 311)

Thus, the essential defect in aphasia, according to Jackson, consisted of a loss of this ability to "propositionise," that is, to use words in the service of thought. At the same time, the capacity to use words as a form of emotional expression might well be retained. The capacity for propositional speech is an intellectual, not a narrowly linguistic, ability, and consequently the aphasic patient of necessity "will be lame in his thinking" since "speech is a PART of thought" (Jackson, 1874).

A somewhat different formulation of aphasia as a cognitive disorder was reflected in the concept of "asymbolia," introduced by Finkelnburg (1870) to denote a general impairment of symbolic thinking. Such a defect might be manifested in dealing with nonverbal, as well as verbal, types of information, for example, failing to recognize the symbolic import of pantomimed actions, the value of coins, or the meaning of environmental sounds, such as the ring of a doorbell or the bark of a dog. Aphasia could then be regarded as a particular manifestation of asymbolia rather than as simply an instrumental disorder of language.

There was also resistance to accepting a basic assumption associated with the localizational models of the diagram makers, namely, that a limited cortical region, such as Broca's area or Wernicke's area, was the repository of memory-images of speech movements or word sounds. It seemed incomprehensible to some students of brain function that the nervous elements comprising these cortical centers could be endowed with such extraordinary functional properties (Benton, 1976). It was not that these critics believed in the functional equipotentiality of all regions of the hemisphere or denied the facts of clinical localization of lesions, but they were convinced that the diagram makers had fallen into the error of confusing symptom with function. Jackson (1874) made this point succinctly when he warned that "to locate the lesion which destroys speech and to locate speech are two different things."

Finally, the creation by Pitres (1898) of the category of AMNESIC APHASIA, a syndrome characterized by difficulty in naming and in retrieving words in conversation, with essential preservation of the basic expressive and receptive language capacities, posed difficulties for the proposed models (cf. Benton, 1988). Some neurologists (e.g., Mills, 1899) tried to meet the problem by postulating the existence of a "naming" center in the temporal lobe, but this simplistic solution was not taken seriously. Pitres (1895) was also a pioneer in the study of aphasia in polyglots.

An all-but-forgotten early contribution is that of Brissaud (1894) who described dysprosodic speech ("aphasia of intonation") and contrasted it with "aphasia of articulation." Some 50 years later Monrad-Krohn (1947) published his classic study of "altered melody of language." Today dysprosody is an active topic of investigation (Graff-Radford, Cooper, Colsher, & Damasio, 1986; Ross, 1981; Ryalls, 1982; Weintraub, Mesulam, & Kramer, 1981).

Despite the attacks on it, the concept that aphasia was a group of disorders produced by breaks in the connection of objects, events, and ideas with their appropriate verbal signs was the one held by most neurologists as of 1900. However, as will be seen, there was a significant change in thinking over the following 25 years in France and Britain as a result of the influential contributions of Pierre Marie and Henry Head, both of whom were vigorous proponents of the cognitive position and of a unitary theory of the nature of aphasia.

Early Twentieth-Century Developments

Associationist Models

During the early twentieth century, there were further elaborations of the concept that discrete cortical and subcortical centers and their interconnections provided the neurological basis of language functions. Joseph-Jules Dejerine (1849–1917) was a major figure in this development. Among his notable achievements was his demonstration of the anatomical substrate of the syndrome of pure alexia without agraphia and his interpretation of it as a "disconnection syndrome" (see Geschwind, 1965; Lecours & Lhermitte, 1979). S. E. Henschen (1847–1930) undertook a monumental analysis of all the clinicopathological reports in the literature on aphasia and formulated a detailed model that postulated the existence of numerous separate cortical centers for almost every aspect of language function as well as for such allied activities as calculation and musical appreciation and expression (Henschen, 1919–1922). Still another important figure was Karl Kleist (1870–1962), who, on the basis of detailed examination of soldiers with penetrating brain wounds, believed that it was possible to make a precise localization of the cortical regions underlying diverse language performances (Kleist, 1934).

Cognitive Models

The development of explicit cognitive theories of the nature of aphasia was an important feature in the development of thought about the disorder during the first quarter of the twentieth century. In large part this development was due to the contributions of Pierre Marie (1853–1940) and Henry Head (1861–1940). Both of these neurologists viewed aphasia as a single disorder that necessarily incorporated the component of intellectual defect.

The first of Marie's papers on the subject bore the provocative title

"The Left Frontal Convolution Plays No Special Role in Language Function" (Cole & Cole, 1971; Marie, 1906). In it he flatly denied that Broca's area was a center of expressive speech and cited clinical evidence to support this negative conclusion. Specifically, he pointed to cases in which a lesion in Broca's area had caused no speech disturbance and, conversely, cases of Broca's aphasia in which no lesion in Broca's area was found. Subsequent papers in the series vigorously attacked the pluralistic concept of discrete types of aphasic disorder and proposed that there was in fact one basic disorder, the syndrome of disturbed fluent speech expression and impaired understanding of speech known as Wernicke's aphasia. This disorder ALWAYS involved impairment in general intelligence. Marie did not offer an explicit definition of the nature of this impairment. Apparently what he had in mind was the aphasic patient's intellectual passivity and frequent inability to cope with practical tasks that made no obvious demands on the understanding or expression of speech. In consonance with his unitary conception of the nature of aphasia, Marie proposed a single broad localization of the lesion causing the disorder. Later he modified his opinion to some degree, but at the time when he advanced his famous "Revision of the Question of Aphasia," he implicated a single extensive territory that included the posterior parts of the first and second temporal gyri, the supramarginal gyrus, and the angular gyrus.

The work of Henry Head (1926) in England was equally influential in fostering a significant change in attitude about the role of cognitive factors in aphasia. Defining the disorder as a loss of capacity for symbolic formulation and expression, he insisted that it involved an impairment in thinking that was reflected in the patient's nonverbal performances as well as verbal behavior. Consequently, the extensive test battery that he developed for the assessment of aphasic disorder included nonverbal tasks that are not ordinarily considered to be measures of language functions. Head maintained, however, that performance on such tasks as imitating the posture of the confronting examiner, drawing pictures, or setting the hands of a clock involved the manipulation of symbols and concepts and that, therefore, they were valid measures of the fundamental cognitive capacity that was impaired in aphasia.

Another figure deserving mention in this context is Kurt Goldstein (1878–1965), who applied cognitive theory with particular force to the category of amnesic aphasia, with its defining features of impairment in object naming and difficulty in finding words in conversation. Goldstein insisted that these linguistic defects were a direct expression of a loss of the abstract attitude that was also reflected in defective performance on such nonverbal tasks as the sorting of colors and the classification of objects, which also made demands on the capacity for abstract reasoning (Goldstein, 1924). However, his ideas received more attention abroad than in Germany where the Wernicke–Lichtheim model retained its dominant position.

The Modern Period

To divide the history of a topic into periods or stages is necessarily a somewhat arbitrary procedure. I have designated 1935 as the beginning of the "modern period" because this was the year of publication of the comprehensive study by Weisenburg and McBride that generated a substantial amount of new information about aphasia and at the same time provided a methodological model for subsequent investigations.

Cognitive Factors in Aphasia

Weisenburg and McBride (1935) gave an extensive battery of verbal and nonverbal tests to 60 aphasic patients and compared their performances with those of 38 nonaphasic patients with unilateral brain disease and 85 control patients (i.e., without evidence of brain disease). The nonverbal component of their test battery included drawing, visuoperceptual, and block-assembling tasks. They found that, although a majority of the aphasic patients showed inferior performance on varying numbers of the nonverbal tasks, there was considerable interindividual variability: Some patients performed on a defective level on many tests and others performed adequately on all tests. They also found a positive relationship of moderate degree between the extent of the observed cognitive impairment on the nonverbal tests and the estimated severity of the patient's aphasic disability.

Despite their findings that cognitive defects were extraordinarily frequent in aphasic patients, Weisenburg and McBride concluded that aphasia did not necessarily involve impairment in intellectual function since even some severely aphasic patients performed adequately on nonverbal tests. Nor could they support Head's contention that the essential cognitive defect in aphasia was a disturbance of symbolic thinking, since in many instances defective performance did not seem to be related to faulty symbolic understanding or formulation. On the other hand, they emphasized the considerable variation in performance from case to case and ascribed at least a part of this variability to differences in the role of language in the thinking of different individuals. As they phrased it:

> It cannot be doubted that verbal symbols and language formulations have permeated mental functioning to a far greater extent in some persons than in others, and that the more firmly established they are as types of reactions and means of attacking problems the greater will be the consequences of the language disorder. (Weisenburg & McBride, 1935, p. 461)

Thus, the premorbid intellectual makeup of an aphasic patient was invoked as a possible determinant of the cognitive changes observed in association with his or her linguistic disability. Weisenburg and McBride also insisted that the "definition of the changes in intelligence in aphasia must be determined in the individual case, with due regard not only for the decreased efficiency but for the qualitative characteristics of the changes" (p. 462).

Subsequent studies of cognitive function in aphasia generally followed the pattern established by Weisenburg and McBride of comparing the performances of aphasics with those of nonaphasic patients with unilateral brain disease and control patients or normal subjects. These studies produced a broad spectrum of results that did not permit a simple interpretation and that confirmed the position of Weisenburg and McBride that interindividual variability is an overriding feature of the performances of aphasic patients.

A number of studies have utilized the Wechsler–Bellevue Scales (Wechsler, 1944) and the Wechsler Adult Intelligence Scale (Wechsler, 1958) to assess the intelligence of aphasic patients. In line with expectations, the patient's Verbal Scale IQs were generally lower than their Performance Scale IQs. The majority of patients had subnormal Performance Scale IQs as well, testifying to a decline in intellectual function that extended beyond strictly linguistic performances. Alajouanine and Lhermitte (1965) reported that 25% of a group of unselected aphasic patients had a Performance Scale IQ of 79 or lower. Orgass, Hartje, Kerchensteiner, and Poeck (1972) found the mean Wechsler Performance Scale IQ of a group of 30 aphasic patients to be 79, which is far below normal standards. However, interindividual variation was wide, the scores ranging from an IQ of 50, indicative of frank dementia, to an IQ of 113, reflecting intactness of the cognitive skills measured by the performance scale.

Symbolic thinking and abstract reasoning have been studied on the assumption that these capacities are particularly likely to be impaired in patients with aphasic disorder (Bay, 1962, 1964; Goldstein, 1948). Classification tests, such as color and object sorting (Goldstein & Scheerer, 1941), and Raven's Progressive Matrices (1938, 1963) have been among the tasks utilized to investigate the issue. The results have been much the same as those found in studies of nonverbal "intelligence" with the

Wechsler scales. Defective performance was shown by many aphasic patients, whereas most nonaphasic patients with left hemisphere disease performed normally (Basso, De Renzi, Faglioni, Scotti, & Spinnler, 1973; Colonna & Faglioni, 1966; De Renzi, Faglioni, Savoiardo, & Vignolo, 1966; De Renzi, Faglioni, Scotti, & Spinnler, 1972). However, interindividual variability was high, and the correlation between performance level and the severity of the aphasic disorder, as measured by naming ability and level of oral language comprehension, was never high and indeed sometimes absent (Basso et al., 1973). Thus, the general conclusion has been that the inferior performances of some aphasic patients cannot be ascribed simply to their language impairment.

Other types of cognitive deficit have been found to occur with notable frequency in aphasic patients, particularly those with defects in oral and written language comprehension. Among these are impairment in facial discrimination (Benton, 1980; Hamsher, Levin, & Benton, 1979), constructional apraxia (Benton, 1973), and defective grasp of the meaning of pantomimed actions (Duffy, Duffy, & Pearson, 1975; Varney, 1978).

Neurolinguistics

An important development in recent decades has been a concerted effort to describe in precise terms the alterations of speech shown by aphasic patients and to relate these changes to the anatomic substrate of the disorder as well as to the cognitive status of aphasic patients. Dealing with such disturbances as AGRAMMATISM, PARAGRAMMATISM, "word-finding disturbance," and SYNTACTIC APHASIA, this effort obviously required expertise in the field of linguistics. As a consequence, a number of linguists became actively engaged in the undertaking, which has come to be known as NEUROLINGUISTICS.

Although some neurologists and psychologists (e.g., Alajouanine, Ombredane, & Durand, 1939; Kleist, 1934; Ombredane, 1926, 1933; Pick, 1913) had dealt with neurolinguistic problems in earlier years, the seminal figure in the field was Roman Jakobson. His monograph (Jakobson, 1941) comparing the phonemic disturbances in the utterances of aphasic patients to the speech of children and relating both to more general aspects of phonology had a profoundly stimulating effect on subsequent investigative work. Even more important was the fundamental distinction that he made between disorders of "similarity" or selection and disorders of "contiguity" or combination in aphasic speech (Jakobson, 1956). Word-finding difficulties, anomia, and paraphasic utterances reflect impairment of the similarity component in normal speech, that is, application of the appropriate verbal symbol to an idea or intention.

Telegraphic speech and defective syntactic utterances reflect impairment of the contiguity component of normal speech, that is, the temporal organization of words into meaningful, syntactically correct propositions. Jakobson maintained that these two distinctive processes constituted fundamental dimensions along which the speech of aphasics could be classified.

Subsequent research in neurolinguistics followed the lines of Jakobson's thinking and expanded beyond it to address other problems. One important advance was the demonstration of the nature and significance of the fluency–nonfluency dimension in aphasic speech (Benson, 1967; Goodglass, Quadfasel, & Timberlake, 1964; Kerchensteiner, Poeck, & Brunner, 1972; Wagenaar, Snow, & Prins, 1975). This dimension, which had been described by Bouillaud, Jackson, and Wernicke, and which is related in some respects to Jakobson's dichotomy, has been shown to have a bimodal distribution so that a majority of aphasic patients can be validly classified as "fluent" or "nonfluent." Among other linguistic topics that have been the subject of study are agrammatism and paragrammatism (Cohen & Hécaen, 1965; Goodglass & Mayer, 1958), the analysis and measurement of disorders of auditory comprehension (Boller & Dennis, 1979; De Renzi & Vignolo, 1962; Goodglass, Gleason, & Hyde, 1970; Orgass & Poeck, 1966), the stylistic analysis of aphasic speech (Spreen & Wachal, 1973; Wachal & Spreen, 1973), and disturbances in reading (Lesser, 1978; Marshall & Newcombe, 1966; Newcombe & Marshall, 1981). During the past decade these efforts have increased greatly in scope and have led to the establishment of the new field of COGNITIVE NEUROLINGUISTICS.

Anatomical Basis of Aphasia

The extreme localizationist approach to the "anatomy" of the aphasic disorders was carried forth by the California neurologist Joannes Nielsen (1890–1969), whose thinking followed the lines laid down by Henschen (1919–1922) and Poetzl (1928). His monograph (Nielsen, 1936) appeared at a time when concern with identifying the neural mechanisms underlying language function and language disorder had diminished somewhat from that of earlier decades. Interest in the area revived after World War II, however, with the expanded opportunities for study afforded by the large number of casualties produced by that conflict and by advances in the development of neuroradiologic diagnostic procedures.

One topic that engaged the attention of researchers was the question of the relationship between hand preference and hemispheric cerebral "dominance" for language. The rule that the relationship between handedness and the cerebral hemisphere controlling language function was symmetric in nature (i.e., that the "language" hemisphere was opposite in side to the preferred hand) was accepted for many decades after its original formulation in the 1860s. The generalization was first questioned by Chesher (1936), who pointed out that "crossed" aphasia (i.e., following a lesion in the hemisphere IPSILATERAL to the preferred hand) occurred with too high a frequency in left-handed patients to be considered exceptional. Chesher concluded that hemispheric specialization for language in these patients must be different in nature from that in right-handed patients. Subsequent studies by Conrad (1949), Goodglass and Quadfasel (1954), Humphrey and Zangwill (1952), and Russell and Espir (1961) of aphasic and nonaphasic patients with unilateral brain lesions demonstrated conclusively that hemispheric specialization differed markedly in right handers and left handers. For example, Russell and Espir recorded the side of lesion in 189 right-handed and 13 left-handed patients who presented an aphasic disorder after having sustained a unilateral penetrating brain wound. Of the 189 right handers, 186 proved to have a left hemisphere lesion and only 3 (1.6%) had a right hemisphere wound, indicating the rarity of crossed aphasia in right-handed persons. Of the 13 left handers, however, 9 (69%) had left-hemisphere wounds and 4 (31%) had right-hemisphere wounds. Thus, they confirmed the earlier findings of Conrad and others that the traditional rule linking the language hemisphere with hand preference held for right handers but not for left handers, who were at least as likely to be left-hemisphere dominant as right-hemisphere dominant for speech. Furthermore, a number of observers recorded their impression that aphasic disorders tended to be milder and more transient in left handers and inferred from this that some left handers have bilateral representation of language functions (Hécaen & de Ajuriaguerra, 1963; Subirana, 1969), a conclusion that was supported by Milner, Branch, and Rasmussen (1966), who showed that a small proportion of left handers were rendered aphasic after pharmacologic inactivation of EITHER hemisphere by the Wada test (Wada & Rasmussen, 1960).

At the same time, it became clear that the mediation of language function in right-handed persons is not an exclusive property of the left hemisphere and that the right hemisphere also possesses some linguistic capabilities, however limited they may be. Gazzaniga and Sperry (1967; Gazzaniga, 1970) showed that some patients who had undergone section of the corpus callosum for relief of intractable epilepsy could understand the meaning of simple words presented in the left visual field although they were unable to read the words aloud. Since the visuoverbal information was processed by the disconnected right hemisphere, it was reasonable to infer that the successful recognition of the meaning of the words was mediated by neural mechanisms in that hemisphere. Even more convincing evidence that the right hemisphere does possess some capacity to mediate language was furnished by Smith (1966; Burkland & Smith, 1977) in studies of right-handed patients who had undergone complete left hemispherectomy in an effort to arrest the growth of malignant cerebral neoplasm. Although both of the patients studied were severely aphasic postoperatively, they nevertheless showed some ability to respond appropriately to oral and written verbal commands and some expressive speech. Similar findings were reported by Gott (1973) in her study of a 12-year-old girl who had undergone complete left hemispherectomy at the age of 10 years.

A first step toward achieving some degree of understanding of the anatomical basis of hemispheric cerebral dominance for language was made by Geschwind and Levitsky (1970), who demonstrated that the planum temporale, that is, the superior surface of the posterior temporal lobe, is larger on the left side than on the right in a majority of human brains. This morphological asymmetry of an area involved in the mediation of language function was, of course, consistent with the rule of left hemisphere dominance. Wada (1967; Wada, Clarke, & Hamm, 1975; Witelson & Pallie, 1973) found that this hemispheric difference is already evident in infant brains, and subsequent studies showed that there are interhemispheric architectonic differences (Galaburda, Sanides, & Geschwind, 1978) and physiologic differences as well (Gur et al., 1983).

A path-breaking and influential paper by Geschwind (1965), in which agnosic, apraxic, and aphasic disorders were interpreted as products of neural disconnection, provided the impetus for a fresh approach to the anatomical study of aphasic syndromes. Investigative work employing modifications and refinements of his basic approach includes studies of conduction aphasia (Benson et al., 1973; H. Damasio & Damasio, 1980), mixed transcortical aphasia (Geschwind, Quadfasel, & Segarra, 1968), transcortical motor aphasia (Rubens, 1976), and the subcortical aphasias (Cappa & Vignolo, 1979; A. R. Damasio, Damasio, Rizzo, Varney, & Gersh, 1982; Graff-Radford, Eslinger, Damasio, & Yamada, 1984; Mohr, 1983; Naeser, 1983).

References

Alajouanine, T., & Lhermitte, F. (1965). Non-verbal communication in aphasia. In A. V. S. de Rueck & M. O'Connor (Eds.), *Disorders of language*. Boston, MA: Little, Brown.

Alajouanine, T., Ombredane, A., & Durand, M. (1939). *Le syndrome de désintégration phonétique dans l'aphasie*. Paris: Masson.

Andral, G. (1840). *Clinique médicale* (4th ed.). Paris: Fortin, Masson et Cie.

Basso, A., De Renzi, E., Faglioni, P., Scotti, G., & Spinnler, H. (1973). Neuropsychological evidence for the existence of cerebral areas critical to the performance of intelligence tests. *Brain, 96,* 715–728.

Bay, E. (1962). Aphasia and non-verbal disorders of language. *Brain, 85,* 411–426.

Bay, E. (1964). Classifications and concepts of aphasia. In A. V. S. de Rueck & M. O'Connor (Eds.), *Disorders of language.* Boston, MA: Little, Brown.

Benson, D. F. (1967). Fluency in aphasia: Correlation with radioactive scan localization. *Cortex, 3,* 258–271.

Benson, D. F. (1979). *Aphasia, alexia and agraphia.* New York: Churchill-Livingstone.

Benson, D. F., & Geschwind, N. (1971). Aphasia and related cortical disturbances. In A. B. Baker & L. H. Baker (Eds.), *Clinical neurology.* New York: Harper.

Benson, D. F., Sheremata, W. A., Buchard, R., Segarra, J., Price, D., & Geschwind, N. (1973). Conduction aphasia. *Archives of Neurology (Chicago), 28,* 339–346.

Benton, A. L. (1964). Contributions to aphasia before Broca. *Cortex, 1,* 314–327.

Benton, A. L. (1965). J. A. P. Gesner on aphasia. *Medical History, 9,* 54–60.

Benton, A. L. (1973). Visuoconstructive disability in patients with cerebral disease: Its relationship to side of lesion and aphasic disorder. *Documenta Ophthalmologica, 34,* 67–76.

Benton, A. L. (1976). Historical development of the concept of hemispheric cerebral dominance. In S. F. Spicker & H. T. Engelhardt, Jr. (Eds.), *Philosophical dimensions of the neuromedical sciences.* Dordrecht, Holland: Reidel.

Benton, A. L. (1977). The interplay of experimental and clinical approaches in brain lesion research. In S. Finger (Ed.), *Recovery from brain damage: Research and theory.* New York: Plenum.

Benton, A. L. (1980). The neuropsychology of facial recognition. *American Psychologist, 35,* 176–186.

Benton, A. L. (1984). Hemispheric dominance before Broca. *Neuropsychologia, 22,* 807–811.

Benton, A. L. (1988). Pitres and amnesic aphasia. *Aphasiology, 2,* 209–214.

Benton, A. L., & Joynt, R. J. (1960). Early descriptions of aphasia. *Archives of Neurology (Chicago), 3,* 205–221.

Boller, F., & Dennis, M. (1979). *Auditory comprehension: Clinical and experimental studies with the Token Test.* New York: Academic Press.

Bouillaud, J. B. (1825a). Recherches cliniques propers à démontrer que la perte de la parole correspond à la lésion des lobules antérieurs du cerveau. *Archives Générales de Médecine, 8,* 25–45.

Bouillaud, J. B. (1825b). *Traite clinique et physiologique de l'encéphalite.* Paris: Baillière et Fils.

Breasted, J. H. (1930). *The Edwin Smith surgical papyrus.* Chicago, IL: University of Chicago Press.

Brissaud, E. (1894). Sur l'aphasie d'articulation et l'aphasie d'intonation. *Semaine Médicale, 14,* 341–343.

Broca, P. (1863). Localisation des fonctions cérébrales: Siège du langage articulé. *Bulletin de la Société d'Anthropologie, 4,* 200–203.

Broca, P. (1865). Du siège de la faculté du langage articulé. *Bulletin de la Société d'Anthropologie, 6,* 337–393.

Burkland, C. W., & Smith, A. (1977). Language and the cerebral hemispheres. *Neurology, 27,* 627–633.

Cappa, S. F., & Vignolo, L. A. (1979). "Transcortical" features of aphasia following left thalamic hemorrhage. *Cortex, 15,* 121–130.

Chadwick, J., & Mann, W. N. (1950). *The medical works of Hippocrates.* Oxford: Blackwell.

Chesher, E. C. (1936). Some observations concerning the relationship of handedness to the language mechanism. *Bulletin of the Neurological Institute of New York, 4,* 556–562.

Cohen, D., & Hécaen, H. (1965). Remarques neurolinguistiques sur un cas d'agrammatisme. *Journal de Psychologie Normale et Pathologique, 62,* 273–296.

Cole, M. F., & Cole, M. (1971). *Pierre Marie's papers on speech disorders.* New York: Hafner.

Colonna, A., & Faglioni, P. (1966). The performance of hemisphere damaged patients on spatial intelligence tests. *Cortex, 2,* 293–307.

Conrad, K. (1949). Ueber aphasische Sprachstoerungen bei hirnverletzten Linkshaendern. *Nervenarzt, 20,* 148–154.

Creutz, W. (1934). *Die Neurologie des 1.-7. Jahrhunderts n. Chr.: Eine historisch-neurologische Studie.* Leipzig: Thieme.

Crichton, A. (1798). *An inquiry into the nature and origin of mental derangement.* London: T. Cadell, Jr. & W. Davies.

Critchley, M. (1965). Dax's law. *International Journal of Neurology, 4,* 199–206.

Damasio, A. R., Damasio, H., Rizzo, M., Varney, N., & Gersh, F. (1982). Aphasia with nonhemorrhagic lesions in the basal ganglia and internal capsule. *Archives of Neurology (Chicago), 39,* 15–20.

Damasio, H., & Damasio, A. R. (1980). The anatomical basis of conduction aphasia. *Brain, 103,* 337–350.

De Renzi, E., Faglioni, P., Savoiardo, M., & Vignolo, L. A. (1966). The influence of aphasia and of the hemispheric side of lesion on abstract thinking. *Cortex, 2,* 399–420.

De Renzi, E., Faglioni, P., Scotti, G., & Spinnler, H. (1972). Impairment of color sorting behavior after hemispheric damage: An experimental study with the Holmgren skein test. *Cortex, 8,* 147–163.

De Renzi, E., & Vignolo, L. A. (1962). The Token Test: A sensitive test to detect receptive disturbances in aphasics. *Brain, 85,* 665–678.

Duffy, R., Duffy, J., & Pearson, K. (1975). Pantomime recognition in aphasic patients. *Journal of Speech and Hearing Research, 18,* 115–132.

Finkelnburg, F. C. (1870). Niederrheinische Gesellschaft: Sitzung von 21 März 1870 in Bonn. *Berliner Klinischer Wochenschrift, 7,* 449–450, 460–462. (Also published as: Finkelnburg's 1870 lecture on aphasia with commentary, R. J. Duffy & B. Z. Liles [Trans.], *Journal of Speech and Hearing Disorders,* 1979, *44,* 156–168.)

Freud, S. (1891). *Zur Auffassung der Aphasien.* Leipzig & Vienna: Deuticke. (Also published as: *On aphasia,* E. Stengel [Trans.]. New York: International Universities Press, 1953.)

Galaburda, A. M., Sanides, F., & Geschwind, N. (1978). Human brain: Cytoarchitectonic right-left asymmetries in the temporal speech region. *Archives of Neurology (Chicago), 35,* 812–817.

Gazzaniga, M. S. (1970). *The bisected brain.* New York: Appleton.

Gazzaniga, M. S., & Sperry, R. W. (1967). Language after section of the cerebral commissures. *Brain, 90,* 131–148.

Geschwind, N. (1965). Disconnexion syndromes in animals and man. *Brain, 88,* 237–294, 585–644.

Geschwind, N. (1967). Wernicke's contribution to the study of aphasia. *Cortex, 3,* 449–463.

Geschwind, N., & Levitsky, W. (1970). Human brain: Left-right asymmetries in temporal speech region. *Science, 161,* 186–187.

Geschwind, N., Quadfasel, F. A., & Segarra, J. M. (1968). Isolation of the speech area. *Neuropsychologia, 6,* 327–340.

Goldstein, K. (1924). Das Wesen der amnestischen Aphasie. *Schweizer Archiv fuer Neurologie und Psychiatrie, 15,* 163–175.

Goldstein, K. (1948). *Language and language disturbances.* New York: Grune & Stratton.

Goldstein, K., & Scheerer, M. (1941). Abstract and concrete behavior: An experimental study with special tests. *Psychological Monographs, 43,* 1–151.

Goodglass, H. (1988). Historical perspective on concepts of aphasia. In F. Boller & J. Grafman (Eds.), *Handbook of neuropsychology* (Vol. 1). Amsterdam: Elsevier.

Goodglass, H., Gleason, J. B., & Hyde, M. (1970). Some dimensions of auditory language comprehension in aphasics. *Journal of Speech and Hearing Research, 13,* 595–606.

Goodglass, H., & Mayer, J. (1958). Agrammatism in aphasia. *Journal of Speech and Hearing Disorders, 23,* 99–111.

Goodglass, H., & Quadfasel, F. A. (1954). Language laterality in left-handed aphasics. *Brain, 77,* 521–548.

Goodglass, H., Quadfasel, F. A., & Timberlake, W. H. (1965). Phrase length and type and severity of aphasia. *Cortex, 1,* 133–153.

Gott, P. S. (1973). Language after dominant hemispherectomy. *Journal of Neurology, Neurosurgery and Psychiatry, 36,* 1082–1088.

Graff-Radford, N. R., Cooper, W. E., Colsher, P. L., & Damasio, A. R. (1986). An unlearned foreign "accent" in a patient with aphasia. *Brain and Language, 28,* 86–94.

Graff-Radford, N. R., Eslinger, P. J., Damasio, A. R., & Yamada, T. (1984). Nonhemorrhagic infarction of the thalamus; behavioral, anatomic and physiologic correlates. *Neurology, 34,* 14–23.

Gur, R. C., Gur, R. E., Rosen, A. D., Warach, S., Alavi, A., Greenberg, J., & Reivich, M. (1983). A cognitive-motor network demonstrated by positron emission topography. *Neuropsychologia, 21,* 601–606.

Hamsher, K., Levin, H. S., & Benton, A. L. (1979). Facial recognition in patients with focal brain lesions. *Archives of Neurology (Chicago), 36,* 837–839.

Head, H. (1926). *Aphasia and kindred disorders of speech.* London: Cambridge University Press.

Hécaen, H., & de Ajuriaguerra, J. (1963). *Les gauchers: Prévalence manuelle et dominance cérébrale.* Paris: Presses Universitaires de France.

Henschen, S. E. (1919–1922). *Klinische und anatomische Beiträge zur Pathologie des Gehirnes,* 7 vols. Stockholm: Nordiska Bokhandeln.

Humphrey, M. E., & Zangwill, O. L. (1952). Dysphasia in left-handed patients with unilateral brain lesions. *Journal of Neurology, Neurosurgery and Psychiatry, 15,* 184–193.

Jackson, J. H. (1874). On the nature of the duality of the brain. *Medical Press and Circular, 1,* 19, 41, 63. (Reprinted in *Brain,* 1915, *38,* 80–103).

Jackson, J. H. (1878). On affections of speech from disease of the brain. *Brain, 1,* 304–330.

Jakobson, R. (1941). *Aphasie, Kindersprache und allgemeine Lautgesetze.* Stockholm: Almqvist & Wiksell. (Also published as: *Child language, aphasia and language universals,* A. R. Keiler [Trans.]. The Hague: Mouton, 1968.)

Jakobson, R. (1956). Two aspects of language and two types of aphasic disturbances. In R. Jakobsen & M. Halle (Eds.), *Fundamentals of language.* The Hague: Mouton.

Joynt, R. J., & Benton, A. L. (1964). The memoir of Marc Dax on aphasia. *Neurology, 14,* 851–854.

Kerchensteiner, M., Poeck, K., & Brunner, E. (1972). The fluency-nonfluency dimension in the classification of aphasic speech. *Cortex, 8,* 233–247.

Kleist, K. (1934). *Gehirnpathologie.* Leipzig: Barth.

Lecours, A. R., & Lhermitte, F. (1979). *L'aphasie.* Paris: Flammarion.

Lesser, R. (1978). *Linguistic investigations of aphasia.* London: Arnold.

Lichtheim, L. (1885). [On aphasia.] *Brain, 7,* 433–485. (Originally published in *Deutsches Archiv fuer Klinische Medizin,* 1885, *36,* 204–268).

Lordat, J. (1843). Analyse de la parole pour servir à la théorie de divers cas d'alalie et de paralalie. *Journal de la Société de Médicine Pratique de Montpellier, 7,* 333–353, 417–433; *8,* 1–17.

Marcé, L. V. (1856). Sur quelques observations de physiologie pathologique tendant à démontrer l'existence d'un principe coordinateur de l'écriture. *Mémoires de la Société de Biologie, 3,* 93–115.

Marie, P. (1906). La troisième circonvolution frontale gauche ne joue aucun rôle spécial dans la fonction du langage. *Semaine Médicale, 26,* 241–247.

Marshall, J. C., & Newcombe, F. (1966). Syntactic and semantic errors in paralexia. *Neuropsychologia, 4,* 169–176.

Meunier, M. (1924). *Histoire de la médecine.* Paris: La François.

Mills, C. K. (1899). Anomia and paranomia with some considerations regarding a naming center in the temporal lobe. *Journal of Nervous and Mental Disease, 26,* 757–758.

Milner, B., Branch, C., & Rasmussen, T. (1966). Evidence for bilateral speech representation in some non-right handers. *Transactions of the American Neurological Association, 91,* 306–308.

Mohr, J. P. (1983). Thalamic lesions and syndromes. In A. Kertesz (Ed.), *Localization in neuropsychology.* New York: Academic Press.

Monrad-Krohn, G. H. (1947). Dysprosody or altered melody of speech. *Brain, 70,* 405–415.

Naeser, M. A. (1983). CT scan lesion size and lesion locus in cortical and subcortical aphasias. In A. Kertesz (Ed.), *Localization in neuropsychology.* New York: Academic Press.

Newcombe, F., & Marshall, J. C. (1981). On psycholinguistic classifications of the acquired dyslexias. *Bulletin of the Orton Society, 31,* 29–46.

Nielsen, J. M. (1936). *Agnosia, apraxia, aphasia: Their value in cerebral localization.* New York: Harper (Hoeber).

Ogle, W. (1867). Aphasia and agraphia. *St. George's Hospital Reports, 2,* 83–122.

Ombredane, A. (1926). Sur le mécanisme de l'anarthrie et sur les troubles associés due langage intérieur. *Journal de Psychologie Normale et Pathologique, 23,* 940–955.

Ombredane, A. (1933). Le langage. In G. Dumas (Ed.), *Nouveau traité de psychologie* (Vol. 3). Paris: Alcan.

Orgass, B., Hartje, W., Kerchensteiner, M., & Poeck, K. (1972). Aphasie und nichtsprachliche intelligenz. *Nervenarzt, 43,* 623–627.

Orgass, B., & Poeck, K. (1966). Clinical evaluation of a new test for aphasia: An experimental study of the Token Test. *Cortex, 2,* 222–243.

Osborne, J. (1833). On the loss of faculty of speech depending on forgetfulness of the art of using the vocal organs. *Dublin Journal of Medical and Chemical Science, 4,* 157–170.

Pagel, W. (1958). Medieval and Renaissance contributions to knowledge of the brain and its functions. In F. N. L. Poynter (Ed.), *The history and philosophy of knowledge of the brain and its functions.* Oxford: Blackwell.

Pick, A. (1913). *Die agrammatischen sprachstörungen.* Berlin: Springer-Verlag.

Pitres, A. (1895). Etude sur l'aphasie chez les polyglottes. *Revue de Medecine, 15,* 873–899.

Pitres, A. L. (1898). *L'aphasie amnésique et ses variétés cliniques.* Paris: Alcan.

Poetzl, O. (1928). *Die optisch-agnostischen Stoerungen.* Leipzig: Deuticke.

Raven, J. C. (1938). *Progressive matrices.* London: H. K. Lewis.

Raven, J. C. (1963). *Guide to using the coloured progressive matrices.* London: H. K. Lewis.

Ross, E. D. (1981). The aprosodias; functional-anatomic organization of the affective components of language in the right hemisphere. *Archives of Neurology (Chicago), 38,* 561–569.

Rubens, A. (1976). Transcortical motor aphasia. In H. Whitaker & H. A. Whitaker (Eds.), *Studies in neurolinguistics* (Vol. 1). New York: Academic Press.

Russell, W. R., & Espir, M. L. E. (1961). *Traumatic aphasia.* Oxford: Oxford University Press.

Ryalls, J. H. (1982). Intonation in Broca's aphasia. *Neuropsychologia, 20,* 355–360.

Smith, A. (1966). Speech and other functions after left (dominant) hemispherectomy. *Journal of Neurology, Neurosurgery and Psychiatry, 29,* 467–471.

Soury, J. (1899). *Le système nerveux central.* Paris: Carré & Naud.

Spreen, O., & Wachal, R. S. (1973). Psycholinguistic analysis of aphasic language. *Language and Speech, 16,* 130–146.

Subirana, A. (1969). Handedness and cerebral dominance. In P. J. Vinken & G. W. Bruyn (Eds.), *Handbook of clinical neurology* (Vol. 4). Amsterdam: North-Holland.

Trousseau, A. (1865). *Clinque medicale de l'Hôtel-Dieu de Paris* (2nd ed.). Paris: Baillière et Fils.

Varney, N. R. (1978). Linguistic correlates of pantomime recognition in aphasic patients. *Journal of Neurology, Neurosurgery and Psychiatry, 41,* 564–568.

Wachal, R. S., & Spreen, O. (1973). Some measures of lexical diversity in aphasic and normal language performance. *Language and Speech, 16,* 169–181.

Wada, J. A. (1969). Interhemispheric sharing and shift of cerebral speech function. *International Congress Series—Excerpta Medica, 193,* 296–297.

Wada, J. A., Clarke, R., & Hamm, A. (1975). Cerebral hemispheric asymmetry in humans. *Archives of Neurology (Chicago), 32,* 239–246.

Wada, J. A., & Rasmussen, T. (1960). Intra-carotid injection of sodium amytal for the lateralization of cerebral speech dominance. *Journal of Neurosurgery, 17,* 262–282.

Wagenaar, E., Snow, C., & Prins, R. (1975). Spontaneous speech of aphasic patients; a psycholinguistic analysis. *Brain and Language, 2,* 281–303.

Wechsler, D. (1944). *The measurement of adult intelligence* (3rd ed.). Baltimore, MD: Williams & Wilkins.

Wechsler, D. (1958). *The measurement and appraisal of adult intelligence* (4th ed.). Baltimore, MD: Williams & Wilkins.

Weintraub, S., Mesulam, M., & Kramer, L. (1981). Disturbances in prosody; a right hemisphere contribution to language. *Archives of Neurology (Chicago), 38,* 742–744.

Weisenburg, T., & McBride, K. E. (1935). *Aphasia.* New York: Commonwealth Fund. (Reprinted in 1964. New York: Hafner).

Wernicke, C. (1874). *Der aphasische Symptomenkomplex.* Breslau: Cohn & Weigert.

Wernicke, C. (1886). Einige neuere Arbeiten über Aphasie. *Fortschritte der Medizin, 4,* 371–377.

Witelson, S. F., & Pallie, W. (1973). Left hemisphere specialization for language in the newborn: Neuroanatomical evidence of asymmetry. *Brain, 96,* 641–646.

Young, R. M. (1970). *Mind, brain, and adaptation in the nineteenth century.* Oxford: Oxford University Press (Clarendon).

2

Signs of Aphasia

ANTONIO R. DAMASIO

This chapter is a discussion of the clinical presentation of the aphasias, the major types, and the principal signs. A discussion of the neurophysiology and neuroanatomy of language (and, by extension, of the physiopathology of the aphasias) is outside the scope of this text. However, the comments on clinical evidence presented here reflect a particular theoretical perspective which has been discussed elsewhere in detail (A. R. Damasio, 1989a, 1989b, 1989c, 1990; H. Damasio and Damasio, 1989), and which the reader may wish to consult.

By referring to the LOCALIZATION VALUE or CORRELATE of a given sign, I do not imply that the correlated brain locus normally operates to produce the missing function. In the perspective outlined in the articles cited above, language, like other complex psychological functions, depends on the concerted operation of multicomponent neural networks. The neural components are often widely dispersed, in the neuroanatomical sense, and each acts as a partial contributor rather than the purveyor of a whole complicated process. In other words, Wernicke's area (part of which can be conceptualized as a component of a systems-level language network) does *not* normally execute auditory comprehension, although its impairment often leads to auditory comprehension defects.

Aphasia is a disturbance of the complex process of comprehending and formulating verbal messages that results from newly acquired disease of the central nervous system (CNS). We shall begin by analyzing each component of this operational definition.

Newly Acquired Disease. It is important to note that the disease that produces aphasia is both acquired and recent (e.g., cerebral infarction,

27

tumor, or contusion) rather than congenital and long standing (e.g., genetic or environment-induced prenatal cerebral defect). The former befalls individuals previously capable of using language appropriately. The latter may produce developmental language defects in young individuals whose ability to use language will never attain a normal level.

Of the Central Nervous System.   The reference to the CNS is important (although it should be clear that all mental activity and communication stems from the activity of the CNS) because aphasia is not the result of a peculiar utilization of language related to psychogenic or social deviations.

Verbal Messages.   Throughout the chapter I refer to VERBAL COMMU-NICATION and LANGUAGE almost interchangeably. On the other hand, the terms LANGUAGE and SPEECH are not interchangeable. The latter should be reserved for the act of "speaking a verbal message" independently of the process of formulating the message itself. In the definition above, VERBAL MESSAGES is used to call attention to the fact that aphasia relates exclusively to a disturbance in verbal language as opposed, for example, to the language of gestures—body or facial expressions— which is an important component of social communication.

Disturbance of the Process of Comprehending and Formulating Verbal Messages.   Aphasia can affect the comprehension of the language the patient hears spoken or sees written, or both. It can also affect the formulation of oral language production, writing, or both. Often, aphasia disturbs both reception and expression of language, in both visual (written) and auditory (spoken) modes. Yet, each of the several fundamental types of aphasia compromises one of these modes preponderantly. Indeed, in some instances (e.g., in PURE ALEXIA or in PURE WORD DEAF-NESS), only one of those abilities suffers while all others remain unaffected. More about this particular issue later.

The emphasis on the terms COMPREHENDING and FORMULATING is especially pertinent. Aphasics have trouble comprehending verbal messages, that is, deciphering their meaning, as opposed to hearing or seeing those messages. Neither deafness (peripheral or central) nor blindness is the problem. A deaf or blind person cannot comprehend language in the modality of the perceptual impairment, but normally can comprehend the same verbal message when processed by an intact sensory channel, for example, tactile Braille reading in the blind. Aphasics also have trouble formulating verbal messages, for example, selecting the lexical and syntactic items necessary to convey meaning, and deploying them in a relational framework such that meaning is indeed imparted on the receiver of the message. Yet an impediment of phonation that prevents speech production has nothing to do with the formulation of verbal messages (people can still write what they cannot say), just as the loss of the two hands does not interfere with language formulation (people may still speak if they have formulated a message, and they may even write with a pen held between the teeth or the toes).

To characterize the nature of the disturbance, stating what aphasia is not becomes as important as stating what it is. Aphasia is not a disturbance of articulation. Many patients suffer from speech disturbances due to acquired disease of the basal ganglia, the brain stem or cerebellum, or even the left or right side of the cerebral cortex, yet few of those patients will have aphasia. Although their speech sounds are poorly formed or are inappropriately repeated, word selection and sentence structure are grammatically correct, appropriate to the intentions of their author, and understandable to the attentive listener. Although such patients have a speech disturbance, it does not follow that they have a verbal language disturbance: Their language formulation is normal, their communication is linguistically correct, and hence they do not have aphasia.

Patients with mutism, who can be entirely silent, also are not aphasic, although on occasion their absence of speech does conceal an aphasia. Often these patients fail to indicate any desire to communicate by gesture, mimicry, or writing. Consequently, little is known about what they do or do not comprehend, and about what they may or may not want to say (or think, for that matter). However, most mutism patients awake from these peculiar states of apparent indifference and resume language communication showing no evidence of aphasia. When probed about their abnormal behavior, they clearly give testimony to a strange experience of avolition and diminished richness of thought content, but not to any problem with the actual composition of verbal communication. Most such patients have CNS disease in areas of the brain different from those that produce the aphasias, for example, in the supplementary motor area or cingulate gyrus, as opposed to the region surrounding the sylvian fissure. A few have acute psychotic states and no macroscopically detectable brain disease, although they may suffer from profound changes in neurotransmitter systems innervating certain regions of the brain.

Also not aphasic are patients with aphonia that may result from diseases of the larynx and pharynx. They are mute, in the narrow sense of the word, and are suffering from an impediment in their phonatory apparatus that prevents them from speaking. They should be able to comprehend language (and indicate so by nodding or pointing responses), and they should be able to turn their thoughts into language by writing, in addition to being able to mouth words. The exception (other than for malingering) is a conversion reaction, the currently uncommon psychiatric diagnosis of HYSTERICAL APHONIA.

Finally, the language disorder noted in altered states of consciousness is not an aphasia. Any patient with a confusional state will produce disturbed language and fail to comprehend verbal communication; however, such patients have a concomitant disorder of their thought processes that parallels the language disturbance. Unlike the patient with aphasia, who struggles but fails to turn properly organized meanings into language (or tries, without success, to turn the message he or she heard into internal meaning), patients with confusional states communicate their disordered thought processes verbally, with remarkable success. Confusional states are most commonly produced by metabolic disturbances or substance intoxication but can be the result of cerebral tumors (directly or indirectly affecting CNS structures that sustain vigilance).

The picture of a patient with aphasia should begin to emerge now.

1. An aphasic produces some speech, or even abundant speech, which does not conform to the grammatical rules of the language being used. The errors include omission of functor words (such as conjunctions or prepositions), erroneous choice of words (substitution of the intended word for another that may or may not be related in sound or meaning), and disturbance of word order. Although aphasic patients produce some speech, they may not during the initial hours or days of the disease. Even during a phase of speechlessness, however, most aphasic patients attempt to communicate by gesture or facial expression.

2. An aphasic often has difficulty in comprehending a purely verbal command (i.e., a verbal message given thorough auditory or visual means, without accompanying gestures, facial expressions, or meaningful emotional intonation). The errors of comprehension may range from an almost complete inability to understand any but the most elementary questions, to mild defects that surface when complex sentences are presented (e.g., sentences with double negatives or dependent clauses).

3. An aphasic is alert to person and environment and enters the situation of being medically examined in appropriate fashion. He or she is intent on communicating thoughts regarding his or her own condition and surroundings. Again, there may be exceptions, particularly in the first few hours after an acute brain lesion, in which aphasic patients may appear inattentive and uninterested in communication. In some pa-

tients, well into the chronic stage, a depression may prevent an appropriate relation with examiners and surroundings. In general, however,
as far as we can fathom, the view of the world available to an aphasic is
impoverished by lack of intact verbal processing but is NOT that of a
confused, demented, or psychotic patient. Accordingly, the appearance
of the aphasic patient is not that of an alienated individual. More often
than not, despite the barrier of handicapped communication, the examiner of an aphasic patient can empathize with the patient. The student of
aphasia should develop a keen sensitivity to this important aspect of
aphasia.

The Signs of Aphasia

Naming Disturbances and the
Production of Paraphasias

At the core of language formulation lies the ability to select from the
verbal lexicon a word that conveys the meaning of a given thought. The
selection process is often automatic although we may deliberately search
for the precise lexical item (a process that should be referred to as WORD
FINDING). When word selection fails, the result is either a complete
omission of the intended item or a substitution by an incorrect and
unintended word. The latter is termed PARAPHASIA and probably is the
central sign of aphasia. If an entire word is substituted, the paraphasia is
called VERBAL (or GLOBAL). If the incorrectly selected item belongs to the
same semantic field (e.g., *chair* for *table*), it is termed a SEMANTIC
paraphasia. Too many verbal paraphasias appearing in sentence after
sentence give rise to JARGON SPEECH.

Paraphasias can be entirely novel words which do not exist in the
lexicon of a given language (NEOLOGISTIC paraphasias). The mechanism
for the formation of the new word may be a succession of phoneme
substitutions: a single phoneme substituted or added (e.g., *table*
becomes *trable* or *fable*) is known as a PHONEMIC or LITERAL paraphasia.
Too many phonemic paraphasias produce an unintelligible neologism,
and too many neologistic paraphasias give rise to NEOLOGISTIC JARGON.

Paraphasias can appear in spontaneous speech or in a dialogue, on
repetition of spoken sentences or on reading aloud, on naming tasks,
and in writing; however, they are generally absent in automatic speech
(emotional exclamations, series of numbers, calendar sequences).

One of the most exciting new developments in aphasia research
comes from the systematic investigation of patterns of word-finding and

paraphasic defects, and how they relate to the underlying nonverbal lexical knowledge. Patients with naming defects are not impaired for all categories of words, or for words that denote all categories of knowledge. On the contrary, the defects are more pronounced in some categories than others, and their seeming selectivity reveals some of the underpinnings of lexical organization (see A. R. Damasio, 1990, for review).

Disturbance of Fluency

Although the general characteristics of speech in aphasic patients are not always easily classifiable, they often fall into one of two categories: FLUENT or NONFLUENT. These designations can have slightly different meanings for different authors, but for most aphasiologists, fluent speech is that which approximates normal speech in terms of the rate of word production, the length of each sentence, the melodic contour of the sentences, and the overall ease of the speaking act. In practical terms, it is usually measured by the longest continuous string of words that the patient produces in conversation. Fluent aphasic speech may actually be more abundant than normal speech. Nonfluent speech is the opposite: The rate is low, sentence length is short, melodic contour is lost, production is effortful, and more pauses than actual words may occur in a given time unit.

Judging the quality of articulation is a separate matter from judging fluency. Most patients with fluent speech have normal articulation, although some may have minor difficulties. Many patients with nonfluent speech also have perfect articulation, although some do not. As noted, the ability to articulate speech and the ability to formulate language are different. Even patients with severe nonfluent speech are able to produce perfectly articulated automatized verbal sequences (as in counting or in emotional exclamations).

A measure of fluency may help with clinical classification and provide a rough indication for the localization of lesion. Most patients with fluent aphasias have lesions in the posterior aspect of the perisylvian region, whereas most patients with nonfluent aphasias have lesions in the anterior aspect of the perisylvian region (Benson, 1967).

Disturbances of Repetition

A failure to repeat words or sentences is another hallmark of aphasia. The ability to repeat may be entirely lost, or may be marred by phonemic paraphasias or omissions of sounds and words. Repetition is impaired in

most aphasias, and actually dominates the clinical presentation of conduction aphasia because other pronounced defects are lacking. The impairment of repetition also has localization value. Its presence places the
lesion firmly in the perisylvian region of the dominant hemisphere.
Repetition defects are notably absent in the transcortical aphasias and in
the so-called anomic aphasia, whose correlated lesion is located outside
the perisylvian ring. Patients with the transcortical aphasias may actually repeat only too well, echoing the examiner's words immediately
after they are pronounced, often with little or no comprehension of what
they are parroting. Such a defect is called ECHOLALIA.

Disturbances of Auditory Comprehension

Auditory comprehension can be impaired to variable degrees. Some
patients are able to participate in a colloquial conversation, giving appropriate verbal replies or indicating that they understand the content of
the messages by nodding, pointing responses, facial expression, or gestures. Confronted with laboratory tests, however, they may fail many
items, especially when the questions aim at specifics rather than gener-
alities, and when the linguistic structure is complex rather than transparent. Other patients may be quite impaired even in a simple conversation, let alone in the laboratory tests.

Disturbances of Grammatical Processing

AGRAMMATISM is another important sign of aphasia. It refers to difficulty with generating the syntactic frames into which lexical selections
must be placed, and to a defective utilization of grammatical morphemes. Grammatical morphemes include items such as functor words
(free grammatical morphemes) and the inflectional affixes that mark
tense, aspect, or person when placed at a verb ending (bound grammatical morphemes). For quite some time the impression was that only
patients of the Broca type were agrammatic, but it is now clear that
patients with other aphasia types, namely, the commonly encountered
Wernicke's aphasia, are also agrammatic. Elsewhere in this volume, the
topic of agrammatism is discussed at length.

Disturbances of Reading and Writing

Reading comprehension can be disturbed in much the same way as
auditory comprehension, although the two defects do not necessarily
occur together. Patients with auditory comprehension defects usually

have some reading impairment, but the proportion of patients with both defects is small. On the other hand, reading impairment can appear in pure form without impairment of auditory comprehension or writing. In most cases of aphasia, however, reading, writing, and auditory comprehension all are impaired, although rarely to the same degree.

Apraxia

Many aphasic patients also present with apraxia, forms of which, from practical and clinical standpoints, can be considered yet another sign of aphasia. APRAXIA may be defined as a disorder of the execution of learned movement that cannot be accounted for by either weakness, incoordination, sensory loss, or impaired comprehension or attention to commands. Theoretically, however, it should be clear that apraxia can appear in isolation, without aphasia, and that its many varieties and mechanisms justify a separate entity status. The presence of apraxia should be investigated in all aphasic patients, as it may interfere with the performance of acts requested through verbal command. Students of aphasia should be aware of the fact that patients do not "complain" of apraxia and that, except for the extreme forms of ideational apraxia, the phenomenon is neither immediately disruptive to the patient's life nor evident to the examiner. The reader is referred to Geschwind (1975) for a comprehensive view of the phenomenon.

Classifications of Aphasia

Classifications are a necessary evil. Attempting to review the classification systems of aphasia is foolhardy. The variety of criteria used over the past 100 years may disorient the reader at first. The diversity of the nomenclature is exasperating. The seeming conflict between systems that include as many as eight different varieties of aphasia and those that limit themselves to two or three is a source of puzzlement. Yet, the student of aphasia should realize that diversity and conflict reflect an evolution of the science of the aphasias and are more apparent than real. From the practical standpoint, few of the many available classification systems have survived. Current researchers and clinicians in leading aphasia centers use but one or two of the more recent systems. Furthermore, some of the apparently discrepant systems are not really so, since they derive from different points of view in relation to the phenomena of aphasia. For instance, Weisenburg and McBride's (1935) classic designations of EXPRESSIVE, RECEPTIVE, and MIXED aphasia reflect a clinical vantage point. Luria's (1966) nomenclature—for example, EFFERENT and AFFERENT MOTOR, or DYNAMIC—reflects a physiological approach. On the other hand, Jakobson's (1964) description of CONTIGUITY (or combination) and SIMILARITY (or selection) defects is the product of a psycholinguistic point of view. The systems do not conflict but rather complement each other. Be that as it may, a modern researcher or clinician should have a working knowledge of the different classification systems, from Wernicke's (1874) to Geschwind's (1965). This knowledge should be complemented with a conversant use of one modern classification system: the proper definition of each of its categories, their anatomical and physiological significance, and their prognostic implications.

The system generally associated with the Boston school of aphasia is perhaps the most useful. It can be used in conjunction with most forms of laboratory and bedside assessment and does not necessarily require the use of the Boston Diagnostic Aphasia Examination (BDAE). The Boston classification comprises all of the frequently encountered aphasias for which there is an established and accepted anatomical correlation. The nomenclature utilizes a combination of eponyms, clinically descriptive terms, and physiologically based terms and is not especially mysterious (see Goodglass & Kaplan, 1972, 1983).

The following paragraphs contain descriptions of the aphasias most frequently encountered in clinical practice. I refer to them as "types" because each description corresponds to the averaged mental representation that an experienced observer forms, out of many comparable exemplars, bringing together signs that are salient over different epochs after the onset of aphasia. The reasons why signs cluster in fairly distinct patterns are largely biological. Damage to certain neural units tends to produce, fairly consistently, a given sign of dysfunction. By the same token, the reason why the precise cluster of signs varies from individual to individual—a sign may be missing from the usual combination, or some sign may be far more or less pronounced than usual—is largely neuroanatomical. The precise lesion placement varies from individual to individual because of individual variations of normal neural and vascular anatomy, combined with variations of neuropathologic dynamics. Furthermore, there are individual variations in the assignment of components of normal psychological function, to separate anatomical components of neural networks.

Despite these sources of variance, the consistency with which certain signs do cluster, over and over again, is astonishing. As a consequence, we consider the aphasia typology discussed below to be useful to clinicians in sorting diagnostic and management issues and in communicating among themselves in effective ways. On the other hand, aphasia types or even finer etched aphasia syndromes are generally NOT helpful in establishing groups of patients for research, and are of little use as a basis for neurophysiological reasoning. Research purposes are best served by making separate signs as the variable with which neuroanatomical information or the result of cognitive experiments are connected.

Major Aphasia Types

Wernicke's Aphasia

Wernicke's aphasia is perhaps the least controversial of the aphasia types. Speech is fluent and well articulated, with frequent paraphasias (both verbal and literal). Syntactic structure appears less disturbed than in Broca's aphasia (see below), but it is reasonable to say that BOTH Wernicke's and Broca's aphasics exhibit some form of agrammatism. Aural comprehension is defective. Repetition of words and sentences is also defective. In general, both reading and writing are disturbed.

Most patients may have no other evidence of neurological disease as right hemiparesis is infrequent or transient; right visual field defects are not the rule. Thus, the diagnosis rests almost solely on the language signs, and the accuracy of the diagnosis is mandatory: Because a patient with acute Wernicke's aphasia may sound "confused," the unskilled examiner may take a psychiatric rather than neurological diagnostic approach. Even assuming that the mistake is eventually corrected, the delay can be disastrous.

Patients with Wernicke's aphasia seem to be less easily frustrated than those with Broca's aphasia; however, a tendency for paranoid ideation is more evident in Wernicke patients than in Broca's. It should be recalled that these are among the few neurological patients who can develop a major paranoid syndrome and become homicidal.

This complex syndrome, which combines both output and input disturbances, is also known as RECEPTIVE aphasia, from Weisenburg and McBride's (1935) classification, and as SENSORY aphasia, as Wernicke himself (1874) called it, with appreciable modesty but little physiological sense. Kleist (1934) aptly called it WORD DEAFNESS, but the term is rarely used, whereas Brain (1961) named it PURE WORD DEAFNESS, an inaccurate designation, since patients with Wernicke's aphasia are indeed word deaf but clearly not in pure form. (Patients with pure word deafness do exist, however; they are unable to understand speech and to repeat words, but they speak fluently and WITHOUT paraphasias). Head (1926) called it SYNTACTIC aphasia, a rather useless designation.

Broca's Aphasia

The existence of Broca's aphasia is currently well established, yet some of the major controversies in the history of aphasia have revolved around its nature and pathological correlation. The first patient described by Broca in 1861 did not have what came to be known as Broca's aphasia, and it is clear that the degree of involvement of Broca's area and of the surrounding frontal operculum produce considerably different degrees of aphasia (Mohr et al., 1978). What currently is called Broca's aphasia can be defined as the opposition of Wernicke's aphasia. It is characterized by nonfluent speech, few words, short sentences, and many intervening pauses. The words that do appear are produced with labor and often with distorted sounds. The melodic contour is flat. Syntactic structure is more disturbed than in Wernicke's aphasia. The general appearance of speech is telegraphic, due both to the selective deletion of many functor words and to disturbances of canonical word order. On the other hand, aural comprehension is relatively intact in colloquial conversation, although formal testing often discloses a defective performance. Repetition of words and sentences is impaired. Broca's aphasia should be distinguished from APHEMIA, an articulatory disorder caused by generally small lesions underneath the motor cortices or in the vicinity of the basal ganglia (Schiff, Alexander, Naeser, & Galaburda, 1983).

Unlike patients with Wernicke's aphasia, the patient with Broca's aphasia invariably presents with a right-sided motor defect (often a complete hemiparesis more marked in the upper extremity and face). As a consequence, patients with Broca's aphasia are less vulnerable to misdiagnosis. Their presentation is clearly neurological. On the other hand, they are often depressed and may respond to testing failures with "catastrophic" reactions (sudden weeping and refusal to proceed with examination) more frequently than do Wernicke's aphasics.

Broca's aphasia also has been known as EXPRESSIVE (Weisenburg & McBride, 1935) and MOTOR (Goldstein, 1948; Wernicke, 1874) aphasia. For a time it was refused the status of aphasia and called ANARTHRIA (Marie, 1906) and, later, DYSARTHRIA (Bay, 1965). Head (1926) called it VERBAL aphasia.

Conduction Aphasia

The speech of conduction aphasics is fluent but usually less abundant than that of Wernicke's. Commonly there are minor defects in aural comprehension, although understanding of colloquial conversation is intact. The impairment in repetition of words and sentences dominates. The defect takes many forms. Usually, patients repeat words with phonemic paraphasias, but often they omit or substitute words, and they may fail to repeat anything at all if function words rather than nouns are requested. Comprehension of the defectively repeated sentences is good. Similarly, patients comprehend the sentences that they read aloud with numerous paraphasias.

Conduction aphasics often have some accompanying motor signs (paresis of the right side of the face and of the right upper extremity), but recovery is good. The syndrome has been known as CENTRAL aphasia, Goldstein's (1948) curious designation, and as AFFERENT MOTOR aphasia, Luria's term. Luria (1966) attempted to break down the condition, giving it a motor component (AFFERENT MOTOR) and an auditory one (ACOUSTIC AMNESIC). Kertesz (1979) proposed a comparable distinction (EFFERENT CONDUCTION and AFFERENT CONDUCTION).

Transcortical Sensory Aphasia

Patients with transcortical sensory aphasia (TSA) have fluent and paraphasic speech (global paraphasias predominate over phonemic) and a severe impairment in aural comprehension. Yet their repetition is intact (occasionally echolalic), setting them clearly apart from Wernicke's aphasics. The distinction is important since the localization of the lesion is different (see chapter 3 on localization). This underscores the need to test repetition in every aphasic patient.

TRANSCORTICAL was the original designation of Goldstein (1948), and it has held well through the years, both for TSA and for transcortical motor aphasia, some cases of which Luria preferred to call DYNAMIC aphasia (Luria & Tsevtkova, 1968).

Transcortical Motor Aphasia

Patients with transcortical motor aphasia (TMA) have intact repetition, as do patients with TSA, and can have echolalia as well. However, their speech is nonfluent and troubled by phonemic and global paraphasias, perseveration, and loss of connective words. In our experience, auditory comprehension is also impaired when tested formally, although patients can often carry on a simple conversation at bedside.

Patients with TMA should be distinguished from those with mutism on several counts. First, patients with TMA are inclined to communicate and do so, within their verbal limitations. Patients with mutism do not and are as impoverished in nonverbal as in verbal communication. Second, the speech of TMA patients is clearly aphasic, characterized by unquestionable phonetic, lexical, and syntactic errors, whereas patients with mutism either produce no speech at all or utter a few short but linguistically correct sentences. Again, the distinction is important because the localization of the lesion is different.

Global Aphasia

As the name implies, global aphasics present with an almost complete loss of ability to comprehend or formulate verbal communication. Propositional speech may be reduced to a few words, the remainder of verbal communication consisting of emotional exclamations and serial utterances. Auditory comprehension is often reduced to a variable number of nouns and verbs, while the comprehension of functor words or of syntactically organized sentences is virtually negligible.

Hemiplegia accompanies most, but not all, global aphasias. In global aphasia without hemiplegia, the defects are less pronounced and the recovery is better (Tranel, Biller, Damasio, Adams, & Cornell, 1987).

Anomic Aphasia

Pure anomic aphasia occurs rarely. It is important to distinguish it from anomia as a sign of aphasia, because the latter is present in practically all aphasias. Anomic aphasia is characterized by a pervasive impairment of word finding, but intact repetition and speech that is fluent, well articulated, and grammatically correct. The neuroanatomical basis of anomic aphasia is currently being elucidated (H. Damasio, 1989; H. Damasio & Damasio, 1989; Graff-Radford et al., in press; Tranel, Damasio, & Damasio, 1988). Different entities and conceptual–lexical categories are impaired or spared in a dissociated manner (e.g., patients are far better at naming entities that are man-made than natural, and subgroupings within those broad classes reveal further dissociations). Such disparities, along with the theoretical formulations necessary to account for them, provide an important source of evidence for studies of lexical representation. The terms AMNESIC (amnestic) aphasia, NOMINAL aphasia, and VERBAL AMNESIA are synonymous.

Alexia with Agraphia

Alexia with agraphia is extremely rare. More often than not, patients with both alexia and agraphia have signs of Wernicke's aphasia or transcortical sensory aphasia. In the absence of aphasia, they generally have signs of parietal lobe dysfunction. Naturally, the diagnosis of alexia with agraphia applies only when the disturbances of reading and writing predominate over the aphasic or parietal symptomatology. The fact that this syndrome can be associated with impaired as well as intact repetition, and with a greater or smaller extent of accompanying signs, suggests that a large segment of parietal and temporal lobe structures, both cortical and subcortical, is engaged in the complex processes of reading and writing. The anatomical significance of this entity is considerably smaller than that of alexia WITHOUT agraphia (pure alexia).

Alexia without Agraphia (Pure Alexia)

As the designation implies, patients presenting alexia with agraphia become unable to read while they continue to be able to write, spontaneously or to dictation. Many such patients can also copy writing, although they do so with difficulty. Speech, auditory comprehension, and repetition are intact. Oral spelling of words (or its converse, the construction of words spelled orally) is normal. Reading in the tactile mode is also normal. Whatever visual reading they can do is of single letters. The patient often can read aloud the letters of a word, one by one, and then reconstitute the word from the spelled out components.

Although neither writing nor oral language impairments are present, most patients have some form of accompanying impairment of visual function (see A. R. Damasio & Damasio, 1983, for review). It can be a right homonymous hemianopia (the field of vision to the right of the vertical median is blind) or a right hemiachromatopsia (loss of color perception without true blindness in the right hemifield). Most patients also have color anomia, a disturbance of naming colors with otherwise normal color perception. Some present with optic ataxia, a disturbance in the visual guidance of hand movements.

First described by Dejerine (1892), the syndrome was long forgotten and even denied, but was revived by Geschwind (1965), who used it as a cornerstone for his theory of disconnection syndromes.

Pure Word Deafness

Patients with pure word deafness have a profound loss of auditory comprehension and a complete impairment of repetition, yet they produce normal fluent speech, mostly without paraphasias. It could be argued that pure word deafness, like pure alexia, is not a true aphasia, since language formulation itself is not affected. From a physiopathological standpoint, both conditions reflect the inability of verbal information to reach structures capable of processing it into meaning. Inner language operations as well as exteriorization of well-formulated language remain intact. There are reasons, however, why the two conditions should be discussed along with the aphasias. First, they resemble aphasias from the standpoint of the communication impairment they produce. Second, anatomical and physiological knowledge derived from studying these two "input" disorders has contributed importantly to the understanding of the aphasias.

"Atypical" Aphasias

A considerable number of aphasia cases fail to conform to any of the types described above. This happens for a variety of neurobiological, neuropsychological, and cultural reasons. Perhaps the most frequently encountered atypical exemplars are ascribed to a so-called nonstandard cerebral dominance disposition (right cerebral dominance for language in a left hander or right hander, or "ambidominance" in a left hander). But another important source of atypical aphasias is damage in a noncortical sector of language networks. The lesion can be located in the deep nuclear gray masses (basal ganglia or thalamus) and may involve white matter in the vicinity (e.g., the anterior limb of the internal capsule). As an example, aphasia can arise following nonhemorrhagic infarction that damages the left head of the caudate and the anterior limb of the internal capsule (A. R. Damasio, Damasio, Rizzo, Varney, & Gersh, 1982; H. Damasio, Eslinger, & Adams, 1984; Naeser et al., 1982). Damage to left thalamus caused by either hemorrhagic (Alexander & Lo Verme, 1980; Hier & Mohr, 1977) or nonhemorrhagic infarction (Graff-Radford, Damasio, Yamada, Eslinger, & Damasio, 1985) also causes aphasia.

Acknowledgments

This work was supported by NINCDS grant PO1 NS19632.

References

Alexander, M. P., & Lo Verme, S. R. (1980). Aphasia after left hemispheric intercerebral hemorrhage. *Neurology, 30,* 1193–1202.

Bay, E. (1964). Principles of classification and their influence on our concepts of aphasia. In A. V. S. de Rueck & M. O'Connor (Eds.), *Disorders of language.* Boston, MA: Little, Brown.

Benson, D. F. (1967). Fluency in aphasia: Correlation with radioactive scan localization. *Cortex, 3,* 373–394.

Brain, W. R. (1961). *Speech disorders.* London: Butterworth.

Broca, P. (1861). Remarques sur le siège de la faculte du langage articule, suivies d'une observation d'aphémie (perte de la parole). *Bulletin de la Societe d'Anatomie (Paris), 36,* 330–357.

Damasio, A. R. (1989a). The brain binds entities and events by multiregional activation from convergence zones. *Neural Computation, 1,* 123–132.

Damasio, A. R. (1989b). Concepts in the brain. *Mind and Language, 4,* 24–28.

Damasio, A. R. (1989c). Time-locked multiregional retroactivation: A systems level model for some neural substrates of recall and cognition. *Cognition, 33,* 25–62.

Damasio, A. R. (1990). Category-related recognition defects as a clue to the neural substrates of knowledge. *Trends in Neurosciences, 13,* 95–98.

Damasio, A. R., & Damasio, H. (1983). The anatomic basis of pure alexia. *Neurology, 33,* 1573–1583.

Damasio, A. R., Damasio, H., Rizzo, M., Varney, N., & Gersh, F. (1982). Aphasia with nonhemorrhagic lesions in the basal ganglia and internal capsule. *Archives of Neurology (Chicago), 39,* 15–20.

Damasio, A. R., Damasio, H., Tranel, D., & Anderson, S. W. (1990). Category-related recognition defects: Neuropsychological profiles and neural correlates. *Journal of Clinical and Experimental Neuropsychology, 12,* 80.

Damasio, H. (1989). Neuroimaging contributions to the understanding of aphasia. In F. Boller & J. Grafman (Eds.), *Handbook of neuropsychology* (Vol. 2, pp. 3–46). Amsterdam: Elsevier.

Damasio, H., & Damasio, A. R. (1989). *Lesion analysis in neuropsychology.* New York: Oxford University Press.

Damasio, H., Eslinger, P., & Adams, H. P. (1984). Aphasia following basal ganglia lesions: New evidence. *Seminars in Neurology, 4,* 151–161.

Dejerine, J. (1892). Des différentes variétés de cecité verbale. *Memoires de la Societé de Biologie, Ser. 9, 4,* 61–90.

Geschwind, N. (1965). Disconnexion syndromes in animals and man. *Brain, 88,* 237–294, 585–644.

Geschwind, H. (1975). The apraxias: Neurological mechanisms of disorders of learned movement. *American Scientist, 63,* 188–195.

Goldstein, K. (1948). *Language and language disturbances.* New York: Grune & Stratton.

Goodglass, H., & Kaplan, E. (1972). *Assessment of aphasia and related disorders.* Philadelphia, PA: Lea & Febiger.

Goodglass, H., & Kaplan, E. (1983). *Assessment of aphashia and related disorders* (2nd ed.). Philadelphia, PA: Lea & Febiger.

Graff-Radford, N. G., Damasio, A. R., Hyman, B. T., Hart, M., Tranel, D., Damasio, H., Van Hoesen, G. W., & Rezai, K. (1990). Progressive aphasia in a patient with Pick's disease: A neuropsychological, radiological and anatomical study. *Neurology, 40,* 620–626.

Graff-Radford, N. G., Damasio, H., Yamada, T., Eslinger, P., & Damasio, A. R. (1985). Nonhemorrhagic thalamic infarction: Clinical, neurophysiological and electrophysiological findings in four anatomical groups defined by CT. *Brain, 108,* 485–516.

Head, H. (1926). *Aphasia and kindred disorders of speech.* Cambridge: Cambridge University Press.

Hier, D. B., & Mohr, J. P. (1977). Incongruous oral and written naming. Evidence for a subdivision of the syndrome of Wernicke's aphasia. *Brain and Language, 4,* 115–126.

Jakobson, R. (1964). Towards a linguistic typology of aphasic impairments. In A. V. S. de Rueck & M. O'Connor (Eds.), *Disorders of language.* Boston, MA: Little, Brown.

Kertesz, A. (1979). *Aphasia and associated disorders.* New York: Grune & Stratton.

Kleist, K. (1934). *Gehirnpathologie.* Leipzig: Barth.

Luria, A. R. (1966). *Higher cortical functions in man.* New York: Basic Books.

Luria, A. R., & Tsevtkova, L. (1968). The mechanisms of dynamic aphasia. *Foundations of Language, 4,* 296–307.

Marie, P. (1906). Revision de la question de l'aphasie: La troisième circonvolution frontale gauche ne joue aucun rôle special dans la fonction du langage. *Semaine Medicale, 21,* 241–247.

Mohr, J. P., Pessin, M. S., Finkelstein, S., Funkenstein, H. H., Duncan, G. W., & Davis, K. R. (1978). Broca's aphasia: Pathologic and clinical. *Neurology, 28,* 311–324.

Naeser, M. A., Alexander, M. P., Helm-Estabrooks, N., Levine, H. L., Laughlin, S. A., & Geschwind, N. (1982). Aphasia with predominantly subcortical lesion sites. *Archives of Neurology (Chicago), 39,* 2–14.

Schiff, H. G., Alexander, M. P., Naeser, M. A., & Galaburda, A. M. (1983). Aphemia: Clinical-anatomic correlations. *Archives of Neurology (Chicago), 40,* 720–727.

Tranel, D., Biller, J., Damasio, H., Adams, H. P., & Cornell, S. (1987). Global aphasia without hemiparesis. *Archives of Neurology (Chicago), 44,* 304–308.

Tranel, D., Damasio, H., & Damasio, A. R. (1988). Dissociated verbal and nonverbal retrieval and learning following left anterotemporal damage. *Neurology, 38,* 322.

Weisenburg, T., & McBride, K. (1935). *Aphasia.* New York: Commonwealth Fund.

Wernicke, C. (1874). *Der aphasische symptomencomplex.* Breslau: Cohn & Weigert.

3

Neuroanatomical Correlates of the Aphasias

HANNA DAMASIO

This chapter complements Chapter 2 on types and signs of aphasia. It makes use of the same theoretical and practical framework (see A. R. Damasio, 1989a, 1989b, 1989c; H. Damasio & Damasio, 1989). The aim is to provide an overview of the neuroanatomical correlates of the major aphasia types. A discussion of the physiopathological basis of aphasia signs and types is outside the scope of this chapter. Naturally, this text should not be regarded as a discussion of the neural basis of language processes, although information on the neuroanatomical correlates of the aphasias is critical to experimental work that aims at understanding language's neural underpinnings. All the cautions expressed in Chapter 2, regarding syndromes, types, and signs, apply here as well. Most importantly, the description of consistent neural correlates and the emphasis on reliable lesion localization, given certain signs, should not be confused with an attribution of specific functions to the areas of damage.

The history of cerebral localization of the aphasias begins with Broca's discovery of a relation between a disturbance of language and damage to the lower posterolateral aspect of the left frontal lobe (Broca, 1861a, 1861b). Broca was not only calling attention to the asymmetry of the brain in relation to language, in what became the first modern study in cerebral dominance, but preparing the ground for further correlations between acquired aphasia and cerebral lesions. The next historical step came with Wernicke's (1874) report of the association between the symptom complex of Wernicke's aphasia and damage to the posterior aspect

ACQUIRED APHASIA, SECOND EDITION

of the first left temporal gyrus. The notion of left cerebral dominance for language acquired strength, and the concept that varied pathological behaviors could be related to different brain lesions was established. Wernicke proceeded to predict the anatomical lesion responsible for a third aphasia type, conduction aphasia. The lesion, he thought, would fall between those found in Wernicke's and Broca's aphasias, most probably in the insular region. It is currently apparent that, in essence, his prediction was correct.

The next important step came with Dejerine's descriptions of ALEXIA and AGRAPHIA (1891) and ALEXIA WITHOUT AGRAPHIA (1892). His studies established a connection between written language and specific brain regions, as Broca's and Wernicke's had established similar links for aural languages. Alexia with agraphia was associated with damage to the left parietal lobe, in structures interposed between Wernicke's area and the visual association cortices. On the other hand, alexia without agraphia was found to follow a lesion in the left occipital lobe which damaged exclusively visual association cortices. The location of the lesion was such, he proposed, that it prevented access of visual information to those structures of the parietal and temporal lobe with which impairments of reading, writing, and aural comprehension had previously been associated. The lesion had to be strategically located at a crossroads of visual information traffic. It interrupted the flow of information from the right to the left visual cortices, by means of damaging either the corpus callosum proper or its outflow (the forceps major). It also severed crucial connections between the left visual cortex itself and left parietal and temporal language cortex.

A further step in the anatomical mapping of the aphasias should be noted. Wernicke, and later Goldstein (see Goldstein, 1948), reported on the appearance of peculiar forms of aphasia associated with lesions different from the ones described before then, and hallmarked by a lack of impediment in verbal repetition. These were designated transcortical motor and transcortical sensory; their anatomical correlates were located anteriorly and posteriorly to the ones associated with the other varieties of aphasia. For transcortical motor aphasia, the lesion was in frontal lobe structures rostral to Broca's area. For transcortical sensory aphasia, damage was found in parietal and occipitotemporal structures posterior to Wernicke's area. (Figure 3.1 illustrates the gross localization of these fundamental syndromes of aphasia.)

During the decades that followed, knowledge of aphasia localization was consolidated. Numerous case reports of all the principal types of aphasia, accompanied by more or less expert descriptions of clinical

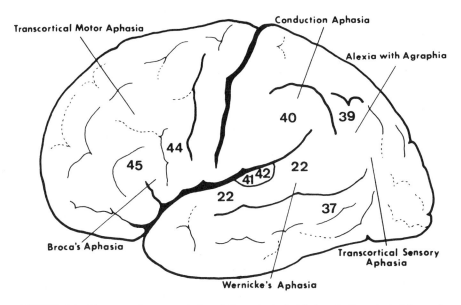

FIGURE 3.1. *Diagrammatic representation of the major loci of lesions in the principal types of aphasia. Brodmann's areas 44 and 45 correspond to the classic Broca's area, and area 22 to Wernicke's area. Areas 41 and 42 correspond to the primary auditory cortex; these are located in the depth of the sylvian fissure and cannot be seen in a lateral view of the brain. Area 40 is the supramarginal gyrus, and area 39 is the angular gyrus. Area 37, principally located in the posterior sector of the second and third temporal gyrus, does not have correspondence in gyral nomenclature.*

symtpomatology, confirmed the values of the discoveries of the founding fathers of aphasiology. Occasionally such case reports have given rise to conflicting evidence, but rarely if ever have such conflicts shattered the foundations provided by Broca, Wernicke, Dejerine, and Goldstein. On the contrary, mapping of earlier days has been refined, rendering knowledge on the anatomical correlates of the aphasias even more complex.

In 1965 Geschwind drew on this remarkable body of morphological evidence to interpret the aphasias and associated disorders in modern anatomical and physiological terms. In the years that followed, stimulated by Geschwind's seminal monograph, researchers reassessed the anatomical correlation of the various aphasic syndromes. New tools were added, as well: the radionuclide brain scan made its appearance, permitting new anatomical insights, and the Boston Aphasia Research Center's classification categories became widely accepted, making comparison of cases from different centers somewhat easier. The notion of fluency as a useful variable for correlation was also introduced. Using radionuclide brain scans, Benson (1967) demonstrated a consistent association between nonfluent speech and prerolandic lesions. The nonfluent aphasias were those of the Broca and transcortical motor types. Within the limits of brain scan resolution, they correlated as expected with left frontal lobe lesions. The fluent aphasias included Wernicke's, conduction, and transcortical sensory, which tended to cluster in the posterior left quadrant. For a variety of reasons, some exceptions to this pattern were found; however, the adherence to this rule was more impressive than the departure from it. Only a partially conflicting study came to light (Karis & Horenstein, 1976), whereas a more extensive study corroborated the results of Benson (Kertesz, Lesk, & McCabe, 1977).

The advent of computerized tomography (CT) in 1973 changed the panorama of the anatomical study of higher behavior in the human and was particularly beneficial for the field of aphasia. CT provided the possibility of studying with considerable anatomical detail not only a large variety of cerebral lesions but also the surrounding intact cerebral tissue. The first study of CT correlations with aphasia came from Naeser and Hayward (1978). Their localization of Broca's, Wernicke's, conduction, and global aphasis conformed to classical anatomical localizations. Kertesz, Harlock, and Coates (1979) replicated Naeser and Hayward's findings, adding data on the differences produced by acute and chronic stages of aphasia. Later, by establishing a correspondence between gross brain anatomy and Brodmann's cytoarchitectonic map, other authors attempted to further the anatomical information of CT studies by developing templates of the CT cuts (Basso, Lecours, Moraschini, & Vanier, 1985; H. Damasio, 1983, 1989; H. Damasio & Damasio, 1989; Gado, Hanaway, & Frank, 1979; Hayward, Noeser, & Zatz, 1977; Kertesz et al., 1979; Luzzatti, Scotti, & Gattoni, 1979; Matsui & Hirano, 1978; Mazzocchi & Vignolo, 1979; Poeck, De Bleser, & von Keyerlingk, 1984). Using bony structures and the ventricular system as landmarks, the lesions seen in the CT scan were plotted into the best-fitting templates and then read as a three-dimensional reconstruction.

In the 1980s the advent of magnetic resonance (MR) further improved the detection of structural abnormalities in the living human brain and permitted an unprecedented detail of anatomical characterization *in vivo* (H. Damasio, 1980; H. Damasio & Damasio, 1989). Emission tomography, either of the single photon or positron emission varieties, has allowed us to study brain activity during language processing (H. Damasio, Rezai, Eslinger, Kirchner, & Van Gilder, 1986; Petersen, Fox, Posner, Minton, & Raichle, 1988).

Fluent Aphasias

Conduction Aphasia

The anatomical correlates of conduction aphasia have been documented with postmortem studies (Benson et al., 1973) and with CT and MR scan studies (H. Damasio, 1989; H. Damasio & Damasio, 1980, 1989; Kertesz et al., 1979; Naeser & Hayward, 1978; Rubens & Selnes, 1986). Conduction aphasia is associated with left perisylvian lesions involving the primary auditory cortex (areas 41 and 42), a portion of the surrounding association cortex (area 22), and to a variable degree the insula and its subcortical white matter as well as the supramarginal gyrus (area 40). Not all of these regions need to be damaged in order to produce this type of aphasia. In some cases without involvement of auditory and insular regions, the compromise of area 40 is extensive (H. Damasio, 1989). In others, the supramarginal gyrus may be completely spared and the damage limited to insula and auditory cortices (H. Damasio & Damasio, 1980) or even to insula alone (Rubens & Selnes, 1986). It is important, however, to note that the area of damage does not involve the posterior sector of the superior temporal gyrus or Wernicke's area (see Figures 3.2 and 3.3).

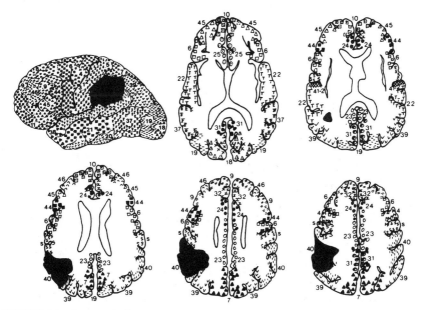

FIGURE 3.2. *Computerized tomographic template from a patient with conduction aphasia (LR 194). The lesion was limited to the left supramarginal gyrus.*

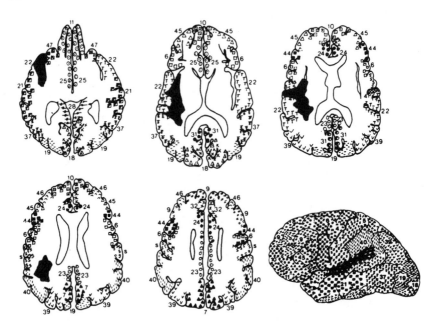

FIGURE 3.3. *Computerized tomographic template from a patient with conduction aphasia (RF 089) in whom the lesion involved the left auditory cortex* AND *the insula. The cortex of the spramarginal gyrus remained intact. The crosshatched area represents the area of damage that cannot be seen in the lateral surface of the brain.*

Wernicke's Aphasia

The core of the lesions in Wernicke's aphasia maps to the posterior region of the left superior temporal gyrus. A typical example is shown in Figure 3.4. This has been the case since Wernicke's original description in 1886, and no significant changes have been introduced by more recent investigations (H. Damasio, 1989; Kertesz et al., 1979; Knopman, Selnes, Niccum, & Rubens, 1984; Mazzochi & Vignolo, 1979; Naeser & Hayward, 1978; Selnes, Knopman, Niccum, & Rubens, 1985; Selnes, Knopman, Niccum, Rubens, & Larson, 1983; Selnes, Niccum, Knopman, & Rubens, 1984). But it also became clear that the lesions often extend into the second temporal gyrus and into the nearby parietal region (the lower segment of the supramarginal and angular gyri). Figure 3.5 shows an example of such a case. It is important to note that, as with conduction aphasia, the extent of damage in the different brain areas may vary and that this may be related to the profile of linguistic disability. For instance, the overall severity of auditory comprehension deficit may be related to the extent of damage in the primary auditory cortices (areas 41 and 42), and the severity of visual naming deficit may well depend on the extent

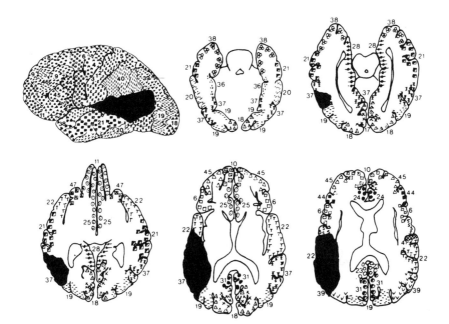

FIGURE 3.4. *Magnetic resonance template from a patient with Wernicke's aphasia (WG 988). The lesion involved the posterior sector of the left superior and middle temporal gyri but did not extend into the parietal lobe.*

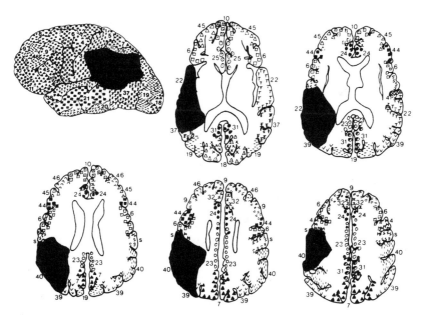

FIGURE 3.5. *Computerized tomographic template from a patient with Wernicke's aphasia (MS 319). The lesion involved the left superior temporal gyrus and most of the inferior parietal lobule (both supramarginal and angular gyri).*

of damage to the middle and inferior temporal gyrus (in areas 20, 21, and 37). Furthermore, paraphasic errors may be more or less prominent in certain categories of names (e.g., animals vs. manipulable man-made tools), depending on whether the damage extends mostly into lower and anterior temporal regions or, on the contrary, into the parietal region (for further examples, see H. Damasio, 1980; H. Damasio & Damasio, 1989).

Anomic Aphasia

As indicated in chapter 2 the enigmatic anatomical correlates of anomic aphasia are now elucidated. We have accumulated a large number of instances of anomic aphasia of both progressive (Graff-Radford et al., 1990) and nonprogressive (A. R. Damasio, Damasio, Tranel, & Anderson, 1990) varieties and have concluded that damage to left anterior temporal cortices is essential (see Figure 3.6). Whether anomic aphasia can arise out of a middle and interior temporal lesion alone, without involvement in structures anterior to it, remains unclear at this

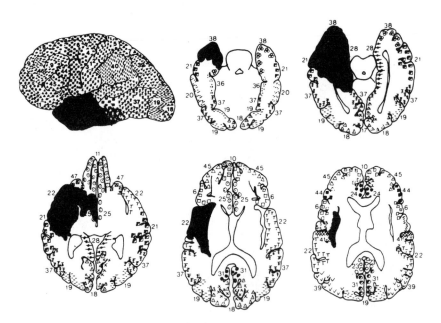

FIGURE 3.6. *Magnetic resonance template from a patient with anomic aphasia (LR 488). The damage is limited to the anterior half of the left temporal lobe and the insula. Note that it does not extend into Wernicke's area, area 37, or the inferior parietal lobule.*

point. The exact role of the mesial component in these lesions, namely, the involvement of the hippocampus, is also the topic of current study.

Transcortical Sensory Aphasia

The neuroanatomical correlates of this type of aphasia became clear only after the advent of CT (H. Damasio, 1989; Kertesz et al., 1979). The posterior segment of area 22 in the superior temporal gyrus (or Wernicke's area) is never entirely damaged in this type of aphasia. The same applies to the primary auditory cortices (areas 41 and 42). The lesions can be seen in the posterior sector of the middle temporal gyrus (area 37) and in the angular gyrus (area 39) or in the white matter underlying these cortices (Figure 3.7).

Comparing the three main types of fluent aphasia, it is evident that there are some areas of anatomical overlap. Nevertheless, the core of each anatomical pattern is distinctive. Along a rostro–caudal axis, the anatomical core of Wernicke's aphasia seems to occupy the midsector, with involvement of the planum temporale (the posterior portion of area

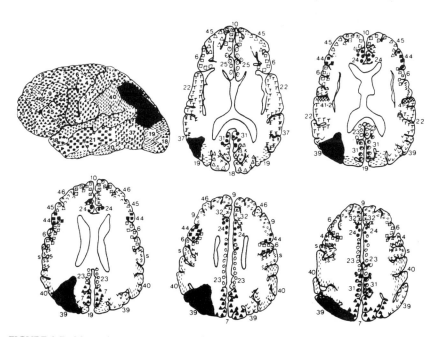

FIGURE 3.7. *Magnetic resonance template from a patient with transcortical sensory aphasia (LH 1356). The lesion involved the left angular gyrus and the posterior sector of the supramarginal gyrus. Note that the temporal lobe is spared.*

22, contained in the sylvian fissure) plus some anterior and posterior extension. The core of conduction aphasia is more anterior and superior, often extending into the insula. Overlap with Wernicke's loci takes place in the anterior portions of area 22. The core for transcortical sensory aphasia occupies the more posterior sector, encompassing area 37, and extending into visual association cortex and angular gyrus. Overlap takes place in the more posterior portion of area 22. Just as importantly, none of these three anatomical loci overlap with those for the nonfluent aphasias, discussed in the next section.

Nonfluent Aphasias

Broca's Aphasia

Broca's aphasia, associated with lesions in the left frontal operculum, began with Paul Broca's description in 1861 and has not survived without controversy (the most notorious debates occurred at the beginning of the century between Dejerine and Pierre Marie at the Societe de Medicine in Paris [1908]). The advent of modern imaging methods has clarified several of the questions raised then, and parcellation of both the clinical findings and the underlying deficits have been attempted (H. Damasio, 1989; H. Damasio & Damasio, 1989; Kertesz et al., 1979; Mohr et al., 1978; Naeser & Hayward, 1978; Schiff, Alexander, Naeser, & Galaburda, 1983; Tonkonogy & Goodglass, 1981). In general, it is fair to say that lesions in Broca's aphasia may encompass not only the frontal operculum (areas 44 and 45), but also premotor and motor regions immediately behind and above, in addition to extending into underlying white matter and basal ganglia as well as the insula. As might be expected, the extension of damage into these many different regions correlated with diverse accompanying deficits and with the extent of recovery. I will illustrate this point with two examples.

Case 1 is that of a 40-year-old, right-handed woman, with a thrombotic infarction. Initially she had a complete inability to utter single words or sentences but had remarkably intact aural comprehension and gestural communication. A right central facial paresis completed the neurological picture. Speech improved rapidly to a nonfluent halting discourse in which connectives were missing. Repetition of sentences was impaired, as was writing. The CT scan showed a small area of gray matter enhancement, suggestive of a lesion in the left frontal lobe, that would involve (a) areas 45 and 44 (Broca's area); (b) the portion of area 6 immediately above (the so-called Exner's area); and (c) the nearby facial motor region. Subcortical extension was minimal (see Figure 3.8). This patient continued to recover so well that a year later she had only minimal signs of impairment. Her speech is now slow but grammatically correct. An MR obtained 7 years poststroke showed a stable area of encephalomalacia in precisely the same location as mentioned above, and emission tomography studies performed with a language activating task demonstrated increased signal intensity both in the intact lower left frontal operculum and the opposite hemisphere (see H. Damasio, 1989).

Case 2 represents the other extreme of Broca's aphasia. A 76-year-old right-handed man suffered a thrombotic infarction. In the acute phase, he had minimal speech output, inability to repeat words or sentences, a defect in aural comprehension, impaired reading and writing, and right-sided neglect. The CT scan of this man also showed a lesion in the left frontal lobe, but it included far more than Broca's area. Areas 45 and 44 were involved, but the lesion extended into area 6, as well as into the motor cortex and the anterior segment of the insula. Furthermore, it extended deep into the white matter reaching close to the anterior horn of the left lateral ventricle, damaging part of the head of the caudate

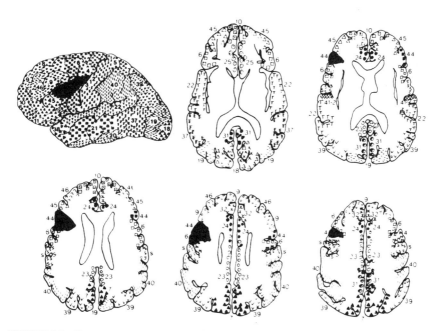

FIGURE 3.8. *Computerized tomographic template from a patient with Broca's aphasia (MW 018). The lesion involved only the superior sector of Broca's area (area 44) and the premotor region (area 6) immediately above it.*

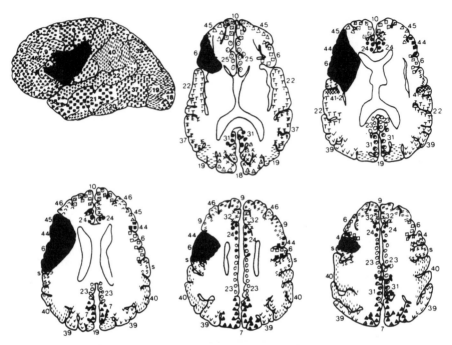

FIGURE 3.9. *Magnetic resonance template from a patient with Broca's aphasia (JP 1172). The lesion involved most of Broca's area (areas 44 and 45), as well as motor and premotor regions (areas 6 and 4), above and behind the frontal operculum, as well as the underlying white matter, the insula, and part of the basal ganglia.*

nucleus as well as part of the lenticular nucleus (see Figure 3.9). It should be noted, however, that regardless of being an extensive lesion, it did not reach posteriorly into the temporal lobe region; that is, it never overlapped areas related to the fluent aphasias. The evolution of this case was quite different from the previous one. Speech, as it emerged, was nonfluent, with the usual characteristics of Broca's aphasia. Recovery was modest in comparison with the first case.

Transcortical Motor Aphasia

The principal difference between transcortical motor aphasia and Broca's aphasia is in verbal repetition, which is possible in the former and impaired in the latter. Patients with transcortical motor aphasia often have echolalia in the setting of an otherwise nonfluent speech. Lesions are almost invariably located outside Broca's area, either anteriorly or superiorly, either deep in the left frontal substance or in the

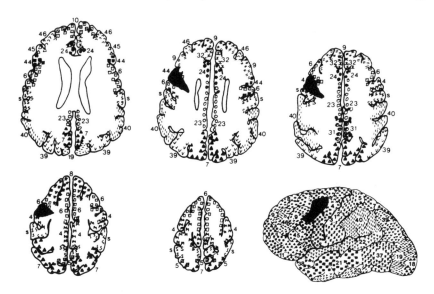

FIGURE 3.10. *Magnetic resonance template from a patient with transcortical motor aphasia (RW 680). The lesion involved left premotor and motor cortices, just above Broca's area.*

cortex. Figure 3.10 shows the MR template of such a case. The lesion is small and located just above the frontal operculum. It barely touches area 44 and extends superiorly into premotor and motor cortex. In other cases it may also be small and located deep in the white matter of the left frontal lobe, lying close to the anterior horn of the left lateral ventricle. In those cases, it does not involve cortical areas, but it most certainly disrupts connections between mesial structures of the frontal lobe, namely the supplementary motor area, and structures of Broca's area and the motor area (see H. Damasio, 1989).

Mutism

The syndromes of mutism are not, in the strict sense, part of the aphasias. In mutism, speech output is minimal or absent at all times, unlike the aphasias, in which it is only absent during the acute phase. However, the place of mutism in a discussion of localization of the aphasias is justified because mutism is often mistaken for transcortical motor aphasia and even for Broca's aphasia. Just as the clinical differences are clear, however, so are the anatomical correlates. Patients with mutism are aspontaneous both in relation to their nonexistent speech and in relation to other motor behaviors, for example, gestural communication and motor drive toward new stimuli. However, if stimulated enough, they can repeat words and sentences normally, and their comprehension of aural and written language is intact. The recovery of these patients is also different from that of patients with Broca's aphasia or transcortical motor aphasias, since the improvement is usually faster (in fact it can be sudden) and proceeds into grammatically correct speech with normal fluency without an intervening agrammatical stage. True mutism is associated with lesions in the mesial aspect of the frontal lobe, which involves the supplementary motor area (the mesial portion of area 6), its connections, and the nearby anterior cingulate (area 24).

Figure 3.11 shows an example of a patient with mutism. The lesion appears in the very high portion of the left frontal lobe, above the level of the lateral ventricles. The core of damage involves the cortex and white matter immediately underneath in the mesial portion of area 6. The nearby anterior cingulate cortex and its connections are involved. In other cases, the damage can extend to involve motor areas mainly in their mesial aspect (corresponding to the cerebral representation of the lower limb) but also in their lateral portion (related to upper limb representation). This generally correlates with the presence or absence of paralysis of the foot and leg or of the arm. However, the lesions do not

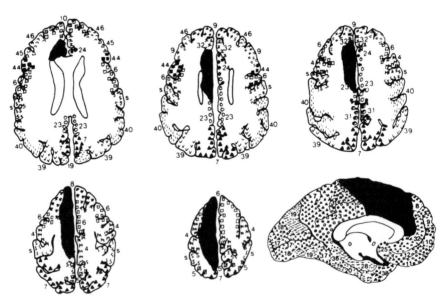

FIGURE 3.11. *Magnetic resonance template from a patient with akinetic mutism (DM 414). The lesion involved the left anterior cingulate gyrus, the supplementary motor area, and the mesial motor region.*

extend into the frontal regions, which we have previously seen affected
in the aphasias.

Global Aphasia

The typical lesion in a patient with standard global aphasia involves
the whole left perisylvian region, affecting all areas whose damage correlates with the aphasias. Figure 3.12 shows the lesions of such a case.

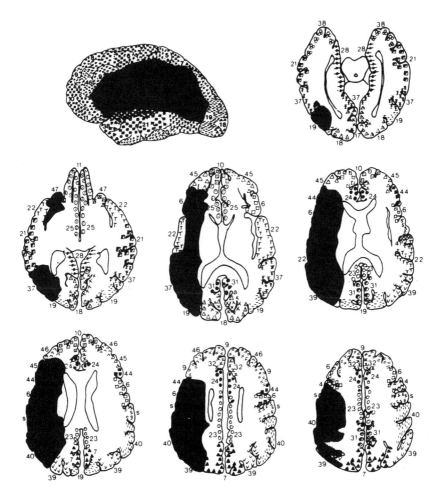

FIGURE 3.12. *Magnetic resonance template from a patient with global aphasia and hemiparesis
(VD 1266). The lesion involved most of the cortices and subcortical white matter supplied by the left
middle cerebral artery.*

The damage is the result of an infarction in the territory of the middle
cerebral artery. All the perisylvian language areas are involved. The
damage extends from areas 45 and 44 anteriorly; to the insula; to auditory areas 41, 42, and 22; to area 40; and in part to areas 39 and 37. The
motor and somatosensory areas 4, 3, 1, and 2 are also involved. The
damage, however, is not limited to the cortex: There is involvement of
the underlying white matter, as well as of part of the lenticular and the
caudate nuclei.

A similar clinical picture can be seen with the combination of two
lesions in the left hemisphere, one anterior and one posterior (Tranel,
Biller, Damasio, Adams, & Cornell, 1987). This is illustrated in Figure
3.13. In this case the anterior lesion involves the superior sector of area
44 as well as the underlying white matter and extends into area 6 immediately above. The posterior lesion involves the angular gyrus together
with the caudal sector of the supramarginal gyrus and the superior
sector of area 37 and the white matter underlying these cortices. However, the insula, basal ganglia, and temporal lobe are spared, as are the
motor cortices.

The patient had a global aphasia with severe impairment in all lin-

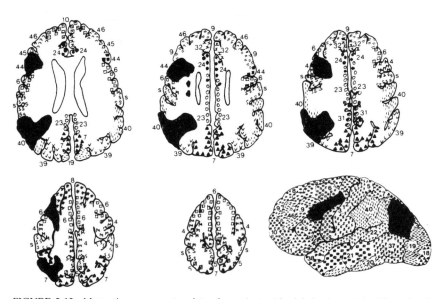

FIGURE 3.13. *Magnetic resonance template of a patient with global aphasia but without hemiparesis (JM 656). In this patient there were two lesions in the left hemisphere, one in the superior
sector of the frontal operculum and premotor cortex immediately above and another in the angular
gyrus.*

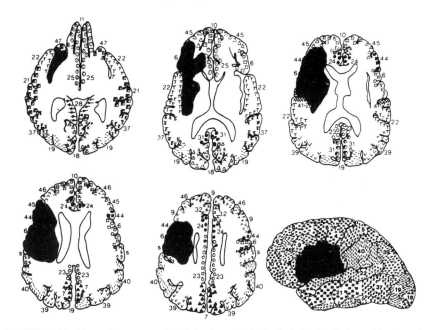

FIGURE 3.14. *Magnetic resonance template of a patient who had global aphasia and hemiparesis (BD 638) in the acute stage. Later the aphasia changed and was best characterized as a severe Broca's. Note that the lesion involved the left frontal operculum (areas 44 and 45), the premotor and motor cortices immediately behind and above Broca's area, as well as the insula and basal ganglia, but spared completely the temporal and parietal lesions.*

guistic abilities, but did *not* have hemiplegia. Another difference relates to recovery. In a case such as that shown in Figure 3.13, the language-related cortices are not damaged to the same extent as in the case shown in Figure 3.12, and recovery is far superior. These patients may not recover to normal speech and language but they certainly do not remain severe global aphasics.

Another anatomical pattern seen in global aphasia is that of a patient with a lesion in the left frontal operculum, underlying white matter, basal ganglia, insula, and even part of the parietal operculum, but sparing the temporal lobe. Such patients also tend to recover and, in the chronic stable state, come to resemble a Broca's aphasia (Figure 3.14).

Alexia without Agraphia (Pure Alexia)

Alexia without agraphia is not an aphasic disorder as such, since speech output and aural comprehension are intact. The condition is associated with a remarkably consistent anatomical localization (A. R.

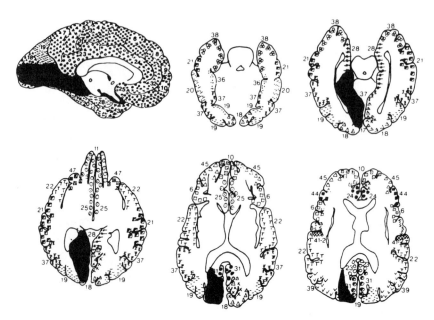

FIGURE 3.15. *Computerized tomographic template of a patient with alexia without agraphia (PA 321). The lesion involved the mesial sector of the left occipital lobe, the mesial occipitotemporal junction, and the white matter in the paraventricular region (where the forceps major courses), but spared the corpus callosum proper.*

Damasio & Damasio, 1983). Figure 3.15 shows a case of alexia without agraphia. The lesion extends from the occipital cortex deep into the white matter, reaching the left lateral ventricle at the level of the trigone and occipital horn (the paraventricular area). It involves the primary visual cortex (area 17) and part of the visual association cortices (areas 18 and 19). It extends into the mesial occipitotemporal function involving mesial area 37 and the posterior sector of the parahippocampal gyrus. The corpus callosum is intact, but the lesion disrupts interhemispheric connectional systems that course through the splenium of the corpus callosum, in the forceps major, and interlock the visual cortices. Thus, even if the corpus callosum proper does not show any damage, its outflow is compromised.

Atypical Aphasias

The advent of the modern neuroimaging techniques led to the identification of the left basal ganglia as the lesion correlate for a group of aphasias known as "atypical" for lack of a better term. These aphasias are generally of the fluent type, in some way resembling Wernicke's aphasia. Yet, unlike typical fluent aphasias, these are also characterized by disturbances of articulation and, even more deviantly, a right hemiparesis is present (A. R. Damasio, Damasio, Rizzo, Varney, & Gersh, 1982; H. Damasio & Damasio, 1989; H. Damasio, Eslinger, & Adams, 1984; Naeser et al., 1982).

The lesions are located deep in the left hemisphere and invariably include portions of the caudate nucleus and putamen and the anterior limb of the internal capsule. They often occur in younger individuals due to embolic events, where an embolus becomes lodged in the proximal segment of the middle cerebral artery at the level of the lenticulostriate arteries which supply the head of the caudate, the anterior limb of the internal capsule, and the lenticular nucleus.

Another atypical aphasic syndrome, with strong resemblance to transcortical sensory aphasia, can occur with infarcts in the left thalamus when the anterior nuclei are involved (Graff-Radford, Damasio, Yamada, Eslinger, & Damasio, 1985). In neither of these cases is there cortical damage in acute or chronic stages.

Conclusion

In conclusion, a large variety of acquired aphasic syndromes and of closely associated disturbances (mutism, pure alexia) can be correlated with damage to relatively specific brain lesions, located throughout the left cerebral hemisphere. More than 100 years of study of anatomoclinical correlations, using autopsy material as well as CT and MR scans, have proven that, in spite of the inevitable individual variability, the correlation between aphasia types and locus of cerebral damage is surprisingly consistent. Naturally, there are numerous exceptions. They can be found, in particular, in left-handed subjects, whose cerebral dominance for language is varied, and even in a minority of right-handed subjects who have right cerebral dominance for language (lesions within right hemispheres give rise to crossed aphasias).

The value of these consistent correlations for clinical diagnoses is unquestionable. But it should be clear that such correlations per se provide only limited information about the physiopathology of aphasia and the neurophysiology of language.

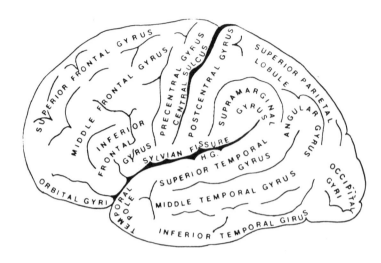

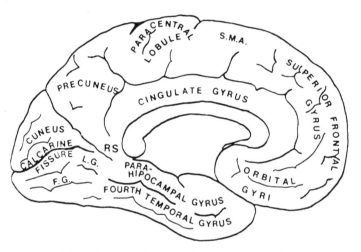

FIGURE 3.16. *Left hemisphere, lateral and mesial aspects, with identification of major fissures, and gyri. Note that the insula cannot be seen on a lateral view since it is buried in the depth of the sylvian fissure, in its anterior portion, and is covered by the frontal operculum (the more posterior and inferior portion of the inferior frontal gyrus and the inferior portion of the precentral gyrus), and that Heschl gyri also cannot be seen because they occupy the superior surface of the superior temporal gyrus, buried inside the sylvian fissure. F.G., fusiform gyrus; H.G., Heschl gyri (seen only in the superior surface of the superior temporal gyrus); L.G., lingual gyrus; R.S., retrosplenial area; S.M.A., supplementary motor area.*

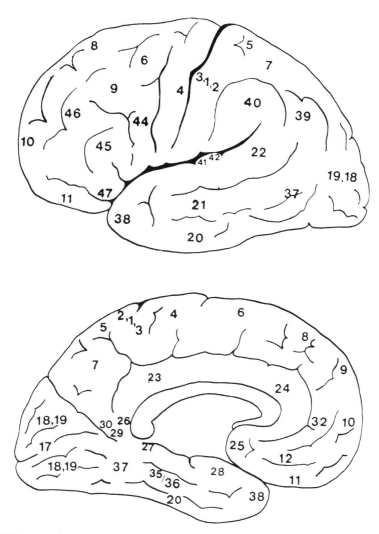

FIGURE 3.17. *Left hemisphere, lateral and mesial view with Brodmann's cytoarchitectonic nomenclatures. Note that areas 41 and 42, corresponding to Heschl gyri, are not actually seen in this view because they occupy the superior surface of the superior temporal gyrus, inside the sylvian fissure.*

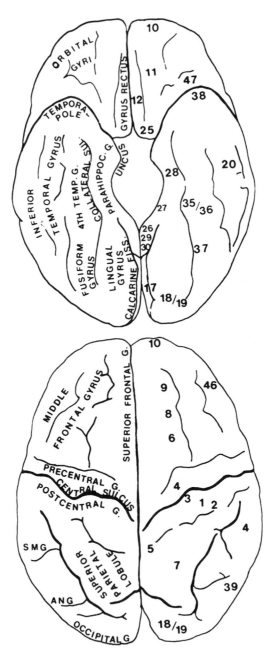

FIGURE 3.18. *Inferior and superior views of both hemispheres. On the left-hand side of each view the major gyri and fissures are marked, and on the right-hand side Brodmann's cytoarchitectonic fields are shown.*

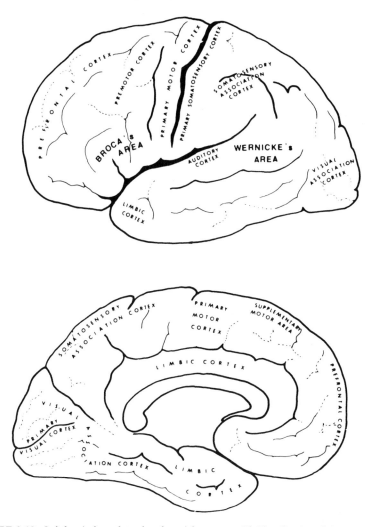

FIGURE 3.19. *Left hemisphere, lateral and mesial aspects, with identification of the major functional areas. Note that the auditory cortex occupies both the lateral aspect of the superior temporal gyrus and the superior aspect, inside the sylvian fissure (not seen in this lateral view) where the transverse temporal gyri (the primary auditory areas) and the planum temporale are located.*

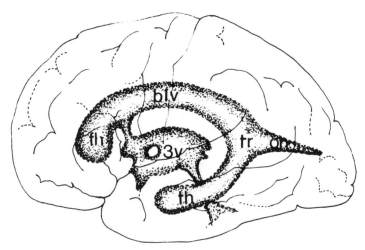

FIGURE 3.20. *Left hemisphere with the ventricular system. fh + blv + tr + oh + th = left lateral ventricle; fh, frontal horn; blv, body; tr, trigone; oh, occipital horn; th, temporal horn; 3v, third ventricle, which connects with both lateral ventricles through the foramina of Monro (the left one is marked with an arrow) and continues caudally into the aqueduct (double arrow).*

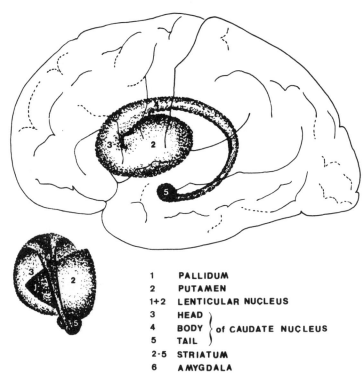

1	PALLIDUM
2	PUTAMEN
1+2	LENTICULAR NUCLEUS
3	HEAD ⎫
4	BODY ⎬ of CAUDATE NUCLEUS
5	TAIL ⎭
2-5	STRIATUM
6	AMYGDALA

FIGURE 3.21. *Left hemisphere with the basal ganglia seen in lateral view. The insert shows the basal ganglia seen from the occipital pole.*

Acknowledgments

This work was supported by NINCDS grant PO1 NS19632.

References

Basso, A., Lecours, A. R., Moraschini, S., & Vanier, M. (1985). Anatomoclinical correlations of the aphasias as defined through computerized tomography: Exceptions. *Brain and Language, 26,* 201–229.

Benson, D. F. (1967). Fluency in aphasia: Correlation with radioactive scan localization. *Cortex, 3,* 373–394.

Benson, D. F., Sheremata, W. A., Buchard, R., Segarra, J., Price, D., & Geschwind, N. (1973). Conduction aphasia. *Archives of Neurology (Chicago), 28,* 339–346.

Broca, P. (1861a). Portée de la parole. Ramollisement chronique et destruction partielle du lobe antérieur gauche du cereveau. *Bulletin de la Societe d'Anthropologie (Paris), 2,* 219.

Broca, P. (1861b). Remarques sur le siège de la faculté du langage articule, suivies d'une observation d'aphémie. *Bulletin de la Societe d'Anatomie (Paris), 2,* 330–357.

Damasio, A. R. (1989a). The brain binds entities and events by multiregional activation from convergence zones. *Neural Computation, 1,* 123–132.

Damasio, A. R. (1989b). Concepts in the brain. *Mind and Language, 4,* 24–28.

Damasio, A. R. (1989c). Time-locked multiregional retroactivation: A systems level model for some neural substrates of recall and cognition. *Cognition, 33,* 25–62.

Damasio, A. R., & Damasio, H. (1980). Prosopagnosia: Anatomical basis and neurobehavioral mechanism. *Neurology, 30,* 390.

Damasio, A. R., & Damasio, H. (1983). The anatomic basis of pure alexia. *Neurology, 33,* 1573–1583.

Damasio, A. R., Damasio, H., & Chui, H. (1980). Neglect following damage to frontal lobe or basal ganglia. *Neuropsychologia, 18,* 123–132.

Damasio, A. R., Yamada, T., Damasio, H., & McKee, J. (1980). Central achromatopsia: Behavioral, anatomical, and physiologic aspects. *Neurology, 30,* 1064–1071.

Damasio, A. R., Damasio, H., Rizzo, M., Varney, N., & Gersh, F. (1982). Aphasia with nonhemorrhagic lesions in the basal ganglia and internal capsule. *Archives of Neurology (Chicago), 39,* 15–20.

Damasio, A. R., Damasio, H., Tranel, D., & Anderson, S. W. (1990). Category-related recognition defects: Neuropsychological profiles and neural correlates. *Journal of Clinical and Experimental Neuropsychology, 12,* 80.

Damasio, H. (1983). A computed tomographic guide to the identification of cerebral vascular territories. *Archives of Neurology (Chicago), 40,* 138–142.

Damasio, H. (1989). Neuroimaging contributions to the understanding of aphasia. In *Handbook of neuropsychology* F. Boller & J. Grafman (Eds.), (Vol. 2, pp. 3–46). Amsterdam: Elsevier.

Damasio, H., & Damasio, A. R. (1979). "Paradoxic" extinction in dichotic listening: Possible anatomic significance. *Neurology, 29,* 644–653.

Damasio, H., & Damasio, A. R. (1980). The anatomical basis of conduction aphasia. *Brain, 103,* 337–350.

Damasio, H., & Damasio, A. R. (1989). *Lesion analysis in neuropsychology.* New York: Oxford University Press.

Damasio, H., Eslinger, P., & Adams, H. P. (1984). Aphasia following basal ganglia lesions: New evidence. *Seminars in Neurology, 4,* 151–161.

Damasio, H., Rezai, K., Eslinger, P., Kirchner, P., & Van Gilder, J. (1986). SPET patterns of activation in intact and focally damaged components of a language-related network. _Neurology, 36,_ 316.

Dejerine, J. (1891). Sur un cas de cecité verbale avec agraphie, suivi d'autopsie. _Memoires Societe Biologique, 3,_ 197–201.

Dejerine, J. (1892). Contribution à l'étude anatomo-pathologique et clinique des différentes variétés de cecité verbale. _Memoires Societe Biologique, 4,_ 61–90.

Gado, M., Hanaway, J., & Frank, R. (1979). Functional anatomy of the cerebral cortex by computed tomography. _Journal of Computer Assisted Tomography, 3,_ 1–19.

Geschwind, N. (1965). Disconnexion syndromes in animals and man. _Brain, 88,_ 237–294, 585–644.

Goldstein, K. (1948). _Language and language disturbances._ New York: Grune & Stratton.

Graff-Radford, N., Damasio, H., Yamada, T., Eslinger, P., & Damasio, A. R. (1985). Non-hemorrhagic thalamic infarction: Clinical, neurophysiological and electrophysiological findings in four anatomical groups defined by CT. _Brain, 108,_ 485–516.

Graff-Radford, N. G., Damasio, A. R., Hyman, B. T., Hart, M., Tranel, D., Damasio, H., Van Hoesen, G. W., & Rezai, K. (1990). Progressive aphasia in a patient with Pick's disease: A neuropsychological, radiological and anatomical study. _Neurology, 40,_ 620–626.

Hayward, R. W., Naeser, M. A., & Zatz, L. M. (1977). Cranial computed tomography in aphasia. _Radiology, 123,_ 653–660.

Karis, R., & Horenstein, S. (1976). Localization of speech parameters by brain scan. _Neurology, 26,_ 226–230.

Kertesz, A., Harlock, W., & Coates, R. (1979). Computer tomographic localization, lesion size, and prognosis in aphasia and nonverbal impairment. _Brain and Language, 8,_ 34–50.

Kertesz, A., Lesk, D., & McCabe, P. (1977). Isotope location of infarcts in aphasia. _Archives of Neurology (Chicago), 34,_ 590–601.

Knopman, D. S., Selnes, O. A., Niccum, N., & Rubens, A. B. (1984). Recovery of aphasia: Relationship to fluency, comprehension and CT findings. _Neurology, 34,_ 1461–1470.

Luzzatti, C., Scotti, G., & Gattoni, A. (1979). Further suggestions for cerebral CT-localization. _Cortex, 15,_ 483–490.

Matsui, T., & Hirano, A. (1978). _An atlas of the human brain for computerized tomography._ Tokyo: Igaku-Shoin Ltd.

Mazzocchi, F., & Vignolo, L. A. (1979). Localization of lesions of aphasia: Clinical CT scan correlations in stroke patients. _Cortex, 15,_ 627–654.

Mohr, J. P., Pessin, M. S., Finkelstein, S., Funkenstein, H. H., Duncan, G. W., & Davis, K. R. (1978). Broca's aphasia: Pathologic and clinical aspects. _Neurology, 28,_ 311–324.

Naeser, M. A., Alexander, M. P., Helm-Estabrooks, N., Levine, H. L., Laughlin, S. A., & Geschwind, N. (1982). Aphasia with predominantly subcortical lesion sites. _Archives of Neurology (Chicago), 39,_ 2–14.

Naeser, M. A., & Hayward, R. W. (1978). Lesion localization in aphasia with cranial computed tomography and the Boston Diagnostic Aphasia Exam. _Neurology, 28,_ 545–551.

Petersen, S. E., Fox, P. T., Posner, M. I., Minton, M., & Raichle, M. E. (1988). Positron emission tomography studies of the cortical anatomy of single-word processing. _Nature (London), 331,_ 585–589.

Poeck, K., De Bleser, R., & von Keyerlingk, D. G. (1984). Computed tomograph localization of standard aphasic syndromes. _Advances in Neurology, 42,_ 71–89.

Rubens, A., & Selnes, O. (1986). _Aphasia with insular cortex infarction._ Proceedings of the Academy of Aphasia Meeting, Nashville, TN.

Schiff, H. B., Alexander, M. P., Naeser, M. A., & Galaburda, A. M. (1983). Aphemia: Clinico-anatomic correlations. _Archives of Neurology (Chicago), 40,_ 720–727.

Selnes, O. A., Knopman, D. S., Niccum, N., & Rubens, A. B. (1985). The critical role of Wernicke's area in sentence repetition. *Archives of Neurology (Chicago), 17,* 549–557.

Selnes, O. A., Knopman, D. S., Niccum, N., Rubens, A. B., & Larson, D. (1983). Computed tomographic scan correlates of auditory comprehension deficits in aphasia: A prospective recovery study. *Archives of Neurology (Chicago), 13,* 558–566.

Selnes, O. A., Niccum, N., Knopman, D. S., & Rubens, A. B. (1984). Recovery of single word comprehension: CT-scan correlates. *Brain and Language, 21,* 72–84.

Tonkonogy, J., & Goodglass, H. (1981). Language function, foot of the third frontal gyrus, and rolandic operculum. *Archives of Neurology (Chicago), 38,* 486–490.

Tranel, D., Biller, J., Damasio, H., Adams, H. P., & Cornell, S. (1987). Global aphasia without hemiparesis. *Archives of Neurology (Chicago), 44,* 304–308.

Wernicke, K. (1874). *Der aphasische symptomkomplex.* Breslau: Cohn & Weigert.

4

Assessment of Aphasia

OTFRIED SPREEN and ANTHONY RISSER

This chapter focuses on the currently available methods of the assessment of aphasia. To view the development of assessment methods in context, a brief historical introduction is necessary. In addition, we attempt to establish a frame of reference for reviewing available methods by describing what appears to us to be key requirements for an acceptable method in general and for the examination of brain-damaged populations in particular. We then review the strengths and weaknesses of each currently available method. We finish with a discussion of the choice of methods in clinical work, with special reference to the widely differing problems, ranging from purely research-oriented questions to questions of measuring day-to-day improvement during therapy and assessing communicative ability in the home or occupational setting.

Historical Introduction

Even the earliest records of medical knowledge make reference to language disorders after brain damage (Benton, 1964). Accounts of simple clinical examinations were often included in such reports, but it was not until the second half of the nineteenth century (specifically since the publications of Broca; Joynt, 1964) that aphasia was explored more systematically. Case reports by Wernicke (1874/1908) and contemporaries contained detailed descriptions of examination procedures for individual patients, often extending over three or more printed pages. Whereas some of these examinations were probably standard procedure in certain hospitals, others were invented on the spot to explore individual features of a specific syndrome of aphasia. Understandably, the reports focused on the patient's specific disorder rather than on the examination procedure.

The clinical examination as developed in the late nineteenth century has been modified and augmented, but it has remained the essential tool of the clinical neurologist. Such examinations are exemplified in the writings of Jackson (1915) and Pick (1913). The standard repertoire of many clinical examinations includes such routine procedures as the Paper Test of Pierre Marie (1883), the Hand–Eye–Ear Test of Henry Head (1926), and Geschwind's (1971) "no ifs, ands, or buts" repetition as a simple task with high multiple demands on the patient's understanding, processing, and repetition ability.

The clinical examination has a number of disadvantages, which gradually led to the development of more generally applicable and standardized assessment instruments. Clinical examinations tend to vary from one place to another, both in content and in the way in which they are administered; what is considered abnormal remains the subjective judgment of the clinician; and the examinations are difficult to replicate and compare. Early attempts to produce a more standardized examination were published by Head (1926), who insisted on a detailed "clinical protocol." Another examination procedure was published by Froeschels, Dittrich, and Wilheim (1932).

The first comprehensive battery of psychological and educational achievement tests for aphasic patients was used by Weisenburg and McBride (1935) in a 5-year study of 60 aphasic patients. Schuell (Schuell, Jenkins, & Jiménez-Pabón, 1964) called this study a landmark because it was the first to use control subjects, to compare aphasic with non-aphasic brain-damaged subjects, and to use standardized methodology. Several other batteries were developed in the 1950s by Wepman (1951), Eisenson (1954), Wepman and Jones (1961), and Schuell (1955), partly as a result of intensive treatment efforts with World War II veterans. Benton (1964) reviewed the development of assessment procedures and noted the work done in various centers, criticizing that none of the procedures had been published in "usable form." The descriptions of procedures were insufficient, no standardization information was presented, and neither exact criteria for scoring nor detailed guides for interpretation were included. He compared the state of the art with the "pre-Binet stage" in intelligence testing: "We are today where intelligence testing was in 1900" (p. 263).

The situation has changed in the 25 years since Benton's review. Instruments have been published that present detailed administration and scoring criteria and that, at least in part, provide information on standardization and interpretation procedures. Our review deals primarily with these more recently developed assessment techniques. Other reviews have been presented by Darley (1979), Kertesz (1979), and Skenes and MacCauley (1985).

Purposes of Assessment and Testing

Assessment procedures vary greatly, depending on the examiner's goal. It is important to consider this goal in evaluating and choosing specific procedures. Obviously, little is gained by administering a lengthy and difficult test battery designed for patients with mild language deficits to a bedridden patient with severe or global aphasia or by limiting an evaluation to a screening test of organicity in a patient with known brain damage. Matching the assessment procedure to the patient requires a flexible and knowledgeable approach to assessment and testing. Four general types of evaluation purposes may be distinguished: (a) screening or clinical procedures, (b) diagnostic evaluation, (c) descriptive assessment for counseling and rehabilitation, and (d) progress evaluation.

Screening.   Screening refers to a typically brief and cursory examination to detect the presence of a disorder. Three types of aphasia screening may be identified: (a) the bedside clinical examination; (b) screening tests per se; and (c) tests of specific aspects of language functioning that are sensitive to the presence of aphasia. The latter are used as part of a broader, specificity-based evaluation.

The BEDSIDE CLINICAL EXAMINATION, as discussed above, is a clinical evaluation in the tradition of classical neurology (see Benson, 1979b; Strub & Black, 1977) and historically has been the primary method of assessing aphasia. Currently, it permits a brief and practical evaluation of language disorders of medical inpatients during the acute stage and remains a standard tool for many attending physicians, neurologists, and speech clinicians. The skilled clinician obviously makes maximal use of his or her communicative interactions with the patient to rule out aphasia, establish a diagnosis, or reach a decision that a more comprehensive diagnostic assessment is warranted.

SCREENING TESTS, such as the one described for Halstead–Reitan examinations (Reitan, 1984; Wheeler & Reitan, 1962), reflect the once-popular application arising out of clinical psychology in the 1950s of screening individuals for the presence or absence of "organicity" (a loose term referring to any form of damage to the nervous system affecting psychological functions), particularly in high-risk groups and in conjunction with psychiatric evaluations. In relation to aphasia, some relatively brief and highly sensitive screening tests are available, but testing for the purpose of screening has lost its attractiveness and usefulness since the 1950s. One reason is that the accuracy of screening devices is limited, usually around 80% (Spreen & Benton, 1965). Another reason is that in clinical practice such cursory "detective work" is rarely necessary, since most patients are referred with an established clinical impression of aphasia, a known organic etiology, and neuroradiological localization. Finally, the information obtained from such instruments offers poor specificity (i.e., there are many reasons why a nonaphasic patient might fail a language screening test) and reveals little to indicate how severe a problem the detected aphasia is in the daily life of the patient. Thus, screening tests have been all but abandoned. Reitan's test remains useful only in the context of a larger neuropsychological evaluation extending far beyond the language area (discussed in more detail below).

Finally, SPECIFIC-FUNCTION TESTS that explore a highly sensitive aspect of language functioning are easily incorporated into comprehensive evaluations, such as the neuropsychological evaluation, to "screen" (explore) the nature of language functioning and determine the need for additional and/or ancillary testing to better describe an observed deficit. The Token Test has proven itself to be the most durable and broadly employed of such specific-function tests; subtests of established aphasia batteries also are employed in this manner, such as the Neurosensory Center Comprehensive Examination for Aphasia (NCCEA) Word Fluency ("F-A-S") task. These tasks (and others) are described later.

Diagnostic Evaluation. Diagnostic evaluation refers to an overall assessment of a patient's language performance to arrive at both a diagnostic statement and a detailed description of areas of associated strengths and weaknesses. Because of the comprehensive nature of this examination, it is suitable for patients who are medically stable in the acute to postacute period of their recovery and for initial and/or follow-up evaluations of patients with subjective complaints of language problems. Diagnostic assessments tend to elicit brief samplings of performance in many different areas and may not necessarily be of use to the speech clinician interested in a detailed exploration of a particular problem. When the evaluation is confined to performances on language and aphasia-related tasks, the diagnostic impression may either refer to the type of aphasia present (i.e., classification) or go beyond the description of the functional deficit and arrive at speculative conclusions about the nature and location of the underlying brain disorder itself (i.e., localization). Impressions from a broader cognitive (neuropsychological) evaluation include the type of aphasia as only one of a number of differentially diagnosable neurobehavioral syndromes, such as dementia, confusional states, amnestic syndrome, attentional disorder, and so forth, in order to determine the full spectrum of the patient's deficits.

Most test authors advocate a particular package or battery of diagnostic tests which, in their view, produces a comprehensive overview of significant aspects of language behavior in the aphasic patient. As a result, fixed batteries are the almost inevitable choice of the clinician looking for a comprehensive diagnostic instrument. Unfortunately, such batteries also reflect the particular school of thought as well as the bias of the test author. For this reason, becoming fully familiar with the theoretical positions of test authors is imperative, although Marshall (1986) pointed out that most batteries that use classification schemes rely on a Wernicke/Lichtheim model, and that between 41% and 50% of patients remain unclassified by such models. Another disadvantage of the fixed battery approach is that including additional examination procedures and interpreting them in relation to the battery itself is difficult because each instrument has been standardized and validated on somewhat differing populations. Nevertheless, such a flexible approach (i.e., adding and elaborating in certain areas, especially if deficits are found) may be the best choice for the speech clinician looking for additional information beyond a classification.

Descriptive Assessment.   For the purpose of counseling and rehabilitation, a descriptive assessment would seem to be the most sensible approach to take in aphasia evaluation, choosing, when warranted, a variety of assessment procedures—a comprehensive diagnostic battery, a functional communication scale, and a number of ancillary and additional tests. Counseling and rehabilitation pose different questions than can be answered from a strictly diagnostic assessment. In particular, it is important to gain as much information as possible about areas of functional strength, as well as about the presence of deficits, since this allows better-reasoned advice of what treatment activities to pursue, what vocational options remain open to the patient, and what actual communicative level the patient can attain. The clinical context often will define the appropriate balance between diagnostic and descriptive modalities in assessment.

Often the ability of patients to name objects or construct sentences from the materials presented in the evaluation setting is not most important, but rather the ability to communicate and to make themselves understood in everyday environments. For this reason, the assessment shifts in emphasis from a strict testing situation to the observation of communicative behavior (often expressed in terms of ratings or levels of success). A bridging of test contexts is necessary in order to compare the relation between specific language behaviors and deficits with the general ability to communicate. Descriptive assessment in the rehabilitation setting also involves (a) making predictions of recovery and of response to treatment and (b) measuring the ability of the patient to process, learn, and remember new material and, hence, be able to actively participate in and benefit from individualized treatment programs.

Progress Evaluation. Closely related to descriptive assessment, progress evaluation permits an evaluation of spontaneous recovery when initial evaluations are repeated in follow-up fashion or when day-to-day or week-to-week progress is charted in treatment settings. The clinician caring for a patient would like to be able to chart changes accurately over time rather than rely on subjective judgments or enthusiastic endorsements of the usefulness of therapy made by the patient or relatives. No formal tests have been developed specifically for this purpose, mainly because such progress assessments have to be tailor-made for each individual and his or her current level and range of deficit. Additionally, criteria need to be established, on an individual basis, as to what will qualify as significant progress, as this likely would vary on a case-by-case basis depending upon patients' premorbid characteristics. Ad hoc assessments may be formulated for tests of entire domains of language functioning or for specific features of modification of singular language behaviors. For this reason, therapists may prefer to "lift" whole sections of an existing test in the appropriate area of deficit and amplify such tests with additional material of their own choosing in order to establish a baseline of performance at the beginning of therapy. Repeated examinations after specified periods of training will then allow a plotting of any change over time and, if a criterion is specified, a determination of whether significant progress has been attained.

The methodology for the development of progress-evaluation or criterion-based techniques during therapy has been well established by authors in the behavior modification field (e.g., Lahey, 1973). The "test–teach–test" approach in both education and speech therapy has the advantage of being directly relevant to the material being taught or the language problem under training; no inferences from a general sampling of language behavior in test batteries are necessary. The approach has the disadvantage of not allowing observations about the broader, more general progress of the patient; however, skilled clinicians will perform comprehensive follow-up diagnostic evaluations for this purpose (at least by the time of discharge from the treatment setting).

Psycholinguistic Evaluation of Aphasic Language

While some of the formalized testing methods to be discussed in the following sections (e.g., the assessment of communicative abilities in daily living) make use of conversational speech in a natural setting with limited structure, some studies have attempted to analyze conversational speech of aphasic patients in a setting that makes no specific demands on the patient. Ideally, one could monitor and record a patient's utterances on audio- or videotape in the course of a day in the hospital or at home. The main goal of such studies is not, however, an assessment of communicative abilities but a more detailed study from a psycholinguistic point of view. Studies of use and abuse of syntax; grammar; word choice; frequency of word usage, pauses, and hesitations; speed of utterance; and so forth, can be conducted with such "free-speech" samples. The alternative approach is to focus on each aspect of psycholinguistic analysis individually and construct an experimental setting that allows an analysis of the types of errors produced by an aphasic patient.

Both the open-ended free-speech and the experimental approach have been used extensively in research with aphasia (Goodglass & Blumstein, 1973; Spreen, 1968). Insofar as these studies represent experiments rather than attempts to assess the aphasic patient's deficit, such studies are not reviewed here. However, some of these studies have led to conclusions about the nature of the deficit in specific types of aphasia and can be translated into suitable methods of assessment. We will briefly describe these studies, and point out their potential application in the development of assessment techniques.

The first comprehensive studies of a psycholinguistic nature were conducted by Wepman and collaborators (Fillenbaum, Jones, & Wepman, 1961; Jones, Goodman, & Wepman, 1963; Spiegel, Jones, & Wepman, 1965; Wepman, Bock, Jones, & Van Pelt, 1956; Wepman & Jones, 1964). Part of this work is based on conversational speech by 50 aphasic speakers in response to the task of making up stories for the Thematic Apperception Test. Various linguistic parameters were calculated, including grammatical form class usage, grammatical correctness, intelligibility, and word-finding problems (the latter three problems correspond to the syntactic, semantic, and pragmatic types of aphasia in

Wepman's terminology). The studies involved complex calculations as well as judgments by linguistically trained researchers; they cannot be readily translated into more directly accessible forms of assessment.

The second major project was conducted by Howes and collaborators (Howes, 1964, 1966, 1967; Howes & Geschwind, 1964) and involved a detailed analysis of conversational speech of 5000 words of each of more than 80 aphasic and nonaphasic speakers. The analysis concentrated on lexical diversity (i.e., the frequency of word usage in aphasic versus nonaphasic speakers) and also distinguished between "fluent" and "nonfluent" speakers, who were viewed as similar to Wernicke's and anomic aphasics and to classical Broca's aphasics, respectively. Benson (1967) attempted to develop a simplified and clinically useful rating scale system based on the information of Howes's study and adding some additional rating dimensions. The ratings used a 3-point scale and involved rate of speaking, prosody, pronunciation, phrase length, effort, pauses, press of speech, perseveration, word choice, paraphasia, and verbal stereotypes. These 11 characteristics were related to radioactive brain scan localization. It was found that anterior lesions tended to produce speech with low verbal output, dysprosody, dysarthria, considerable effort, and predominant use of substantive nouns, whereas posterior lesions produced speech that was normal or near normal on all these features but showed paraphasia, press of speech, and a lack of substantive words.

A third study with a comprehensive analysis of conversational speech of a minimum of 1000 words from 50 aphasic and 50 normal speakers was conducted by Spreen and Wachal (1973; Wachal & Spreen, 1973) using a computer–scorer interaction analysis of various psycholinguistic aspects of spoken language. Crockett (1972, 1976) designed 5-point rating scales for 17 characteristics of speech—including rate of speech, prosody, pronunciation, hesitation, phrase length, effort, pauses, press of speech, perseveration, word choice, paraphasia, communication, naming, grammar, use of interstitial connectives, understanding of spoken language, and use of inflection, tense or gender, and neologisms—in an attempt to translate psycholinguistic speech characteristics into basic rating scale dimensions. Interrater agreement among five judges was satisfactory after some training, and a carefully worded description of each characteristic was given.

Another analysis of "procedural discourse" was performed by Ulatowska, Doyel, Stern, and Haynes (1983), who showed that aphasics showed reduction in complexity and amount, but not in terms of sentential grammar, discourse grammar, and subjective ratings of content and clarity.

Although Benson's (1967) and Crockett's (1972, 1976) translation of psycholinguistic aspects of aphasic speech appeared to be quite successful within the limited scope of the research problems under investigation, further use of this approach has been limited. Some of the ratings have been incorporated into the Boston Diagnostic Aphasia Examination (BDAE). Kerschensteiner, Poeck, and Brunner (1972) used a similar rating system for the study of conversational speech, and Voinescu, Mihajlescu, and Lugoji (1987) rated the communicative value of 27 stimuli in a standard interview to measure progress in the treatment for aphasia. Recently, Shewan (1988) attempted to develop a system to describe and quantify aphasic subjects' connected language in describing pictures, using phonological, semantic, and syntactic components, as well as general parameters of output, such as number of utterances, time, length, articulation, repetition, and paraphasia. The Shewan Spontaneous Language Analysis also received some psychometric support, indicating adequate intrajudge, interjudge, and test–retest reliability, and validity based on clinical judgment of severity of connected language impairment. Other experimental studies include Ryalls and Reinvang's (1986) investigation of the lateralization of linguistic tones (phonemic tone-contrasted pairs); Blumstein, Goodglass, Statlander, and Biber's (1983) study of syntactic comprehension; and DeWolfe, Rausch, and Fedirka's (1985) development of a word-ordering task in which sentences with jumbled word order were reordered by the patient into grammatically correct sentences. Finally, Paul and Cohen (1982) attempted to demonstrate a reciprocal relationship between normal language disorder and language dissolution in aphasia.

These studies demonstrate clearly that the somewhat elusive aspects of speaking style can be translated into scales that are readily understood and usable. Perhaps one reason for the infrequent use of such ratings has been that most have been developed in the context of a relatively complex research rather than in the context of an assessment-oriented project. Another reason may be that psycholinguistic aspects of aphasic speech are rather complex in themselves and not readily understood without prior linguistic training; hence, the clinically oriented examiner tends to shy away from psycholinguistic evaluations and use the relatively more concrete standard testing and assessment methods.

Construction Principles of Aphasia Tests

As pointed out earlier, a distinction can be made between the relatively informal (though frequently well-structured and systematically executed) clinical examination and more formal tests. Both clinical examination and tests may examine the same areas of difficulty; the distinction lies in the quantification of the test examination and in the opportunity to compare quantitative scores with reference norms. Hence, a test could be defined as a clinical examination that meets a number of psychometric requirements.

The following section describes the psychometric requirements for a well-constructed test to establish the information that should be critically evaluated before a test is put to use in daily practice. It should be stated beforehand, however, that hardly any test in the area of aphasia assessment fully meets the stringent psychometric requirements often demanded by the psychometric specialist and by associations concerned with standards of testing (American Psychological Association, 1985). The reason for this is that most tests in the field of aphasia have been developed in individual laboratories in the context of clinical work and are not generally adopted by a large number of services and institutions. At the same time, the demand for such tests remains small (as compared, e.g., to tests of general intelligence). Hence, the collection of norms and the conduct of validity and reliability studies proceeds slowly and is almost entirely dependent on the resources of the test authors and their collaborators. In other words, test development is demanding in terms of both time and money. Aphasia tests are not best-sellers; as a result, development has been less than optimal in most instances and completely neglected in others.

General Requirements for Tests

The most frequently stated requirements for tests of any kind are demonstrated validity, reliability, and standardization (Anastasi, 1988; Nunnally, 1978). We will point out briefly the importance of each of these in general and then with specific reference to the field of aphasia.

STANDARDIZATION

Standardization refers to the test administration itself, which should be constant from patient to patient and from one examiner to another. If test administration and the conditions under which the test is administered are kept as controlled as possible, measurement error can be kept to a minimum. Any deviation from a standard administration procedure (e.g., prompting if the patient cannot respond readily, extending the time limits for answering) will inevitably produce more variability in test scores, and hence undesirable variance when the scores of patients or groups of patients are compared. The clinician may be tempted to use the test material to explore how much a patient may improve as a result of simple aids given during the testing. However justified such a procedure, it should be understood that test results achieved under such modified conditions are no longer comparable to the published norms; that is, they contain an undesirable degree of measurement error. Exploration of the impact on performance of the use of aids and cues on a nonstandard, ad hoc basis is often referred to as "testing the limits" and frequently is used for descriptive rather than diagnostic purposes.

Standardization also refers to the establishment of norms against which the performance of an individual patient can be compared. Norms essentially are a range of scores obtained from a reference group, including the mean score, standard-deviation values, and the distribution of scores from the highest to the lowest scoring subject in that group. These are often expressed in percentile ranks or in relation to a normal distribution score in terms of z scores, t scores, and so forth. Such converted scores indicate a given patient's score in relation to the distribution. For example, a score at the 90th percentile indicates a performance better than 90% of the reference population. If the test is constructed for a variety of populations, separate standardization procedures have to be conducted. For example, if scores tend to vary greatly with age, sex, educational level, or socioeconomic status, separate norms have to be established. Occasionally, additional norms can be avoided by using correction scores for these factors, but this may be impractical if more than two of these factors interact with each other. Norms are usually produced for a group of healthy men and women without neurological impairment or aphasia, which allows the examiner to see where a given person's performance lies in the distribution of scores. Clinically, the examiner can determine whether a patient's performance is within normal limits, is a borderline performance, or is clearly defective (i.e., a performance less than the 1st percentile). Norms developed for normal subjects may not be sufficient for the evaluation of the aphasic patient; this issue is discussed later in the context of specific requirements for tests of aphasia.

RELIABILITY

Reliability refers to the demonstration that on repeat administration after a reasonable time interval and under the same conditions similar results will be obtained for the same subject. Reliability is often demonstrated by giving an alternate form of the test during the same or at a subsequent session, by comparing alternate (odd-numbered and even-numbered) items of the test, by subdividing the test, or by measuring item interrelationships by other means. Generally, reliability is best demonstrated with normal, healthy subjects, since the measurement error in patient populations and the likelihood of change in performance due to changes in the patient's condition are high. Test scoring often involves a certain amount of judgment on the part of the test administrator. For example, if the patient is asked to describe the use of a hairbrush, the response *for hair* may be judged to be unsatisfactory by one scorer and satisfactory by another. In practice, interscorer differences can be reduced to a minimum if the test manual contains sufficient scoring instructions and samples of how a given item can be scored. One form of expressing scoring reliability is to give test records to two or more independent scorers and compute a correlation coefficient between scorers. Such interscorer reliability is highly desirable, since poor reliability of this type will obviously not only affect the general reliability of the test but also introduce measurement error into studies of validity and other psychometric properties.

VALIDITY

Validity is probably the most crucial requirement for any test. It refers to the demonstration that a test measures what it claims. Validity can be demonstrated in a variety of ways; typically, a distinction is made between predictive (or criterion-related), content, and construct validity. Of the three forms, the demonstration that a test is a valid "predictor" of whether a patient is aphasic is the most popular, but of limited value in several ways. The demonstration of validity relies entirely on the fact that the aphasic patient's performance can be discriminated from that of normal subjects on the basis of test results; in other words, the demonstration of validity comes close to the screening problem described earlier. Such a demonstration relies on the clinical judgment made for the aphasic group but neglects the fact that the discrimination between aphasics and normals could result from entirely irrelevant (for aphasia) or trivial test items. In the ideal case, other contrast groups in addition to healthy, normal subjects (i.e., brain-damaged patients without aphasia) should be used. The question of validity for predicting membership in a specific subgroup of aphasics, for example, Broca's aphasia, will be addressed later.

Construct validity is often demonstrated by investigating the correlation of a new test with another test of known validity. However, since few tests in the aphasia field have known validity, an alternative form of validity examination—the demonstration of factorial construct validity—is frequently used. In this case, factor analytic statistical techniques are used to show whether the tests in a given battery all contribute to a major factor of common variance that represents language functions.

Content validity refers to the adequacy of sampling from the domain of behaviors to be measured. In the case of testing for aphasia, for example, measuring verbal fluency alone would not be sufficient, because it does not appear to sample language behavior adequately (unless, of course, it could be shown that other expressive and receptive language functions all correlate highly and uniformly with word fluency). In other words, test items should be based on sound reasoning and should not be trivial or selectively biased. The content should also agree with the content area as defined by other researchers. The range and diversity of the content of a test can also be explored by factor analysis.

Specific Requirements for Tests with Brain-Damaged and Aphasic Patients

In addition to the general requirements for the construction of tests described in the previous section, several specific problems frequently occur in tests that are designed primarily for use with brain-damaged patients and specifically with aphasics. These problems arise in relation to the range of item difficulty, the need to clarify the nature of specific deficits revealed by the tests, the overlap of examinations for aphasia with measures of intelligence, the usefulness of a test in conjunction with recovery and therapy, and the overall conceptualization of the nature of aphasia.

RANGE OF ITEM DIFFICULTY

Range of item difficulty is usually determined by selecting from a range of "very easy" to "very difficult" items. In a well-constructed test, items should be homogeneously distributed; that is, the difficulty range (expressed in percentage of subjects passing each item) should rise in a linear fashion from the first to the last item. This principle of homogeneity of item distributions is relatively easy to follow if we are dealing with a test for a normal population that is reasonably well defined (e.g., all first-grade children in selected, representative parts of the country). The principle can also be followed fairly well for a language test constructed to test normal adults. However, if aphasic subjects are used, most items would be far too difficult for a majority of the patients. As a result, most aphasic subjects would have scores in the bottom range of the distribution or even at a percentile of zero. Consequently, aphasia tests must shift the difficulty of item distribution toward the lower or "easy" end to make it possible to discriminate between mild, moderate, and severe levels of aphasia and to determine aphasic subtypes. In other words, the range of item difficulty will have to be determined by the target population of aphasics, not by the general, healthy population. This shift inevitably produces a "ceiling" effect if the test is applied to normal subjects; normal subjects will usually score at or near the 100% correct range. It is, of course, possible to include items that are easy enough to discriminate between different degrees of aphasia as well as items difficult enough for a normal population; such a test, however, would be extremely lengthy and impractical. In short, for a test to be adequate in discriminating aphasics of different degrees, we will have to abandon the notion that this test can generally be useful for other populations with reasonably normal language behavior.

CLARIFICATION OF DEFECTS

Clarification of specific defects found in aphasics is necessary in many cases, especially in cases of multiple disorders (e.g., aphasia and motor disorder, aphasia and sensory disorder). For example, if a patient cannot provide the name of an object, we cannot automatically ascribe this deficit to an aphasic disorder. It is possible that the patient has difficulty recognizing the object visually or that some form of agnosia is present. If the patient cannot name an object placed in his or her hand, it is possible that sensory loss, inadequate motoric ability to handle the object, or inadequate stereognostic or kinesthetic recognition is responsible. Similarly, reading tasks, which are frequently part of an aphasia assessment, can be influenced by inadequate form discrimination and other factors. In a clinical examination, such alternative explanations are frequently obvious and quickly excluded by appropriate informal tests. It is important, however, to systematically check for such associated deficits, since the test profile produced at the end of standardized testing with many standard batteries may easily be misinterpreted if used in a "blind evaluation" or by an inexperienced examiner. Some aphasia batteries have included supplementary tests for associated deficits and developed clear rules as to when a supplementary test should be used. Such supplementary tests should also follow standard psychometric principles if they are to be used routinely. The inclusion of supplementary tests (see, e.g., Benton, 1967, 1969) may expand the field of examination far beyond the area of aphasia. A comprehensive neuropsychological evaluation can provide such a broad-based examination of aphasic patients.

OVERLAP WITH INTELLIGENCE TESTS

The overlap of assessment of aphasia with measures of intelligence has often gone unnoticed, but it deserves special consideration in the context of item selection and in the context of our discussion of other defects found in association with aphasia. We do not intend to enter into the discussion of whether language-mediated behavior does or does not form an integral part of the cognitive ability of the individual or whether the presence of aphasia must of necessity affect the intellectual ability of the patient. Rather, it should be stressed that in the examination of aphasia the demands on the general intellectual abilities of the patient should be kept to a minimum; in addition, previously acquired knowledge of specific concepts and terms should influence the assessment of aphasia as little as possible.

The problem does not generally arise with the "easy" items used in aphasia tests, but when items for the "difficult" level are constructed, the separation of what is strictly language and what is intelligence becomes blurred. For example, naming tasks can be advanced to any level of difficulty by adding rare words and concepts that are likely to be found only in the vocabulary of the college-educated person of above-average intelligence. Tasks requiring definitions invariably tend to place higher value on abstract, elegant wording and penalize the uneducated, less intelligent subject. Tasks requiring oral arithmetic reasoning and the finding of superordinate concepts and similarities are, in fact, part of most recognized standard intelligence tests presently in use. For this reason, tests must be carefully scrutinized for content that exceeds the basic examination of language abilities. If such content cannot be avoided because of the range of item difficulties, the test must contain separate norms for patients of different ranges of intellectual and educational background or must apply adequate corrections for such factors.

USE IN MEASURING RECOVERY

The use of tests in the context of recovery and therapy pose two problems. The first is essentially an additional validity problem, that is, whether or not a test is suitable for the measurement of recovery with or without therapy. Tests adequate for the measurement of recovery may be slightly different in content from tests that merely indicate the presence or type of aphasia and may require more items in certain difficulty ranges to allow the measurement of even small steps in recovery. A related question may be the ability of a test to predict recovery, which must be established independently of or in addition to other validation procedures.

The second related problem deals with the ability of patients to relearn or compensate for what they have lost. This is a neglected aspect of aphasia assessment. Most tests merely measure the status quo but deliberately exclude any practice or learning during the testing procedure. As pointed out earlier, providing cues to a patient during diagnostic evaluations usually is seen as contributing to measurement error and hence must be avoided at all costs. If a test were to be designed to provide information on the relearning capacity of the patient, an entirely different approach to item construction would have to be taken. This approach would systematically include a variety of short learning trials with different kinds of cues in order to investigate whether the patient's language performance benefits, at least within the immediate testing situation. It should be obvious that the inclusion of such procedures in the assessment of aphasia would dramatically change the usual form of testing, affect retest reliability, and presumably add to the length of the test. Yet it is our impression that the benefits of such tests will outweigh the additional problems of test construction and validation and that such tests will be a major concern of test development in the future. Informal assessment of a patient's relearning capacity has, of course, been available for quite some time, and specific rules for such procedures have been developed in detail. This question will be addressed further in the last part of this chapter.

CONCEPTUALIZATION OF THE NATURE OF APHASIA

The conceptualization of the nature of aphasia is one recurrent theme underlying many of the considerations outlined in this section. The selection of tests is directly influenced by whether we see aphasia as a specific disorder of selected abilities or as a pervasive disturbance of communication, and by whether we conceive of aphasia as unitary in nature or as consisting of many "subtypes." Benton (1967) in his discussion of this problem pointed out that the choice of a model of language functioning determines what kind of test we construct or use. He indicated that the problem is similar to the one posed by the conceptualization of intelligence; it is similar also in the sense that no common agreement exists. Although Benton at that time still expressed some hope for the possibility of achieving a consensus, the development of research in aphasia (and in test construction) would seem to suggest that we have reached an impasse similar to that reached in the conceptualization (and testing) of intelligence. As a result, two approaches to test construction should be recognized as equally reasonable at this time:

1. To construct tests on the basis of one of the currently accepted conceptions of aphasia. This "taxonomic" or diagnostic approach ensures that the test measures all aspects viewed as important in a specific theoretical approach but makes it probable that the test will not be widely used as long as different conceptualizations of aphasia are held by other works in the field.

2. To approach the problem pragmatically, avoid specific conceptualizations, and construct a test that contains a wide variety of probes

of all abilities usually described by researchers of widely differing theoretical viewpoints. This pragmatic approach, also described by Benton and quite commonly used in the field of intelligence testing, will not be fully satisfactory to any of the prevailing schools but may gain wider acceptance if the test instrument is otherwise well constructed and of demonstrated use in clinical practice. One drawback of this shotgun approach to test construction is the possibility of including redundant and/or highly specific material that may be irrelevant to the assessment of aphasia. This problem can be solved by future factor analytic investigations as long as the range of material is sufficiently wide to allow such conclusions.

Both approaches have been applied in the construction of currently used tests. In the following description of individual tests, we make specific reference to the conceptual framework used in each for the information of the reader unfamiliar with a given instrument.

Current Methods for the Assessment of Aphasia

The following review of assessment procedures is given in an attempt to survey current and readily available methods and to provide sufficient introductory information for readers unfamiliar with some of the procedures to choose those methods most likely to meet their needs. Table 4.1 lists, in alphabetical order, the tests that will be reviewed and each test's primary source, from which the test may be obtained. Information on the test procedure itself, the choice and range of assessment, the psychometric properties of the test, the theoretical position of the test authors, and the most likely areas of use of each test will be described. We begin with descriptions of published clinical assessment procedures, then discuss brief tests that are screening tests or may address only specific aspects of aphasia. Rating procedures and other measures of actual conversational speech in a communication setting will be considered next. Finally, comprehensive tests will be described. A short section on tests specifically designed for children is added.

Clinical Examination

The clinical examination, historically the primary method of assessing aphasia, remains the standard tool of the clinical examiner, especially the neurologist as well as many speech clinicians. The advantage of the

TABLE 4.1
Aphasia Assessment Instruments

Full title	Abbreviation used in text	Source
Aphasia Language Performance Scales	ALPS	Keenan and Brassell (1975)
Aphasia Screening Test	AST	Reitan (1984)
Appraisal of Language Disturbances	ALD	Emerick (1971)
Auditory Comprehension Test for Sentences	ACTS	Shewan (1980)
Boston Diagnostic Aphasia Examination	BDAE	Goodglass and Kaplan (1983)
Boston Naming Test	–	Kaplan et al. (1983)
Communicative Abilities in Daily Living	CADL	Holland (1980)
Functional Communication Profile	FCP	M. T. Sarno (1969)
Minnesota Test for Differential Diagnosis of Aphasia	MTDDA	Schuell (1965, 1973)
Multilingual Aphasia Examination	MAE	Benton and Hamsher (1989)
Neurosensory Center Comprehensive Examination for Aphasia	NCCEA	Spreen and Benton (1977)
Pantomime Recognition	–	Benton et al. (1983)
Phoneme Discrimination	–	Benton et al. (1983)
Porch Index of Communicative Ability	PICA	Porch (1973)
Reporter's Test	–	De Renzi (1980)
Sklar Aphasia Scale	SAS	Sklar (1973)
Sound Recognition Test	SRT	Spreen and Benton (1974)
Token Test	–	Many versions, see text
Western Aphasia Battery	WAB	Kertesz (1982)

clinical examination lies in its flexibility, brevity, and suitability for even severely physically impaired patients, since the examiner can conduct a cursory examination at the bedside during acute recovery and follow up any errors made by the patient by further exploration with additional tasks, while skipping quickly across areas of strength where there is no obvious impairment.

Numerous versions of the clinical examination have been recorded, in formal descriptions within the contexts of a mental status examination in neurology (Strub & Black, 1977), a general neurological examination (Poeck, 1974), and specifically designed clinical examinations (Benson, 1979b), as well as in individual case descriptions (e.g., Geschwind & Kaplan, 1962). Luria (1966) provided a detailed description of the clinical examination. The clinical examination usually includes:

1. An evaluation of spontaneous or conversational speech, observing specifically the fluency of output, effort, articulation, phrase length, dysprosody, paraphasias, and tendencies to omit words.
2. Repetition, including the standard repetition of digits and building to the repetition of multisyllabic words, complex sentences, or verbal sequences.
3. Comprehension of spoken language. For the patient with major motor impairment, it is necessary to restrict the examination to questions that can be answered with yes or no or, if speaking is impaired, by pointing.
4. Word finding, usually by asking for the names of common objects and object parts both with and without prompting. Frequently the initial phoneme is offered as a cue, or an open-ended statement is provided to allow the word to be produced in appropriate embedding.
5. Reading, usually from a newspaper or a magazine.
6. Writing, starting with the patient's own name and proceeding to dictated and spontaneous writing (e.g., "Describe your job.").

Because the clinical examination varies greatly in form as well as detail from one setting to another, we do not attempt a comparative evaluation of different examination methods. Clinical examination skills must be acquired under close supervision in a clinical setting.

In a reevaluation of her Short Examination for Aphasia, Schuell (1966) carefully debates the merits of the clinical examination in comparison to the comprehensive test. She stresses that only a comprehensive test can assess all aspects of "aphasia, [which] deals with one of the most complex and perhaps the only unique function of the human brain" (Schuell, 1966, p. 138).

Screening Tests

The following tests have been deliberately designed to screen for the presence or absence of aphasia within a limited time period. They are described here as short screening tests since they do not claim to provide a detailed description of the aphasic disorder but to check for and focus the direction on the problem if aphasia is present.

APHASIA SCREENING TEST (AST)

The Reitan (1984; Heimburger & Reitan, n.d., Wheeler & Reitan, 1962) version of this screening device is designed to determine whether the patient can perform such simple tasks as spelling a word or naming an object. The AST procedures are such that the clinician should elicit the patient's best possible performance. A large array of language function is briefly assessed by one or two items each. For example, the patient is required to draw a shape, name it, and spell it; to read (e.g., "See the black dog"); to do a single pencil-and-paper and a single "in-head" arithmetic problem; and to demonstrate object use and picture drawing.

The test takes approximately 20 min to complete. The test manual provides many illustrative examples of performances. As stated in the introduction of this chapter, screening tests of this type have seen little use recently because they provide very limited information and tend to show only limited accuracy. The test is usually given within the context of a complete neuropsychological test battery intended to assess the full range of psychological deficits after brain damage (Meier, 1974). Inter-rater reliability has been reported as high (Barth et al., 1984). The screening efficiency of the test as a single measure (discrimination between aphasic and nonaphasic brain-damaged patients) has been reported as 80% correct (Krug, 1971). Ernst (1988) reported normative data for elderly subjects.

It should be noted that Barth (1984), Goldstein and Shelly (1984), and Werner, Ernst, Townes, Peel, and Preston (1987) reported significant correlation between the AST and IQ as well as educational level in large neuropsychiatric populations. In a study by Snow (1987), only 1 of 33 items of the AST differentiated between right- and left-hemisphere lateralized tumor and stroke patients.

APHASIA LANGUAGE PERFORMANCE SCALES (ALPS)

The ALPS (Keenan & Brassell, 1975) was designed to address the following questions: "What is the patient's best level of performance in each language modality, and how can we best use this information to plan effective therapy?" (p. 3). The authors considered the ALPS to be a "significant departure" from psychometric objectivity in aphasia assessment. The endpoint of this psychometric trend, according to the ALPS authors, is such that examiners "are encouraged, in short, to divest themselves in their own personality, to suppress their individual responses to each change in their environments, and to behave rather like machines" (p. 31).

The ALPS is composed of four 10-item scales: listening, talking, reading, and writing. Item arrangement in each scale is in terms of difficulty. For each scale, a correct response is defined as that which the tester might expect from a normal adult. A correct or self-corrected response is given full credit (1 point); a correct response that requires prompting is given half credit (½ point). The tester is free to begin each scale at whichever level he or she feels the patient will be competent. A scale is terminated upon two consecutive failures. Criteria for determining normal performance, the need for prompting, and the point in the subscale at which the patient will be competent are at the discretion of the tester. The number of correctly completed items is used as a score for each section and is directly translated into a scale of impairment. The authors have provided an arbitrarily determined descriptive scale of impairment for each section, ranging from "profoundly impaired" for a scale score of 0–1 to "insignificant impairment" for a scale score of 9.5–10.

Normative data are not provided. Given the subjective nature of the ALPS administration, however, normative data would be, for all intents and purposes, of little value.

The ALPS would seem to fall into the gray area between clinical and psychometric screening assessment: Although systematized to a greater degree than many personal clinical examinations, the ALPS falls short of being a standard and comprehensive test instrument. The authors disclaimed any psychometric intentions in creating the ALPS. Hence, the interested clinician would do well by weighing the positive and negative aspects of the ALPS against his or her own personal, informal clinical assessment rather than attempting, as the authors did, to contrast the ALPS with psychometrically established comprehensive aphasia examinations.

SKLAR APHASIA SCALE (SAS)

The SAS (revised SAS; Sklar, 1973) provides a brief assessment of the aphasic patient's abilities along four dimensions: auditory decoding, visual decoding, oral encoding, and graphic encoding. Each of the four subtests is represented by five areas that are each composed of five items. The SAS is constructed within the framework of a decode (input), transcode (process), and encode (output) model of language communication and its disabilities. Items on the SAS were chosen solely for their ability to sample verbal behavior; other items were omitted in deference to neuropsychological and neurological assessments of the patient.

Each response on the SAS is scored on a 5-point scale: a "correct" response (0), a correct though "retarded" response (1), a correct though "assisted" response (2), a "distorted" response (3), and an "erased" response (i.e., no response) (4). An impairment score for each subtest is obtained by finding the mean value of the four subtest impairment scores (0 = no impairment to 100 = full impairment). Five categories of the severity of total impairment are provided. The test author stated that the total impairment index may be used prognostically in terms of potential benefit of therapy if modified by both the recency of the impairment and the patient's overall state of health.

SAS items were standardized on a sample of 20 adults ranging in age from 29 to 78 years. The test author reported high correlations between SAS performance and performance on Eisenson's aphasia examination, Schuell's short version based upon the Minnesota Test for Differential Diagnosis of Aphasia (MTDDA), and the Halstead–Wepman aphasia screening test in a sample of 12 aphasic patients.

The SAS is a brief aphasic examination designed to elicit relevant information on a patient's abilities along four dimensions of decoding and encoding. Although reliability data are not presented, the test author presented five studies examining the validity of the SAS as an instrument to assess language ability in aphasics. The test author stated that the impairment index derived from SAS performance has prognostic significance; however, such prognostication is based on only a very simple index score (e.g., an aphasic performing with a score of 70 having a better prognosis than an aphasic scoring 15), and psychometric evaluations of SAS prognostic significance have not yet been presented.

Other screening tests have been developed by Fitch and Sands (1987), Lecours, Mehler, Parente, and Beltrami (1988), and Orzeck (1964; Inglis & Lawson, 1981), but have so far found only limited use.

Tests of Specific Aspects of Language Behavior

Several tests have been constructed for the detailed assessment of a specific function (e.g., language comprehension only; see also the detailed review of auditory comprehension tests by Boller, Kim, & Mack, 1977). Such tests usually make no claim to cover all aspects of aphasia but provide a relatively thorough assessment of the function in question. Because such functions are usually central to the aphasic disorder, however, these tests may also provide a reasonable discrimination between aphasic and nonaphasic patients in general. Some of these tests have been used as screening devices because of their good discrimination, although this was not necessarily the intent of the authors.

TOKEN TEST

The Token Test was introduced as a brief test by De Renzi and Vignolo in 1962 to examine subtle auditory comprehension deficits in aphasic patients, by having patients respond gesturally to the tester's verbal command. Since its inception, the original Token Test has been widely used, has been modified (De Renzi, 1980; De Renzi & Faglioni, 1978), and functions as a subtest in some aphasia batteries (e.g., Benton & Hamsher, 1978, 1989; Spreen & Benton, 1977). The original test has spawned many variants, for example, short forms (Boller & Vignolo, 1966; Spellacy & Spreen, 1969; Van Harskamp & Van Dongen, 1977), a concrete-objects version (Martino, Pizzamigilo, & Razzano, 1976), a format with both auditory and visual presentation of commands (Kiernan, 1986), a Token Test "battery" (Brookshire, 1978); and a version with expanded linguistic examination (McNeal & Prescott, 1978). The many versions available have led to natural confusion as to what a "Token Test" performance actually represents.

The Token Test is a brief and portable test that, in most versions, is composed of 20 plastic token stimuli of two sizes (large and small), two shapes (square and round), and five colors. Tokens are laid out in front of the patient, typically in a standard 4 × 5 matrix. The test comprises a variable number of sections that generally increase in their linguistic complexity (e.g., from "Point to a square" to "Pick up the small green square" to "Put the small red square on the large blue circle"). The McNeal and Prescott (1978) version provides the most complex commands.

Some authors have reported age (Emery, 1986) and level of education (De Renzi, 1980; De Renzi & Faglioni, 1978) differences on certain versions of the Token Test. Gallaher (1979) reported day-to-day retest reliabilities for one version of the Token Test and its subsections to be greater than .90. Validation studies have shown the Token Test to be a strong and accurate discriminator between the performance of aphasic patients and that of normal hospitalized adults (De Renzi, 1980), nonaphasic right-hemisphere damaged adults (Boller & Vignolo, 1966; Swisher & Sarno, 1969), and nonaphasic diffuse and focal brain-damaged adults (Orgass & Poeck, 1966). Morley, Lundgren, and Haxby (1979) found the Token Test to discriminate particularly well between normals and aphasics with high levels of ability in comparison with discriminations on the Boston Diagnostic Aphasia Examination (BDAE) comprehension section and the Porch Index of Communicative Ability (PICA). Poeck, Kerschensteiner, and Hartje (1972) also demonstrated independence of Token Test performance and the fluency–nonfluency dimension in aphasic patients. Cohen, Kelter, and Shaefer (1977) and Cohen, Lutzweiler, and Woll (1980) examined construct validity and other aspects of Token Test validity. The memory component of Token Test performance was examined by Lesser (1976), Cohen, Gutbrod, Meier, and Romer (1987), and Gutbrod, Mager, Meier, and Cohen (1985), who concluded that the test measures deficits in the short-term storage of highly specific information in aphasics. In contrast, Riedel and Stud-dert-Kennedy (1985) claimed that a general cognitive deficit is responsi-ble for poor Token Test performance.

The Token Test has maintained consistent popularity as both a clinical and an investigative test instrument, and has been examined for use as a therapeutic tool (Holland & Sonderman, 1974; West, 1973). Two major compilations of work with the Token Test are available (Boller & Dennis, 1979; McNeal & Prescott, 1978). At least three English-language versions are commercially available (Benton & Hamsher, 1989; McNeal & Pres-cott, 1978; Spreen & Strauss, 1991).

The Token Test's advantages lie in sound discriminative validity, por-tability, and brief administration time. Brookshire's (1973) early advice remains notable, that is, that the clinician keep in mind that, although it is a sensitive indicator of comprehension deficits, the Token Test relies on a limited stimulus array. Other tests of auditory comprehension (e.g., the Auditory Comprehension Test for Sentences [ACTS]) may be used to supplement or replace the Token Test. Other comprehension tests devel-oped in recent years include Lexical Understanding with Visual and Semantic Distractors (LUVS; Bishop & Byng, 1984), which focuses on semantic comprehension, and an object-manipulation test designed to measure syntactic comprehension (Caplan, 1987).

REPORTER'S TEST

De Renzi employed the stimuli and most of the commands from the Token Test (De Renzi & Faglioni, 1978) to construct the Reporter's Test, a screening test for expressive deficits in aphasic patients (De Renzi, 1980; De Renzi & Ferrari, 1979). The Reporter's Test was designed to meet two specific goals: (a) to elicit organized speech, and (b) to limit the range of what the patient is expected to say. Whereas picture description tasks (e.g., BDAE or the Western Aphasia Battery [WAB]) adequately fulfill the first goal, they fail on the second. The patient is required to act as a "reporter" on this task; that is, the patient must report the actions of the tester to an imaginary third person. For example, if the tester were to touch the large red circle stimulus, the patient must verbalize the rele-vant information necessary for a third person to reproduce the tester's action ("Touch the large red circle."). The Reporter's Test begins with several sample items to acquaint the patient with the task. The test comprises five sections; the first four sections are taken from parts 2–5 of the Token Test.

De Renzi (1980) reported initial findings for the Reporter's Test in discriminating 24 aphasic patients from 40 hospitalized, nonaphasic, nonbrain-damaged controls. In this study, an actual third person sat next to the aphasic patient and performed as the aphasic instructed. Scoring was on a pass–fail basis; partial credit was given for correct performances after repetition. Years of education, but not age, were significantly related to performance; for this reason, scores were corrected to account for education. Using a cutting score expected to produce 5% false positives, a 97% overall hit rate was obtained. Classification accuracy was higher for the Reporter's Test than for four other tests of verbal expression: visual naming, oral fluency, sentence repetition, and story telling.

De Renzi and Ferrari (1979) described aphasic performance employing both pass–fail scoring and weighted scoring (1 point for each bit of information on a trial but without particular credit for repetition). Aphasic patients, nonaphasic left-brain–damaged patients, and nonaphasic right-brain–damaged patients were described. Using the pass–fail scoring system, a cutting score of 18.35 resulted in a 92% hit rate, yielding 10% false positives in the sample of nonaphasic left-brain–damaged patients and 15% false positives in the right-brain–damaged sample. Sample classification on the Reporter's Test again proved superior to that on tests of visual naming, word fluency, sentence repetition, and story telling. Score corrections for educational level are provided. Using the weighted scoring system, a cutting score of 54 resulted in an 82% hit rate; while yielding 15% false positives in the nonaphasic left-brain–damaged group. The authors recommended the use of both scoring systems to offset the weaknesses of each: low classification for the weighted system and overly severe evaluation using pass–fail scoring.

A critical assessment of the utility of the Reporter's Test in a clinical setting must await detailed normative data as well as data indicating test reliability and validity. De Renzi recommended that it be used following the Token Test, so that the patient is acquainted with the stimuli and the required commands. The test has yet to show the same broad appeal and use as has the Token Test.

WORD FLUENCY TESTS

Word fluency tests provide fast, efficient assessments of verbal fluency in aphasic patients. The task is one of controlled word association to a specific letter of the alphabet or to some category, such as animals or foods; the test does not measure fluency of conversational speech. The patient is required to produce as many words as possible within a given time period. Deficits in aphasic patients are common, but defective controlled word association also may be observed in patients with dementia and in patients with anterior left hemisphere lesions. Several standardized tests of word fluency are available. The first word fluency test, by

Spreen and Benton (1977), is a subtest of the NCCEA. Others have been created by Benton and Hamsher (1978, 1989) in the Multilingual Aphasia Examination (MAE), by Wertz (1979), and by Goodglass and Kaplan (1983) in the BDAE.

Spreen and Benton's version requires the patient to say as many words as possible that begin with the letters F, A, and S within 1-min time periods. Proper names and words that differ only in suffix are excluded; performance is gauged in terms of the sum of admissible words in all three trials. Normative data, as well as corrections for age and level of education, are available in the NCCEA test manual (Spreen & Benton, 1977; Spreen & Strauss, 1991).

The letters employed in the NCCEA version are of the "easy" level, as defined by Borkowski, Benton, and Spreen (1967). Borkowski et al. examined the number of associations by normal adult females for 24 of the 26 letters of the alphabet. The number of associations was related with the difficulty level, as defined by both the Thorndike–Lorge (1944) count ($r = .80$) and the number of words per letter in *Webster's New Collegiate Dictionary* ($r = .74$). The authors also reported that a heterogeneous sample of brain-damaged patients performed less well than normal adults at all levels of brain difficulty, lending validity to the testing method. Patients with low IQ scores were better differentiated with easy-level letters, whereas patients with high IQ scores were better distinguished with more difficult levels.

Interscorer reliability is near perfect; one-year test–retest reliability has been reported as .70 (Snow & Tierney, 1988). Concurrent validity has been established in several studies, generally indicating better validity for letters than for concrete categories (Coelho, 1984). Correlation with age is .19, with education .32, with Wechsler Adult Intelligence Scale (WAIS) Verbal IQ .14 and with Performance IQ .29 (Yeudall, Fromm, Reddon, & Stefanyk, 1986). The test contributed mainly to Factor 1 (reading–writing) in a factor analytic study with child data (Crockett, 1974); this finding is probably due to the still-developing spelling skills at that age. In children with closed head injury, 15% of those with mild and 35% of those with moderate and severe injury scored below the 6th percentile for age and sex (Ewing-Cobbs, Levin, Eisenberg, & Fletcher, 1987). Adults with closed head injuries had mean scores of less than 28 (M. T. Sarno, Buonaguro, & Levita, 1986), similar to means found for nonaphasic brain-damaged patients, whereas aphasics ranged from 0 to 46 with a mean of 11.5 words (Spreen & Benton, 1977). Alzheimer's and Huntington's disease patients did not show reduced word fluency, but did show more intrusions (wrong letters), perseverations, and variations (*fish, fishy, fishing*) (K. Adams, personal communication, 1988). Miller and

Hague (1975) and Murdoch, Chenery, Wilks, and Boyle (1987), however, did find reduced word fluency in Alzheimer's disease patients, whereas patients with depression mimicking dementia showed little change compared with normals (Kronfol, Hamsher, Digre, & Waziri, 1978).

Benton and Hamsher's (1978, 1989) MAE version differs from the NCCEA in using three letters of progressively increasing associative difficulty. Otherwise, the testing format is quite similar. Two equivalent versions are available for repeated or follow-up administrations. Normative and validational data and age and level of education corrections are provided in the MAE manual.

Wertz's (1979) format, like that of the NCCEA, employs all easy-level letters (i.e., *S, T, P,* and *C*), However, proper names are permitted, and age and level of education corrections are not employed. Normative data have been provided by Wertz and Lemme (1974) and Wertz, Keith, and Custer (1971). Standardized instructions for Wertz's format are available in the protocol manual of the Veteran's Administration (1973). Wertz et al. (1971) reported correlations of word-fluency performance with PICA overall and verbal dimensions, and with performance on the last section of the Token Test format that they used in their study.

The BDAE (Goodglass & Kaplan, 1983) makes use of Animal Fluency, a format with a tradition of use in child evaluation settings.

Tests of word fluency are quick and simple. The versions described here have proven discriminative validity. Reliability data, however, are lacking. Word fluency tests may not be very sensitive in distinguishing at lower levels of ability, but they are capable of screening for the presence of less severe disability.

"IOWA GROUP" TESTS

In addition to developing two full-scale aphasia batteries (described below), Benton and his colleagues have developed a number of specific-function tests for use in the evaluation of aphasic patients. Some of these tests are described briefly.

The SOUND RECOGNITION TEST (SRT) (Spreen & Benton, 1974; Spreen & Strauss, 1991) affords the examination of auditory object recognition by requiring the identification of familiar sounds. The original format of the SRT involved two equivalent forms of 13 items apiece. Three modes of administration were described: verbal response, pointing to one of four written multiple-choice names per trial, and pointing to one of four multiple-choice line drawings per trial. Varney (1980, 1984a) modified the format such that all 26 items are presented and multiple-choice pointing to line drawings is employed as the response format. Spreen and Benton (1974) described norms for normal adult and child controls and the performances of brain-damaged adults; Varney (1980) described normative information for his modified SRT. Impairments in sound recognition are typically limited to aphasic patients and frequently associated with aural comprehension deficits. Aphasics with aural comprehension deficits in the acute stage of recovery from CVA but with normal sound recognition show rapid and near complete recovery of aural comprehension deficits, although patients with acute aural comprehension and sound recognition defects show a much poorer outcome (Varney, 1984a). Defects in sound recognition are associated with a number of lesion sites, none of which appear specific for the manifestation of the defect (Varney & Damasio, 1986).

The PANTOMIME RECOGNITION test (Benton, Hamsher, Varney, & Spreen, 1983), presented on videotape (¾-in. format), shows a male pantomiming different activities (e.g., using a telephone). The patient is presented with four multiple-choice responses: one correct, one semantic error, one neutral error, and one odd error. Defective pantomime recognition is an infrequent finding, observed most frequently in aphasic patients, and appears to be related to associated defects in reading comprehension. Demented patients also may perform defectively on the task.

The PHONEME DISCRIMINATION test (Benton et al., 1983) is a brief test of the accurate discrimination of phonemic sounds. The test developed from basic theory of the relation between oral language comprehension in aphasic patients and the underlying factors that might be related with this level of comprehension, such as phonemic decoding and sequential sound perception. The test consists of 30 pairs of one- or two-syllable nonsense words on audiotape. The patient has to indicate whether the pair members are the same or different. Practice or pretraining is encouraged to determine if the patient can make same–different responses with reliability. Normative data and performances by samples of 100 aphasic left-hemisphere–damaged and 16 nonaphasic right-hemisphere–damaged patients are reported in the test manual. Comparisons of the performances of the aphasic patients on the Phoneme Discrimination test and on the MAE Aural Comprehension test also are reported (see also Varney & Benton, 1979). Varney (1984b) presented longitudinal data on the Phoneme Discrimination test in the context of evaluation of additional measures of comprehension.

AUDITORY COMPREHENSION TEST FOR SENTENCES (ACTS)

The ACTS (Shewan, 1980) is an examination of auditory comprehension and represents the clinical version of an earlier experimental instrument (Shewan & Canter, 1971). Sentences are spoken by the tester, and the patient must point to one of four visual displays to indicate which correctly represents the spoken sentence. Four preliminary training tri-als are permitted, which also serve as a screening device to determine which patients are too impaired to perform the entire task. These initial trials are followed by the 21 test items, which vary along parameters of (a) sentence length, (b) vocabulary difficulty, and (c) syntactic complex-ity. Pass–fail and qualitative error-analysis scoring are possible; the use of each system is made easy by the clear and concise ACTS response sheet. The test manual states that an average of 10–15 min is required to complete the ACTS.

An ACTS score of 18 of 21 (i.e., approximately 2 *SD*s below the mean) is considered to be the lower bound of normal limits for adults with at least an elementary school education. Shewan (1980) reported an ACTS internal consistency correlation coefficient of .82, as well as a test–retest reliability coefficient of .87. Two statements of validity are provided in the manual. First, a correlation of .80 was obtained between the ACTS and an 8-point clinical rating of functional auditory-verbal comprehen-sion. Second, when compared with established tests, a correlation of .52 between the ACTS and the BDAE auditory comprehension section and one of .89 with the WAB comprehension section were obtained. The lower ACTS–BDAE correlation was attributed to the wider range of abilities assessed in the BDAE than in the ACTS.

Information regarding the ACTS standardization sample of 150 apha-sics and 30 normal adult controls is provided in the test manual. The aphasic sample comprised 134 cases of cerebrovascular accidents, 10 cases of trauma, and 6 postsurgical cases. Means and standard devia-tions of the performance of various aphasic syndrome groups (Wer-nicke's, Broca's, and amnesic, as diagnosed clinically), as well as typical profiles, are included. As might be expected, Wernicke's aphasics per-formed the poorest, followed in turn by Broca's aphasics, aphasics with anomia, and normal controls. Qualitative features of group differences are discussed in the manual. The ACTS (along with the WAB) has been used to examine recovery over time and the differential impact of treat-ment in a subtyped sample of 100 aphasics (Shewan & Kertesz, 1984); improvements in performance over time were similar for treated and untreated patients.

The ACTS is brief, is easy to administer and score with an excellent response sheet, and requires simple nonverbal responses by the patient. It exhibits reliability, validity, and a good deal of promise as a test of comprehension for sentence-length material with systematic variations in sentence length, difficulty, and complexity. The test manual contains cautions in evaluating obtained performance, such as differences be-tween the ACTS standardization sample and the clinician's referral base, as well as educational and cultural influences on test performance.

Rating Scales

Rating scales take a position somewhat in between the clinical assessment and psychometric tests. The clinician who assigns a label of "mild," "moderate," or "severe" to the symptoms of a patient is actually involved in a basic rating of severity. Ratings are frequently used (a) as a summary judgment of severity of any given symptom or syndrome and (b) as a specific judgment of aspects of a patient's behavior that cannot be readily measured. The first application refers to a complex process that weighs all the information on a given patient. A specific example is a professional's judgment in an indemnity suit in court; the professional may even be asked to specify whether the impairment affects 20% or 50% of the patient's ability before the onset of illness. The second application is of more specific interest in the context of this discussion. In this case, some aspect of the patient's speech behavior—for example, fluency of expression or ability to communicate in the home setting—is rated on a scale of levels or points. Several comprehensive batteries— the BDAE, MAE, and WAB—include qualitative rating scales as part of their set of subtests. Usually, a rating scale does not exceed 7 points (from "normal" to "very severe"), since it has been demonstrated that rating scales with more than 7 points do not enhance the accuracy of the ratings but merely provide a false impression of greater accuracy.

Rating scales should be subjected to careful interjudge reliability studies. Such reliability improves with very careful description of each rating point. For example, instead of marking the lowest point as "normal" and the highest as "very severe," each point should be illustrated in as much detail as possible with examples and descriptions. Rating scales are no substitute for psychometric testing, but they are extremely valuable if the information being rated cannot be readily tested or is too complex to be documented in test item scores. Ratings of communicative ability in the home or in a conversational setting are often made by an informant (e.g., a relative or a member of the nursing staff) rather than by the clinician who sees the patient only in a highly structured, isolated, and somewhat artificial examining or therapy situation. The Functional Communication Profile (M. T. Sarno, 1969) is a standardized rating scale of such communicative features.

Communication Profiles

A distinction between selective language behavior on aphasia batteries and the patient's attempt to communicate in everyday environments has intuitive value to the speech clinician. Sarno's Functional

Communication Profile (FCP; M. T. Sarno, 1969; Taylor, 1965) was the first standardized attempt to assess the functional usefulness of language ability in the everyday life of the aphasic patient. The Communicative Abilities in Daily Living (CADL; Holland, 1980) was the second psychometric measure to index the degree of disability faced by the patient in attempting to communicate in daily life. A more recent functional communication measure, the Communicative Effectiveness Index (Lomas et al., 1989), relies mainly on the patient's communicative interaction with spouses or significant others. The rating of functional language and verbal processing skills in daily living has also become a common constituent dimension in the many geriatric rating scales (see review by DeBettignies & Mahurin, 1989) and in available mental competency batteries (e.g., the Cognitive Competency Battery; Wang, Ennis, & Copland, 1986), but these somewhat omnibus measures for use with the elderly generally lack the suitable standardization and item range for use with aphasic patients.

The FCP and the CADL defer obtaining pure, isolated samples of specific language behaviors (as obtained by diagnostic tests of aphasia) in favor of sampling complex communicative behaviors, such as abilities to communicate on the telephone, handle money, read newspapers and product labels, and ask for, correct, and impart significant information to and from others. As such, the information gauged on these profiles is a unique contribution to the overall assessment of the aphasic patient, providing the clinician with descriptive information about the communicative status of the patient, which can be considered as a second dimension of information not directly obtained from formal diagnostic testing procedures (M. T. Sarno, 1984a).

FUNCTIONAL COMMUNICATION PROFILE (FCP)

The FCP (M. T. Sarno, 1969; Taylor, 1965) is designed to measure natural language use in everyday communication, as distinguished from language elicited in the typically structured test setting. The FCP attempts to index the aphasic patient's ability to employ language in common situations, relative to the patient's estimated premorbid level of ability. "Normal" performance on the profile is defined by the clinician's skilled estimation of the patient's previous language ability based on available evidence (e.g., education level, occupation, interviews with family members, available objective documentation). The effectiveness of a clinician-based rating scale of this type is directly related to the experience and skill of the user; therefore, the FCP is not recommended for use by testing technicians or clinicians with limited experience, or in settings where few adult aphasics are likely to be seen. Its usefulness also may be very limited in situations where little premorbid information is available.

The clinician's primary role is to create an informal rapport with the patient wherein the clinician can observe the patient's natural communicative behavior without resorting to formal testing. Forty-five behaviors are rated on a 9-point scale of current ability as a proportion of estimated former ability. The scale ranges from "normal" (100%) to "absent" (0%) ability. Examples of functional abilities include abilities to indicate yes and no, to read newspaper headlines, and to make change. The 45 behaviors are clustered into five categories: Movement, Speaking, Understanding, Reading, and Miscellaneous (e.g., calculation and writing) abilities. Overall cluster scores are obtained by determining the mean rating of the items in a cluster.

Despite the subjective clinical nature of the scoring system, M. T. Sarno (1969) reported interrater reliability coefficients larger than .87 for each of the five FCP categories. Reliability was determined for three judges using a sample of 20 right-hemiplegic patients with language symptoms of at least 2 months' duration.

Psychometric test improvements may or may not be accompanied by functional, useful improvements in communication. Gains on psychometric testing do not automatically imply improved functional abilities, and conversely functional gains may not alter diagnostic classification. The distinction between functional ratings and psychometrically isolated language functioning was examined by J. E. Sarno, Sarno, and Levita (1971). Measurements of improvement were determined by comparing original and follow-up performances on the NCCEA Visual Naming and Identification by Sentence (i.e., Token Test) subtests and the FCP Speaking and Understanding subscales. Only a modest relationship was found between the original and follow-up scores on each of the two speech measures (i.e., NCCEA Visual Naming and FCP Speaking), and no correlation was found between score changes on the two comprehension measures (NCCEA Identification by Sentence and FCP Understanding). On the other hand, M. T. Sarno and Levita (1981) reported some concordance between NCCEA Token Test performance and FCP Understanding in the examination of global aphasics at 1-year follow-up examinations. Differences between male and female aphasics and between patients with closed head injury and stroke (with similar postonset times) were found to be minimal (M. T. Sarno, Buonaguro, & Levita, 1985, 1987).

The information obtained using the FCP is not designed to replace a comprehensive examination of the aphasic patient's language abilities and disabilities. Its goal is to provide information about natural language capacity, an area not readily tested by a standard diagnostic examination (e.g., M. T. Sarno, 1984a). The information yielded by a properly administered FCP may well be more easily translatable into a description of the patient's everyday capabilities than the information provided by a standard comprehensive examination. When properly used, the FCP may provide information on the functional consequences of the patient's aphasic condition that is not otherwise (except anecdotally) available. Repeated FCP administration may provide information on the recovery process of functionally relevant communicative ability (Sands, Sarno, & Shankweiler, 1969; M. T. Sarno, Buonaguro, & Levita, 1985; M. T. Sarno & Levita, 1979).

COMMUNICATIVE ABILITIES IN DAILY LIVING (CADL)

The CADL (Holland, 1980) also was designed to measure the communicative ability of the aphasic patient. Its purpose, like that of the FCP, is to provide additional information regarding functional language communicative ability in the overall assessment of the aphasic patient. Much of the test involves patient performance during simulated, cued-context daily activities, such as dealing with a receptionist, communicating with a doctor, driving, shopping, and making telephone calls. Given its inherent focus on communicative ability, rather than on language ability per se, accurate communication via oral, written, gestural, or any other modality of transmission is acknowledged as significant. The "staged" quality of some sets of items requires a certain acting ability on the part of the examiner and may not always be successful with patients who refuse or cannot enter into such simulated interactions. Caution must also be exercised with apraxic patients, although the test may serve as a supplementary instrument in such a population (Wertz et al., 1981).

The CADL is composed of 68 items, which are scored as either "correct" (2 points), "adequate" (1 point), or "wrong" (0 points) on the basis of the patient's attempt to communicate. For example, at one point the tester asks the patient, "Your first name is _____, right?" (filling in a fictitious name). If the patient's response includes both a negative response ("No," headshake, written response, etc.) and his or her correct name, 2 points are allotted. If the patient simply replies with a negative response without further elaboration, the response is considered adequate but not fully appropriate and is scored 1 point. If the patient responds affirmatively, perseverates, echoes the question, responds incoherently, or simply does not respond, no points are allotted. Requests for repetition are considered to be legitimate communicative statements and are not penalized. However, if the patient fails to respond within 5 sec, only partial credit (1 point) is allowed for a correct response. Given the generally slowed psychomotor and information-processing speed that frequently accompanies acquired brain damage, one wonders whether this time restriction is overly strict and does not indeed violate one of the goals of the CADL, which is to rate communication success regardless of transmission method. Normative data in the form of sample means and standard deviations, cutoff scores, and item analyses are presented in the CADL test manual.

Test standardization, reliability, and validity information from two principal studies are provided in the test manual. In the initial study, 80 aphasic patients were assessed on an earlier 73-item version of the CADL, the BDAE, the FCP, and the PICA, and were observed during a 4-hr period to examine the frequency, appropriateness, and type of communicative behavior the patients employed in everyday life. The internal consistency of the CADL was .97. Item–scale correlations of at least .40 were present for 68 of the 73 test items, indicating test consistency. An interrater reliability coefficient of .99 was obtained for two scores testing a subsample of 20 patients. Concurrent validity was manifested, as the CADL correlated .93 with the PICA, .87 with the FCP, and .84 with the BDAE. Criterion validity was assessed by determining the relationship between the patients' CADL performance and their behavior during the 4-hr observation period; significant correlations between .60 and .64 were obtained between the test and the observational measures. Construct validity was demonstrated, as level of CADL performance varied with BDAE aphasic subtype classification. Global aphasics showed the poorest CADL performance. Wernicke's aphasics performed more satisfactorily than did the global aphasics, but less well than did Broca's aphasics. Anomic aphasics performed with the highest levels of performance for aphasic groups.

In the second study, normative data were collected on 130 aphasic patients and 130 normal adults. Age, sex, living situation (i.e., home vs. institution setting), education, and occupation were examined. Better CADL performances were recorded for nonaphasics compared with aphasics, home-setting individuals compared with institutionalized individuals, and younger individuals compared with older individuals. CADL performances were not influenced either by education or by occupation. Females performed slightly better than males. Aphasic patients, as a group, showed more heterogeneity in performance than did the normal group. Global aphasics again performed the poorest of aphasic groups, whereas anomic aphasics showed the best performances. Lower intermediate scores by mixed aphasics and Wernicke's aphasics and higher intermediate scores by Broca's aphasics and conduction aphasics were noted.

The CADL score is simply the sum of points earned on the 68 items and, as such, is less subjective than the scoring on the FCP; in addition, there are 10 interrelated performance categories (e.g., Social Convention, Sequential Relationships, Humor–Metaphor–Absurdity). The CADL test manual presents error profiles for each type of aphasic subtype. The test author stated that the CADL requires 35–45 min to complete. Two test protocols and a recorded cassette tape of a third protocol are provided in the manual for training purposes.

The clinician has a choice between the CADL and the FCP for the measurement of functional communication. None of the diagnostic test batteries discussed later in this chapter provides direct measurement of functional communication. Either the FCP or the CADL would make a useful addition to aphasia assessment for the descriptive assessment evaluation modality discussed at the beginning of this chapter, in association with a comprehensive diagnostic battery. There are likely to be individual situations in which each test might be maximally efficient, and the reasonable clinician should consider gaining a working knowledge of both tests.

Comprehensive Examinations

Comprehensive examinations of the aphasic patient's language ability seek to obtain a diverse sampling of performance at different levels of task difficulty along all dimensions of function that the test author deems relevant to language disability. Examples of dimensions common to most of these tests include naming, oral expression, auditory comprehension, repetition, reading ability, and writing ability. Other dimensions vary according to the theoretical orientations of the authors.

As test instruments, comprehensive examinations vary widely in purpose, structure, utility, and adequacy. Some tests, for example, are constructed to examine lesion localization and to provide prognostic information regarding a defined set of standard anatomically based aphasic syndromes. Proponents of such tests see the data generated from such endeavors as forming the diagnostic anchors at a given level of brain-behavior knowledge. Others are concerned with eliciting behavior that will provide more descriptive information without subscribing to a specific taxonomic system. The value of taxonomic classification has been questioned by Marshall (1986) and Caramazza (1984). Marshall pointed out that in traditional taxonomic classification attempts with larger patient populations, only 59% (Benson, 1979a), 20–30% (Albert, Goodglass, Helm, Rubens, & Alexander, 1981; Prins, Snow, & Wagenaar, 1978), or 49% (Reinvang, 1985) could be placed into one of the specific aphasic syndromes. Both Marshall (1986) and Caramazza (1984) suggested the use of a more descriptive approach to aphasia assessment in considering psycholinguistic parameters.

For practical purposes, we limit the current review to instruments designed for and/or primarily used in English. Tests developed and available mainly in other languages (e.g., the Aachen Aphasia Battery; Willmes, Poeck, Weniger & Huber, 1983; Willmes & Ratajezak, 1987) have been omitted. Tests available in translations or designed as multilingual instruments will be mentioned in the section on bilingualism later in this chapter.

A common denominator of these test instruments is the need for adequate training and practice before the examination can be effectively employed. The choice of an assessment instrument is a serious decision for the clinician that not only involves personal preferences but also takes into consideration the clinical setting, the type of referrals that the clinician can expect, the stated intentions of the test instrument, as well as the adequacy of the examination as an at least minimally reliable, valid, and useful test instrument.

APPRAISAL OF LANGUAGE DISTURBANCE (ALD)

The author of the ALD (Emerick, 1971) views aphasia as an impairment of symbol functioning subsequent to cortical damage and characterized by one or more of the following symptoms: input disturbances via the modal channels, central processing disturbances, and output disturbances via modal channels. The stated purpose of this examination is to provide a systematic inventory of the patient's communicative abilities by examining input modalities, central processing, and output modalities to allow the clinician to determine the best avenues of reception and expression to initiate therapy.

The ALD has three primary sections: (a) eight input–output pathways (e.g., aural to oral, aural to visual, aural to gesture, visual to oral, and visual to graphic); (b) a central language comprehension section in which matching, sorting and arranging, and manding (a Skinnerian term referring to requesting or demanding) are examined; and (c) a section on related factors, including tactile recognition, arithmetic, and an oral examination for signs of paralysis or other abnormality. The structure of the test follows closely the input–processing–output language model developed by Osgood and Sebeok (1965).

Normative data for the test are not reported, nor are formal validity studies available. The test manual is brief and frequently lacking in detail. According to the manual, material and procedures were developed on the basis of "intensive scrutiny of 75 aphasic patients." Fifty-six of these patients were retested after an interval of 2 weeks to 5 months, resulting in a reliability coefficient of .74 (.81 for a subsample of 39 neurologically stable patients). Interscorer reliability for 39 neurologically stable patients was .86.

There are several limitations to the usefulness of the ALD. First, many items considered as part of the assessment of central language processing are of questionable value. For example, two of the three matching tasks, given the test author's conception of aphasia, might well be more parsimoniously labeled "visual–gesture" avenue tasks rather than "central language comprehension." Second, many tasks in this section and the related-function section are more adequately covered in other examinations. For example, the single object assembly item and the single verbal arithmetic problem would be more adequately assessed using such common test instruments as the Wechsler intelligence tests. Third, the Peabody Picture Vocabulary Test (PPVT; Dunn, 1965) is to be completed as part of the central language comprehension section; however, no instructions for incorporating PPVT test results into the ALD are provided. No decision rules are provided that would guide the reader in identifying subtypes of aphasia. Emerick (1971) stated this explicitly, stressing that "it is far more useful clinically to simply identify what the patient can and cannot do" (p. 5).

At present, the paucity of adequate psychometric studies, the brief and often uninformative test manual, and questionable test construction (i.e., the central language comprehension section and the rather rigid adherence to a schematic model of language) offset any positive value that the ALD might possess relative to the other comprehensive examinations reviewed in this chapter.

BOSTON DIAGNOSTIC APHASIA EXAMINATION (BDAE)

The original BDAE (Goodglass & Kaplan, 1972) has been revised (Goodglass & Kaplan, 1983). The primary focus of the BDAE, which remains one of today's more popular aphasia examinations (e.g., Beele, Davies, & Muller, 1984), is the diagnosis of classic anatomically based aphasic syndromes. This diagnostic goal is attained by comprehensive sampling of language components that have previously proven themselves valuable in the identification of aphasic syndromes.

Goodglass and Kaplan stated that the design of their instrument is based on the observation that various components of language function may be selectively damaged by central nervous system (CNS) lesions; this selectivity is an indication of (a) the anatomical neural organization of language, (b) the localization of the lesion causing the observed deficit, and (c) the functional interactions of various parts of the language system. A number of studies have validated this stated purpose (e.g., Naeser, Hayward, Laughlin & Zatz, 1981; Naeser & Hayward, 1978; Naeser, Mazurski, Goodglass & Peraino, 1987).

The BDAE is divided into five language-related sections: conversational and expository speech, auditory comprehension, oral expression, understanding written language, and writing. Each section is composed of a variety of subtests. Each subtest attempts to measure a specific function in as purely isolated a fashion as possible.

The detailed manner of examination of conversational and expository speech in the BDAE remains an important and relatively unique aspect of this test. A "speech characteristics profile," indexing verbal prosody (melodic line), fluency, articulation, grammatical level, paraphasias, and word-finding difficulty, is derived from a sample of free conversation and from a sample of narrative speech in the description of a line drawing (the "Cookie Theft" card). Repetition and auditory comprehension also are rated, but are derived from subtest performances. Finally, an overall rating of symptom severity, the "severity rating scale," is determined from conversational speech samples, ranging from "no usable speech or auditory comprehension" (a score of 0) to "minimal discernible speech handicaps" apparent to the listener (a score of 5). The reliability of the speech characteristics profile was examined in the original BDAE employing three judges who rated 99 patients' tape-recorded speech samples. The lowest correlation coefficients of .78 and .79 were obtained for word-finding difficulties and paraphasias, respectively. The other dimensions had coefficients of at least .85.

The speech characteristics profile and the severity rating are central to diagnostic decision making with the BDAE; particularly important is the differential fluency–nonfluency dimension. More detailed diagnoses may incorporate corroborative information from the profile sheet delineating subtest performance. Knowledge of the classification system employed by the "Boston school" approach is necessary to adequately interpret the BDAE (e.g., Benson, 1979a). The test manual provides BDAE profiles for classic and rarer aphasic subtypes. These subtype profiles appear to be based on the profile and the severity rating; expected subtest performances for aphasic subtypes are described but are not accompanied by clear objective diagnostic rules.

Auditory comprehension is examined by (a) word recognition in six distinct semantic categories: objects, letters, geometric forms, actions, colors, and numbers; (b) body-part identification; (c) commands; and (d) complex ideational material requiring yes–no responding.

Oral expression is gauged on 12 diverse subtests that include oral agility, naming, recitation, automatized sequences, repetition of words and phrases, and sentence reading. A subtest of controlled oral word fluency–Animal Naming—also is included in this section. Articulation and the presence of various types of paraphasias are recorded.

Understanding written language is assessed by four subtests, including associative skills that either underlie reading or are by-products of the reading process (e.g., phonetic associations and word–picture matching).

Writing is assessed through mechanics, recall of written symbols, word finding, and written formulation.

Supplementary language and nonlanguage tests that may be of use in a given clinical setting are included in the test manual. Among the supplementary language tests are additional (and useful) auditory comprehension tasks with psycholinguistic delineation. The Boston Naming Test (Kaplan, Goodglass, & Weintraub, 1983) is cited as a BDAE language supplement to the revised version. A nonverbal "spatial-quantitative" test battery, also known as the Parietal Lobe Battery, is described in the manual, along with performance features of the standardization sample; performance of normal participants was originally described by Borod, Goodglass, and Kaplan (1980).

The original BDAE was standardized on a sample of 207 aphasic patients with relatively distinct cerebrovascular lesions and isolated, well-defined symptoms. Although standardization on such a large ample of patients is psychometrically useful, the clinician whose referrals do not reflect this select sample (i.e., referrals with a different bias in symptomatology and severity, or those who may have diffuse lesions such as those seen in traumatic brain damage, or referrals from a different socioeconomic background) may not be able to reference his or her patients directly to the BDAE sample. The revised BDAE was standardized on a new sample of 242 aphasic patients. As in the original sample, selective aphasias produced by a single cerebrovascular accident predominate. However, the authors reported that the new standardization sample was less selectively chosen from the patient population available to them and, therefore, includes more patients with larger lesions and more severe aphasic symptoms. Subtest comparisons from the original and new standardization samples, listed in Table 2 of the BDAE manual, show that the new sample generally performed more poorly as a group than did the original sample.

Performances by a sample of 147 normal adult controls on all but seven BDAE subtests are reported in the test manual and also had been reported in 1980 by Borod et al. Their results are reproduced in Table 8 of the BDAE manual showing, among other features, cutoff scores for normal performances that are 2 *SD*s below group mean performances. Age and education factors are delineated in the 1980 report.

The test manual provides a good overview to the psychometric properties of the revised and the original BDAE. It describes good internal consistency for all the test measures that contain a series of scorable items. Test–retest reliability has yet to be reported. Factor analyses related to the BDAE subtest structure and discriminant analyses are described. Percentile data have replaced z scores for description of subtest performances.

Many studies using the BDAE have been published. As with other aphasia test instruments, the BDAE has both strong and weak points. Favorable features include its comprehensive sampling of behavior, its standardization based on a large sample of aphasic patients, its attempt at a qualitative analysis of speech, and its portability. Unfortunately, some of these strengths also reflect weaknesses of the test, namely the time-consuming length of administration, the selective nature of the standardization sample, and the fact that the utility of a qualitative analysis is directly related to the skill and experience of the professional performing the rating. Reinvang and Graves (1975) attempted to clarify decision rules regarding the classification of the aphasias. The BDAE as a whole and the oral apraxia score were also related to a specifically designed articulation task (Sussman, Marquardt, Hutchinson, & Mac-Neilage, 1986). Dyadic interaction measures, on the other hand, did not correlate well with the BDAE, or with the FCP or the CADL (Behrmann & Penn, 1984). Helm-Estabrooks and Ramsberger (1986) and Davidoff and Katz (1985) reported that the BDAE measured progress in therapy; Selnes, Niccum, Knopman and Rubens (1984) found word reading and Knopman, Selnes, Niccum and Rubens (1984) found confrontation naming of the BDAE strikingly improved after 6 months of recovery. Brookshire and Nicholas (1984) noted that the BDAE auditory comprehension subtest was not an adequate predictor of auditory paragraph comprehension using independent standardized material, and in a second study (Nicholas, MacLennan, & Brookshire, 1986) they demonstrated that both aphasic and healthy subjects were able to answer a similarly high number of questions about paragraph reading without having actually read the passage, suggesting a high passage dependency of this test. This dependency applied not only to the BDAE, but to similar tests in the MTDDA and WAB as well.

The ultimate usefulness of the BDAE must be determined by the needs of the individual clinician. The ability to operationally define classic aphasia syndromes subsequent to a delineated cerebrovascular accident using this reliable, valid diagnostic instrument is of certain and durable importance to many clinicians and clinical researchers. The new standardization sample with larger "dirtier" cerebrovascular lesions resulting in more severe symptoms is important for fairer interpretation of test results in more diverse poststroke clinical settings. Clinicians who may be looking for a comprehensive evaluation of aphasic performances that has prognostic value, who are looking for an evaluation that can be used to develop an individual intervention program, or who work with a patient population with predominantly non-CVA etiologies might have to look elsewhere for a test instrument. Finally, in broader cognitive or neuropsychological evaluations, it is improbable that the FULL BDAE—unlike, for example, the MAE (Benton & Hamsher, 1989)—can be considered for inclusion in comprehensive evaluations, given its length and the diversity of its behavioral sampling. We have found, however, that a number of individual subtests are valuable additions to neuropsychological evaluations, such as the use of Animal Naming to replace word-fluency tests in testing illiterate patients or those with limited educational backgrounds. The Boston Naming Test may also be used as a stand-alone test, for example, to evaluate recognition-cued word-retrieval skills in the elderly (LaBarge, Edwards, & Knesevich, 1986). The BDAE authors clearly and very fairly describe the primary goals of their test, facilitating such decisions.

MINNESOTA TEST FOR DIFFERENTIAL DIAGNOSIS
OF APHASIA (MTDDA)

The MTDDA (Schuell, 1955, 1973) still ranks among the more popular batteries (Beele et al., 1984). It is a comprehensive examination designed to observe the level at which language performance is impaired in each of the principal language modalities at different levels of task difficulty. To Schuell, the goal of a careful and comprehensive description of impairment in the aphasic patient is to provide a guide for effective therapeutic intervention.

The current version of the MTDDA is the result of numerous systematic revisions of the original experimental version of the late 1940s. Hundreds of aphasics were examined. The author employed empirical factor analytic techniques (Schuell, Jenkins, & Carroll, 1962) as well as clinical experience to construct and revise the test. The construction of the MTDDA reflects Schuell's theoretical consideration of aphasia as a unitary reduction of available language that crosses all language modalities and that may or may not be complicated by perceptual or sensorimotor involvement, by various forms of dysarthria, or by other sequelae of brain damage (Schuell, 1974b; Schuell & Jenkins, 1959; Schuell et al., 1964).

The MTDDA is composed of five sections: auditory disturbances (represented by 9 subtests); visual and reading disturbances (9 subtests);

speech and language disturbances (15 subtests); visuomotor and writing disturbances (10 subtests); and numerical relations and arithmetic processes (4 subtests). Within each section, subtest order generally is arranged from the least to the most difficult. Each section may be started at an estimated level of difficulty corresponding to the patient's ability (the "Binet method") and then continued to a point where the patient fails 90% or more of the items. Most items are scored either "correct" or "incorrect." Both the test manual (Schuell, 1965) and the companion monograph (Schuell, 1973) describe supplementary tests that should be considered for each section as well as the factor and intercorrelation structure for the sections of the test.

The auditory disturbance subtests include examinations of discrimination, retention span, and comprehension for vocabulary, sentences, and paragraphs. The visual and reading subtests include examinations of form and letter matching, matching printed words to pictures, matching printed to spoken words, reading comprehension for sentences and paragraphs, and oral reading of words and sentences. The speech and language subtests include 4 subtests that deal with speech movements and articulation and 11 that deal with language, ranging from overlearned serial tasks to retelling a paragraph. Tasks of intermediate difficulty in this section include sentence completion, responding to questions, naming, and providing sentences. The visual and writing subtests include 5 dealing with the reproduction and recall of visual forms and 5 dealing with written language, including spelling, producing sentences, writing sentences to dictation, and writing a paragraph. The 4 numerical and arithmetic subtests deal with functional arithmetic ability, minimizing the influence of education on performance. These tasks include coin values, clock setting, and simple computations in the four basic arithmetic operations: addition, subtraction, multiplication, and division.

Differential diagnosis of aphasia with the MTDDA identifies five aphasic syndromes: simple aphasia; aphasia with visual involvement; aphasia with sensorimotor involvement; aphasia with scattered findings compatible with generalized brain damage; and irreversible aphasic syndrome (Schuell, 1974a). Schuell (1966, 1973) also added two additional "minor syndromes": mild aphasia with persistent dysfluency (dysarthria) and aphasia with intermittent auditory imperception. Definitions, language features ("signs"), and MTDDA test discriminations are provided in the monograph (Schuell, 1973). However, as Zubrick and Smith (1979) pointed out, the MTDDA was not designed to deal with broader issues of aphasic differential diagnosis: distinguishing aphasia from nonaphasic disorders that may manifest language disturbance (e.g., memory loss, dementia, severe hearing loss, and confusional state). The test has been successfully used to measure language recovery after stroke and to show that language recovery is relatively independent of intelligence (David & Skilbeck, 1984).

The length of the MTDDA is one feature that may present a problem for the user of the test. Short forms (Schuell, 1957) and "very short" forms (Powell, Bailey, & Clark, 1980) of the MTDDA have been created, although Schuell herself was not impressed with the role of short examinations in the diagnosis of aphasic disorders, as described earlier in this chapter. The large number of subtests include many functions that exceed what some authors would consider the assessment of speech and language functions and range into material that has been a traditional component of many standard intelligence tests. Schuell's factor analysis may on closer inspection seem to reflect a major first "general" factor that is closely related to the *g* obtained in factor analyses of intelligence tests. Schuell and Jenkins (1959), however, consider this factor a general language factor, supporting their assumptions about the unitary nature of language.

In sum, the MTDDA is an extensive examination of many facets of speech and language functioning. The test represented a major breakthrough in the development of comprehensive aphasia test instruments that met the requirements of both standardization and objectivity. Great care has been taken in its construction, employing both clinical expertise and empirical technique. Potential users of the MTDDA should consider whether its length will be prohibitive in their clinical settings. Potential users need to examine the congruence of the theoretical bases of the MTDDA relative to their own conceptions of the nature of aphasic deficits and balance its breadth against practical needs.

MULTILINGUAL APHASIA EXAMINATION (MAE)

The benefits to aphasiologists of having equivalent versions of a single aphasia examination for several language communities has been well stated by Benton (1967, 1969). The MAE (for the revised English version, see Benton & Hamsher, 1989) has developed through the efforts of Benton and his North American and European collaborators to meet the requirements of such an examination (Benton & Hamsher, 1978). Chinese, French, German, Italian, Portuguese, and Spanish versions of the test are being prepared. The different language versions of the MAE are functionally equivalent in content rather than simply translations of an identical test. For example, Controlled Oral Word Association, the subtest of word fluency, uses letters that have corresponding levels of difficulty in each language (e.g., all letters that have corresponding level of difficulty across language communities) rather than employing identical letters. Hence, performance of the task in each language is functionally equivalent.

The MAE, a shortened and highly modified relative of the NCCEA, is composed of seven subtests: Visual Naming, Sentence Repetition, Controlled Oral Word Association (i.e., word fluency), Spelling, a version of the Token Test, Aural Comprehension of words and phrases, and Reading Comprehension of words and phrases. Two MAE rating scales are included. The first is a rating scale of speech articulation based upon verbal performance throughout the test session. Ratings range from 0 ("speechless or usually unintelligible speech") to 8 ("normal speech"). The second rating scale encodes writing praxis, scored when possible by performance on a task of writing to dictation (from the MAE Spelling subtest and/or the NCCEA Writing to Dictation subtest); scores range from 0 ("illegible scrawl") to 8 ("good penmanship").

A practical and distinctive feature of the MAE is that alternate English versions of Sentence Repetition, Controlled Oral Word Association, Spelling, and Token Test are available when a repeat assessment of the patient is warranted. Hermann and Wyler (1988) provided a research example of the utility of MAE alternate forms in an examination of language behavior prior to and after temporal lobectomy in epileptic patients. Visual Naming requires naming of line drawings (whole objects and object details), which is more difficult than naming of actual objects. Controlled Oral Word Association is composed of three letters progressively increasing in their associative difficulty. The spelling subtest is actually a "minibattery" that employs any combination of three modalities: oral spelling, writing to dictation, or block-letter spelling. The Token Test is composed of 22 commands at two levels of complexity and is scored in pass–fail fashion. Aural and Reading Comprehension are administered in a multiple-choice format. Scoring adjustments for age and educational level are provided in the manual for those subtests that require them.

The MAE test manual (Benton & Hamsher, 1989) does not provide much basic psychometric information; however, it does provide standardized test instructions, normative information (in the form of percentiles) from a sample of 360 normal Iowa adults (aged 16 to 69 years) without a history or evidence of neurological disability. A second validational sample of 50 aphasic patients is included, which may also be employed to discern aphasic subtypes.

Because the Visual Naming subtest may be especially sensitive to cultural experience, separate normative data have been obtained for urban inner-city Black residents (Roberts & Hamsher, 1984). Controlled Oral Word Association was included in a cognitive battery normed on healthy elderly adults aged 65 to 84 years; there was no suggestion of significant performance decrement over the age span (Benton, Eslinger, & Damasio, 1981). Normative information for children recently has become available (Schum, Sivan, & Benton, 1989) and is included in the new 1989 test manual. Research has shown that performance failure on the MAE Token Test is a sensitive indicator of the presence of acute confusional states (delirium) in nonaphasic medical inpatients (Lee & Hamsher, 1988). Levin and colleagues (Levin et al., 1976; Levin et al., 1981) have employed the MAE to examine the linguistic performances of patients with closed head injuries, documenting the high frequency of naming errors, defective associative word finding, and impaired comprehension of nonredundant aural commands (i.e., Token Test), and revealing their correlation with the severity of brain injury. Current research is examining the use of both MAE performance and clinical features of the aphasic's language (e.g., paraphasias in conversational speech, *conduite d'approche*) in order to provide an MAE differential diagnosis of aphasic subtypes (K. Hamsher, personal communication).

In sum, it is hoped that the successful deployment of the MAE in a number of language communities will facilitate direct cross-community comparisons of case and sample data. Regardless of this research goal, clinical use of the English-language MAE does suggest that it is an effective diagnostic instrument requiring a relatively brief (typically under 45 min) administration time. In addition, use in general clinical practice of individual MAE subtests (viz., Visual Naming, Token Test, Controlled Oral Word Association) can serve as a good exploratory examination as to the presence of language deficits in order to document performance status and to determine the need for further delineation with additional testing.

NEUROSENSORY CENTER COMPREHENSIVE EXAMINATION
FOR APHASIA (NCCEA)

The NCCEA (Spreen & Benton, 1977; Spreen & Strauss, 1991) is designed to provide a comprehensive assessment of language comprehension, language production, reading, and writing. Other stated goals of the NCCEA are to provide subtests that are sufficiently complex that the clinician can obtain a relatively exact measure of performance level; to standardize and score performances such that necessary corrections for age, sex, and education can be made; to include nonlinguistic subtests to ensure valid interpretation of performance deficits on language tests as either linguistic in nature or due to other dysfunction; and to include specific subtests that could be employed to investigate research questions in aphasiology (Benton, 1967).

The NCCEA is composed of 20 subtests that focus on the language functions stated above and 4 "control" subtests of visual and tactile functioning. Use of the control subtests is indicated when performance deficits on certain subtests need to be differentiated as either language related or visual or tactile in nature. The test is designed to yield a description of the patient's profile of abilities and disabilities. The order of subtests provides a meaningful grouping into tests of name finding (subtests 1–4), immediate verbal memory (5–7), verbal production and fluency (8 and 9), receptive (decoding) ability (10 and 11), reading (12–15), writing (17–19), and articulation (20). Eight of the 20 language subtests and 3 of the 4 control subtests require the use of four arrays of eight common objects. These objects are arranged in order of difficulty from least to most difficult. The four sets are matched for item difficulty. The four trays of objects rotated throughout the test are equivalent in mean and distribution of difficulty for aphasic patients (mean percent correct is approximately 63% for all trays) and young children (mean acquisition age of names approximately 5:8 years). Three object substitutions were made in 1987 to eliminate outdated items. NCCEA subtests include stimulus presentations in either the visual, auditory, or tactile modality. The remaining subtests measure visual object naming, description of object use, tactile object naming for each hand, sentence repetition, sentence construction, object identification by name, oral reading of names and sentences, oral reading of names and sentences for meaning, object name writing, writing to dictation, copying sentences, and articulation. Unlike other aphasia test instruments, provisions for collapsing performance on several subtests into category or modality performances are not provided in the test manual.

Several subtests provide a set of items for initial testing as well as a second set of items for use only if errors occurred in the first set. This feature tends to shorten administration time for the examination of areas in which a patient has no difficulties. The second set of items then provides more detailed quantitative information on problem areas. Isolated errors due to poor attention or other irrelevant causes will be reduced in importance if the second set of items is passed correctly.

The range of item difficulty is limited. In an attempt to avoid highly specialized or low-frequency words, the authors used only very common objects for their object naming, identification, and similar tasks. As a result, the test has a rather low ceiling on some of the subtests, with the effect that very mild aphasic symptoms in highly educated patients may be missed. Other subtests, however, are "open-ceiling" tests for which this limitation does not apply.

Scores on the NCCEA are determined by response correctness. Incorrect responses and mispronounced correct responses are recorded verbatim, as are unusual features of the patient's performance, to yield qualitative performance information. An individual's performance on the NCCEA, when corrected for the influences of age and educational level as instructed, can be converted into percentile scores to yield relative levels of performance on each subtest and can be ranked on three profile sheets. These profile sheets allow the clinician to compare the patient's performance to that of samples of normal adults (Profile A), aphasic patients (B), and nonaphasic brain-damaged patients (C). The aphasic and the nonaphasic brain-damaged samples consist of consecutive referrals for neuropsychological evaluation in acute-care hospital settings.

Since the development of the NCCEA, a number of studies have investigated its properties and its practical usefulness. Because it was designed primarily for the examination of patients with aphasia or aphasia-type complaints, patients without language problems and normal controls tend to obtain ceiling scores. As a result, the test cannot be used to measure language ability in normal individuals, although language development in children has been successfully measured with most subtests up to a ceiling age ranging from 8 to 13 years (Gaddes & Crockett, 1975). Because of the low ceiling of the naming tasks, the Visual Naming subtest can be supplemented by use of the Boston Naming Test.

An empirical study with 353 children aged 5:5 to 13:5 (Crockett, 1974) found that seven factors described the content of the NCCEA in that population: reading/writing, verbal memory, name finding, auditory comprehension, syntactic fluency, reversal of digits, and repeating digits.

One-year retest reliability in older adults for selected subtests has been reported as satisfactory (Word Fluency, .70; Visual Naming, .82; Token Test, .50; Snow & Tierney, 1988).

Construct validity was examined in two studies by Crockett (1976, 1977). The first study examined the discrimination of groups of aphasic patients based on ratings of verbal productions, and divided on the basis of the Howes/Geschwind two-type and the Weisenburg/McBride three-type typologies. Neither of the two models showed significant multivariate differences. The second study demonstrated significant differences on the NCCEA between four types of aphasia empirically derived from ratings of verbal production by hierarchical grouping analysis. Two of these four types appeared to be similar to Howes 2 types, a third appeared to reflect Schuell's single dimension of language disorder, and the fourth seemed to be characterized primarily by memory impairment.

Concurrent validity with the WAB was demonstrated by Kertesz (1979). Concurrent validity for changes in language functions during therapy was reported by Kenin and Swisher (1972) for the overall FCP score.

Predictive validity was established in a study by Lawriw (1976), who also presented a successful cross-validation between patient groups from Iowa City, New York City, and Victoria, British Columbia. Kenin and Swisher (1972) and Ludlow (1977) investigated patterns of recovery from aphasia; improvement was best reflected in writing from copy and tests of comprehension, whereas expressive performance showed least improvement. Single-word reception or production was more readily recovered than that of longer verbal units. The authors mentioned that reading, writing, and oral production items were not sufficiently difficult for patients at an advanced stage of recovery. In contrast, Ewing-Cobbs et al. (1987) reported that a striking percentage of a sample of 23 children and 33 adolescents with closed head injuries exhibited clinically significant language impairment on the NCCEA. Visual Naming, Sentence Repetition, Word Fluency, and Writing to Dictation best discriminated between mild and moderate/severe closed head injury in children and adolescents. M. T. Sarno (1984c) described significant differences between aphasic, dysarthric/subclinical, and subclinical aphasic patients on Visual Object Naming, Sentence Repetition, Word Fluency, and the Token Test. Patients with Alzheimer's disease scored significantly lower in the areas of verbal expression, auditory comprehension, repetition, reading, and writing compared with age-matched nonneurological controls (Murdoch et al., 1987).

The 1977 NCCEA normative data for an aphasic reference group are based on 206 unselected referrals to neuropsychological hospital–clinic services in Iowa City, New York City, and Victoria. Although the concept of "averaging" across aphasic patients disregards the different types of aphasia, this procedure allows the profiling of individual patients against this reference group; that is, an individual patient's subtype will stand out more clearly. However, if patients from another referral source (e.g., patients in rehabilitation or patients with residual aphasia) are seen, the reference group may no longer be appropriate. Similarly, Profile C is based on a population of patients with brain lesions referred to a neuropsychological service excluding patients with diagnosed aphasia. Other patient groups (e.g., those with dementia of the Alzheimer type) may provide a very different referral base.

Normative data for most subtests remain stable through the age span up to age 64. Results of individual studies with some of the tests (Montgomery, 1982) show only a minor decline of 1 or 2 points, which has been incorporated into the age and education correction rules. A study by Tuokko (1985) of elderly subjects in Vancouver, British Columbia, for example, showed a mean for Visual Naming of 16 for subjects below 60 years to hold up to age 79, and a drop to a mean of 15.44 for subjects 80 years and older. Similarly, Description of Use showed a ceiling score of 16 for subjects below 60 and up to age 74; the mean for subjects of ages 75 to 80 and older was 15.78. Tactile Naming (right hand) showed a mean of 15.66 for subjects below 60 and up to age 79, and of 14.89 for subjects 80 years and older. Tactile Naming (left hand) showed a mean of 16 for subjects under 60, and means between 15.14 and 15.57 for subjects between the ages of 60 and 79, but a mean of 12.44 for subjects 80 years and older.

Normative data for children between 6 and 13 are presented. The norms were merged from Gaddes and Crockett (1975) and Hamsher (1980) since the differences between these two sources (Victoria and Milwaukee) were minimal. No sex differences were found on 11 of the 20 subtests; on the remaining subtests, sex differences were transient around ages 6 and 7 when girls did slightly better on the writing and reading tasks, except for Word Fluency on which girls were more productive between ages 9 and 13, and Spelling of Written Names on which boys were poorer at ages 7, 9, 10, and 11.

The test has also been adapted into Italian, Japanese, and Spanish. A detailed description of the rationale and the details of test construction are not available, although the manual provides some of this information.

In summary, the NCCEA provides a comprehensive assessment of language functions for aphasic patients without the use of a specific model of language and without specifying a specific approach to delineating diagnostic types of aphasias. Psychometric development of the test since its original version in 1969 has been slow, but a fair number of validation studies has accumulated. The development of three different profile sheets for score evaluation is a distinct asset. On the other hand, the low ceiling of some of the subtests suggests that some aspects of language function in mildly or borderline aphasic patients cannot be adequately measured.

PORCH INDEX OF COMMUNICATIVE ABILITY (PICA)

The PICA (Porch, 1967, 1973) is designed to assess verbal, gestural, and graphic responsiveness subsequent to brain damage. Unlike classificatory instruments, the PICA is designed to categorize the nature of the aphasic patient's ability to respond, modality of response, and quality of response to task demands. A prime use of the PICA has been in assessing patient performance on multiple occasions postonset to determine the recovery of language ability. The PICA is composed of 18 subtests: 4 verbal, 8 gestural, and 6 graphic. A high degree of homogeneity among the subtests is established through the repeated use of 10 common, everyday objects of equal difficulty (e.g., a key, a cigarette) for a majority of the subtests. Subtest order is arranged so as to introduce minimal information during the earlier subtests that would be needed to perform later subtests. The use of many items of equal difficulty was employed to examine fluctuations in patient subtest performance over time. Similar to other aphasia tests, subtests were created to conform with a model of language functioning involving several possible input modalities, a central processor for incoming information and outgoing responses, and several possible output modalities (see ALD).

The PICA author stresses the need to have formally trained examiners (preferably by means of workshops about the instrument) in order for the test to have full usefulness. (Information about these workshops is provided by the test's publisher.) Examiners benefit from training in scoring responses. A persistent problem in recording responses to test items involves assessing and quantifying the given response as one of a wide variety of potential responses. As a compromise between two possible extremes (i.e., longhand notation of the characteristics of the response and simple pass–fail or normal–subnormal dichotomous scoring), the PICA uses a 16-point multidimensional scoring system, an attempt by the author to integrate the strengths of the two approaches while minimizing their weaknesses.

A given response to a PICA test item is evaluated along five relevant and basic dimensions: accuracy, responsiveness, completeness, promptness, and efficiency. A scoring system that considers all possible permutations of these five dimensions is, for all practical purposes, impossible and meaningless. Hence, 16 categories have been identified that represent various relevant combinations of these five dimensions, resulting in a 16-point ranked scale from "no response" (a score of 1) to "complex response" (a score of 16). For example, any attempt by the patient to perform on the task is scored at least a 6; all accurate responses are scored at least an 8. Additional points are given for a correct response after repeated instructions, for self-corrected responses, responsive ease, completeness, promptness, and efficiency. Porch (1967) reported the viability of the rank ordering of the 16 categories by providing empirical evidence available in the clinical literature as well as by pointing out the high agreement between PICA category ordering and the ranking of categories by 12 speech pathologists.

The individual item scores (180 possible) are transformed into an overall performance score, several modality scores, and individual subtest scores, for evaluative purposes. The overall performance score is considered as the best single index of the patient's general communicative ability. Modality scores yield information of the relative capacity of verbal, gestural, and graphic communicative ability. Subtest means provide further information on specific performances. Use of mean values require that statistical and conceptual assumptions of equal intervals between category levels be met. Whether this assumption is legitimate for the PICA has been the subject of a good deal of debate (e.g., see Martin, 1977; McNeil, 1979). Although single item responses can be categorized on the 16-point scale (i.e., a score of 12 represents an incomplete response), mean values cannot be so categorized. Hence, mean scores cannot categorize the method by which the patient generally communicates, but can only represent a performance level relative to either normative values or the patient's other derived scores.

Data indicating that the PICA shows high interrater reliability as well as high test–retest reliability are provided in volume 1 of the test manual (Porch, 1967). The construct validity of the PICA is addressed logically, but not statistically, in the test volume: Both the model of language functioning upon which the PICA is structured and the behaviors categorized in the scoring system have been noted in aphasiological literature. Holland (1980) reported concurrent validity of the PICA as .93 with the CADL scale, .86 with the FCP, and .88 with the BDAE. Lendrum and Lincoln (1985) found that the PICA given at 4 weeks postonset successfully predicted recovery at 6 months.

Percentile data from normative samples of 280 left hemisphere damaged patients and 100 bilaterally damaged patients are presented in volume 2 of the test manual (Porch, 1973). Percentiles for all principal transformed scores are provided. In addition to providing relative information for these transformed scores, percentiles are also utilized to determine a given patient's "aphasia recovery curve," employing the overall test percentile, the mean percentile of the nine highest scored subtests, and the mean percentile of the nine lowest scored subtests. Predictions on the scope of recovery can be attempted from this curve; a recovery ceiling is assumed when the three percentiles coincide (Porch, Collins, Wertz, & Friden, 1980).

The underlying factor structure of the PICA has been addressed by Clark, Crockett, and Klonoff (1979a, 1979b). Three definable factors emerged from a factor analysis of Porch's original standardization sample ($N = 150$). The first factor was formed by the four verbal subtests, representing a pure dimension of verbal competence. Factor two represented five of the six graphic subtests. Factor three represented the eight gestural and the other graphic subtest; however, only four of the eight gestural subtests were principally defined by this factor. A higher order factor analysis of the factor intercorrelation matrix indicated the presence of a general language impairment factor. PICA subtests showed loadings on this general factor as a function of task difficulty. A factor analysis of a second sample revealed five distinct factors: verbal competence, graphic expression, gestural demonstration of verbal and reading competency, basic gestural function, and graphic copying of geometric forms. The first four of these factors were highly intercorrelated, suggesting the presence of a general language impairment factor. These two studies suggested the presence of a basic general impairment factor for language; they also suggested a needed revision in the PICA subtest structure (3 or 5 distinct areas of interest rather than 18) and provided empirical evidence for the diversity of subtests subsumed under the gestural modality (Martin, 1977). DiSimoni, Keith, Holt, and Darley (1975) also found a high degree of redundancy among PICA subtests and concluded that a shortened form of the test may be more useful DiSimoni, Keith, and Darley (1980) described a short version of the PICA.

In sum, the PICA is a very well-developed and standardized test instrument that has been extensively employed in rehabilitative settings to track recovery postonset (a topic discussed in detail in the test manual). The two-volume test manual is exemplary. The multidimensional scoring system has become the most criticized aspect of the test. Both rank order of the categorized behaviors (McNeil, Prescott, & Chang, 1975) and assumptions of equal interval scaling made by Porch (Martin, 1977) have been criticized. A well-written comprehensive critique of the PICA is provided by Martin (1977). Two further shortcomings of the PICA include the paucity of sampling auditory comprehension and the misleading labeling of several subtests as gestural when they entail other specific behaviors. McNeil (1979) suggested that such criticisms should not turn clinicians away from considering the PICA as a test instrument, but rather should make them more cautious interpreters of PICA findings.

WESTERN APHASIA BATTERY (WAB)

The WAB (Kertesz, 1979, 1982) is a close relative of the BDAE and shares with it the diagnostic goal of classifying aphasia subtypes and rating the severity of the aphasic impairment. The examination, designed for both clinical and research use, comprises four language and three performance domains. Syndrome classification is determined by the pattern of performance on the four language subtests, which assess spontaneous speech, comprehension, repetition, and naming. Weighted performance on these language subtests yields an overall measure of aphasic severity: the Aphasia Quotient (AQ). Stepwise regression has shown that, of the AQ constituents, the Information Content rating is most highly correlated with the AQ (Crary & Rothi, 1989). The three performance areas—reading and writing, praxis, and construction—yield a second summary measure: the Performance Quotient (PQ). Finally, the AQ and the PQ are summed to form a Cortical Quotient (CQ). Based on the language subtest performances of 150 aphasic patients with various etiologies (mostly cerebrovascular accident), criteria for classification of eight aphasic syndromes are described; these syndromes are global, Broca's, Wernicke's, anomic, conduction, isolated, transcortical motor, and transcortical sensory.

Spontaneous speech is assessed in terms of the patient's speech both in response to questioning (e.g., "How are you today?") and in a description of a line drawing, much as in the BDAE. Speech is rated on two 10-point rating scales: information content and fluency (the fluency scale incorporates both grammatical competence and the presence of paraphasias). Comprehension is assessed by yes–no questions that may be answered in either verbal or nonverbal fashion, by word recognition, and by performance to sequential command. Repetition is composed of 15 items that are scored either as correct, in phonemic error (partial credit), or as an error. Naming is composed of object naming (without cuing or, if necessary, with tactile and/or phonemic cuing), word fluency (animals), sentence completion, and responsive speech. Test items were selected to provide a wide enough range of difficulty for assessing all grades of severity.

An uncommon feature of this test's structure is the dissociation from language performance of reading and writing abilities, which, along with nonverbal measures, form part of the PQ. In a more recent report, Shewan (1986) reunited the spoken language section (i.e., the AQ tests) with reading and writing as part of a scale called the Language Quotient (LQ), and provided a detailed account of reliability and validity for this addition to the original WAB format. The LQ is weighted so that 60% reflects spoken language performance and 40% reflects written language performance. Shewan's report emphasized the relation between the LQ measure and the severity of the aphasic disorder.

WAB standardization information and reliability and validity data were provided by Kertesz and Poole (1974) and then updated by Kertesz (1979) and Shewan and Kertesz (1980). The WAB clearly meets standard rules of test construction, although it is ranked last in a review of nine aphasia tests based on criteria reported by Skenes and McCauley (1985). The WAB manifests good internal consistency and high interrater and intrarater reliabilities. High test–retest reliability has been reported for a sample of 38 chronic aphasic patients. Successful criterion validity has been described by the author. Aphasics were differentiated from non–brain-damaged adults in their WAB performance; the AQ distinguished the aphasics from the non–brain-damaged controls. Construct validity was assessed on a sample of 15 patients who were examined on both the WAB and the NCCEA; there were high correlations between corresponding subtests ranging from .82 for spontaneous speech subtests to .95 for comprehension subtests. One recent study examined the validity of cutoff scores on the CQ (Fromm & Holland, 1989). The authors stated that the language subtests can be administered in approximately 1.5 hr, but that the full WAB might require at least two test sessions to complete. The test manual is far less detailed than Kertesz's book (1979), which still remains a good detailed introduction to the WAB.

The WAB has established itself as a useful classificatory research instrument. A strong research role for the WAB is helped by its inclusive objective classification rules and its summary measures (i.e., AQ, PQ, and CQ), which aid interpretation of group data. Studies have included novel cluster analytic taxonomies of aphasic syndromes of different etiologies over time (Kertesz & Phipps, 1980), the evolution of aphasic syndromes over the course of recovery (Kertesz, 1981) and during therapy (Lesser, Bryan, Anderson, & Hilton, 1986; Shewan & Kertesz, 1984), the relation between aphasia and nonverbal intelligence (Kertesz & McCabe, 1975), the relation between language and praxis (Gonzales-Rothi & Heilman, 1984; Kertesz & Hooper, 1982), comparative diagnostic classifications between a Portuguese version of the WAB and a Portuguese aphasia examination (Ferro & Kertesz, 1987), and the efficacy of aphasia treatment (Shewan & Kertesz, 1984).

Like the BDAE, the WAB offers a method of assessing spontaneous speech, a useful feature for any aphasia test battery. The WAB method of measuring spontaneous speech, however, appears to be less comprehensive than the BDAE method; for example, fluency, grammatical competence, and the extent of paraphasic errors are combined into a single scale on the WAB, whereas they are assessed independently on the BDAE. Shewan and Donner (1988) also noted that the WAB spontaneous speech subtest does not provide comprehensive information compared with other tests designed to evaluate this aspect of language. The repetition test does not appear to be as encompassing or as well structured as other repetition tasks (e.g., NCCEA's Sentence Repetition). In terms of measuring controlled associative fluency, the WAB is like the BDAE in assessing animal naming, in contrast to the NCCEA and the MAE.

In sum, the primary use of the WAB, like the BDAE, is diagnostic: the classification of aphasic performances into traditional aphasic syndrome subtypes. Explicit decision rules about which classification applies in an individual case are provided, although the test operates on the assumption that all cases can clearly be classified as one of eight basic types. Such clear-cut classification is, of course, implicit in cluster analytic research but has little meaning for the "mixed" aphasias that occur much more often in clinical practice than this classification system suggests. In our 1985 review of the WAB, we stated that the WAB, as the newest clinically available and adequately constructed aphasia battery, "has added to the selection of aphasia batteries at a level in keeping with the requirements of the contemporary field" (Risser & Spreen, 1985, p. 468), but we did not feel as if the WAB was novel or had broken any new ground in aphasia assessment, such as by including a direct measure of functional communication in the battery of tests.

Assessment of Aphasia in Children

The complex topic of aphasia in children is addressed in another chapter of this book. In the context of this chapter, we deal with the assessment of aphasia only briefly, since a full discussion of the specific assessment problems in childhood would not fit within the space limitations and, more importantly, would deal with a topic that has found only limited attention in the aphasia assessment field.

The major obstacle encountered in designing assessment methods for children is that language ability increases with chronological age in the normal child and there is relatively high variability from child to child within a given age level. Full language competency is not reached until 12 to 14 years of age (depending on definition of competency); after this age, further development takes place in terms of increased vocabulary, grammatical complexity, awareness of rules of generative grammar, and so on. For these reasons, any assessment method for children requires the establishment of normative data for each year (or half year) of age; because of the somewhat different rates of growth of language abilities in girls and boys, separate norms for each sex are also required. Obviously, the construction of suitable tests for children requires much more extensive psychometric work, especially for standardization, than does the construction of tests for adults; however, validity and reliability must also be fully established for each age level and cannot be taken for granted on the basis of studies involving children from all age levels.

Several tests of normal language development in children are available, such as the Illinois Test of Psycholinguistic Abilities (ITPA; Kirk,

McCarthy, & Kirk, 1968), but very few assessment techniques have been constructed or restandardized for children for the specific purpose of aphasia assessment (see review by Eisenson, 1972).

Among the brief or specific-purpose assessment methods, several adaptations of the sentence repetition method have been attempted. One experimental technique which used 24 sentences that vary according to grammatical complexity in congenitally aphasic children, was reported by Bliss and Peterson (1975). Adaptations of the word fluency examination usually change from words starting with a given letter to animal names or similar categories for children who cannot be expected to have sufficient knowledge of spelling. DiSimoni (1978) published an adaptation of the Token Test for Children, standardized with 1304 children from preschool age 3 to grade 6 (age 12:6) from a mixed suburban population. The test manual also reviews several other studies investigating the scoring criteria as well as aspects of concurrent validity with other tests of auditory comprehension, including the Illinois Test of Psycholinguistic Abilities (ITPA) and the Peabody Picture Vocabulary Test (a test widely used with normal children). The Token Test has also been investigated in relation to socioeconomic status of the home, an important aspect of language development in children as a discriminator between aphasic and brain-damaged children (Gutbrod & Michel, 1986), and in relation to speech training in language-delayed children (Alexander & Frost, 1982). Syntactic comprehension in children was also examined with the Token Test and the BDAE Auditory Comprehension subtest, and compared with adult forms of aphasia (Naeser, Mazurski, Goodglass, & Peraino, 1987). Other tests of auditory comprehension not specifically designed for the assessment of aphasia but potentially useful are the Assessment of Children's Language Comprehension (Foster, Giddon, & Stark, 1973) and Carrow's (1972) Test for Auditory Comprehension of Language (Tallal, Stark, & Mellits, 1985).

Comprehensive examinations for children available at this time include the already mentioned ITPA (which has been used for aphasia assessment in some studies, e.g., Paul & Cohen, 1984), the Reynell Developmental Language Scales (Reynell & Huntley, 1971), the Northwestern Syntax Screening Test (Arndt, 1977; L. L. Lee, 1970), and the Utah Test of Language Development (Mecham, Jex, & Jones, 1967); no specific studies for children with acquired aphasia are available for these tests. Adaptations for children of comprehensive examinations for aphasia in adults have been presented for the NCCEA, the MAE (Schum et al., 1989), the children's revision of the AST (Tramontana & Boyd, 1986), and the PICA. The NCCEA adaptation (Gaddes & Crockett, 1975) merely provides norms for children between ages 6 and 13 for each of the NCCEA subtests, but it has not been used in research studies with aphasic children. The presented norms show an acceptable gradual increase of scores with age for some subtests, whereas other subtests show a rapid increase within a limited age span, after which the test scores remain at ceiling level. The Porch Index of Communicative Ability in Children (PICAC; Porch, 1979) contains a "basic battery" for 3- to 6-year-olds and an "advanced battery" for 6- to 12-year-olds. With the exception of some floor effects, score progression with age is satisfactory and reliability data are provided, but thus far no validity studies with aphasic children have been reported. As with the PICA, the multidimensional scoring system poses some problems and requires extensive training.

Numerous other assessment procedures aimed at the general intellectual development of the child, but including one or more measures of language development, are available. They will not, however, be reviewed in this context, nor can the numerous available tests of articulation for children be considered here.

Assessment of Aphasia in Clinical Practice

This final section presents some general concepts and considerations regarding the assessment of aphasia in clinical practice. In particular, we discuss the decision-making process before, during, and after the clinical assessment of questions of diagnosis, treatment planning, and prediction of recovery. Such decisions cannot be replaced by any assessment procedure, no matter how well constructed and "comprehensive" a test battery may be, but remain the responsibility of the clinician in consultation with related professionals involved with the individual patient.

Brookshire (1973) raised three major questions usually posed in aphasia assessment:

1. Does the patient have a speech or language disorder?
2. Are these speech or language defects treatable?
3. Can recovery of speech and language ability realistically be expected?

We would add to the first question the more basic supplementary question: What is the nature of the speech or language deficit? All four questions overlap with the various purposes of assessment described in the introductory section of this chapter: screening, diagnostic evaluation, descriptive assessment for counseling and rehabilitation, and progress evaluation.

Decisions About the Presence or Absence of Aphasia

In clinical practice, some patients are referred with an obvious diagnosis of aphasia of a moderate or severe degree. In a fair number of patients presenting with mild or questionable language disorders, however, a decision that rules out aphasia should be made before proceeding to other questions. On the surface, it would seem that well-validated tests of a more comprehensive nature, or even of a screening type, would be sufficient to determine whether aphasia is present. It should be remembered, however, that no test has a discrimination accuracy of 100% and that the gray area of false-positive and false-negative decisions encountered by any given test lies of necessity in the borderline area between mild (or residual) aphasic features and normal language. Relying solely on cutoff points provided by test authors in patients with borderline impairment would, in effect, not be much better than random guessing.

The presence of defective language performances, however, need not indicate the presence of an aphasic disorder. Significant nonaphasic language changes or deficits may be observed in other neuropsychological syndromes, such as dementia or acute confusion, and even in psychopathology. Because the traditional aphasia subtypes are best seen when the etiology is a nonhemorrhagic cerebrovascular accident, language deficits may display different features when there are different etiologies, such as diffuse and severe traumatic brain injury. Experience in acute medical-care and rehabilitation settings suggests to us that the terms "aphasia," "expressive aphasia," and "receptive aphasia" tend to be overused as descriptions of language behaviors that a review of the medical history and a formal evaluation reveal to be language manifestations of other disorders, such as acute confusion or psychopathology.

The clinician must use informed judgment to arrive at his or her own diagnosis that significant language changes are present and that they actually represent an aphasic disorder. Language disorders are frequently seen in the context of dementing diseases and may be described by many linguistic parameters, although not necessarily as aphasic disorders (e.g., Bayles, 1984; Bayles, Boone, Tomoeda, Slauson, & Kaszniak, 1989; Bayles & Tomoeda, 1983; Fromm & Holland, 1989). Non-defective language changes may be observed in the population of the normal, healthy elderly (e.g., Obler, Nicholas, Albert, & Woodward, 1985). Language and communication deficits are common after traumatic head injury, again in the absence of frank aphasia (e.g., Hagen, 1981; Levin et al., 1976; Marquardt, Stoll, & Sussman, 1988; M. T. Sarno, Buonaguro, & Levita, 1986). These topics are given fuller consideration in other chapters of this volume.

Premorbid Language Function and Intelligence

One major consideration is making an informed diagnosis is the determination or estimation of a given patient's language ability and intelligence before the onset of illness. The two factors, intelligence and language, are closely but not perfectly related. Since test results before the onset of illness are rarely available, a careful evaluation of the patient's educational history, occupational background, language, and reading and writing habits must be made; relatives may be consulted with regard to this information and their judgment may be invited as to whether any language impairment is noticeable to them. The judicious clinician often can arrive at a reasonable estimate of premorbid level of intellectual functioning by obtaining demographic information, such as educational level, occupation, age, sex, and race (Barona, Reynolds, & Chastain, 1984; Hamsher, 1984). Such estimates of premorbid functioning are quite limited in the context of premorbid illiteracy (Lecours, Mehler, Parente, & Caldeira, 1987).

Additional information may be provided by concurrently administered tests of general intelligence. Gross discrepancies between IQ tests and aphasia tests usually suggest selective language impairment. However, it must be remembered that many IQ tests rely heavily on tests involving verbal functions; only the so-called nonverbal component of IQ tests is useful in this regard. Once this information has been collected, an expected level of language function may be determined. Some tests allow a score correction based on the premorbid educational level to be added before interpretation; many other tests leave this consideration open.

A related but more difficult consideration concerns the sociocultural habits of the normal home and job environment of the patient. The need for verbal expression varies greatly from one setting to another, and ethnic influences particularly tend to affect such factors as verbal fluency, general fund of information, vocabulary, articulation (and intelligibility), and prosody.

Bilingualism

Patients whose first language is not English pose a special problem in the assessment of aphasia. For such patients (e.g. Spanish-Americans, French-Canadians), the judgment of premorbid language ability in English becomes difficult. Moreover, the matter of a differential impairment in the two languages requires investigation. Various theories have proposed that the "older," the "more affectively favored," the "most frequently used" language is less affected by aphasia, whereas other studies point out either that little difference actually exists between languages (Albert & Obler, 1978) or that the language environment during recovery from brain damage is the crucial factor. It is usually sensible to refrain from any such generalization and to establish premorbid language competence and assess impairment for both languages.

Frequently, the examination in the second language is carried out by using the same assessment methods with or without the use of an interpreter. Although this provides seemingly close comparability of the assessment in the two languages, such comparability may be tenuous at best. Frequently, an "instant" translation of this type only poorly approximates the difficulty level of vocabulary and grammar because of basic differences in the frequency of word use and grammatical structure in the languages. The MAE described earlier addresses these prob-

TABLE 4.2
Tests Available in Transitions or Adaptations

Test	Languages
Multilingual Aphasia Examination	Chinese, French, German, Italian, Portugese, Spanish
Bilingual Aphasia Test	French and other languages (Pardis, 1987)
Boston Diagnostic Aphasia Examination	Norwegian (Reinvang & Graves, 1975)
Western Aphasia Battery	Portugese
Communicative Abilities in Daily Living	Italian, Japanese (Pizzamiglio, 1984; Sasanuma, 1989)
Boston Naming Test	Spanish (Taussig, Henderson, & Mack, 1988)
Word Fluency	Spanish (Taussig, Henderson, & Mack, 1988)

lems and attempts to provide fully equivalent forms in several languages. A bilingual test, however, can be used to best effect only when the test administrator is fluent in the two languages. More broadly, any translated or interpreted verbal performance on aphasia evaluation is subject to bias on the part of the translating resource, whether technical (i.e., quality of translation) or interpersonal (i.e., a family member who, despite best intentions, may "normalize" the aphasic patient's speech).

Individual tests have been deliberately constructed for the assessment of bilinguals. Translations and adaptations of several other tests are available, but mainly are still in an experimental state or without adequate psychometric studies (see Table 4.2). Unless adequate adaptations are available, it is far more preferable to use tests developed in foreign countries. Two examples of well-developed foreign language tests are the Aachen Aphasia Battery (in German and Italian; De Bleser, Denes, Luzatti, & Mazzucchi, 1986) and the Standard Language Test of Aphasia (in Japanese; Kusunoki, 1985).

Motivational, Affective, and Attentional Considerations

Language is not an isolated cognitive function. Patients who still show the acute aftereffects of brain damage are frequently apathetic, drowsy, and uncooperative. Patients may show considerable emotional reaction to their neurological impairments. Depressed mood, for example, is frequently observed during the phase of neurological stabilization, when patients begin to realize the full extent of their disabilities. These emotional reactions are seen across most neurological presentations and, therefore, are not limited to patients with aphasia or with left-hemisphere lesions (e.g., Gass & Russell, 1986). Other patients frankly deny their deficits and are unwilling to submit to testing procedures. Patients with accompanying acute confusion, another frequent manifestation of newly onset neurological disease, may be too disoriented or agitated to yield valid performances (e.g., Lipowski, 1980). Confused patients typically show impaired levels of verbal comprehension, regardless of whether they are aphasic, complicating evaluation for aphasia. For these reasons, it is quite common that willingness or ability to communicate is drastically reduced and test performances are defective due to lack of motivation, attentional defects, or changes in consciousness. Assessment then calls on the judgment of the clinician rather than blind reliance on test results.

The Nature of the Speech and Language Deficit

After a general diagnosis of aphasia is made, the description of the exact nature of the deficit becomes of paramount importance. What exactly is it that the patient can or cannot do? What degree of impairment is present in each of the areas under examination? A description of areas of strength is as important as the description of the areas of deficit, since the approach to treatment relies on both types of information.

Information about the nature of the deficit continually influences the process of assessment. As we find out about a specific area of weakness, a more detailed description of that area and related deficits will be required. Special testing procedures may be added to gather this information. Occasionally, it is necessary to continue the examination in this fashion after the initial assessment results have been reviewed.

The stress on diagnostic types of aphasia has led many test authors to develop a test pattern for each type either empirically or descriptively. As was pointed out earlier, the range of types of aphasia described varies from test to test, depending on the theoretical orientation of the authors. It is perhaps obvious from the preceding text that fitting a patient into a particular type on the basis of test results is of only limited preliminary diagnostic value. Types of aphasia have been related to location of lesion as well as to rate and stage of recovery, but, as with the borderline between aphasic and normal language function, the gray area between types presents serious problems. Perfect fit for individual patients into such types is rare, and general impairment defying any typology is the norm rather than the exception. For these reasons, the description of the nature of the language deficit must proceed beyond typology and produce an individual language profile for each patient.

Comprehensive Assessment

The focus in this chapter has been on an assessment of aphasia rather than on a general evaluation of a patient's deficits. The need to refer to results from general intelligence tests has already been mentioned, as have affective considerations. Similarly, the results of other cognitive, perceptual, and motor tests are necessary to fully appreciate the consequences of the underlying neurological disease process that generated the patient's aphasia. Importantly, the ancillary evaluation of basic motor, sensory, and attentional functions is required. Certain language functions are likely to show severe deficits if the patient experiences impairment or distortions of visual perception, hearing, or basic ability to maintain attention. Patients are not likely to produce valid responses on tactile naming if impairment of motor functions or stereognosis is present. Comprehension may be impaired by attentional losses as well as by language deficits. Some aphasia test authors have built in supplementary tests for such functions that are automatically administered if the patient fails on specific language tasks; in other tests, the clinician must ascertain the patient's basic abilities without such guidance (requiring considerable training and experience). In multidisciplinary settings, clinical neuropsychologists may be available to provide comprehensive evaluations of cognitive status that may be interpreted in conjunction with results from aphasia tests. Regardless of the employed route, the description of the aphasic deficit will be clearly modulated if an examination is not restricted to features of language performance and if ancillary and additional deficits are formally considered (e.g., Benton, 1982). Neuropsychological evaluation can also be employed in order to explore the presence of acquired deficits in new learning and memorization and to appreciate the residual learning capacities of aphasic patients, features of considerable importance in treatment planning and community reentry.

Recovery and Treatment of the Aphasic Disorder

Another chapter in this volume is devoted to a discussion of the treatment of aphasia; however, since many patients are referred for evaluation mainly to explore treatment options, the issue should be considered briefly in relation to assessment. Increasing numbers of research studies are addressing the question of recovery from aphasia and the most effective ways to evaluate recovery (e.g., Kertesz, 1981; Lendrum & Lincoln, 1985; M. T. Sarno & Levita, 1981; Shewan & Kertesz, 1984). As discussed elsewhere in this book, some general facts (e.g., better recovery in younger, in female, in left-handed, and in less severely impaired patients or those with relatively recent onset) have been recognized, but are not without some controversy. One goal of clinical research has been to discern assessment findings with predictive (prognostic) value or with associative value relative to the recovery process (e.g., Naeser, Helm-Estabrooks, Haas, Auerbach, & Srinivasan 1987; Varney, 1984b).

Obviously, if exploring treatment options is the purpose of an assessment, the choice of assessment instruments will differ from the choice made for diagnostic purposes. However, many of the features described in earlier parts of this section still need to be considered (e.g., the presence of concurrent neuropsychological, sensory, or perceptual deficits; the patient's motivational status) for their impact on the recovery process and for identification of treatment modalities. Situational circumstances, family support, and other factors also may have to be assessed.

Most important in this context is an actual assessment of the patient's relearning capacity. None of the existing aphasia assessment procedures provides an adequate opportunity to judge this capacity. For this reason, the clinician may resort to self-made tasks carefully calibrated in difficulty to the residual capacity of the patient. For a simple, informal assessment of relearning, a brief series of items (e.g., word finding to pictures or objects, description of use, comprehension of words or sentences) can be used and repeated until all items are fully learned; the measure in this case would be the number of trials needed to reach criterion (e.g., full comprehension of five items). A repetition of the same procedure on the following day will indicate the patient's "gain" or "carryover," that is, how many fewer trials are needed for relearning the same items. Under some circumstances, existing test material can be used as training material.

Conclusion

Choice of Tests

No formal battery of tests can be recommended as sufficiently comprehensive to arrive at an optimal description of the nature of the speech and language deficit for an individual patient. In clinical practice, we, as well as many other clinicians, tend to use a flexible approach for which a comprehensive test battery is only the beginning. Complete reliance on a given test battery tends to introduce an element of rigidity that may result in failure to fully explore the patient's problem.

An optimal description may be gained by using one of the more comprehensive, well-validated instruments described in the preceding pages. The choice of instrument will depend on the purposes of the assessment, as well as on individual preference and theoretical orientation. The comprehensive test chosen should be supplemented with other test procedures: specific-purpose tests (or parts of another comprehensive battery), a functional communication assessment, a clinical examination of specific problems, and, if possible, specially constructed tasks suitable for retraining, as discussed earlier.

The approach advocated here requires full knowledge of all available instruments as well as clinical skills and judgment. Although parts of the examination are likely to be conducted by a trained psychometrist in many settings, the full involvement of the experienced clinician is necessary. Although computerized test administration and scoring are becoming available for many tests, the need for the clinician to carefully evaluate such scores and interpret the test protocol remains.

Other considerations in the choice of assessment methods are (a) psychometric adequacy of a test, (b) portability of the test material, and (c) time requirements. In the first part of this chapter, psychometric requirements for a well-constructed test were stated explicitly. Obviously, the more a test meets the ideals of a psychometrically well-developed test, the more likely it is that valid and reliable results are obtained. Attention should also be paid to research conducted with a given instrument, since this provides additional information about the test's validity and about making specific decisions concerning diagnosis, treatment, and prognosis. Portability tends to be of no major concern in a hospital-based clinic or evaluation service, but does become a problem if bedside examinations are frequently carried out. In this latter case, one would prefer a handy portfolio of pictures rather than a suitcase full of objects, even though any pictured items tend to lose some value on a "reality" dimension. Time is a crucial consideration in many facilities with heavy patient loads; however, the time requirements should be carefully weighed against the amount of information gleaned from a given test. Brevity is no virtue if crucial information is not collected. In fact, the approach advocated in this chapter suggests that time requirements should be of secondary importance, and that experimental variants and additional exploratory procedures that may be of benefit in the long run should be used in the assessment process. If, on the other hand, brief screening is the only goal of assessment, then many of the short forms or screening devices deserve consideration.

A last point should be mentioned: Assessment is not an end in itself, but must be considered in relation to its potential value to the patient and the treatment and management of the patient's deficits. As Messick (1980) pointed out, the adequacy of a test is not dictated solely by psychometric soundness. Rather the concept of construct validity should include the "ethics" of assessment; that is, it must provide a rational foundation for predictiveness and relevance as well as take into account the implications of test interpretation per se.

Interpretation of Assessment Results

Every clinician has his or her own model of how best to survey a summary sheet of assessment results, with and without frequent glances at the actual test records and notes on the behavior of the patient during testing. Many of the comprehensive tests provide, of course, their own grouping of the test information and hence a suggested approach to interpretation (e.g., summary scores for assessment dimensions such as auditory comprehension and verbal expression). Other authors leave the approach to interpretation open to the clinician using the test. Our own approach (and that of many other clinicians) tends to be "syndromatic" in the sense that we tend to focus on the most seriously defective scores in the assessment record and scan the record for related information and corroborative test findings. For example, if the patient's most serious problem is on a test of word finding, we scan all related test results, as well as information about the patient's ability to find words in conversational settings, for higher order performance on verbal and nonverbal memorization/new learning tests and so forth. This allows a better description of the deficit, that is, whether the deficit is generalized or specific to the test setting, whether it is related to a specific sensory modality, whether it is a secondary manifestation of a nonaphasic amnestic or attentional disorder, and so forth. Additional assessment procedures may well be necessary to fully evaluate this first "syndrome."

We then proceed to the next syndrome that appears to be reasonably independent of the first and again search for associated task failures and other corroborative evidence. In this fashion, we can move toward the least deviant score on the assessment record, keeping in mind the estimated premorbid intelligence of the patient. Such syndromes may or may not be related to each other; they may or may not reflect a "classical type" of aphasia with localizing significance. Our primary purpose is to gain a detailed picture of the patient's deficits in order of severity and in the context of other deficits.

We then proceed in the opposite direction, searching for the highest score in the test record or the best preserved function until the information in the assessment record is exhausted.

Finally, we reexplore the noted syndromes by evaluating the actual behavior of the patient on individual tests or other assessment procedures, as well as on follow-up tests given after the initial interpretation of test findings. Typically, this step results in a fuller description of the patient's performance. Interpretation of findings in the broader neurobehavioral context of the patient's level of adjustment to his or her current deficits, the patient's awareness of his or her deficits, family cohesiveness and ability to provide support, and a clinician's appreciation for individualized community reentry needs all are likely to influence the clinician's understanding of the patient. For instance, we would no longer be describing "anomia for visually presented real objects," but can now include details of whether this deficit is part of a fuller diagnostic syndrome, what the associated impairments are, how the deficit affects the patient and his or her family, and how remediative treatment might approach the deficit by building on strengths and working on weaknesses.

The approach described here is highly idiosyncratic in a deliberate attempt to avoid preconceived models of language and brain functions. However, until a more generally accepted model of language disorders and generally accepted standards of procedure for generally accepted standard questions are developed—and little progress has yet been made in that direction—this outline of objective procedures for interpretation may provide the fullest utilization of assessment results at the present state of knowledge.

References

Albert, M. L., Goodglass, H., Helm, N. A., Rubens, A. B., & Alexander, M. P. (1981). *Clinical aspects of aphasia*. New York: Springer.

Albert, M. L., & Obler, L. K. (1978). *The bilingual brain: Neuropsychological and neurolinguistic aspects of bilingualism*. New York: Academic Press.

Alexander, D. W., & Frost, B. P. (1982) Decelerating synthesized speech as a means of shaping speed of auditory processing of children with delayed language. *Perceptual and Motor Skills, 55,* 783–792.

American Psychological Association. (1985). *Standards for educational and psychological tests*. Washington, DC: APA Press.

Anastasi, A. (1988). *Psychological testing* (5th ed.). New York: Macmillan.

Arndt, W. B. (1977). A psychometric evaluation of the Northwestern Syntax Screening Test. *Journal of Speech and Hearing Disorders, 42,* 316–319.

Aten, J. L., Caligiure, M. P., & Holland, A. (in press). Efficacy of communication therapy for aphasic patients. *Journal of Speech and Hearing Disorders*.

Barona, A., Reynolds, C. R., & Chastain, R. (1984). A demographically based index of premorbid intelligence for the WAIS-R. *Journal of Consulting and Clinical Psychology, 52,* 885–887.

Barth, J. T. (1984). Interrater reliability and prediction of verbal and spatial functioning with a modified scoring system for the Reitan-Indiana Aphasia Screening Examination. *International Journal of Clinical Neuropsychology, 6,* 135–138.

Bayles, K. A. (1984). Language and dementia. In A. Holland (Ed.), *Language disorders in adults* (pp. 209–244). San Diego, CA: College-Hill Press.

Bayles, K. A., Boone, D. R., Tomoeda, C. K., Slauson, T. J., & Kaszniak, A. W. (1989). Differentiating Alzheimer's patients from the normal elderly and stroke patients with aphasia. *Journal of Speech and Hearing Disorders, 54,* 74–87.

Bayles, K. A., & Tomoeda, C. K. (1983). Confrontation naming in dementia. *Brain and Language, 19,* 98–114.

Beele, K. A., Davies, E., & Muller, D. J. (1984). Therapists' views on the clinical usefulness of four aphasia tests. *British Journal of Disorders of Communication, 19,* 169–178.

Behrman, M., & Penn, C. (1984). Non-verbal communication of aphasic patients. *British Journal of Disorders of Communication, 19,* 155–168.

Benson, D. F. (1967). Fluency in aphasia: Correlation with radioactive scan localization. *Cortex, 3,* 373–394.

Benson, D. F. (1979a). Aphasia. In K. M. Heilman & E. Valenstein (Eds.), *Clinical neuropsychology*. New York: Oxford University Press.

Benson, D. F. (1979b). *Aphasia, alexia and agraphia*. New York: Churchill-Livingstone.

Benton, A. L. (1964). Contributions to aphasia before Broca. *Cortex, 1*, 314–327.

Benton, A. L. (1967). Problems of test construction in the field of aphasia. *Cortex, 3*, 32–53.

Benton, A. L. (1969). Development of a Multilingual Aphasia Battery: Progress and problems. *Journal of the Neurological Sciences, 9*, 39–48.

Benton, A. L. (1982). Significance of nonverbal cognitive abilities in aphasic patients. *Japanese Journal of Stroke, 4*, 153–161.

Benton, A. L., Eslinger, P. J., & Damasio, A. R. (1981). Normative observations in neuropsychological test performances in old age. *Journal of Clinical Neuropsychology, 3*, 33–42.

Benton, A. L., & Hamsher, K. (1978). *Multilingual Aphasia Examination*. Iowa City, IA: Benton Laboratory of Neuropsychology.

Benton, A. L., & Hamsher, K. (1989). *Multilingual Aphasia Examination* (2nd ed.). Iowa City, IA: AJA Associates Inc.

Benton, A. L., Hamsher, K., Varney, N. R., & Spreen, O. (1983). *Contributions to neuropsychological assessment*. New York: Oxford University Press.

Bishop, D., & Byng, S. (1984). Assessing semantic comprehension: Methodological considerations, and a new clinical test. *Cognitive Neuropsychology, 1*, 233–243.

Bliss, L. S., & Peterson, D. M. (1975). Performance of aphasic and nonaphasic children on a sentence repetition task. *Journal of Communication Disorders, 8*, 207–212.

Blumstein, S., Goodglass, H., Statlander, S., & Biber, C. (1983). Comprehension strategies determining reference in aphasia: a study of reflexivization. *Brain and Language, 18*, 115–127.

Boller, F., & Dennis, M. (1979). *Auditory comprehension: Clinical and experimental studies with the Token Test*. New York: Academic Press.

Boller, F., Kim, Y., & Mack, J. L. (1977). Auditory comprehension in aphasia. In H. Whittaker & H. A. Whittaker (Eds.), *Studies in neurolinguistics* (Vol. 3). New York: Academic Press.

Boller, F., & Vignolo, L. A. (1966). Latent sensory aphasia in hemisphere-damaged patients: An experimental study with the Token Test. *Brain, 89*(Pt. 4), 815–830.

Borkowski, J. G., Benton, A. L., & Spreen, O. (1967). Word fluency and brain damage. *Neuropsychologia, 5*, 135–140.

Borod, J. C., Goodglass, H., & Kaplan, E. (1980). Normative data on the Boston Diagnostic Aphasia Examination, Parietal Lobe Battery, and the Boston Naming Test. *Journal of Clinical Neuropsychology, 2*, 209–215.

Brookshire, R. H. (1973). *An introduction to aphasia*. Minneapolis, MN: BRK Publishers.

Brookshire, R. H. (1978). A Token Test battery for testing auditory comprehension in brain-injured adults. *Brain and Language, 6*, 149–157.

Brookshire, R. H., & Nicholas, L. E. (1984). Comprehension of directly and indirectly stated main ideas and details in discourse by brain-damaged and non-brain-damaged listeners. *Brain and Language, 21*, 21–36.

Caplan, D. (1987). Discrimination of normal and aphasic subjects on a test of syntactic comprehension. *Neuropsychologia, 25*, 173–184.

Caramazza, A. (1984). The logic of neuropsychological research and the problem of patient classification in aphasia. *Brain and Language, 21*, 9–20.

Carrow, E. (1972). Auditory comprehension of English by monolingual and bilingual preschool children. *Journal of Speech and Hearing Research, 15*(2), 407–412.

Clark, C., Crockett, D. J., & Klonoff, H. (1979a). Factor analysis of the Porch Index of Communication Ability. *Brain and Language, 7*, 1–7.

Clark, C., Crockett, D. J., & Klonoff, H. (1979b). Empirically derived groups in the assessment of recovery from aphasia. *Brain and Language, 7,* 240–251.

Coelho, C. A. (1984). *Word fluency measures in three groups of brain injured subjects.* Paper presented at the meeting of the American Speech-Language-Hearing Association, San Francisco, CA.

Cohen, R., Gutbrod, K., Meier, E., & Romer, P. (1987). Visual search processes in the Token Test performance of aphasics. *Neuropsychologia, 25,* 983–987.

Cohen, R., Kelter, S., & Shaefer, B. (1977). Zum Einfluss des Sprachverstaendnisses auf die Leistungen im Token Test. *Zeitschrift fuer Klinische Psychologie, 6,* 1–14.

Cohen, R., Lutzweiler, W., & Woll, G. (1980). Zur Konstruktvaliditaet des Token Tests. *Nervenarzt, 51,* 30–35.

Crary, M. A., & Rothi, L. J. G. (1989). Predicting the Western Aphasia Battery Aphasia Quotient. *Journal of Speech and Hearing Disorders, 54,* 163–166.

Crockett, D. J. (1972). *A multivariate comparison of Schuell's, Howes', Weisenburg and McBride's, and Wepman's types of aphasia.* Unpublished doctoral dissertation, University of Victoria.

Crockett, D. J. (1974). Component analysis of within correlations of language-skill tests in normal children. *Journal of Special Education, 8,* 361–375.

Crockett, D. J. (1976). Multivariate comparison of Howes' and Weisenburg and McBride's models of aphasia on the Neurosensory Center Comprehensive Examination for Aphasia. *Perceptual and Motor Skills, 43,* 795–806.

Crockett, D. J. (1977). A comparison of empirically derived groups of aphasic patients on the Neurosensory Center Comprehensive Examination for Aphasia. *Journal of Clinical Psychology, 33,* 194–198.

Darley, F. L. (Ed.). (1979). *Evaluation of appraisal techniques in speech and language pathology.* Reading, MA: Addison-Wesley.

David, R. M., & Skilbeck, C. E. (1984). Raven IQ and language recovery following stroke. *Journal of Clinical Neuropsychology, 6,* 302–308.

Davidoff, M., & Katz, R. (1985). Automated telephone therapy for improving comprehension in aphasic adults. *Cognitive Rehabilitation, 3,* 26–28.

DeBettignies, B. H., & Mahurin, R. K. (1989). Assessment of independent living skills in geriatric populations. *Clinics in Geriatric Medicine, 5,* 461–475.

De Bleser, R., Denes, G. F., Luzatti, C., & Mazzucchi, A. (1986). L'Aachener Aphasie Test (AAT): I. Problemi e soluzioni per una versione italiana del Test e per uno studio crosslinguistico dei disturbi afasici. *Archivio di Psicologia, Neurologia e Psichiatria, 47,* 209–237.

De Renzi, E. (1980). The Token Test and the Reporter's Test: A measure of verbal input and a measure of verbal output. In M. T. Sarno & O. Hook (Eds.), *Aphasia: Assessment and treatment.* Stockholm: Almqvist & Wiksell, New York: Masson.

De Renzi, E., & Faglioni, P. (1978). Normative data and screening power of a shortened version of the Token Test. *Cortex, 14,* 41–49.

De Renzi, E., & Ferrari, C. (1979). The Reporter's Test: A sensitive test to detect expressive disturbances in aphasics. *Cortex, 15,* 279–291.

De Renzi, E., & Vignolo, L. A. (1962). The Token Test: A sensitive test to detect receptive disturbances in aphasics. *Brain, 85,* 665–678.

DeWolfe, A. S., Rausch, M. A., & Fedirka, P. J. (1985). A word-ordering test to differentiate between aphasia and schizophrenia. *Journal of Communication Disorders, 18,* 49–58.

DiSimoni, F. (1978). *The Token Test for Children: Manual.* Hingham, MA: Teaching Resources Corporation.

DiSimoni, F. G., Keith, R. L., & Darley, F. L. (1980). Prediction of PICA overall score by short versions of the test. *Journal of Speech and Hearing Research, 23,* 511–516.

DiSimoni, F. G., Keith, R. L., Holt, D. L., & Darley, F. L. (1975). Practicality of shortening the Porch Index of Communicative Ability. *Journal of Speech and Hearing Research, 18,* 491–497.

Dunn, L. (1965). *Peabody Picture Vocabulary Test: Manual.* Circle Pines, MN: American Guidance Service.

Eisenson, J. (1954). *Examining for Aphasia: A manual for the examination of aphasia and related disturbances.* New York: Psychological Corporation.

Eisenson, J. (1972). *Aphasia in children.* New York: Harper.

Emerick, L. L. (1971). *The Appraisal of Language Disturbance: Manual.* Marquette: Northern Michigan University.

Emery, O. B. (1986). Linguistic decrement in normal aging. Special issue: Language, communication and the elderly. *Language and Communication, 6,* 47–64.

Ernst, J. (1988). Language, grip strength, sensory-perceptual, and receptive skills in a normal elderly sample. *Clinical Neuropsychologist, 2,* 30–40.

Ewing-Cobbs, L., Levin, H. S., Eisenberg, H. M., & Fletcher, J. M. (1987). Language functions following closed-head injury in children and adolescents. *Journal of Clinical and Experimental Neuropsychology, 9,* 575–592.

Ferro, J. M., & Kertesz, A. (1987). Comparative classification of aphasic disorders. *Journal of Clinical and Experimental Neuropsychology, 9,* 365–375.

Fillenbaum, S., Jones, L. V., & Wepman, J. M. (1961). Some linguistic features of speech from aphasic patients. *Language and Speech, 4,* 92–108.

Fitch, J. F., & Sands, E. (1987). *Bedside evaluation and screening test of aphasia.* Rockville, MD: Aspen Publishers.

Foster, R., Giddon, J., & Stark, J. (1973). *Assessment of children's language comprehension* (1973 rev.). Palo Alto, CA: Consulting Psychologists Press.

Froeschels, E., Dittrich, O., & Wilheim, I. (1932). *[Psychological elements in speech]* (E. Ferre, Trans.). Boston, MA: Expression.

Fromm, D., & Holland, A. L. (1989). Functional communication in Alzheimer's Disease. *Journal of Speech and Hearing Disorders, 54,* 535–540.

Gaddes, W. H., & Crockett, D. J. (1975). The Spreen-Benton aphasia tests, normative data as a measure of normal language development. *Brain and Language, 2,* 257–280.

Gallaher, A. J. (1979). Temporal reliability of aphasic performance on the Token Test. *Brain and Language, 7,* 34–41.

Gass, C. S., & Russell, A. W. (1986). Minnesota Multiphasic Personality Inventory correlates of lateralized crebral lesions and aphasic deficits. *Journal of Consulting and Clinical Psychology, 54,* 359–363.

Geschwind, N. (1971). Current concepts: Aphasia. *New England Journal of Medicine, 284,* 654–656.

Geschwind, N., & Kaplan, E. (1962). A human cerebral deconnection syndrome. *Neurology, 12,* 675–685.

Goldstein, G., & Shelly, C. (1984). Relationship between language skills as assessed by the Halstead-Reitan battery and the Luria-Nebraska language-related factor scales in a non-aphasic patient population. *Journal of Clinical Neuropsychology, 6,* 143–156.

Gonzales-Rothi, L. J., & Heilman, K. M. (1984). Acquisition and retention of gestures by apraxic patients. *Brain and Cognition, 3,* 426–437.

Goodglass, H., & Blumstein, S. (1973). *Psycholinguistics and aphasia.* Baltimore, MD: Johns Hopkins Press.

Goodglass, H., & Kaplan, E. (1972). *The assessment of aphasia and related disorders.* Philadelphia, PA: Lea & Febiger.

Goodglass, H., & Kaplan, E. (1983). *The assessment of aphasia and related disorders* (2nd ed.). Philadelphia, PA: Lea & Febiger.

Gutbrod, K., Mager, B., Meier, E., & Cohen, R. (1985). Cognitive processing of tokens and their description in aphasia. *Brain and Language, 25,* 37–51.

Gutbrod, K., & Michel, M. (1986). Zur klinischen Validitaet des Token Tests bei hirngeschaedigten Kindern mit und ohne Aphasie. *Diagnostica, 32,* 118–128.

Hagen, C. (1981). Language disorders secondary to closed head injury: Diagnosis and treatment. *Topics in Language Disorders, 5,* 73–87.

Hamsher, K. (1980). *Percentile rank norms for children on the NCCEA.* Milwaukee: University of Wisconsin Medical School, Department of Neurology.

Hamsher, K. (1984). Specialized neuropsychological assessment methods. In G. Goldstein & M. Hersen (Eds.), *Handbook of psychological assessment* (pp. 235–256). New York: Pergamon.

Head, H. (1926). *Aphasia and kindred disorders of speech.* New York: Macmillan.

Heimburger, R. F., & Reitan, R. M. (n.d.). *Testing for aphasia and related disorders.* Indianapolis: Indiana University Medical Center.

Helm-Estabrooks, N., & Ramsberger, G. (1986). Treatment of agrammatism in long-term Broca's aphasia. *British Journal of Disorders of Communication, 21,* 39–45.

Hermann, B. P., & Wyler, A. R. (1988). Effects of anterior temporal lobectomy on language function: A controlled study. *Annals of Neurology, 23,* 585–588.

Holland, A. L. (1980). *Communicative abilities in daily living: manual.* Baltimore, MD: University Park Press.

Holland, A. L., & Sonderman, J. C. (1974). Effects of a program based on the Token Test for teaching comprehension skills to aphasics. *Journal of Speech and Hearing Research, 17,* 589–598.

Howes, D. (1964). Application of the word-frequency concept to aphasia. In A. V. S. de Rueck & M. O'Connor (Eds.), *Disorders of language.* Boston, MA: Little, Brown.

Howes, D. (1966). A word count of spoken English. *Journal of Verbal Learning and Verbal Behavior, 5,* 572–606.

Howes, D. (1967). Some experimental investigations of language in aphasia. In K. Salzinger & S. Salzinger (Eds.), *Research in verbal behavior and some neurophysiological implications.* New York: Academic Press.

Howes, D., & Geschwind, N. (1964). Quantitative studies of aphasic language. In D. M. K. Rioch & E. A. Weinstein (Eds.), *Disorders of communication.* Baltimore, MD: Williams & Wilkins.

Inglis, J., Lawson, J. S. (1981). Sex differences in the effects of unilateral brain damage on intelligence. *Science, 212,* 693–695.

Jackson, J. H. (1915). On the physiology of language. *Medical Times and Gazette, 2,* 275. (Reprinted in *Brain,* 1968, *38,* 59–64).

Jones, L. V., Goodman, M. F., & Wepman, J. M. (1963). The classification of parts of speech for the characterization of aphasia. *Language and Speech, 6,* 94–107.

Joynt, R. J. (1964). Paul Pierre Broca: His contribution to the knowledge of aphasia. *Cortex, 1,* 206–213.

Kaplan, E., Goodglass, H., & Weintraub, S. (1983). *The Boston Naming Test.* Philadelphia, PA: Lea & Febiger.

Keenan, J. S., & Brassell, E. G. (1975). *Aphasia language performance scales.* Murfressboro, TN: Pinnacle Press.

Kenin, M., & Swisher, L. P. (1972). A study of patterns of recovery in aphasia. *Cortex, 8,* 56–68.

Kerschensteiner, M., Poeck, K., & Brunner, E. (1972). The fluency-nonfluency dimension in the classification of aphasic speech. *Cortex, 8,* 233–247.

Kertesz, A. (1979). *Aphasia and associated disorders: Taxonomy, localization, and recovery.* New York: Grune & Stratton.

Kertesz, A. (1981). Evolution of aphasic syndromes. *Topics in Language Disorders, 5,* 15–27.

Kertesz, A. (1982). *Western Aphasia Battery.* New York: Grune & Stratton.

Kertesz, A., & Hooper, P. (1982). Praxis and language: The extent and variety of apraxia in aphasia. *Neuropsychologia, 20,* 275–286.

Kertesz, A., & McCabe, P. (1975). Intelligence and aphasia: Performance of aphasics on Raven's Coloured Progressive Matrices (RCPM). *Brain and Language, 2,* 387–395.

Kertesz, A., & Phipps, J. (1980). The numerical taxonomy of acute and chronic aphasic syndromes. *Psychological Research, 41,* 179–198.

Kertesz, A., & Poole, E. (1974). The aphasia quotient: The taxonomic approach to measurement of aphasic disability. *Canadian Journal of Neurological Science, 1,* 7–16.

Kiernan, J. (1986). Visual presentation of the Revised Token Test: Some normative data and use in modality independence testing. *Folia Phoniatica, 38,* 25–30.

Kirk, S. A., McCarthy, J., & Kirk, W. (1968). *The Illinois Test of Psycholinguistic Abilities* (rev. ed.). Urbana: Illinois University Press.

Knopman, D. S., Selnes, O. A., Niccum, N., & Rubens, A. B. (1984). Recovery of naming in aphasia: Relationship to fluency, comprehension and CT findings. *Neurology, 34,* 1461–1470.

Kronfol, Z., Hamsher, K., Digre, K., & Waziri, R. (1978). Depression and hemispheric function changes associated with unilateral ECT. *British Journal of Psychiatry, 132,* 560–567.

Krug, R. S. (1971). Antecedent probabilities, cost efficiency, and differential prediction of patients with cerebral organic conditions or psychiatric disturbances by means of a short test for aphasia. *Journal of Clinical Psychology, 27,* 468–471.

Kusunoki, T. (1985). A study on scaling of Standard Language Test of Aphasia (SLTA): A practical scale based on a three-factor structure. *Japanese Journal of Behaviormetrics, 12* (23), 8–12.

LaBarge, E., Edwards, D., & Knesevich, J. W. (1986). Performance of normal elderly on the Boston Naming Test. *Brain and Language, 27,* 380–384.

Lahey, B. B. (Ed.). (1973). *The modification of language behavior.* Springfield, IL: Thomas.

Lawriw, I. (1976). *A test of the predictive validity and a cross-validation of the Neurosensory Center Comprehensive Examination for Aphasia.* Unpublished master's thesis, University of Victoria.

Lecours, A. R., Mehler, J., Parente, M. A., & Beltrami, M. C. (1988). Illiteracy and brain damage. III. A contribution to the study of speech and language disorders in illiterates with unilateral brain damage. *Neuropsychologia, 26,* 575–589.

Lecours, A. R., Mehler, J., Parente, M. A., & Caldeira, A. (1987). Illiteracy and brain damage. 1. Aphasia testing in culturally contrasted populations (control subjects). *Neuropsychologia, 25,* 231–245.

Lee, G. P., & Hamsher, K. (1988). Neuropsychologic findings in toxicometabolic confusional states. *Journal of Clinical and Experimental Neuropsychology, 10,* 769–778.

Lee, L. L. (1970). A screening test for syntax development. *Journal of Speech and Hearing Disorders, 35,* 103–112.

Lendrum, W., & Lincoln, N. B. (1985). Spontaneous recovery of language in patients with aphasia between 4 and 34 weeks after stroke. *Journal of Neurology, Neurosurgery and Psychiatry, 48,* 743–748.

Lesser, R. (1976). Verbal and non-verbal memory components in the Token Test. *Neuropsychologia, 14,* 79–85.

Lesser, R., Bryan, K., Anderson, J., & Hilton, R. (1986). Involving relatives in aphasia: An application of language enrichment therapy. *International Journal of Rehabilitation Research, 9,* 259–267.

Levin, H., Grossman, R. G., & Kelly, P. J. (1976). Aphasic disorders in patients with closed head injury. *Journal of Neurology, Neurosurgery and Psychiatry, 39,* 1062–1070.

Levin, H., Grossman, R. G., Sarwar, M., & Meyers, C. A. (1981). Linguistic recovery after closed head injury. *Brain and Language, 12,* 360–374.

Lipowski, Z. J. (1980). *Delirium: Acute brain failure in man.* Springfield, IL: Thomas.

Lomas, J., Pickard, L., Bester, S., Elbard, H., Finlayson, A., & Zoghaib, C. (1989). The Communicative Effectiveness Index: Developmental and psychometric evaluation of a functional communication measure for adult aphasia. *Journal of Speech and Hearing Disorders, 54,* 113–124.

Ludlow, C. L. (1977). Recovery from aphasia: A foundation for treatment. In M. Sullivan & M. S. Kommers (Eds.), *Rationale for adult aphasia therapy.* Omaha: University of Nebraska Medical Center.

Luria, A. R. (1966). *Higher cortical functions in man.* New York: Basic Books.

Marie, P. (1883). De l'aphasie, cecité verbale, surdite verbale, aphasie motire, agraphie. *Revue Medicale, 3,* 693–702.

Marquardt, T. P., Stoll, J., & Sussman, H. (1988). Disorders of communication in acquired cerebral trauma. *Journal of Learning Disabilities, 21,* 340–351.

Marshall, J. C. (1986). The description and interpretation of aphasic language disorder. *Neuropsychologia, 24,* 5–24.

Martin, A. D. (1977). Aphasia testing: A second look at the Porch Index of Communicative Ability. *Journal of Speech and Hearing Disorders, 42,* 547–561.

Martino, A. A., Pizzamiglio, L., & Razzano, C. (1976). A new version of the Token Test for aphasics: A concrete objects form. *Journal of Communication Disorders, 9,* 1–5.

McNeil, M. R. (1979). Porch Index of Communicative Ability. In F. L. Darley (Ed.), *Evaluation of appraisal techniques in speech and language pathology.* Reading, MA: Addison-Wesley.

McNeil, M. R., & Prescott, T. E. (1978). *Revised Token Test.* Baltimore, MD: University Park Press.

McNeil, M. R., Prescott, T. E., & Chang, E. C. (1975). A measure of PICA ordinality. In R. H. Brookshire (Ed.), *Clinical aphasiology, conference proceedings.* Minneapolis, MN: BRK Publishers.

Mecham, M. J., Jex, J. L., & Jones, J. D. (1967). *Utah test of language development.* (rev. ed.). Salt Lake City: Communication Research Associates.

Meier, M. J. (1974). Some challenges for clinical neuropsychology. In R. M. Reitan & L. A. Davison (Eds.), *Clinical neuropsychology: Current status and applications.* New York: Wiley.

Messick, S. (1980). The validity and ethics of assessment. *American Psychologist, 35,* 1012–1027.

Miller, E., & Hague, F. (1975). Some characteristics of verbal behavior in presenile dementia. *Psychological Medicine, 5,* 255–259.

Montgomery, K. M. (1982). *A normative study of neuropsychological test performance of a normal elderly sample.* M.A. thesis, University of Victoria.

Morley, G. K., Lundgren, S., & Haxby, J. (1979). Comparison and clinical applicability of auditory comprehension scores on the behavioral neurology deficit evaluation, Boston Diagnostic Aphasia Evaluation, Porch Index of Communicative Ability and Token Test. *Journal of Clinical Neuropsychology, 1*(3), 249–258.

Murdoch, B. E., Chenery, H. J., Wilks, V., & Boyle, R. S. (1987). Language disorders in dementia of the Alzheimer type. *Brain and Language, 31,* 122–137.

Naeser, M. A., Hayward, R. W., Laughlin, S. A., & Zatz, L. M. (1981). Quantitative CT scan studies in aphasia: I.Infarct size and CT numbers. *Brain and Language, 12,* 140–164.

Naeser, M. A., & Hayward, R. W. (1978). Lesion localization in aphasia with cranial computed tomography and the Boston Diagnostic Aphasia Examination. *Neurology, 28,* 545–551.

Naeser, M. A., Helm-Estabrooks, N., Haas, G., Auerbach, S., & Srinivasan, M. (1987). Relationship between lesion extent in 'Wernicke's area' on computed tomographic scan and predicting recovery of comprehension in Wernicke's aphasia. *Archives of Neurology (Chicago), 44,* 73–82.

Naeser, M. A., Mazurski, P., Goodglass, H., & Peraino, M. (1987). Auditory syntactic comprehension in nine aphasia groups (with CT scans) and children: Differences in degree but not order of difficulty observed. *Cortex, 23,* 359–380.

Nicholas, L. E., MacLennan, D. L., & Brookshire, R. H. (1986). Validity of multiple sentence reading of comprehension tests for aphasic adults. *Journal of Speech and Hearing Disorders, 51,* 82–87.

Nunnally, J. (1978). *Psychometric theory.* New York: McGraw-Hill.

Obler, L. K., Nicholas, M., Albert, M. L., & Woodward, S. (1985). On comprehension across the adult lifespan. *Cortex, 21,* 273–280.

Orgass, B., & Poeck, K. (1966). Clinical validation of a new test for aphasia: An experimental study of the Token Test. *Cortex, 2,* 222–243.

Orzeck, A. Z. (1964). *The Orzeck Aphasia Evaluation.* Los Angeles, CA: Western Psychological Services.

Osgood, C. E., & Sebeok, T. A. (Eds.). (1965). *Psycholinguistics: A survey of theory and research problems.* Bloomington: Indiana University Press.

Paradis, M. (1987). *The assessment of bilingual aphasia.* Hillsdale, NJ: Erlbaum.

Paul, R., & Cohen, D. J. (1982). Communication development and its disorders: A psycholinguistic perspective. *Schizophrenia Bulletin, 8,* 279–293.

Paul, R., & Cohen, D. J. (1984). Outcomes of severe disorders of language acquisition. *Journal of Autism and Developmental Disorders, 14,* 405–421.

Pick, A. (1913). Die agrammatischen Sprachstoerungen. Studien zur psychologischen Grundlegung der Aphasielehre. Part 1. In A. Alzheimer & M. Lewandowsky (Eds.), *Monographien aus dem Gesamtgebiet der Neurologie und Psychiatrie* (Vol. 7). Berlin: Springer.

Pizzamiglio, L. (1984). Capacita communicative di pazienti afasici in situazioni di vita quotidiana: Addatamento italiano. *Archivio di Psicologia, Neurologia e Psichiatria, 45,* 187–210.

Poeck, K. (1974). *Neurologie* (3rd ed.). Berlin: Springer.

Poeck, K., Kerschensteiner, M., & Hartje, W. (1972). A quantitative study on language understanding in fluent and nonfluent aphasia. *Cortex, 8,* 299–304.

Porch, B. E. (1967). *Porch index of communicative ability: Theory and development* (Vol. 1). Palo Alto, CA: Consulting Psychologists Press.

Porch, B. E. (1973). *Porch index of communicative ability: Administration, scoring, and interpretation* (Vol. 2). Palo Alto, CA: Consulting Psychologists Press.

Porch, B. E. (1979). *Porch index of communicative ability in children: Vol. 1. Theory and development.* Palo Alto, CA: Consulting Psychologists Press.

Porch, B. E., Collins, M., Wertz, R. T., & Friden, T. P. (1980). Statistical prediction of change in aphasia. *Journal of Speech and Hearing Research, 23,* 312–321.

Powell, G. E., Bailey, S., & Clark, E. (1980). A very short form of the Minnesota Aphasia Test. *British Journal of Social and Clinical Psychology, 19,* 189–194.

Prins, R. S., Snow, C. E., & Wagenaar, E. (1978). Recovery from aphasia: Spontaneous speech versus language comprehension. *Brain and Language, 6,* 192–211.

Reinvang, I. (1985). *Aphasia and brain organization.* New York: Plenum.

Reinvang, I., & Graves, R. (1975). A basic aphasia examination: Description with discussion of first results. *Scandinavian Journal of Rehabilitation Medicine, 7,* 129–135.

Reitan, R. M. (1984). *Aphasia Screening Test.* Tucson, AZ: Reitan Neuropsychology Laboratory.

Reynell, J., & Huntley, R. M. (1971). New scales for the assessment of language development in young children. *Journal of Learning Disabilities, 4,* 549–557.

Riedel, K., & Studdert-Kennedy, M. (1985). Extending formant transition may not improve aphasics' perception of stop consonant place of articulation. *Brain and Language, 24,* 223–232.

Risser, A. H., & Spreen, O. (1985). The Western Aphasia Battery Test: Review. *Journal of Clinical and Experimental Neuropsychology, 7,* 463–470.

Roberts, R. J., & Hamsher, K. (1984). Effects of minority status on facial recognition and naming performance. *Journal of Clinical Psychology, 40,* 539–545.

Ryalls, J., & Reinvang, I. (1986). Functional lateralization of linguistic tones: Acoustic evidence from Norwegian. *Language and Speech, 29,* 389–398.

Sands, E., Sarno, M. T., & Shankweiler, D. (1969). Long-term assessment of language function in aphasia due to stroke. *Archives of Physical Medicine and Rehabilitation, 50,* 202–222.

Sarno, J. E., Sarno, M. T., & Levita, E. (1971). Evaluating language improvement after completed stroke. *Archives of Physical Medicine and Rehabilitation, 52,* 73–78.

Sarno, M. T. (1969). *The Functional Communication Profile: Manual of directions.* New York: New York University Medical Center, Institute of Rehabilitation Medicine.

Sarno, M. T. (1984a). Functional measurement in verbal impairment secondary to brain damage. In C. V. Granger & G. E. Gresham (Eds.), *Functional assessment in rehabilitation medicine* (pp. 210–222). Baltimore, MD: Williams & Wilkins.

Sarno, M. T. (1984b). Verbal impairment after closed head injury: Report of a replication study. *Journal of Nervous and Mental Disease, 172,* 475–479.

Sarno, M. T. (1984c). Verbal impairment after closed head injury. Report of a replication study. *Journal of Nervous and Mental Disease, 172,* 475–479.

Sarno, M. T., Buonaguro, A., & Levita, E. (1985). Gender and recovery from aphasia after stroke. *Journal of Nervous and Mental Disease, 173,* 605–609.

Sarno, M. T., Buonaguro, A., & Levita, E. (1986). Characteristics of verbal impairment in closed head injured patients. *Archives of Physical Medicine and Rehabilitation, 67,* 400–405.

Sarno, M. T., Buonaguro, A., & Levita, E. (1987). Aphasia in closed head injury and stroke. *Aphasiology, 1,* 331–338.

Sarno, M. T., & Levita, E. (1979). Recovery in treated aphasia in the first year post-stroke. *Stroke, 10,* 663–670.

Sarno, M. T., & Levita, E. (1981). Some observations on the nature of recovery in global aphasia after stroke. *Brain and Language, 13,* 1–12.

Sasanuma, S. (1989). Aphasia rehabilitation in Japan. In M. T. Sarno & D. E. Woods (Eds.), *Aphasia rehabilitation in Asia and the Pacific region* (Monograph No. 45). New York: World Rehabilitation Fund.

Schuell, H. (1955). *Minnesota test for differential diagnosis of aphasia* (res. ed.). Minneapolis: University of Minnesota.

Schuell, H. (1957). A short examination for aphasia. *Neurology, 7,* 625–634.

Schuell, H. (1965). *Differential diagnosis of aphasia with the Minnesota Test.* Minneapolis: University of Minnesota Press.

Schuell, H. (1966). A re-evaluation of the short examination for aphasia. *Journal of Speech and Hearing Disorders, 31,* 137–147.

Schuell, H. (1973). *Differential diagnosis of aphasia with the Minnesota Test* (2nd ed.). Minneapolis: University of Minnesota Press.

Schuell, H. (1974a). Diagnosis and prognosis in aphasia. In L. F Sies (Ed.), *Aphasia, theory and therapy.* Baltimore, MD: University Park Press.

Schuell, H. (1974b). A theoretical framework for aphasia. In L. F. Sies (Ed.), *Aphasia, theory and therapy*. Baltimore, MD: University Park Press.

Schuell, H., & Jenkins, J. J. (1959). The nature of language deficit in aphasia. *Psychological Review, 66,* 45–67.

Schuell, H., Jenkins, J. J., & Carroll, J. B. (1962). A factor analysis of the Minnesota Test for Differential Diagnosis of Aphasia. *Journal of Speech and Hearing Research, 5,* 350–369.

Schuell, H., Jenkins, J. J., & Jiménez-Pabón, E. (1964). *Aphasia in adults, diagnosis, prognosis, and treatment*. New York: Harper.

Schum, R. L., Sivan, A. B., & Benton, A. (1989). Multilingual Aphasia Examination: Norms for children. *Clinical Neuropsychologist, 3,* 375–383.

Selnes, O. A., Niccum, N. E. , Knopman, D. S., & Rubens, A. B. (1984). Recovery of single word comprehension: CT-scan correlates. *Brain and Language, 21,* 72–84.

Shewan, C. M. (1980). *Auditory Comprehension Test for Sentences*. Chicago, IL: Biolinguistics Clinical Institutes.

Shewan, C. M. (1986). The Language Quotient (LQ): A new measure for the Western Aphasia Battery. *Journal of Communication Disorders, 19,* 427–439.

Shewan, C. M. (1988). The Shewan Spontaneous Language Analysis (SSLA) system for aphasic adults: Description, reliability, and validity. *Journal of Communication Disorders, 21,* 103–138.

Shewan, C. M., & Canter, G. L. (1971). Effects of vocabulary, syntax, and sentence length on auditory comprehension in aphasic patients. *Cortex, 7,* 209–225.

Shewan, C. M., & Donner, A. P. (1988). A comparison of three methods to evaluate change in the spontaneous language of aphasic individuals. *Journal of Communication Disorders, 21,* 171–176.

Shewan, C. M., & Kertesz, A. (1980). Reliability and validity characteristics of the Western Aphasia Battery (WAB). *Journal of Speech and Hearing Disorders, 45,* 308–324.

Shewan, C. M., & Kertesz, A. (1984). Effects of speech and language treatment on recovery from aphasia. *Brain and Language, 23,* 272–299.

Sidman, M. (1971). The behavioral analysis of aphasia. *Journal of Psychiatric Research, 8,* 413–422.

Skenes, L. L., & McCauley, R. J. (1985). Psychometric review of nine aphasia tests. *Journal of Communication Disorders, 18,* 461–474.

Sklar, M. (1973). *Sklar Aphasia Scale* (rev. ed.). Los Angeles, CA: Western Psychological Services.

Snow, W. G. (1987). Aphasia Screening Test performance in patients with lateralized brain damage. *Journal of Clinical Psychology, 43,* 266–271.

Snow, W. G., & Tierney, M. C. (1988). *One-year test-retest reliability of selected neuropsychological tests in older adults*. Paper presented at the meeting of the International Neuropsychological Society, New Orleans, LA.

Spellacy, F., & Spreen, O. (1969). A short form of the Token Test. *Cortex, 5,* 390–397.

Spiegel, D. K., Jones, L. V., & Wepman, J. M. (1965). Test responses as predictors of free-speech characteristics in aphasia patients. *Journal of Speech and Hearing Research, 8*(4), 349–362.

Spreen, O. (1968). Psycholinguistic aspects of aphasia. *Journal of Speech and Hearing Research, 11,* 467–477.

Spreen, O., & Benton, A. L. (1965). Comparative studies of some psychological tests for cerebral damage. *Journal of Nervous and Mental Disease, 140,* 323–333.

Spreen, O., & Benton, A. L. (1974). *Sound Recognition Test*. Victoria, BC: University of Victoria.

Spreen, O., & Benton, A. L. (1977). *Neurosensory Center Comprehensive Examination for Aphasia* (1977 rev.). Victoria, B.C.: University of Victoria, Neuropsychology Laboratory.

Spreen, O., & Wachal, R. S. (1973). Psycholinguistic analysis of aphasic language: Theoretical formulations and procedures. *Language and Speech, 16,* 130–146.

Spreen, O., & Strauss, E. (1991). *A Compendium of Neuropsychological Tests.* New York: Oxford University Press.

Strub, R. L., & Black, F. W. (1977). *The mental status examination in neurology.* Philadelphia, PA: Davis.

Sussman, H., Marquardt, T., Hutchinson, J., & MacNeilage, P. (1986). Compensatory articulation in Broca's aphasia. *Brain and Language, 27,* 56–74.

Swisher, L. P., & Sarno, M. T. (1969). Token Test scores of three matched patient groups: Left brain-damaged with aphasia; right brain-damaged without aphasia; non-brain-damaged. *Cortex, 5,* 264–273.

Tallal, P., Stark, R. E., & Mellits, D. (1985). The relationship between auditory temporal analysis and receptive language disorder: evidence from studies of developmental language disorders. *Neuropsychologia, 23,* 527–534.

Taussig, I. M., Henderson, V. W., & Mack, W. (1988). *Spanish translation and validation of a neuropsychological battery: Performance of Spanish- and English-speaking Alzheimer's disease patients and normal comparison subjects.* Paper presented at the Gerontological Society meeting, San Francisco, CA.

Taylor, M. L. (1965). A measurement of functional communication in aphasia. *Archives of Physical Medicine and Rehabilitation, 46,* 101–107.

Thorndike, E. L., & Lorge, T. (1944). *The Teacher's Book of 30,000 Words.* New York: Columbia University.

Tramontana, M. G., & Boyd, T. A. (1986). Psychometric screening of neuropsychological abnormality in older children. *International Journal of Clinical Neuropsychology, 8,* 53–59.

Tuokko, H. (1985). *Normative data for elderly subjects* (unpublished manuscript). Vancouver: University of British Columbia.

Ulatowska, H. K., Doyel, A. W., Stern, R. F., & Haynes, S. M. (1983). Production of procedural discourse in aphasia. *Brain and Language, 18,* 315–341.

Van Harskamp, F., & Van Dongen, H. R. (1977). Construction and validation of different short forms of the Token Test. *Neuropsychologia, 15,* 467–470.

Varney, N. R. (1980). Sound recognition in relation to aural language comprehension in aphasic patients. *Journal of Neurology, Neurosurgery and Psychiatry, 43,* 71–75.

Varney, N. R. (1984a). Phonemic imperception in aphasia. *Brain and Language, 21,* 85–94.

Varney, N. R. (1984b). The prognostic significance of sound recognition in receptive aphasia. *Archives of Neurology (Chicago), 41,* 181–182.

Varney, N. R., & Benton, A. L. (1979). Phonemic discrimination and aural comprehension among aphasic patients. *Journal of Clinical Neuropsychology, 1,* 65–73.

Varney, N. R., & Damasio, H. (1986). CT scan correlates of sound recognition defect in aphasia. *Cortex, 22,* 483–486.

Veteran's Administration Cooperative Study on Aphasia: Protocol Manual (1973). Washington, DC: Veteran's Administration.

Voinescu, I., Mihailescu, L., & Lugoji, G. (1987). Communication value of a standard interview: A functional subtest to assess progress in treated aphasics. *Neurologie et Psychiatrie, 25,* 221–237.

Wachal, R. S., & Spreen, O. (1973). Some measures of lexical diversity in aphasic and normal language performance. *Language and Speech, 16,* 169–181.

Wang, P. L., Ennis, K. E., & Copland, S. L. (1986). *The Cognitive Competency Test: Manual.* Toronto: Mount Sinai Medical Center.

Weisenburg, T. H., & McBride, K. E. (1935). *Aphasia.* New York: Commonwealth Fund.

Wepman, J. M. (1951). *Recovery from aphasia.* New York: Ronald Press.

Wepman, J. M., Bock, R. D., Jones, L. V., & Van Pelt, D. (1956). Psycholinguistic study of aphasia: A revision of the concept of anomia. *Journal of Speech and Hearing Disorders, 21,* 468–477.

Wepman, J. M., & Jones, L. V. (1961). *Studies in aphasia: An approach to testing.* Chicago, IL: Education-Industry Service.

Wepman, J. M., & Jones, L. V. (1964). Five aphasias: A commentary on aphasia as a regressive linguistic phenomenon. In D. M. Rioch & E. A. Weinstein (Eds.), *Disorders of communication.* Baltimore, MD: Williams & Wilkins.

Wernicke, C. (1908). The symptoms complex of aphasia. In A. Church (Ed.), *Diseases of the nervous system.* New York: Appleton. (Original work published 1874).

Werner, M. H., Ernst, J., Townes, B. D., Peel, J., & Preston, M. (1987). Relationship between IQ and neuropsychological measures in neuropsychiatric populations: Within laboratory and cross-cultural replications using WAIS and WAIS-R. *Journal of Clinical and Experimental Neuropsychology, 9,* 545–562.

Wertz, R. T. (1979). Word fluency measure. In F. L. Darley (Ed.), *Evaluation of appraisal techniques in speech and language pathology.* Reading, MA: Addison-Wesley.

Wertz, R. T., Keith, R. L., & Custer, D. D. (1971, November). *Normal and aphasic behavior on a measure of auditory input and a measure of verbal output.* Paper presented at the American Speech and Hearing Association Convention, Chicago, IL.

Wertz, R. T., & Lemme, M. L. (1974). *Input and output measures with adult aphasics* (Final report). Washington, DC: Research and Training Center 10, Social Rehabilitation Services.

Wertz, R. T., Collins, M. J., Weiss, D., Kurtzke, J. F., Friden, T., Brookshire, R. T., Pierce, J., Holtzapple, P., Hubbard, D. J., Porch, B. E., West, J. A., Davis, L., Matovitch, V., Morley, G. K., & Resurreccion, E., (1981). Veterans Administration cooperative study on aphasia: A comparison of individual and group treatment. *Journal of Speech and Hearing Research, 24,* 580–594.

West, J. A. (1973). Auditory comprehension in aphasic adults: Improvement through training. *Archives of Physical Medicine and Rehabilitation, 54,* 78–86.

Wheeler, L., & Reitan, R. M. (1962). The presence and laterality of brain damage predicted from responses to a short aphasia screening test. *Perceptual and Motor Skills, 15,* 783–799.

Willmes, K., & Ratajczak (1987). The design and application of a data- and method-based system for the Aachen Aphaisa Test. *Neuropsychologia, 25,* 725–733.

Willmes, K., Poeck, K., Weniger, D., & Huber, W. (1983). Facet theory applied to the construction and validation of the Aachen Aphasia Test. *Brain and Language, 18,* 259–276.

Yeudall, L. T., Fromm, D., Reddon, J. R., & Stefanyk, W. O. (1986). Normative data stratified by age and sex for 12 neuropsychological tests. *Journal of Clinical Psychology, 42,* 918–946.

Zubrick, A., & Smith, A. (1979). Minnesota Test for Differential Diagnosis of Aphasia. In F. C. Darley (Ed.), *Evaluation of appraisal techniques in speech and language pathology.* Reading, MA: Addison-Wesley.

5

Phonological Aspects of Aphasia

SHEILA E. BLUMSTEIN

The theory of language divides the linguistic system into components or levels. These levels include phonology, syntax, and semantics. Within each level, linguistic primitives define the basic elements of the system. The nature of these elements, their organization, and the interaction of the levels constitute the theory of grammar. Implicit in the theory is the notion that the levels of language are in effect semiautonomous; that is, although these levels are independent of each other, they have to be inextricably linked during the communication process. For example, the sounds of language can be studied independently of meaning, yet they gain their linguistic significance ONLY because they convey meaning.

In this chapter, we will focus on the phonological component of the linguistic system in relation to adult aphasia. It is a useful heuristic to study aphasia in relation to each of the components of the grammar; however, it is important to emphasize that the components of the grammar are never entirely isolable. Perhaps more importantly, aphasia rarely evidences a deficit selective to only one linguistic component. Thus, studying phonology in aphasia does not imply that the patient is normal in other linguistic abilities. In fact, as noted in the course of this chapter, the language behavior of aphasics shows clearly how the components of the grammar do interact in language processing.

The study of the phonological component affords in many ways a view of the effects of brain damage on language that other components cannot. In particular, phonology is embedded in physical reality: speech. At the levels of both production and perception, speech is the primary interface with the linguistic code. In production, an idea is ultimately realized as a set of physiological events, and in perception, meaning is extracted from the acoustic waveform. Thus, unlike the other

ACQUIRED APHASIA, SECOND EDITION

linguistic levels, which by their very nature are abstract, phonology relates to a physical reality. Moreover, the phonological component is the
only linguistic level that can be studied in isolation from the others. For
example, the perception of phonemic contrasts, such as /pa/ versus
/ba/, can be examined independently of word meaning. Thus, it is possible to determine the extent to which a speech perception deficit may be
selectively impaired independently of its relation to the semantic content of a word.

In this chapter, we will focus on a number of areas that relate to
phonological processing in aphasia. We will first investigate speech production in order to characterize the nature of the speech deficits found
in aphasia and to attempt to provide some insight into the underlying
mechanisms responsible for these deficits. Specifically, we will focus
on the dichotomy between phonological and phonetic disintegration in
aphasia. We then turn to speech perception and explore the nature of
the input deficits found in aphasia and suggest their possible underlying
bases. We consider how speech perception deficits may relate to auditory processing deficits on the one hand, and auditory comprehension
deficits on the other. Taken together, such study should provide a characterization of phonological processing in aphasia, a study that requires
the interface of both speech production and speech perception.

The Phonological Component: A Model

Before a discussion of these areas, it may be useful to briefly elaborate
a model of the phonological component of a grammar and review its
primitives and their theoretical organization. The sounds of speech can
be divided into two types of representation. The first is the phonemic
level, which characterizes the minimal sound units that contrast meaning. For example, in English, the sounds /p/ and /b/ are phonemes
because they can be used to differentiate words in the language, for
instance, *pear* versus *bear*. Phonology not only is concerned with the
study of the individual phonemes of the language, but also attempts to
characterize how they combine in the language system. One can determine a grammar of phonology that specifies the combination of speech
sounds for a particular language. In English, for example, some combinations of sounds are allowable sequences, for instance, *brick* or the
nonsense syllable *blick*, whereas others, such as *bnick*, are not.

Although the phonemes are the minimal meaningful sound units of
language, they are further divisible into smaller components or distinctive features (Chomsky & Halle, 1968; Jakobson, Fant, & Halle,

1962). These features describe the phonemes in terms of either the articulatory or acoustic characteristics that contribute to the phonemic identity of the segment. Figure 5.1 shows the bundle of distinctive features that characterize the phonemic segments /p/, /b/, and /d/. The phoneme /p/is a consonant (in contrast to a vowel), [+consonantal]; it is produced with a complete closure of the vocal tract followed by an abrupt release, [+stop]; the closure occurs at the lips, [+bilabial]; and the vocal cords do not begin to vibrate until after the release of the stop closure, [−voice]. The phoneme /b/ shares the distinctive feature characteristics of /p/, except the voicing feature. For /b/, the vocal cords vibrate at the release of the stop consonant, and thus it is described as [+voice]. In contrast to both /p/ and /b/, /d/ is produced with a closure at the alveolar ridge, [−bilabial], and, as a result, is different from /b/ in place of articulation. Note also that /d/ is different from /p/ not only in place of articulation but also in voicing. Implicit in distinctive feature theory is the notion that sounds that are contrasted by a single feature are more alike articulatorily, acoustically, and psychologically than are sounds contrasting by several distinctive features. Thus, /p/ and /b/, distinguished by one distinctive feature, are more "similar" than are /p/ and /d/, distinguished by two features.

The phonological component of a grammar then consists of a characterization of the phonemes, rules for their combination, and distinctive feature specifications for the individual phonemes. Up to this point, the grammar has specified only the segments of speech. However, segments are embedded in a larger framework comprising stress and intonation patterns. Both stress and intonation form a part of what linguists call speech prosody or suprasegmentals, as they are melodic features of speech that span the domain of individual speech segments. The intonation or melody pattern of a sentence indicates to the listener, among other things, whether the sentence is a statement, question, or imperative.

Theoretically, linguists consider the phonological grammar to represent a central mechanism that subserves both speech production and

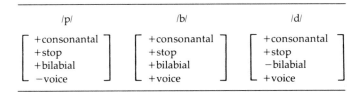

FIGURE 5.1. *Distinctive feature attributes of several phonemes in English.*

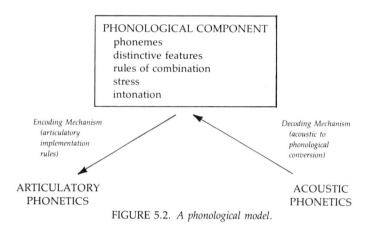

FIGURE 5.2. *A phonological model.*

speech perception. That is, the phonemes, features, organizational properties of segments, and suprasegmentals form the abstract grammar ultimately encoded in articulatory terms for speech production and decoded from the acoustic waveform for language comprehension. Figure 5.2 shows a schematic of the organization of such a model. Note that for production, the abstract phonological entities must be realized PHONETICALLY by means of articulatory implementation rules and that the acoustic signal must be encoded in terms of these abstract properties for comprehension. By PHONETIC is meant all of the detail required to realize the abstract phonological properties in terms of their actual production or perception. For example, the phoneme /p/ can occur in a number of phonological environments—in initial position as in *pill* and in a consonant cluster after /s/ in *spill*. The actual PHONETIC realization of the phoneme /p/ is different depending upon its environment. In initial position, the /p/ is aspirated, whereas after /s-/, it is not; that is *pill*, /pɪl/ → [pʰɪl]; *spill*, /spɪl/ → [spɪl]. Thus, the study of phonology includes an analysis of the abstract properties of speech sounds, and phonetics includes the detailed physical characteristics of these speech sounds specified in terms of their articulatory parameters for production or in terms of their acoustic properties for perception.

Speech Production

Phonological Patterns of Dissolution

Clinical evidence shows that nearly all aphasic patients produce phonological errors in their speech output. Paul Broca was first to focus on the loss of articulatory capacity due to impairment of "la mémoire des moyens de co-ordination que l'on emploie pour articuler les mots" (cited in Taylor, 1958, p. 126).[1] In the ensuing 60 years, such aphasiologists as Hughlings Jackson (see Taylor, 1958), Froschels (1915), Head (1926), and Critchley (1952) noted that patients of nearly all clinical types make phonemic errors in their speech. These errors can be characterized according to four main types:

1. Phoneme substitution errors, in which a target phoneme is substituted for a different phoneme of the language, for example, *teams* → /kimz/.
2. Simplification errors, in which a target phoneme or syllable is lost, thus simplifying the phonological structure of the word, for example, *brown* → /bawn/.
3. Addition errors, in which a target phoneme or syllable is added to the word, for example, *papa* → /paprə/.
4. Environment errors, in which a target phoneme is replaced by or transposed with neighboring sounds, for example, *Crete* → /trit/, *degree* → /gədriz/.

It is interesting that despite the clinical diversity of aphasic patients, all of these error types can be found across aphasic groups. Thus, the presence of such errors does not serve as a clinical diagnostic tool. Nevertheless, the absolute numbers of such errors does seem to vary across groups, suggesting potential differences in severity of impairment (see Blumstein, 1973). Of more importance, the PATTERN of errors rather than simply their presence provides a means of characterizing and hopefully understanding the nature and bases of speech production deficits in aphasia.

For the most part, phonological studies have focused on the patterns of speech obtained for a particular diagnostic group. The groups studied have included primarily anterior and posterior patients. The reasons for the particular dichotomy made between these groups of patients correspond largely to their remarkably different clinical characteristics. Anterior aphasics and especially a subgroup of these, Broca's aphasics, show a profound expressive deficit in the face of relatively preserved auditory language comprehension. Speech output is nonfluent in that it is slow, labored, and often dysarthic, and the melody pattern seems flat. Furthermore, speech output is agrammatic. This agrammatism is characterized by the omission of grammatical words, such as *the* and *is*, as well as the substitution of grammatical inflectional endings marking number,

---

[1] "the memory of the means of coordination that one uses to pronounce words."

tense, and so forth. Naming to confrontation is generally fair to good, and repetition is as good as or better than spontaneous speech output.

In contrast to the nonfluent speech output of the anterior patient, the posterior patient's speech output is fluent. Among the posterior aphasias, Wernicke's and conduction aphasias are perhaps the most studied in relation to phonology. The characteristic features of the language abilities of Wernicke's aphasia include well-articulated but paraphasic speech in the context of severe auditory language comprehension deficits. Paraphasias include literal paraphasias (sound substitutions), verbal paraphasias (word substitutions), or neologisms (productions that are phonologically possible but have no meaning associated with them). Speech output, although grammatically full, is often empty of semantic content and is marked with the overuse of high-frequency "contentless" nouns and verbs, such as *thing* and *be*. The patient also has a moderate to severe naming deficit, and repetition is also severely impaired. Another frequent characteristic of this disorder is LOGORRHEA, or a press for speech.

Conduction aphasia refers to the syndrome in which there is a disproportionately severe repetition deficit in relation to the relative fluency and ease of spontaneous speech production and to the generally good auditory language comprehension of the patient. Speech output contains many literal paraphasias and some naming errors. In addition, these patients often evidence a moderate confrontation naming deficit.

As might be expected, because of the clinical observation that anterior aphasics have a severe ouput deficit, most studies have focused on this group. It is important to note that in this discussion results from studies concerning apraxia of speech and the speech output of Broca's aphasics are considered together. There has been an active dialogue in the literature between those who see apraxia of speech as a nonaphasic and selective articulatory deficit (Aten, Darley, Deal, & Johns, 1975; Johns & LaPointe, 1976) and those who consider apraxia of speech as part of a larger language or aphasic disorder (Buckingham, 1979; Martin, 1974, 1975). Whether apraxia of speech is a linguistically based disorder (i.e., affecting the phonological and consequently the linguistic system) or simply an articulatory disorder is difficult to determine from the obtained data. To dissociate these two possibilities, it is necessary to demonstrate that the patterns of articulatory errors are different from those of phonological errors, and, as we will see, similar patterns are derived regardless of whether the patient is labeled apraxic or aphasic. In reality, it would not be surprising to find similar patterns of phonological disintegration whether the errors are articulatory or linguistically based, primarily because theoretical linguistic assumptions are derived from the intrinsic nature or organization of the PHONETIC properties of speech in relation to their linguistic function. Thus, what is articulatorily simple is phonologically or linguistically simple, and what is articulatorily complex is also linguistically complex.

Turning to the patterns of speech output in anterior aphasics, common patterns of deficits are found. In particular, anterior aphasics make many more consonant than vowel errors (Keller, 1978; Trost & Canter, 1974). Of the consonant errors, a greater number of substitution errors occur than any other type (Blumstein, 1973; Dunlop & Marquardt, 1977; Klich, Ireland, & Weidner, 1979; Trost & Canter, 1974). Furthermore, patients have greater difficulty with consonants produced in initial than in final position, for example, *pete* versus *beep*. Moreover, simplification errors occur most commonly in the environment of consonant clusters and thus reflect an overall reduction in the complexity of the syllable structure.

The patterns of substitution errors can be studied in two ways. First, a phonemic analysis can be done in which the particular phoneme targets and their substitutions are listed. Such analyses have generally shown tremendous variability and inconsistency across patients (Shankweiler & Harris, 1966; Trost & Canter, 1974). Namely, it is impossible to predict what particular phonemes the patients will produce incorrectly, when those errors will occur, and exactly what phonemes will be substituted. As a result, several researchers have considered the errors to be unsystematic and random.

Nevertheless, further analysis reveals distinct patterns of dissolution. This analysis procedure considers the phonological RELATION between the target and substituted phoneme. Thus, the substitution of a /b/ for a /p/ represents not the substitution of one whole sound unit for another, but rather the replacement of the voiced feature with the voiceless feature. As discussed earlier, linguistic theory makes implicit assumptions and predictions about the possible relations among the sounds of a language, and these have direct application to the types of speech production errors found in aphasia. Thus, phoneme substitutions should occur more commonly among sounds sharing a number of feature dimensions, for example, /p/–/b/ versus /t/–/w/. Moreover, sound substitutions should be characterized more commonly by single feature changes than by several feature changes. For example, /p/ → /b/ represents a single feature change of voicing, whereas /p/ → /z/ represents a change of the features of voicing, place of articulation (labial vs. alveolar), and manner (stop vs. fricative).

Roman Jakobson was the first researcher to suggest and ultimately apply these theoretical principles to the study of aphasia and child language (Jakobson, 1968). Further studies have shown a remarkable uniformity in that, overall, many more single feature substitution errors are found than errors of several features (Blumstein, 1973; Martin & Rigrodsky, 1974; Trost & Canter, 1974). With regard to vowel errors, patterns of dissolution similar to those obtained for consonants can be found. Namely, substitution errors are the most common error type, and most errors reflect single feature substitutions (Keller, 1975, 1978; Trost & Canter, 1974).

Nevertheless, as already indicated, despite this systematicity and regularity, the particular occurrence of an error cannot be predicted (Blumstein, 1973; Hatfield & Walton, 1975). Moreover, substitution errors are not unidirectional; that is, voiced consonants can become voiceless and voiceless consonants can become voiced. Thus, the patterns of errors reflect statistical tendencies: When errors occur, they tend to be single feature substitutions, they more likely affect some features than others, and they tend to go more in one direction than another. In this sense, then, the performance of the patients is variable, but it is NOT random, as it follows specific phonological principles.

These results suggest that the patient has not "lost" the ability to produce either particular phonemes or to instantiate particular features. Rather, his or her speech output mechanism does not seem to be able to consistently encode the correct underlying phonemic (i.e., feature) representation of the word. As a consequence, the patient may produce an utterance that is articulatorily correct but that deviates phonologically from the target word; for example, for *team*, the patient produces /kim/. On other occasions, he or she may produce the same target correctly from both an articulatory and phonological point of view; for example, for *team*, he or she produces /tim/.

In general, the pattern of results that have emerged are stable across different languages (French: Bouman & Grünbaum, 1925; Lecours & Lhermitte, 1969; German: Bouman & Grünbaum, 1925; Goldstein, 1948; English: Blumstein, 1973; Green, 1969; Turkish: Peuser & Fittschen, 1977; Russian: Luria, 1966; Finnish: Niemi, Koivuselka-Sallinen, & Hanninen, 1985) and across testing procedures (naming: Trost & Canter, 1974; repetition: Cohen, Dubois, Gauthier, Hécaen, & Angelergues, 1963; Kagan, 1977; reading: Bouman & Grünbaum, 1925; Dunlop & Marquardt, 1977; spontaneous speech: Blumstein, 1973). However, it is important to emphasize that differences have emerged in a number of studies. These differences are often subtle, and are difficult to evaluate because research methodologies have varied across studies, as have the classification schemas for the various error types and the phonetic feature systems used in analyzing the data (Burns & Canter, 1977; Canter, Trost, &

Burns, 1985; Kohn, 1985; Martin, Wasserman, Gilden, & West, 1975; Nespoulous, Joanette, Beland, Caplan, & Lecours, 1987; Trost & Canter, 1974). For example, Trost and Canter (1974) found different distributions of error types using a naming task and a repetition task; that is, subjects produced a greater proportion of responses that could not be judged phonemically in a naming task than in repetition. Such differences are not at all surprising, considering the nature of these test paradigms. Failure to name reflects more than phonological output problems; rather, word-finding deficits can interact with the phonological disorder. In contrast, in repetition, an auditory model of the word is provided and therefore problems of word retrieval are controlled. However, a different variable is introduced in a repetition task; namely, the patient must be able to PERCEIVE correctly the auditory model. Thus, a repetition error could reflect a perceptual error, a production error, a memory deficit (the auditory model must be held in short-term store before it is repeated), or a combination of these three. It is important then in testing a patient that the nature of the task and its demands on the linguistic system be carefully considered and that the behavior of the patient be viewed in relation to the methodology used to elicit the stimuli.

To this point, only the behavior of anterior patients has been reviewed. However, a number of studies have investigated the phonologial patterns of posterior aphasics as well. Clinically, of course, anterior and posterior patients represent contrasting speech output behaviors. The slow, labored, often dysarthric speech pattern of the anterior patient is opposed to the fluent, easily articulated, and facile output of the posterior patient. In fact, early researchers characterized the speech production patterns of anterior aphasics in terms of phonetic disintegration (Alajouanine, Ombredane, & Durand, 1939) and the patterns of posterior aphasics in terms of phonemic disintegration (Luria, 1966). Despite these differences, the speech production behavior of posterior patients breaks down into categories similar to the patterns of the anterior patients. In particular, more consonant than vowel errors are produced, substitution errors are among the most common error types, syllable structure of words is often simplified, and phonemic substitution errors tend to involve single feature substitutions more often than substitutions of more than one feature (Blumstein, 1973; Burns & Canter, 1977; Degiovanni et al., 1977; Dubois Hécaen, Angelergues, Chatelier, & Marcie, 1964; Green 1969; Halpern, Keith, & Darley, 1976). Nevertheless, similar to the results of studies with anterior aphasics, several investigations have reported different patterns of results comparing performance of groups of posterior patients and comparing performance of anterior and posterior patients. As discussed, however, these differences are generally subtle and may be attributed to the varying tasks and methods of analysis employed in the various studies (e.g., Canter et al., 1985; Nespoulous et al., 1987).

In summary, phonological analysis of aphasic speech production indicates similar patterns of dissolution for both anterior and posterior aphasics. These errors can be characterized in terms of the frequency of phoneme substitution errors in which the relation between target word and actual production is distinguished primarily by single distinctive feature contrasts, simplification errors in which the complexity of a phonological form is reduced, the occurrence of intrusions of sounds or syllables, and the influence of neighboring sounds on the final speech output. The stability of these patterns is evidenced by their occurrence across the different phonological systems in natural language. Nevertheless, it is important to emphasize that different experimental tasks as well as differences in the type and complexity of the stimuli and the phonetic feature systems used can contribute to variations among the basic patterns elucidated here.

Phonetic Patterns of Dissolution

As indicated in the previous section, an analysis of the phonological patterns of aphasic speech failed to clearly differentiate among the various clinical types of aphasia. As a whole, these results would suggest that similar mechanisms are responsible for the speech production patterns of aphasic patients. Yet from a clinical point of view, such a conclusion does not seem warranted. Phonological analyses fail to capture what seems to be a qualitative distinction between the anterior and posterior aphasic. This distinction had been alluded to in the previous section under the rubric of phonetic versus phonemic disintegration. It is just this distinction, however, that the phonological analyses have ignored. In particular, the speech production characteristics of anterior aphasics are slow and labored and contain numerous PHONETIC distortions. These characteristics were not considered in the phonological investigations, where only errors that affected the PHONEMIC representation of the target word were considered. Thus, if a patient attempted to say *pear* and said [p^{hhh}ær], overly aspirating the initial consonant, this production would not be considered a phonological error, as the phonemic representation of the phonetic output was correct.

A long-held observation is that some patients, particularly anterior aphasics, produce phonetic errors. The implied basis for these errors is one of articulatory implementation; that is, the commands to the articulators to encode the word are inappropriate, poorly timed, and so forth. Perhaps the first researchers to investigate the nature of phonetic disintegration using instrumental measures were Alajouanine et al. (1939). Three principles were postulated to account for the patterns of consonant production they found in their patients: (a) paralytic, characterized by articulatory weakness; (b) dystonic, characterized by articulatory movements excessive in force and duration; and (c) apraxic, characterized by gross difficulty in forming articulatory movements to command and some difficulty upon imitation. Spectrographic analyses have supported the earlier findings (Lehiste, 1968). It is important to emphasize that in both of these studies patients classified either as having apraxia of speech or as anterior aphasics displayed similar patterns of behavior. These results suggest that anterior aphasics may have a speech production pattern qualitatively different from that of posterior aphasics when phonetic errors are also considered. Perhaps more importantly, it may be that the basis for many of the PHONOLOGICAL errors in anterior patients is actually phonetic in nature; that is, phonological errors, such as /p/ → /b/, may represent extreme phonetic distortions that are perceived by the listener in terms of a change in phonetic category from the target.

A number of studies have explored the phonetic patterns of speech by investigating the acoustic properties or the articulatory parameters underlying the production of particular phonetic dimensions. The dimensions investigated include voicing in stop consonants and fricatives, place of articulation in stops and fricatives, and the nasal and stop manner of articulation. Together, patterns of deficits emerge that provide some insight into the underlying basis of these impairments for aphasic patients. In particular, studies of speech production in anterior patients have shown that these patients have difficulty producing phonetic dimensions that require the timing of two independent articulators. These findings have emerged in the analysis of two phonetic dimensions, voicing and nasality, both requiring the integration of two articulators. In the case of the feature voicing, the dimension studied is voice-onset time— that is, the timing relation between the release of a stop consonant and the onset of glottal pulsing. For voiceless consonants, such as /p/, the vocal cords do not begin to vibrate until about 30 msec after the stop consonant is released, whereas for voiced consonants, such as /b/, vocal cord vibration begins either at the release of the consonant or some 10s of milliseconds after the release of the consonant. The production of nasal consonants also requires appropriate timing between two articulators—in this case, the release of the consonant and velum opening. For /m/, the velum must be open at the release of the consonant so that air may escape from both the oral and nasal cavities as the consonant is released. If the velum is not sufficiently open, air will be unable to escape through the nose and will consequently escape only through the oral cavity, resulting in the corresponding stop consonant /b/. Results of analyses of the production of both the voicing and nasal phonetic dimensions have shown that anterior patients evidence significant deficits (Blumstein, Cooper, Goodglass, Statlender, & Gottlieb, 1980; Blumstein, Cooper, Zurif, & Caramazza, 1977; Freeman, Sands, & Harris, 1978; Gandour & Dardarananda, 1984a; Itoh, Sasanuma, Hirose, Yoshioka, & Ushijima, 1980; Itoh et al., 1982; Itoh, Sasanuma, & Ushijima, 1979; Shewan, Leeper, & Booth, 1984). These patterns emerge not only in English and Japanese for which voice-onset time serves to distinguish voiced and voiceless stop consonants, but also in Thai for which voice-onset time serves to distinguish three categories of voicing in stop consonants. All of these studies have used acoustic measurements and have inferred that the basis for the deficit is phonetic and involves articulatory timing. More direct measures of articulatory timing using fiber optics (Itoh, Sasanuma, Tatsumi, & Kobayashi, 1979; Itoh, Sasanuma, & Ushijima, 1979), computer-controlled X-ray microbeams (Itoh et al., 1980), and electromyography (Shankweiler, Harris, & Taylor, 1968) have also shown that the timing relation among the articulators is impaired. Taken together, these results support the conclusion that motor programming for the synchronization of different articulators is impaired (Itoh, Sasanuma, &Ushijima, 1979) and, furthermore, that there is a reduction in the capacity for independent movement of the articulators (Lehiste, 1968; Shankweiler et al., 1968).

Nevertheless, these patients also show normal patterns of production, which suggest that their disorder affects only particular types of articulatory maneuvers rather than the articulatory implementation of particular phonetic features. In particular, these patients are able to maintain the distinction between voiced and voiceless stops on the basis of the duration of the preceding vowel (Baum, Blumstein, Naeser, & Palumbo, 1990; Duffy & Gawle, 1984). Moreover, they do not show a systematic relation between the ability to realize the voicing dimension by means of voice-onset time and vowel duration (Tuller, 1984). Thus, these patients do not have a disorder affecting the articulatory implementation of the feature voicing, but a disorder affecting particular articulatory maneuvers, namely, the timing or integration of movements of two independent articulators. Consistent with this view is the finding that anterior aphasics maintain formant frequency characteristics of different vowels despite increased variability in their productions (Kent & Rosenbek, 1983; Ryalls, 1981, 1986, 1987).

Although anterior aphasics show a disorder in temporal coordination, their disorder does not seem to reflect a pervasive timing impairment. Their fricative durations do not differ significantly from those of normals (Harmes et al., 1984), and they maintain the intrinsic duration differences characteristic of fricatives varying in place of articulation; for example [s] and [š] are longer than [f] and [θ] (Baum et al., 1990). Although overall vowel duration is longer for anterior aphasics than for normals (see Ryalls, 1987, for review), these patients do maintain differences in the intrinsic durations of vowels—for example, tense vowels [i] and [e] are longer than lax vowels [I] and [E]—and they maintain the phonemic vowel length distinction in Thai (Gandour & Dardarananda, 1984b).

In addition to an impairment in the timing of independent articulators, difficulties for anterior aphasics have also emerged with laryngeal control. They have shown impairments in the production of voiced fricatives (Baum et al., 1990; Harmes et al., 1984; Kent & Rosenbek, 1983) and in particular aspects of the production of stop consonants (Shinn & Blumstein, 1983). These studies indicate that anterior aphasics seem to have impairments in the implementation of laryngeal gestures affecting voicing in consonant production, as well as those spectral parameters requiring the interaction of the laryngeal system and the supralaryngeal vocal tract system (Baum et al., 1990).

The timing problem described for anterior aphasics has been defined solely with respect to the production of individual segments and their underlying features. Kent and Rosenbek (1983) suggested that this problem is a manifestation of a broader impairment in the integration of articulatory movements from one phonetic segment to another. Individual segments are not produced in the stream of speech as though they were "beads on a string" (i.e., individual units isolated from the sounds around them). Rather, the sounds of speech exert considerable influence on each other. For example, the production of [s] and its consequent acoustic characteristics vary depending upon whether [s] is followed by the vowel [i] or [u]. The study of coarticulation explores the nature of such effects in the production of speech. It provides insight not only into the question of the dynamic aspects of speech production, but also into the size of the planning units that can be programmed in the production of syllables or words.

Recent investigations on coarticulation effects indicate that anterior patients produce relatively normal anticipatory coarticulation. For example, in producing the syllable [su], they anticipate the rounded vowel [u] in the production of the preceding [s] (Katz, 1988). Nevertheless, they seem to show a delay in the time it takes to produce these effects (Ziegler & von Cramon, 1985, 1986), and they may show some deficiencies in their productions (Tuller & Story, 1986; but see Katz, 1987, for discussion). Moreover, these patients have shown lengthening of formant transitions of consonants, suggesting difficulties in integrating articulatory gestures for a consonant into those for a vowel (Kent & Rosenbek, 1983). Taken together with the results for consonant production, it is clear that a fundamental characteristic of the speech production disorder of anterior aphasics is phonetic in nature and involves at the very least, a deficit in the timing and integration of articulatory movements. Furthermore, comparison of these patterns of speech with those of posterior patients has revealed that Broca's aphasics can be qualitatively distinguished from Wernicke's aphasics on the basis of their speech production. In particular, voice-onset time analyses have shown that Broca's aphasics display the timing deficits described here, whereas Wernicke's aphasics show minimal impairment (Blumstein et al., 1980).

Many of the phonological errors described in the preceding section probably reflected deficits of articulatory programming rather than planning. However, it is not clear whether the various types of errors and characteristics of segment production found in anterior aphasics can be attributed solely to articulatory deficits. Some of the voicing and nasal errors could well have reflected incorrect phoneme selection (i.e., inappropriate phoneme choice), as well as articulatory implementation problems. Moreover, it is difficult to attribute many of the error types—such as errors of simplification, addition, and sequencing, as well as consonant substitutions for place of articulation—to articulatory programming deficits. Thus, anterior aphasics may evidence both a phonological deficit, implying a disorder in phoneme selection, as well as a phonetic deficit, implying a disorder in articulatory implementation.

In contrast to the clear-cut phonetic disorder of the anterior aphasics, analysis of the patterns of the phonetic dimensions of posterior aphasics reveals that they may be qualitatively distinguished from anterior aphasics on the basis of their speech production. Posterior aphasics do not display the timing deficits that anterior aphasics manifest in the production of voice-onset time in stop consonants (Blumstein et al., 1980; Gandour & Dardarananda, 1984a; Hoit-Dalgaard, Murry, & Kopp, 1983; Shewan et al., 1984; Tuller, 1984) or in the production of nasal consonants (Itoh & Sasanuma, 1983). Nor do they show the impairments in laryngeal control either for the production of voicing or for those articulatory maneuvers requiring the integration of laryngeal movements and movements of the supralaryngeal vocal tract (Baum et al., 1990; Shinn & Blumstein, 1983). Nevertheless, although clearly distinguished from anterior aphasics, posterior patients do seem to display a subtle phonetic impairment. Most typically, they show increased variability in the implementation of a number of phonetic parameters (Kent & McNeill, 1987; Ryalls, 1986), including vowel formant frequencies (Ryalls, 1986) and vowel durations (Ryalls, 1986; Tuller, 1984). In addition, the absolute duration of their production of voiceless fricatives differs from that of normal individuals (Baum et al., 1990). What is not clear is the nature of the deficit contributing to these patterns of speech production. Several hypotheses may be suggested, but at this point all are speculative. One possibility is that subtle phonetic impairments emerge consequent to brain damage, be it to either the left or the right hemisphere. Alternatively, posterior fibers projecting to the motor/articulatory system may be damaged, or the auditory feedback system normally contributing to the control of the articulatory parameters of speech may be impaired. Further research will be necessary to fully characterize this subclinical deficit.

The Production of Speech Prosody

To this point, the analysis of the speech production patterns in aphasia has focused on segmental features. Another important feature of speech production is its rhythm and melody, called SPEECH PROSODY. The most common area of study in this regard is intonation, which is of interest for several reasons. On the one hand, intonation provides important clues concerning speech planning abilities. That is, several features characterize intonation patterns in declarative sentences in normal speech, and these features interact with syntactic complexity and sentence length. These features include:

1. Terminal falling fundamental frequency (or pitch) in utterance final position; that is, the pitch contour of the last word in a declarative sentence shows a sharp drop in frequency or pitch.
2. Fundamental frequency declination over the full sentence; that is, normally there is a higher fundamental frequency at the beginning and a lower fundamental frequency at the end of the sentence. This so-called declination effect usually occurs over the full range of a declarative sentence.
3. Lengthening of the final word in the sentence (Cooper & Sorenson, 1980).

For the speaker to produce the appropriate pitch contours and word duration, it is necessary for him or her to effectively preplan the sentence, taking into consideration its length and syntactic structure.

Besides studying planning behavior, the study of prosody is particularly important in understanding the nature of the speech production abilities of Broca's or anterior aphasics. As described earlier, one clinical feature of anterior aphasia is slow, labored speech in the context of a flattened intonation contour. It is useful then to see if acoustic investigations substantiate this clinical impression. To date, only a few studies have been conducted, and because only a few patients have been actually tested, the results should be considered preliminary. Nevertheless, they are extremely interesting. Analysis of two-word spontaneous speech utterances and reading in Broca's aphasics has shown that these patients have some rudimentary control over some features of prosody (Cooper, Soares, Nicol, Michelow, & Goloskie, 1984; Danly, de Villiers, & Cooper, 1979). The patient tends to maintain a terminal falling fundamental frequency, which occurs even in utterances in which the pauses between words may reach durations of as long as 7 sec. This suggests that Broca's aphasics do have a linguistic sense of an utterance and that even the very severe agrammatic patient is not simply stringing together lexical items, each one forming a holophrastic utterance. Nevertheless, there is a restriction in the F_o range of Broca's aphasics compared to normals (Cooper et al., 1984; Ryalls, 1982). Thus, the clinical impression that these speakers produce utterances with a flattened intonation is substantiated by these data.

Further analysis revealed a number of systematic problems in the production of prosody in these patients. In the first place, patients do not show utterance final lengthening. In fact, they show systematically longer durations in word initial than final position (Danly et al., 1979; Danly & Shapiro, 1982). Interestingly, this finding does not correlate with the durations of utterances or the occurrence of pauses between words. These results are consistent with the findings of Goodglass and his colleagues that anterior aphasics need primary stress at the beginning of a sentence to initiate speech. Dubbed the stress-saliency hypothesis, it suggests that part of the production problem of the anterior aphasic is an increased threshold for initiating and maintaining the flow of speech (Goodglass, 1968; Goodglass, Quadfasel, & Timberlake, 1964). A second form of evidence of a prosodic deficit in Broca's aphasics is that these patients do not show normal declination patterns in longer utterances. Instead, the declination effect, usually occurring over the entire range of the sentence in normals, is found only in short phrases in Broca's aphasics; that is, the domain of the declination pattern seems to be limited to syntactic phrases, such as noun phrases or verb phrases, and not the sentence as a whole. These findings are consistent with those of Goodglass and his colleagues, who showed that the utterances of Broca's aphasics are characterized syntactically by either noun phrases or verb phrases and rarely the concatenation of the two (Goodglass, Gleason, Bernholtz, & Hyde, 1972). Of interest, Broca's aphasics apparently are "cognizant" at some level of their inability to produce complete sentences and end words with continuation rises in F_o, a signal that the utterance is not yet completed (Danly & Shapiro, 1982).

In summary, the patterns of phonetic disintegration clearly show that anterior aphasics have a different speech production pattern than do posterior aphasics. Phonetic disintegration can best be characterized in terms of a deficit in articulatory implementation, especially in the timing of several articulatory maneuvers and laryngeal control. In addition, the prosodic pattern of Broca's aphasics is also abnormal and reflects rudimentary melodic control over only a restricted syntactic domain. While clearly distinguished from the patterns of phonetic disintegration characterized by anterior aphasics, posterior aphasics display a subclinical subtle phonetic impairment.

Speech Perception

The Perception of Phonemic Contrasts

Like production studies, perception studies have focused mainly on the ability of aphasic patients to perceive phonemic or segmental contrasts, for example, *pear* versus *bear*. These studies have been motivated by two primary rationales. The first is to determine if segmental perception is impaired in aphasia. Such results should speak to the nature of the deficits of phonological processing at the receptive level. The second rationale is to ascertain the degree to which speech perception deficits form the basis for language comprehension deficits. Luria (1966) elaborated this view in greatest detail with respect to Wernicke's aphasia. In particular, he argued that the severe comprehension deficit of these patients reflected the loss of "phonemic" hearing, that is, the ability to distinguish minimal phonological contrasts. He reasoned that if patients could not perceive phonological contrasts, then they would be unable to process words appropriately for meaning, resulting in a severe comprehension disorder. Such a view assumes that segmental perception underlies speech processing and, furthermore, that language processing is hierarchically ordered, with speech analysis occurring before meaning is extracted from the signal itself.

Studies on segmental perception have indeed shown that aphasic patients evidence deficits in processing segmental contrasts. Although such deficits are found in Wernicke's aphasics, they are by no means isolated to this particular group. Nearly all aphasics show some problems in discriminating phonological contrasts (Blumstein, Baker, & Goodglass, 1977; Jauhiainen & Nuutila, 1977; Miceli, Gainotti, Payer-Rigo, 1978; Miceli, Caltagirone, Gainotti, & Caltagirone, & Masullo, 1980) or in labeling or identifying consonants presented in a consonant–vowel context (Basso, Casati, & Vignolo, 1977; Blumstein, Cooper, et al., 1977). In terms of the feature relations of the consonants, the results are consistent with theoretical analyses of distinctive features. Namely, subjects are more likely to make discrimination errors when the test stimuli contrast by a single feature than when they contrast by two or more features (Baker, Blumstein, & Goodglass, 1981; Blumstein, Baker, & Goodglass, 1977; Miceli et al., 1978; Sasanuma, Tasumi, & Fujisaki, 1976). Further, discrimination errors on place contrasts—for example, /pa/ versus /ta/—are generally more common than are voicing contrasts—for example, /pa/ versus /ba/ (Baker et al., 1981; Blumstein, Baker, & Goodglass, 1977; Miceli et al., 1978).

The failure of patients to label or discriminate the sounds of speech has been explored for the most part in the context of natural speech. The use of natural speech in perception experiments has the advantage of providing all the cues necessary to signal a particular phonetic dimension. As a result, however, it is impossible to study the contribution of various components of the acoustic signal to the perception of the phonetic dimensions of speech. Studies of the speech perception abilities of normal individuals have in fact attempted to chart out those aspects of the acoustic signal critical to speech perception (Liberman, Cooper, Shankweiler, & Studdert-Kennedy, 1967). Using synthetic speech, acoustic parameters can be independently manipulated and controlled.

A number of studies have explored the abilities of aphasic patients to perceive phonetic categories when presented with synthetic speech continua that vary in systematic steps along a particular acoustic dimension. These studies have focused on two phonetic dimensions, voicing (Basso et al., 1977; Blumstein, Cooper et al., 1977; Gandour & Dardarananda, 1982) and place of articulation (Blumstein, Tartter, Nigro, & Statlender, 1984). The acoustic dimensions varied were voice-onset time distinguishing [d] and [t], and the frequency of the formant transitions and the burst preceding the transitions distinguishing [b], [d], and [g]. Results have shown that patients have particular difficulties labeling these stimuli. To test labeling ability, subjects may be required to either repeat what they hear or point to a printed card containing the appropriate consonant or syllable. Interestingly, these patients may nonetheless be able to discriminate the same stimuli in a manner similar to normal individuals. This dissociation has been interpreted as reflecting the fact that the perception of the acoustic parameters defining the phonetic categories may be spared in aphasia, but the ability to use these dimensions to categorize the sounds of speech in a linguistically relevant way may be impaired: that is, aphasic patients may have a deficit in the perception of phonetic categories as these categories are used in relation to higher order language processing and, in particular, as speech processing relates to lexical processing.

The Relation Between Speech Perception and Auditory Language Comprehension

The dissociation of discrimination from labeling in speech perception begins to address the question of the relation between speech perception abilities and language comprehension. That is, the failure of Wernicke patients to maintain a stable category label might be the basis for their language comprehension deficits. Nevertheless, a number of studies that have compared speech perception abilities with auditory comprehension in aphasia have failed to show any systematic or strong correlations (Basso et al., 1977; Blumstein, Baker, & Goodglass, 1977; Jauhiainen & Nuutila, 1977; Miceli et al., 1980; for general discussion, see Boller, 1978; Lesser, 1978). Patients with good auditory language comprehension skills have shown impairments in speech processing; conversely, patients with severe auditory language comprehension deficits have shown minimal speech perception deficits.

The failure to show a systematic relation between speech perception and language comprehension could be due to several factors. First, speech perception deficits may in fact underlie language comprehension deficits, but these deficits are revealed only in the context of larger streams of speech. Thus, focusing on the perception of segments in isolated words or syllables may not be a sensitive enough index. Second, the extraction of meaning from the auditory signal may require the perception NOT of segmental cues per se, but rather of auditory patterns for individual words (Klatt, 1980). Thus, investigating segmental cues may not tap the primary perceptual deficit. Third, the underlying deficit in auditory comprehension may reflect an inability to relate sound representation to its appropriate meaning. Such a dissociation would be represented clinically by a deficit in word meaning as well as in speech perception. In this view, however, the word meaning deficit is due not to a speech perception impairment but rather to an interaction of phonology and meaning (Baker et al., 1981; Martin et al., 1975).

Some support for this latter view emerged in a recent study investigating the relation between on-line processing of phonological information and lexical access (Milberg, Blumstein, & Dworetzky, 1988). The study of on-line processing provides a means of exploring the processes that contribute to comprehension by using experimental tasks that require the subject to respond while the processing system is still operating on the linguistic input to ultimately derive a semantic interpretation. By definition these tasks are time-dependent, and typical measures involve reaction time of response to a given stimulus input. In Milberg et al.'s study, subjects were asked to make a lexical decision on the second stimulus of stimulus pairs in which either the first stimulus was semantically related to the second or, alternatively, the first phoneme of the first stimulus (prime) was systematically changed by one or more than one phonetic feature (e.g., *cat–dog, gat–dog, wat–dog*). Results showed that both nonfluent and fluent patients' performance differed from that of normal individuals. Interestingly, although both groups showed a similar sensitivity to phonological features, the aphasic groups showed a differential sensitivity to phonological distortion in ACCESSING the lexicon. Fluent patients showed priming in all phonologically distorted conditions relative to the baseline condition, suggesting a reduced threshold for lexical access. As a result, many more potential word candidates would theoretically be accessed. In contrast, nonfluent patients showed priming only in the undistorted semantically related condition (e.g., *cat–dog*) showing an increased threshold for lexical access. As a result, fewer potential lexical entries would theoretically be accessed. These results suggest that impairments in the use of phonological information to access the lexicon can manifest themselves in different ways in aphasic patients in the absence of a deficit in processing the phonological properties of speech themselves.

Perhaps the only study that has shown a systematic relation between auditory perception ability and language comprehension in aphasia has been that of Tallal and Newcombe (1978). They focused on the auditory perception of rapidly changing acoustic information in both nonverbal and verbal stimuli. For nonverbal stimuli, they explored the ability of right-brain–damaged and left-brain–damaged aphasic patients to determine temporal order of two complex tones separated by various interstimulus intervals. For the speech stimuli, they focused on the perception of place of articulation, a phonetic dimension that seems particularly vulnerable in aphasia. One of the acoustic cues for place of articulation in stop consonants is the rapid motion of formant transitions. Tallal and Newcombe's rationale was that aphasic patients may have a primary deficit in processing rapid acoustic events, and, as a result, the deficit is primarily auditory in nature. In this view, speech deficits are a secondary consequence of this disorder, and language comprehension deficits, as well, may be due to an inability to process auditory stimuli normally. Their results showed a dissociation between performance of left- and right-brain–damaged patients, with aphasics being selectively impaired in the nonverbal and language stimuli. Moreover, they found a correlation between performance on the nonverbal task and the Token Test, a test sensitive to auditory language comprehension deficits (De Renzi & Vignolo, 1962). It is interesting to note that the Token Test requires, in the more complex parts of the test, the ability to sequence (i.e., order) a number of stimuli. The relation between this task and the sequencing deficit of auditory stimuli may be due to the nature of the two tasks (i.e., sequencing) rather than to an auditory impairment affecting language comprehension. In any case, on the basis of the obtained correlation, Tallal and Newcombe concluded that at least part of the comprehension deficit of aphasic patients reflects a disorder in auditory processing of rapid acoustic events. As to the place of articulation dimension, they demonstrated that lengthening the duration of formant transitions from 40 to 80 msec resulted in improved performance for only 3 out of 6 aphasic subjects. In fact, several studies have failed to show systematic improvement in either labeling or discrimination of place of articulation with extended formant transition durations (Blumstein, et al., 1984; Riedel & Studdert-Kennedy, 1985). Thus, although Tallal and Newcombe found a significant relation between processing of nonverbal auditory stimuli and language comprehension, it is not clear that the relation holds as strongly for speech stimuli.

Nevertheless, the hypothesis that auditory processing of rapid acoustic events underlies the language processing deficits of aphasics is an interesting one. A number of studies have shown that brain-damaged patients demonstrate increased thresholds for determining temporal order between two events in both the auditory and the visual modalities (Efron, 1963; Swisher & Hirsh, 1972). Such findings are strongly correlated with aphasia (Bond, 1976; Efron, 1963; Swisher & Hirsh, 1972); however, they are restricted to aphasic patients with left hemisphere lesions (Carmon & Nachson, 1971). In fact, it has been shown that both left and right anterior lobectomy patients with no aphasia show increased thresholds for temporal order judgments in the auditory modality (Sherwin & Efron, 1980). Thus, auditory deficits reflected in an inability to process rapidly presented acoustic events cannot be the primary basis for the language comprehension deficits of aphasic patients. If this were the case, all patients who evidence impairments in temporal order judgments should show an auditory language comprehension deficit. The presence of such deficits in nonaphasic patients militates against such an interpretation.

Nevertheless, the notion of time as a crucial variable in auditory language processing does have some support both in the clinical setting and in some subsequent experimental investigations. In particular, it has been reported that speaking slowly to an aphasic may enhance his or her language comprehension (Schuell, Jenkins, & Jiménez-Pabón, 1964). Several studies have shown that rate of stimulus presentation does enhance word retention (Cermak & Moreines, 1976) and overall language comprehension in aphasia (Albert & Bear, 1974; Bergman, Fiselson, Tze'elon, Mendelson, & Schechter, 1977; Lasky, Weidner, & Johnson, 1976; Weidner & Lasky, 1976). These findings seem to obtain for those patients who are not too severely impaired (Weidner & Lasky, 1976) and seems to interact with the syntactic complexity of the stimuli (Blumstein, Katz, Goodglass, Shrier, & Dworetzky, 1985; Weidner & Lasky, 1976). Furthermore, time alone does not seem to be the crucial variable; that is, comprehension performance is not necessarily enhanced with increased duration of the words themselves or of the pauses between words, but rather seems to hinge on increasing silent intervals at major syntactic breaks (Blumstein et al., 1985).

The Perception of Prosody

Prosodic cues serve a very important function in language processing. At the perceptual level, they provide an organizing framework for the different sentence types of language. For example, a rising intonation indicates a question, and a falling intonation, a statement. Both of these characteristics seem to be nearly universal properties of language (Lieberman, 1967). Stress is another suprasegmental component that is linguistically crucial, since it can serve to differentiate meaning in different lexical items. In English, for example, stress contrasts between *hótdog* and *hotdóg* or *cónvict* and *convíct* distinguish different syntactic classes or categories, that is, nouns and noun phrases or nouns and verbs.

In contrast to the segmental features of language, the perception of prosodic cues (i.e., intonation and stress) seems to be remarkably well preserved in aphasia. Severely impaired aphasics have been shown to retain some ability to recognize and distinguish the syntactic forms of commands, yes–no questions, and information questions when marked by intonation cues (Green & Boller, 1974). This performance is superior to the determination of syntactic forms when marked by syntactic and lexical cues. Nevertheless, the perception of these intonation cues is far from normal, and patients still make many perceptual errors. For example, aphasic patients are unable to use prosody at the sentential level to distinguish declarative from interrogative sentences (Heilman, Bowers, Speedie, & Coslett, 1984).

The perception of word accent in Japanese seems to be less impaired than the perception of segmental cues (Sasanuma et al., 1976), and the perception of stress as a semantic cue distinguishing different lexical items in English is also relatively spared (Blumstein & Goodglass, 1972). Nonetheless, as with the intonation cues, the patient's performance is not completely normal. A number of studies have revealed impairments in the comprehension of lexical/phrasal stress contrasts (e.g., *hótdog* vs *hotdóg*) (Baum, Kelsch, Daniloff, & Daniloff, 1982; Emmorey, 1987), as well as of sentential contrasts (e.g., *he fed her dóg biscuits* vs. *he fed her dog bíscuits*) (Baum et al., 1982). Similar findings emerged for the perception of tone contrasts serving as lexical cues in Thai (Gandour & Daradarananda, 1983) and Chinese (Naeser & Chan, 1980). Interestingly, no differences have emerged in any studies between the performance of anterior and posterior patients, a finding consistent with the results for the perception of phonemic contrasts.

It is interesting that the aphasic patient's performance seems to be relatively better preserved in the processing of prosodic cues than of segmental cues. The reason for this dichotomy could reflect a hierarchical organization of phonological cues, with melody cues being simpler or perceptually more basic. Alternatively, it could reflect the participation of the nondominant hemisphere in the processing of these cues.

In summary, the perception of segmental cues in aphasia is clearly impaired. However, the patterns of disintegration are systematic and reflect the relation of the distinctive feature attributes of the phonemic contrasts. Nevertheless, all aphasic types evidence speech perception deficits, and such deficits do not seem to be the primary basis for the auditory language comprehension deficits found in these patients. Patients may show a dissociation between the ability to discriminate and label phonetic dimensions, suggesting that part of the so-called speech perception deficit reflects an inability to use the sounds of speech in a linguistically relevant way. In addition, aphasic patients show deficits in the processing of temporal order and rapidly changing acoustic events. It is not clear that this reflects an auditory rather than a linguistic basis to language processing problems. However, it does suggest that providing more time for the patient to process syntactically demarcated utterances does enhance their language comprehension. Finally, prosodic cues seem to show less impairment than segmental cues, perhaps reflecting the participation of the nondominant hemisphere in the processing of the suprasegmental dimensions of language.

Conclusion

This chapter attempted to delineate the phonological patterns of aphasic speech and to provide some clues as to the nature of the mechanisms underlying such deficits. All clinical types of aphasia evidence some impairments in both speech production and sleep perception. Nevertheless, careful analyses of the patterns of speech production indicated that the production process can be analyzed into at least two distinct stages, phonological planning and articulatory implementation. All patients show similar patterns of deficit at the first stage; however, the anterior patient is also impaired at the stage of articulatory implementation and, as a result, has both a phonetic and phonological impairment. Prosodic as well as segmental cue are affected in the production of anterior aphasics. The constellation of impairments for anterior aphasics suggests that their phonetic disorder reflects an inability to manipulate particular types of articulatory gestures or articulatory parameters rather than an inability to implement particular phonetic features. They display an impairment in the integration of movement and timing of two independent articulators and an impairment in laryngeal control. Posterior aphasics also show evidence of a subtle phonetic impairment. Qualitatively distinct from the phonetic output disorder of anterior aphasics, the underlying basis for this subclinical deficit is not yet understood.

Analogous to speech production, at least two stages of perception are implicated in ongoing processing. The first involves the extraction of the acoustic properties of speech, and the second, the encoding of the attributes into linguistically significant dimensions. Dissociations between these two levels of perception are found in aphasia in the context of spared discrimination and impaired labeling. Nevertheless, the phonological patterns of perception involving the feature relations among segments is similar across aphasic patients.

Despite the presence of phonological disorders in nearly all aphasics, these impairments do not seem to correlate with the severity of language comprehension deficits. Consequently, speech perception deficits do not seem to form the basis for language comprehension deficits. Similarly, auditory deficits do not seem to underlie comprehension impairments.

What then is the relation between speech perception and language comprehension? It may be that perceptual deficits underlie some language comprehension abilities; however, researchers to date have failed to focus on the appropriate dimensions. For example, ongoing speech processing requires the integration of acoustic events over a fairly long time interval, and current research has generally focused on short intervals, such as, for example, the perception of speech segments. Some support for this view is that increasing the temporal parameters of the speech signal at crucial parts of the signal enhances language comprehension in some patients. Alternatively, impairments in the use of phonological information to access the lexicon could contribute to lexical impairments and ultimately to deficits in auditory language comprehension.

Acknowledgments

Many thanks to M. T. Sarno for her comments on an earlier draft of this paper. This work was supported in part by NIH grants DC00314 to Brown University and DC00081 to the Boston University School of Medicine.

References

Alajouanine, T., Ombredane, A., & Durand, M. (1939). *Le syndrome de la désintégration phonétique dans l'aphasie.* Paris: Masson.

Albert, M., & Bear, D. (1974). Time to understand. *Brain, 97,* 373–384.

Alten, J. L., Darley, F. L., Deal, J. L., & Johns, D. F. (1975). Comments on A. D. Martin's "Some objections to the term apraxia of speech." *Journal of Speech and Hearing Disorders, 40,* 416–420.

Baker, E., Blumstein, S. E., & Goodglass, H. (1981). Interaction between phonological and semantic factors in auditory comprehension. *Neuropsychologia, 19,* 1–16.

Basso, A., Casati, G., & Vignolo, L. A. (1977). Phonemic identification defects in aphasia. *Cortex, 13,* 84–95.

Baum, S. R., Blumstein, S. E., Naeser, M. A., & Palumbo, C. L. (1990). Temporal dimensions of consonant and vowel production: An acoustic and CT scan analysis of aphasic speech. *Brain and Language, 39,* 33–56.

Baum, S. R., Kelsch Daniloff, J., & Daniloff, R. (1982). Sentence comprehension by Broca's aphasics: Effects of some suprasegmental variables. *Brain and Language, 17,* 261–271.

Bergman, M., Fiselson, J., Tze'elon, R., Medelson, L., & Schechter, I. (1977). The effects of message speed on auditory comprehension in patients with cerebral cranial injury. *Scandinavian Journal of Rehabilitation Medicine, 9,* 169–171.

Blumstein, S. E. (1973). *A phonological investigation of aphasic speech.* The Hague: Mouton.

Blumstein, S. E., Baker, E., & Goodglass, H. (1977). Phonological factors in auditory comprehension in aphasia. *Neuropsychologia, 15,* 19–30.

Blumstein, S. E., Cooper, W. E., Goodglass, H., Statlender, S., & Gottlieb, J. (1980). Production deficits in aphasia: A voice-onset time analysis. *Brain and Language, 9,* 153–170.

Blumstein, S. E., Cooper, W. E., Zurif, E., & Caramazza, A. (1977). The perception and production of voice-onset time in aphasia. *Neuropsychologia, 15,* 371–383.

Blumstein, S., & Goodglass, H. (1972). The perception of stress as a semantic cue in aphasia. *Journal of Speech and Hearing Research, 15,* 800–806.

Blumstein, S E., Katz, B., Goodglass, H., Shrier, R., & Dworetzky, B. (1985). The effects of slowed speech on auditory comprehension in aphasia. *Brain and Language, 24,* 246–265.

Blumstein, S. E., Tartter, V. C., Nigro, G., & Statlender, S. (1984). Acoustic cues for the perception of place of articulation in aphasia. *Brain and Language, 22,* 128–149.

Boller, F. (1978). Comprehension disorders in aphasia: A historical review. *Brain and Language, 5,* 149–165.

Bond, Z. S. (1976). On the specification of input units in speech perception. *Brain and Language, 3,* 72–87.

Bouman, L., & Grünbaum, A. (1925). Experimentell-psychologische Untersuchungen sur Aphasie und Paraphasie. *Zeitschrift fur die Gesamte Neurologie und Psychiatrie, 96,* 481–538.

Buckingham, H. W., Jr. (1979). Explanation in apraxia with consequences for the concept of apraxia of speech. *Brain and Language, 8,* 202–226.

Burns, M. S., & Canter, G. C. (1977). Phonemic behavior of aphasic patients with posterior cerebral lesions. *Brain and Language, 4,* 492–507.

Canter, G. J., Trost, J. E., & Burns, M. S. (1985). Contrasting speech patterns in apraxia of speech and phonemic paraphasia. *Brain and Language, 24,* 204–222.

Carmon, A., & Nachson, I. (1971). Effect of unilateral brain damage on perception of temporal order. *Cortex, 7,* 410–418.

Cermak, L., & Moreines, J. (1976). Verbal retention deficits in aphasic and amnesic patients. *Brain and Language, 3,* 16–27.

Chomsky, N., & Halle, M. (1968). *The sound pattern of English.* New York: Harper.

Cohen, D., Dubois, J., Gauthier, M., Hécaen, H., & Angelergues, R. (1963). Aspects du fonctionnement du code linguistique chez les aphasiques moteurs. *Neuropsychologia, 1,* 165–177.

Cooper, W. E., Soares, C., Nicol, J., Michelow, D., & Goloskie, S. (1984). Clausal intonation after unilateral brain damage. *Language and Speech, 27,* 17–24.

Cooper, W. E., & Sorenson, J. (1980). *Fundamental frequency in sentence production.* New York: Springer-Verlag.

Critchley, M. (1952). Articulatory defects in aphasia. *Journal of Laryngology and Otology, 66,* 1–17.

Danly, M., de Villiers, J. G., & Cooper, W. E. (1979). The control of speech prosody in Broca's aphasia. In J. J. Wolf & D. H. Klatt (Eds.), *Speech communication papers presented at the 97th meeting of the Acoustical Society of America.* New York: Acoustical Society of America.

Danly, M., & Shapiro, B. (1982). Speech prosody in Broca's aphasia. *Brain and Language, 16,* 171–190.

Degiovanni, E., Khomsi, A., Bosser, E., Souffront, L., Moller, J. N., & Posson, J. (1977). Approche des troubles de l'integration phonémique chez les aphasiques interet d'analyses sonagraphiques *Revnue d'Oto-Neuro-Ophthamologie, 49,* 141–153.

De Renzi, E., & Vignolo, L. A. (1962). The Token Test: A sensitive test to detect receptive disturbances in aphasia. *Brain, 85,* 665–678.

Dubois, J., Hécaen, H., Angelergues, R., Chatelier, M., & Marcie, P. (1964). Etude neurolinguistique de l'aphasie de conduction. *Neuropsychologia, 2,* 9–44.

Duffy, J., & Gawle, C. (1984). Apraxic speakers' vowel duration in consonant-vowel-consonant syllables. In J. Rosenbek, M. McNeil, & A. Aronson (Eds.), *Apraxia of speech.* San Diego, CA: College-Hill Press.

Dunlop, J. M., & Marquardt, T. P. (1977). Linguistic and articulatory aspects of single word production in apraxia of speech. *Cortex, 8,* 17–29.

Efron, R. (1963). Temporal perception, aphasia, and déjà-vu. *Brain, 86,* 403–423.

Emmorey, K. D. (1987). The neurological substrates for prosodic aspects of speech. *Brain and Language, 30,* 305–320.

Freeman, F. J., Sands, E. S., & Harris, K. S. (1978). Temporal coordination of phonation and articulation in a case of verbal apraxia: A voice-onset time study. *Brain and Language, 6,* 106–111.

Froschels, E. (1915). Zur Behandlung des motorischen Aphasie. *Archives Psychiatrist, 56,* 1–19.

Gandour, J., & Dardarananda, R. (1982). Voice onset time in aphasia: Thai, I.: Perception. *Brain and Language, 17,* 24–33.

Gandour, J., & Dardarananda, R. (1983). Identification of tonal contrasts in Thai aphasic patients. *Brain and Language, 18,* 389–410.

Gandour, J., & Dardarananda, R. (1984a). Voice onset time in aphasia: Thai, II.: Production. *Brain and Language, 23,* 177–205.

Gandour, J., & Dardarananda, R. (1984b). Prosodic disturbances in aphasia: Vowel length in Thai. *Brain and Language, 23,* 206–224.

Goldstein, K. (1948). *Language and language disturbances.* New York: Grune & Stratton.

Goodglass, H. (1968). Studies in the grammar of aphasics. In S. Rosenberg & J. Koplin (Eds.), *Developments in applied psycholinguistics.* New York: Macmillan.

Goodglass, H., Gleason, J. B., Bernholtz, N. A., & Hyde, M. R. (1972). Some linguistic structures in the speech of a Broca's aphasic. *Cortex, 8,* 191–212.

Goodglass, H., Quadfasel, F. A., & Timberlake, W. H. (1964). Phrase length and the type of severity of aphasia. *Cortex, 1,* 133–152.

Green, E. (1969). Phonological and grammatical aspects of jargon in an aphasic patient: A case study. *Language and Speech, 12,* 103–118.

Green, E., & Boller, F. (1974). Features of auditory comprehension in severely impaired aphasics. *Cortex, 10,* 133–145.

Halpern, H., Keith, R. L., & Darley, F. L. (1976). Phonemic behavior of aphasic subjects without dysarthria or apraxia of speech. *Cortex, 12,* 365–372.

Harmes, S., Daniloff, R., Hoffman, P., Lewis, J., Kramer, M., & Absher, R. (1984). Temporal and articulatory control of fricative articulation by speakers with Broca's aphasia. *Journal of Phonetics, 12,* 367–385.

Hatfield, F. M., & Walton, K. (1975). Phonological patterns in a case of aphasia. *Language and Speech, 18,* 341–357.

Head, H. (1926). *Aphasia and kindred disorders of speech,* 2 vols. New York: Hafner.

Heilman, K., Bowers, D., Speedie, L., & Coslett, H. B. (1984). Comprehension of affective and nonaffective prosody. *Neurology, 34,* 917–921.

Hoit-Dalgaard, J., Murry, T., & Kopp, H. (1983). Voice onset time production and perception in apraxic subjects. *Brain and Language, 20,* 329–339.

Itoh, M., & Sasanuma, S. (1983). Velar movements during speech in two Wernicke aphasic patients. *Brain and Language, 19,* 283–292.

Itoh, M., Sasanuma, S., Hirose, H., Yoshioka, H., & Ushijima, T. (1980). Abnormal articulatory dynamics in a patient with apraxia of speech. *Brain and Language, 11,* 66–75.

Itoh, M., Sasanuma, S., Tatsumi, I., & Kobayashi, Y. (1979). Voice onset time characteristics of apraxia of speech. *Annual Bulletin of Logopedics and Phoniatrics, 13,* 123–132.

Itoh, M., Sasanuma, S., Tatsumi, I., Murakami, S., Fukusako, Y., & Suzuki, T. (1982). Voice onset time characteristics in apraxia of speech. *Brain and Language, 17,* 193–210.

Itoh, M., Sasanuma, S., & Ushijima, T. (1979). Velar movements during speech in a patient with apraxia of speech. *Brain and Language, 7,* 227–239.

Jakobson, R. (1968). [*Child language, aphasia, and phonological universals*] (A. R. Keiler, Trans.). The Hague: Mouton.

Jakobson, R., Fant, G., & Halle, M. (1962). *Preliminaries to speech analysis.* Cambridge, MA: MIT Press.

Jauhiainen, T., & Nuutila, A. (1977). Auditory perception of speech and speech sounds in recent and recovered cases of aphasia. *Brain and Language, 4,* 572–579.

Johns, D. F., & LaPointe, L. L. (1976). Neurogenic disorders of output processing: Apraxia of speech. In H. Whitaker & H. A. Whitaker (Eds.), *Studies in neurolinguistics* (Vol. 1). New York: Academic Press.

Kagan, A. A. (1977). Articulatory difficulties of an aphasic with apraxia of speech. *South African Journal of Communication Disorders, 24,* 23–40.

Katz, W. F. (1987). Anticipatory labial and lingual coarticulation in aphasia. In J. Ryalls (Ed.), *Phonetic approaches to speech production in aphasia and related disorders.* Boston, MA: College-Hill Press.

Katz, W. F. (1988). Anticipatory coarticulation in aphasia: Acoustic and perceptual data. *Brain and Language, 35,* 340–368.

Keller, E. (1975). *Vowel errors in aphasia.* Unpublished doctoral dissertation, University of Toronto.

Keller, E. (1978). Parameters of vowel substitutions in Broca's aphasia. *Brain and Language, 5,* 265–285.

Kent, R., & McNeil, M. (1987). Relative timing of sentence repetition in apraxia of speech and conduction aphasia. In J. Ryalls (Ed.), *Phonetic approaches to speech production in aphasia and related disorders.* Boston, MA: College-Hill Press.

Kent, R., & Rosenbek, J. (1983). Acoustic patterns of apraxia of speech. *Journal of Speech and Hearing Research, 26,* 231–248.

Klatt, D. (1980). Speech perception: A model of acoustic-phonetic analysis and lexical access. In R. A. Cole (Ed.), *Perception and production of fluent speech.* Hillsdale, NJ: Erlbaum.

Klich, R. J., Ireland, J. V., & Weidner, W. B. (1979). Articulatory and phonological aspects of consonant substitution in apraxia of speech. *Cortex, 15,* 451–470.

Kohn, S. (1985). *Phonological breakdown in aphasia.* Unpublished doctoral dissertation, Tufts University, Medford, MA.

Lasky, E. Z., Weidner, W. E., & Johnson, J. P. (1976). Influence of linguistic complexity, rate of presentation, and interphrase pause time on auditory-verbal comprehension of adult aphasic patients. *Brain and Language, 3,* 386–395.

Lecours, A. R., & Lhermitte, F. (1969). Phonemic paraphasias: Linguistic structures and tentative hypotheses. *Cortex, 5,* 193–228.

Lehiste, I. (1968). *Some acoustic characteristics of dysarthria.* Switzerland: Biblioteca Phonetica.

Lesser, R. (1978). *Linguistic investigations of aphasia.* London: Arnold.

Liberman, A. M., Cooper, F. S., Shankweiler, D. P., & Studdert-Kennedy, M. (1967). Perception of the speech code. *Psychological Review, 74,* 431–461.

Lieberman, P. (1967). *Intonation, perception, and language.* Cambridge, MA: MIT Press.

Luria, A. R. (1966). *Higher cortical functions in man.* New York: Basic Books.

Martin, A. D. (1974). Some objections to the term apraxia of speech. *Journal of Speech and Hearing Disorders, 39,* 53–64.

Martin, A. D. (1975). Reply to Aten, Darley, Deal, and Johns. *Journal of Speech and Hearing Disorders, 40,* 420–422.

Martin, A. D., & Rigrodsky, S. (1974). An investigation of phonological impairment in aphasia: 2, Distinctive feature analysis of phonemic commutation errors in aphasia. *Cortex, 10,* 329–346.

Martin, A. D., Wasserman, N. H., Gilden, L., & West, J. (1975). A process model of repetition in aphasia: An investigation of phonological and morphological interactions in aphasic error performance. *Brain and Language, 2,* 434–450.

Miceli, G., Caltagirone, C., Gainotti, G., & Payer-Rigo, P. (1978). Discrimination of voice versus place contrasts in aphasia. *Brain and Language, 6,* 47–51.

Miceli, G., Gainotti, G., Caltagirone, C., & Masullo, C. (1980). Some aspects of phonological impairment in aphasia. *Brain and Language, 11,* 159–169.

Milberg, W., Blumstein, S. E., & Dworetzky, B. (1988). Phonological processing and lexical access in aphasia. *Brain and Language, 34,* 279–293.

Naeser, M. A., & Chan, S. W.-C. (1980). Case study of a Chinese aphasic with the Boston Diagnostic Aphasia Examination. *Neuropsychologia, 18,* 389–410.

Nespoulous, J. L., Joanette, Y., Beland, S., Caplan, D., & Lecours, A. R. (1987). Production deficits in Broca's and conduction aphasia: Repetition vs. reading. In E. Keller & M. Gopnik (Eds.), *Motor and sensory processes of language.* Hillsdale, NJ: Erlbaum.

Niemi, J., Koivuselka-Sallinen, P., & Hanninen, R. (1985). Phoneme errors in Broca's aphasia: Three Finnish cases. *Brain and Language, 26,* 28–48.

Peuser, G., & Fittschen, M. (1977). On the universality of language dissolution: The case of a Turkish aphasic. *Brain and Language, 4,* 196–207.

Riedel, K., & Studdert-Kennedy, M. (1985). Extending formant transitions may not improve aphasics' perception of stop consonant place of articulation. *Brain and Language, 24,* 196–207.

Ryalls, J. (1981). Motor aphasia; Acoustic correlates of phonetic disintegration in vowels. *Neuropsychologia, 20,* 355–360.

Ryalls, J. (1982). Intonation in Broca's aphasia. *Neuropsychologia, 20,* 355–360.

Ryalls, J. (1986). An acoustic study of vowel production in aphasia. *Brain and Language, 29,* 48–67.

Ryalls, J. (1987). Vowel production in aphasia: Towards an account of the consonant-vowel dissociation. In J. Ryalls (Ed.), *Phonetic approaches to speech production in aphasia and related disorders.* Boston, MA: College-Hill Press.

Sasanuma, S., Tatsumi, I. F., & Fujisaki, H. (1976). Discrimination of phonemes and word accent types in Japanese aphasic patients. *International Congress of Logopedics and Phoniatrics. 16th,* pp. 403–408.

Schuell, H. R., Jenkins, J. J., & Jiménez-Pabón, J. E. (1964). *Aphasia in adults.* New York: Harper.

Shankweiler, D. P., & Harris, K. S. (1966). An experimental approach to the problem of articulation in aphasia. *Cortex, 2,* 277–292.

Shankweiler, D. P., Harris, K. S., & Taylor, M. L. (1968). Electromyographic study of articulation in aphasia. *Archives of Physical Medicine and Rehabilitation, 49,* 1–8.

Sherwin, I., & Efron, R. (1980). Temporal ordering deficits following anterior temporal lobectomy. *Brain and Language, 11,* 195–203.

Shewan, C. M. (1980). Phonological processing in Broca's aphasics. *Brain and Language, 10,* 71–88.

Shewan, C. M., Leeper, H., & Booth, J. (1984). An analysis of voice onset time (VOT) in aphasic and normal subjects. In J. Rosenbek, M. McNeil, & A. Aronson (Eds.), *Apraxia of speech.* San Diego, CA: College-Hill Press.

Shinn, P., & Blumstein, S. E. (1983). Phonetic disintegration in aphasia: Acoustic analysis of spectral characteristics for place of articulation. *Brain and Language, 20,* 90–114.

Swisher, L., & Hirsh, I. J. (1972). Brain damage and the ordering of two temporally successive stimuli. *Neuropsychologia, 10,* 137–152.

Tallal, P., & Newcombe, F. (1978). Impairment of auditory perception and language comprehension in dysphasia. *Brain and Language, 5,* 13–24.

Taylor, J. (Ed.), (1958). *Selected writings of John Hughlings Jackson* (Vol. 2). New York: Basic Books.

Tikofsky, R. (1965). *Phonetic characteristics of dysarthria.* MI: Office of Research Administration.

Trost, J. E., & Canter, G. J. (1974). Apraxia of speech in patients with Broca's aphasia: A study of phoneme production accuracy and error patterns. *Brain and Language, 1,* 63–79.

Tuller, B. (1984). On categorizing aphasic speech errors. *Neuropsychologia, 22,* 547–557.

Tuller, B., & Story, R. S. (1986). Co-articulation in aphasic speech. *Journal of the Acoustical Society of America, 80,* Suppl. 1, MM17.

Weidner, W., & Lasky, E. (1976). The interaction of rate and complexity of stimulus on the performance of adult aphasic subjects. *Brain and Language, 3,* 34–40.

Ziegler, W., & von Cramon, D. (1985). Anticipatory coarticulation in a patient with apraxia of speech. *Brain and Language, 26,* 117–130.

Ziegler, W., & von Cramon, D. (1986). Disturbed coarticulation in apraxia of speech: Acoustic evidence. *Brain and Language, 29,* 34–47.

6

Lexical Deficits

BRENDA C. RAPP and ALFONSO CARAMAZZA

A Lexical Deficit?

What could it mean to say that a patient has a LEXICAL DEFICIT? A number of different things could be meant by such a term. In this chapter we begin by reviewing several possible interpretations and selecting the only one that, we will argue, can provide an adequate basis for understanding a patient's disorder. We hope to make apparent from this discussion that a pattern of impaired performance can be understood only in the context of a theory that describes the cognitive processes that are required to perform the skills that we are interested in understanding, such skills as naming, reading, writing, and sentence processing. The importance of a theory of this mental machinery or "cognitive structure" will become apparent as we consider actual patterns of patient data and attempt, in each case, to draw conclusions about the nature of the underlying deficit.

One possibility is that lexical deficit refers, in a general manner, to a DEFICIT IN LEXICAL PROCESSING, that is, to any difficulty in processing—reading, spelling, comprehending, and producing—single words. A potential problem with this interpretation is that it would include, in the population of patients with lexical deficits, patients who have difficulty processing words for reasons that may have nothing to do with words themselves. For example, we may have a patient who demonstrates difficulty in matching an orally presented word with a picture, which suggests a deficit in comprehension of the meaning of words. However, this particular patient may not be able to discriminate sounds normally and, as a consequence, would demonstrate impaired performance on the word–picture matching task. Most would agree that, although such a

ACQUIRED APHASIA, SECOND EDITION

deficit might reveal itself as a word comprehension deficit, it would be misleading to conclude that such a patient has a lexical deficit. Therefore, the observation that a patient has difficulty processing words would clearly be insufficient grounds for concluding that a patient has a lexical deficit.

A second possibility is that the production of LEXICAL ERRORS (e.g., producing one word for another, as in reading "table" for *chair* or "chain" for *chair*) should be considered the hallmark of a lexical deficit. As in the case in the previous paragraph, this criterion does not guarantee that lexical errors are produced as a result of a deficit at a level of processing that is specific to words. An example is provided by certain patients with unilateral neglect who have difficulty processing the portion of space contralateral to the site of their lesion (i.e., a left hemisphere lesion might result in difficulty processing the right side of a stimulus). Some of these patients have been reported (Behrmann, Moscovitch, Black, & Mozer, 1990a; Caramazza & Hillis, 1990a; Costello & Warrington, 1987; Ellis, Flude, & Young, 1987; Hillis & Caramazza, in press; Kinsbourne & Warrington, 1962) to make errors such as reading "peach" or "pea" for *pear*, where the right side of the word is deleted or substituted. These errors would clearly be defined as lexical errors, yet one would not want to characterize this problem as a deficit in word processing. These patients make comparable errors with pictures and other spatially arrayed stimuli.

Another difficulty in considering the production of lexical errors as the indicator of a lexical deficit is that a patient could, in fact, have damage to mechanisms specific to word processing and yet NOT produce lexical errors. Thus, for example, a patient, when asked to name pictures, may respond to a picture of a chair by saying /dʃaur/. Although the error would not be classified as a lexical error, it may result from damage to representations of the phonological forms of words, representations that serve to guide subsequent articulatory processes.

Finally, even if we were to ascertain that a patient was having difficulty with words and only words, we could still remain in the dark with respect to the NATURE of the difficulty. For example, we can easily imagine that a patient might produce "peach" for *pear* as the result of confusion regarding the exact meaning of words. However, this error indicates a very different deficit from the one in which the same error is produced—"peach" for *pear*—but the patient clearly understood the meaning of the word and responded with a word with a similar meaning because he or she was unable to actually produce the target word. For the first patient, the evidence suggests an impairment in the system that represents word meaning; for the second, a word production system appears to be implicated. Thus, ideally we would want to know not only that a patient has a deficit restricted to the processing of words, but also which particular aspects of word processing have been affected.

The discussion thus far reveals that it is not possible to understand a deficit if we attempt to interpret DIRECTLY the surface manifestations of the deficit: task performance and error patterns. Deficits to nonlexical mechanisms might affect the processing of words and even result in lexical errors. Furthermore, similar error patterns may result from very different impairments within a system dedicated to the processing of words. It becomes apparent that in order to correctly determine the source, or location within a system, of a deficit, we must know (a) which mechanisms possibly UNDERLIE performance on a particular task, and (b) the functioning and purpose of each mechanism, so that we can determine how damage to any one of them would be reflected in task performance and error patterns. Only then are we in the position to explore possible alternative explanations of the performance pattern of a particular patient, test hypotheses concerning the nature of the deficit, and decide whether the weight of the evidence favors one possible locus of impairment over another.

Consider, for example, the case mentioned above of a patient who makes errors in a word–picture matching task. Only because we have reason to believe that a mechanism that adequately discriminates speech sounds is required in the performance of such a task, we devise tests to determine whether such a mechanism is intact. How we proceed, therefore, is determined by what we believe to be the relevant underlying mechanisms. Our conclusions regarding the nature of the impairment in the patient will depend on the results we obtain from testing the integrity of this, and any other, component that we have assumed is required for performing the task.

Thus, it would appear that we can most usefully think of a lexical deficit as A DEFICIT TO A LEXICAL COMPONENT, that is, as an impairment to one or more of the mechanisms thought to be involved specifically in the processing of words. In order to do so, however, we must have a theory of what the possible lexical components might be, how they might function, and what characteristics of performance we might expect to observe when they are damaged. In other words, we need a theory of the lexical processing system. Such a theory will be useful to the extent to which it can provide us with (a) a description of what is often referred to as the functional architecture of the lexical system, a description of the basic components of the system and how they are interrelated, and (b) a description of the internal structure of the individual components (Caramazza, 1988). We develop these points below to lay the groundwork for a discussion of specific patterns of patient performance which will serve to illustrate the role of a theoretical framework in the interpretation of performance.

A Functional Architecture of the Lexical System

One widely accepted theory of the functional architecture of the lexical system is that it consists of the set of autonomous yet interconnected components depicted schematically in Figure 6.1 (Caramazza, 1988; Morton, 1981; Shallice, 1981). According to this theory, a major distinc-

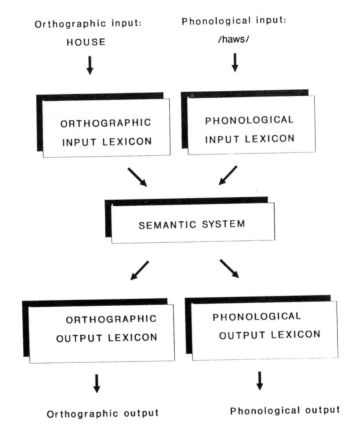

FIGURE 6.1. *A schematic representation of the lexical processing system.*

tion is drawn between input and output components. Input components are those involved in the comprehension of words, whereas output components involve the production of words. A second major distinction is drawn between the modality of input or output—phonological or orthographic—such that each modality is represented separately for input and output. Thus the orthographic input lexicon (OIL), which includes those mechanisms involved in the recognition of written words in reading, is distinguished from the phonological input lexicon (PIL), involved in the recognition of spoken words. Prior to gaining access to these input lexicons, perceptual mechanisms process the stimulus, visual or phonological as the case may be, in order to represent information regarding the letters or phonemes in the stimulus. The modality-specific input lexicons are further distinguished from their corresponding output lexicons, which represent the orthographic and phonological information involved in the production of written and spoken words. These modality-specific lexical components are interconnected through a lexical semantic system that stores the semantic representations for words.

Each lexicon is thought to contain the information necessary to represent a word in a given modality for the purposes of either production or comprehension. Thus, the OIL contains information regarding the familiar letter sequences, that is, GRAPHEMES, corresponding to words. In reading the OIL allows one to recognize that the letter sequences *cloud* and *fish* are familiar words, whereas *clowd* and *fislh* are not. The OIL is said to contain lexical orthographic representations that are activated during reading, whereas the PIL contains the information regarding the phoneme sequences that constitute the words of the language that are activated while listening to speech. The output lexicons contain comparable representations that provide the basis for written and spoken production.

The lexical semantic system is the repository of the meanings of words (Jackendoff, 1983; Miller & Johnson-Laird, 1976). In fact, the phonological and orthographic lexicons can be thought of as providing specific forms to the meaning of a word. Expressing a concept (e.g., four-legged domestic animal that barks) involves activation of semantic knowledge. This semantic representation is then given a phonological shape (/dag/) or an orthographic shape (D-O-G), as needed, based on the information and mechanisms represented in the output lexicons. In comprehension the input lexicons serve to identify an orthographic or phonological form so that its meaning can then be activated in the semantic system and comprehension may occur.

We have claimed that patients' performance is best described in terms of impairment to one or more of the underlying processing components. However, because the integrity of any particular component cannot be examined directly, we must instead examine the available evidence in order to make inferences regarding the condition of the underlying processing system. The evidence that we typically gather is obtained from observing patient performance on different tasks. If, for example, we assume that the task of oral reading involves the OIL, the semantic system, and the phonological output lexicon (POL), then a patient's performance in oral reading might provide information regarding these components. The task of silent reading might involve the first two components but not the third, whereas spontaneous speech might involve the semantic system and the POL but none of the input components. By observing the similarities and differences in a patient's performance on the different tasks, we can make inferences regarding the integrity of the underlying components. It is important to note that, according to such a theory, it is not the case that different components exist to perform different tasks, but rather that each component has a certain FUNCTION and whenever that function is required for any task, the component is utilized. Thus the same phonological output component is recruited in the tasks of oral reading and spontaneous speech, although the former task involves use of the orthographic input lexicon whereas the latter does not. An important consequence of this fact is that we would expect damage to a given component to be reflected in impaired performance on all those tasks that require that component.

We present data from the neurologically impaired patient RGB described by Caramazza and Hillis (1990b) to illustrate what the various components refer to and, at the same time, to show how a theory of cognitive processing can allow us to better understand patterns of impaired performance.

The relevant data regarding RGB's performance are presented in Table 6.1. What is immediately striking about this patient's performance pattern is that a comparable level of impairment occurred *only* in the tasks of oral reading, oral picture naming, and oral tactile naming. For these three tasks the patient must produce a spoken word, that is, phonological output. However, for the first task, the input is orthographic; for the second, pictures serve as stimuli; and for the third, the patient's tactile experience serves as input. The tasks share the semantic processing component as well as a common output mode. The fact that the tasks result in a similar pattern of errors suggests that the patient may have a deficit to some component that the tasks share. In the context of the functional architecture presented above, this indicates a deficit either to the semantic system or to the POL (see Figure 6.2).

TABLE 6.1
Percentage Correct for RGB Across Eight Tasks

Task	Percentage correct
Oral reading	69% (131/191)
Oral naming: pictures	66% (126/191)
Oral naming: tactile	64% (30/47)
Written naming: pictures	94% (179/191)
Writing to dictation	94% (179/191)
Auditory word/picture matching	100% (191/191)
Auditory/printed word matching	100% (47/47)
Written word/picture matching	100% (191/191)

The functional architecture with which we are working makes different predictions for the two possible deficits. According to the interrelationship among the components represented in Figure 6.2, a SELECTIVE deficit in the semantic system should be reflected equally in both phonological and orthographic output processes. Tasks requiring orthographic output include writing to dictation and written naming of objects. Because RGB did not make errors on these tasks comparable to the errors made on tasks requiring phonological output (Table 6.1), we can rule out the hypothesis that a semantic deficit was responsible for the errors observed in oral reading, oral picture naming, and oral tactile naming. Therefore, we can conclude that the probable locus of impairment in this patient was the POL, suggesting that the patient was unable to normally activate certain phonological representations in this component of the lexical system. The implication is that, for RGB, processing prior to the POL was intact; in oral reading, for example, the written form activated a representation in the OIL which allowed the patient to recognize the sequence of letters as familiar and, furthermore, a semantic representation was activated in the semantic system which permitted the patient to understand the meaning of the word he could not produce. Good reading comprehension was reflected in perfect performance on the written word/picture matching task (Table 6.1). The patient's performance was affected only when the semantic representation must activate its corresponding phonological form for output (for reports of other patients with deficits in spoken but not written naming, see Basso, Taborelli, & Vignolo, 1978; Michel, 1979).

The observation that the POL can be damaged without comparable damage to the orthographic output lexicon (OOL) serves to confirm the claim of this particular architecture that there are modality-specific sys-

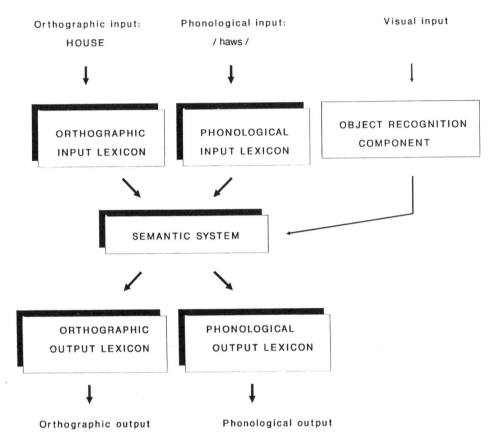

FIGURE 6.3. *The lexical processing system shown in Figure 6.1, including processing components that allow for the mapping of graphemes to phonemes in reading as well as for the assembly of graphemes from phonemes in writing. In addition, output buffers and conversion mechanisms are depicted.*

tems. We have seen that RGB made very few errors in writing the names of pictures or the words that were dictated to him and that he could not name. This pattern of results suggests a relatively intact OOL despite a damaged POL. The fact that observed patterns of performance can find an explanation within a particular theory serves to increase our confidence in the accuracy of the theory.

In addition to the distinction between orthographic and phonological modalities, the architecture of the lexical processing system also distinguishes between input and output mechanisms. Consequently, it predicts that phonological processing may be impaired for output but not for input, or vice versa. In the case of RGB, we have documented an impairment in OUTPUT lexical phonology, coexisting with normal performance on tasks that require intact INPUT lexical phonology. Both writing to dictation and auditory word/picture matching involve phonological input, the recognition of spoken forms. In the first task, the patient must write words presented aurally; in the second, he must match an aurally presented word to a picture. As shown in Table 6.1, RGB performed very well on both of these tasks. This good performance, in the face of poor performance on tasks requiring spoken output, supports the postulated distinction between input and output lexicons.

These results not only provide confirmation for the functional architecture of the lexical system shown in Figure 6.1, but also rule out certain alternative configurations of lexical processing components. For example, one possible theory places the POL prior to the OOL, thus requiring a phonological representation of a word to serve as the basis for retrieving its orthographic representation for spelling. Such an architecture, however, would not account for RGB's pattern of performance. It would predict that errors observed in tasks involving the POL should always be reflected in responses involving the OOL. In RGB's case, however, errors involving phonological output were not reflected in tasks requiring written output.

With this example we hope to have made clear (a) how a functional architecture of the lexical system allows us, on the basis of observed patterns of performance on different tasks, to make inferences about damage to functional components, and (b) how patterns of impaired performance can, in turn, be used to test and develop models of cognitive processes.

Aspects of the Internal Structure of the Functional Components

To this point we have characterized the functioning of the components of the lexical system in the most general of manners, indicating only that the principal lexical components can be classified according to representational type—orthographic, phonological, or semantic—and level of processing—input or output. However, the level of detail at which we can describe these components will determine the level of detail at which we can make predictions regarding the nature of the impairments that will result when a particular component is damaged: the more specific the model, the greater our understanding of patterns of impaired performance. We can, in fact, elaborate further on the structure and function of the lexical components; in this section, we briefly discuss three aspects of the internal structure of the phonological and

orthographic lexical components—differential accessibility, morphological structure, and word class—as well as certain aspects of the semantic
component—semantic categories, abstractness, and representational
format.

Differential Accessibility: Frequency

Normal subjects are faster at recognizing that a string of letters corresponds to a legitimate word of the language when the string corresponds to a frequently occurring word (e.g., *house*) than when a less
frequent sequence (e.g., *enzyme*) is presented (Gordon, 1983; Howes &
Solomon, 1951; Morton, 1969). This finding, usually referred to as a
FREQUENCY EFFECT, holds true with both orthographic representations in
reading and phonological representations in auditory recognition. These
observations have been taken as evidence that the frequency of occurrence of an item in the language is reflected in the ease and speed with
which lexical representations are activated.

We can think of each lexicon as a set of word recognition units, each
unit with a threshold of activation. When appropriate input is presented, the corresponding access unit becomes activated and fires when
activation exceeds the unit's threshold level. Thus, the letter sequence H-
O-U-S-E results in the activation of a stored representation of this letter
sequence in the OIL, while in the PIL the phoneme sequence /haws/
serves as the appropriate input for the phonological representation corresponding to *house*. In the output lexicons, a semantic representation
serves to activate the appropriate output form of an item. For example, a
semantic representation such as "a structure in which people can live"
will activate the phonological form /haws/ in the POL, which subsequently serves as the basis for pronouncing the word. Similarly, in the
OOL, the same semantic representation accesses the orthographic representation of the letter sequence H-O-U-S-E to be used subsequently in
writing or spelling. The activation of a representation is thought to raise
the resting activation level of the unit so that, upon subsequent presentation of the word, the unit reaches threshold more quickly. Frequent
encounters with any given word permanently lowers its threshold, resulting in faster recognition times and, in this way, explaining the frequency effect observed with normal subjects.

According to this account, we might expect that some forms of
damage to a lexicon could affect the integrity of these word recognition
units by elevating the thresholds such that some words will be more
difficult to recognize and others may not be recognized at all. On this
basis, we might expect that the already higher thresholds of low-fre-

quency words may be elevated to such an extent that many of these words will be accessed with much greater difficulty or not at all. This should be reflected in the observation of greater errors with low- than high-frequency items, and is, in fact, observed in patterns of impaired performance. RGB, for example, was able to read 40% of high-frequency words but only 29% of low-frequency words.

Morphological Structure

A number of theoretical and empirical reasons indicate that the representation of lexical items cannot be simply in the form of an unstructured string of phonemes or graphemes (e.g., w+a+l+k+i+n+g), but that the morphological structure of an item must be represented (e.g., WALK+ING). The most compelling reason for believing that morphological structure is represented in the lexicon is that human language is productive, that is, that we can comprehend and produce specific morphologically complex forms that we may not have previously encountered. Thus, although we may have never read the word *chummily*, we know that it must consist of CHUMMY+LY. Because *chummy* and *ly* are represented in the lexicon, we know that *chummily* should mean approximately "like friends + in that manner" or "in a chummy manner." Additional support for the notion that morphological information is represented in the lexicon is the observation that words in graphemic or phonological form are normally understood or produced in a sentence context. In such a context, morphological information is critical for a correct syntactic treatment of the sentence. Thus, for example, to produce the sentence, "I *walk* slowly while my dog *walks* quickly beside me," one must have the knowledge that *walk* (1st person) = WALK, whereas *walk* (3rd person) = WALK+s. If every word we encountered consisted of an undifferentiated string of graphemes or phonemes, such abilities would not be easily accounted for.

These observations have led to the suggestion that lexical information is represented in a morphologically decomposed manner, although the exact manner in which such morphological information is represented is still unresolved. Some researchers would argue that only root forms and derivation and/or inflection are indicated (e.g., CHUM+Y+LY), whereas others would argue that previously encountered stems are also represented (e.g., CHUMMY+LY). In support of the notion of morphological decomposition, there is not only linguistic and psychological evidence from normal language processing (for reviews, see Badecker & Caramazza, 1989; Butterworth, 1983; Henderson, 1989; Taft, 1985), but also findings from impaired performance. Thus, we illustrate below how lexical components can be damaged such that only certain morphological processes are disrupted.

Form Class

In a morphologically decomposed lexicon, there are differences in the representations of words of different parts of speech (i.e., FORM CLASSES). These differences are based, at least in part, on systematic differences in the morphology of different form classes (Caramazza, 1988). For example, in English, nouns can be inflected with an s in forming the plural (*dog, dogs*) or transformed to adjectives in a derivational process that adds AL (*nation, national*); verbs can be inflected with s, ED, ING, and EN (*melts, melted, melting, taken*); adjectives may take the comparative ER and the superlative EST (*big, bigger; small, smallest*); but function words (*on, of, this,* and *that*) are usually uninflected. Consequently, form class information must be represented in order to correctly restrict productivity; for example, we will not form a superlative such as *walkest*.

The claim that form class information forms a part of lexical representation is further supported by the fact that brain damage can selectively affect one form class and not another. A number of reports have described selective deficits of form class. For example, Miceli, Silveri, Villa, and Caramazza (1984) described patients who had greater difficulty in naming verbs than nouns, as well as patients with the reverse order of difficulty. A similar dissociation between verbs and nouns was described by Miceli, Silveri, Nocentini, and Caramazza (1988) for comprehension. These authors also noted that a form class effect in production was not necessarily associated with a similar deficit in word comprehension (for a discussion of similar cases, see Baxter & Warrington, 1985; McCarthy & Warrington, 1985; Zingeser & Berndt, 1988).

Lexical Semantics

Although this is not the place to discuss in detail the difficult and highly debated subject of the internal structure of the lexical semantic system (for a review of some relevant issues, see Jackendoff, 1983; Miller & Johnson-Laird, 1976), certain points, necessary for subsequent discussion of patient data, can be made fairly easily.

The morphological decomposition hypothesis implies that the semantic representation of a morphologically complex item used to address the output components must consist of distinct subsets of features, each specifying the different parts of the lexical item (Miceli & Caramazza, 1988). The semantic representation would include root semantic features, derivational semantic features (where present), and inflectional semantic features. For example, the word *colpevoli* (Italian for *guilty*–plural) might have the semantic representation [(COLPA) (ADJ) (PL)], where COLPA is the semantic component for the root morpheme (COLP–), ADJ is the semantic component for the selection of an adjectival affix (EVOL–), and PL is the semantic component for the selection of the appropriate inflectional plural affix (L). This semantic representation serves to specify the output form addressed and assembled in either the phonological or orthographic output lexicons.

Besides a componential morphological structure, semantic representations may have a componential structure with regards to the meaning of individual morphemes. In other words, the meaning of an item may be represented in terms of semantic features (e.g., the semantic representation for dog may consist of the following features; animal, mammal, domestic, four legs, barks, etc). This characteristic of semantic representations allows for category relationships among lexical items. Words that belong to the same semantic category (e.g., *cat* and *dog*) will share more semantic features than words from different categories (e.g., *dog* and *cheese*).

The fact that items that share semantic features are structurally related to one another is reflected in certain empirical findings with normal subjects. It has been found that processing an item—for example, deciding whether or not DOG constitutes a word—facilitates the subsequent processing of semantically related items—making a decision for CAT (e.g., see Meyer & Schvaneveldt, 1971). Presumably this facilitation is the result of the fact that *dog* and *cat* share certain semantic features and that with the activation of the features of *dog* certain features of *cat* become active. Because a subset of the features of *cat* have been preactivated, the semantic representation corresponding to *cat* will take less time to reach a threshold level of activation when the subject is presented with the word *cat*. This time reduction will be reflected in faster processing times with the word: reading, semantic judgments, lexical decisions, and so forth, will be faster than if *cat* had been preceded by an unrelated word such as *chair*.

Providing additional support for the notion of category relatedness are findings of category-specific impairments. Goodglass, Klein, Carey, and Jones (1966) reported patients who appeared to have disproportionate difficulty with particular semantic categories; Dennis (1976), McKenna and Warrington (1978), and Warrington and McCarthy (1983) reported selective impairments in the comprehension of body-part names; Warrington and McCarthy (1983) presented evidence of a selective impairment in the comprehension of inanimate object names; Warrington and Shallice (1984) reported a selective impairment in the ability to identify living things and foods; and Hart, Berndt, and Caramazza (1985) described a patient with a selective deficit to the category of fruits and vegetables (see also Basso, Capitani, & Laiacona, 1988; Berndt, 1988; Goodglass & Budin, 1988; Hillis & Caramazza, 1990; Sartori & Job, 1988; Semenza & Zettin, 1989; Silveri & Gainotti, 1988; Warrington, 1981a; Warrington & McCarthy, 1987, 1988).

Another type of dissociation observed in impaired performance is one between performance on abstract and concrete words. Some patients have been described who can read concrete words but have difficulty reading abstract words (Marshall & Newcombe, 1966; Patterson & Marcel, 1977; Saffran & Marin, 1977; Shallice & Warrington, 1975), whereas other patients have been better able to define abstract words than concrete words. Warrington and Shallice (1984), for example, described a patient who defined *debate* as "discussion between people, open discussions between group." However, the patient defined *ink* as "food, you put on top of food you are eating, a liquid" (see also Warrington, 1975, 1981b). Although it is unclear how the properties of abstractness and concreteness are represented, this dissociation has been interpreted as indicating that abstractness is a relevant dimension of the organization of semantic information.

Having briefly described the arrangement of the functional components of the lexical system and some aspects of their internal structure, we are now in a position to evaluate the role that such a theory can play in the interpretation of patient's performance. A patient's impairment is often most strikingly reflected in the types of errors produced in performing different tasks. Therefore, we have organized the following discussion in terms of error types: nonword errors, semantic errors, and morphological errors. It is not our intention to provide an exhaustive survey of error types, but instead to use certain error types to illustrate how, within the context of a theory of lexical processing, we can better understand the origin of the errors and the functioning of the system that underlies them. In this context, we raise and discuss issues of current controversy in the field, such as the grouping and classification of patients, the usefulness of syndromes, and the notion of compensatory strategies.

NONWORD ERRORS

Table 6.2 includes errors made by patients JG (Goodman & Caramazza, 1986a) and ML (Hillis & Caramazza, 1989) in written and oral spelling to dictation. Although ML displayed a more severe impairment than JG, each patient performed with comparable accuracy in the written and oral spelling of words: 74% and 65%, respectively, for JG and 25%

TABLE 6.2

Examples of Errors and Accuracy Rates for JG and ML
in Written and Oral Spelling to Dictation

Task	JG	ML
	senate→cenit	dumb→dub
	debt→dete	priest→rpiest
	urge→erg	lamb→llamb
	severe→savier	fabric→frbric
	mercy→mursy	degree→dgree
Written spelling	74% (241/326)	25% (81/326)
Oral spelling	65% (212/326)	36% (15/42)

and 36%, respectively, for ML. Nonword responses, such as those in Table 6.2, constituted the bulk of errors for both patients in the two tasks.

According to the model of lexical processing with which we are working (Figure 6.1), a lexical deficit exclusively to the ability to spell would result from damage to the OOL. The OOL is thought to contain information about the abstract letter sequences that form the basis for written or oral spelling of words. It has been proposed that the representation of the letters is abstract in the sense that letter identities but not specific aspects of the letter form, such as case, font, and name, are represented. Consequently, both written and oral spelling are based on the orthographic information represented in the OOL. The specific form of the output, that is, letter shapes for a written response and letter names for an oral response, is computed at a later stage of processing by allographic and letter name conversion devices, respectively (see Figure 6.3). Data from neurologically impaired patients has confirmed this proposed functional architecture of peripheral spelling processes (Goodman & Caramazza, 1986b; Kinsbourne & Rosenfeld, 1974; Kinsbourne & Warrington, 1965; see Ellis, 1987, for review). Thus, for our purposes, we can assume that damage to the OOL should affect written and oral spelling equally.

If we consider levels of performance, the fact that accuracy in oral and written spelling are comparable is consistent with a deficit to the OOL. However, comparable levels of performance in oral and written naming does not require a deficit to the OOL; such a conclusion would be premature without first ruling out alternative loci suggested by the model of lexical processing. The other major lexical component involved in spelling to dictation is the PIL; thus, it is possible that both patients were impaired in the recognition of spoken words and, for this reason, failed to spell them correctly. We can, however, reject the hypothesis of a

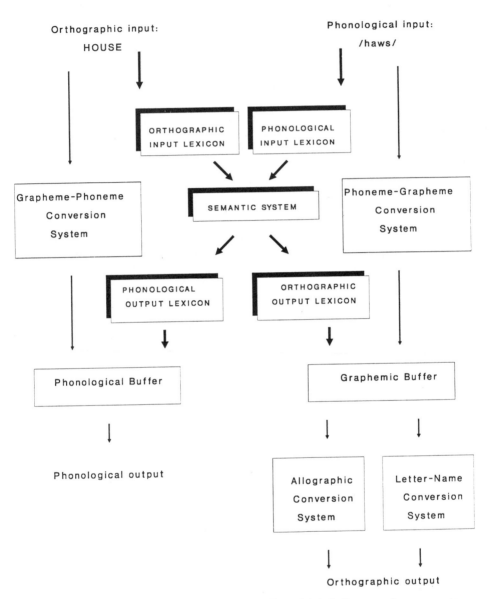

FIGURE 6.3. *The lexical processing system shown in Figure 6.1, including processing components that allow for the mapping of graphemes to phonemes in reading as well as for the assembly of graphemes from phonemes in writing. In addition, output buffers and conversion mechanisms are depicted.*

deficit to the PIL in these patients because they both showed excellent auditory comprehension abilities: JG correctly defined 98% of the words dictated to her, whereas ML scored 100% on the auditory comprehension subtests of the Boston Diagnostic Aphasia Exam (Goodglass & Kaplan, 1972). Furthermore, both patients made errors on a written naming task where they were required to write the name of a pictured object, which therefore did not involve the PIL.

Until this point, the performance patterns of the two patients look quite similar, suggesting an impairment to the OOL. Earlier we discussed that we could expect damage to a lexicon to result in a frequency effect such that performance with low-frequency words would be more impaired than performance with high-frequency words. Table 6.3 presents the performance levels of JG and ML with high- and low-frequency words. JG showed a significant effect of frequency in both oral (χ^2 = 31.94, $p < .001$) and written spelling (χ^2 = 49.18, $p < .001$), whereas ML did not. Thus, these two patients differed with respect to what is often considered to be an indicator of a lexical deficit, suggesting that we might want to explore further before localizing the deficit of both patients to the OOL.

Thus far we have simply examined overall performance levels on a variety of tasks. Another potential source of information regarding the nature of a deficit lies in the FORM OF THE ERRORS that are produced. We will show that a consideration of the form of a patient's errors often provides detailed and specific information regarding the nature of a deficit. We noted that both patients produced nonword responses. Nonetheless, in considering the errors more closely, we noticed that JG's responses, although incorrect, would sound like the target word if pronounced (e.g., SILENCE → sylence); that is, the responses consisted of plausible although incorrect spellings (for descriptions of patients with similar error patterns, see Baxter & Warrington, 1987; Beauvois &

TABLE 6.3

Accuracy in Written and Oral Spelling of High- and Low-Frequency Words for JG and ML

Task	JG	ML
Written Spelling		
High frequency	85% (121/146)	28% (41/146)
Low frequency	46% (67/146)	26% (38/146)
Oral Spelling		
High frequency	89% (130/146)	33% (6/18)
Low frequency	60% (88/146)	39% (7/18)

Derouesne, 1981; Sanders & Caramazza, 1990). In fact, 88% of JG's responses could be categorized as phonologically plausible errors, whereas only 7% of ML's errors were of this type. ML's errors contained substitutions (e.g., HAPPY → fappy), deletions (e.g., JUNK → jnk), transpositions (e.g., TIGER → tgier), and insertions (BOTTLE → bolttlee) of letters that did not result in a plausible phonological rendition of the target word.

It has been suggested that to be able to develop a spelling for unfamiliar words, we must have knowledge of sound–letter relationships (e.g., the sound /f/ may be written as F, GH, PH, etc) (see Cummings, 1988). This information, which we have acquired through our experience with the written language, is often referred to as knowledge of phoneme–grapheme correspondences. The system, which produces a written form corresponding to a phonological input, is often referred to as the phoneme–grapheme conversion system, or PGC system. Thus, if we wished to spell a spoken word whose spelling we did not know, for example, /hɛzɪkæst/, we would probably arrive at spellings such as HEZIKAST, HESICAST, HESYCAST, and HESYCHAST. All would be plausible and could be produced by a system that represents information such as /z/ → s or z, /ɪ/ → I or Y, and so forth. Without having previously encountered the word in its written form and stored a representation for its spelling in the OOL, we would have no way of knowing that the last alternative is, in fact, the correct one.

The form of JG's errors supports the hypothesis that, for those words for which representations in the OOL were damaged, she made use of her knowledge of sound to print correspondences in English to produce a plausible spelling: given a phonological input—the dictated word, for example—she applied phoneme–grapheme rules to arrive at a possible spelling (see Figure 6.3).

It is important to note that, in English, words vary in the degree to which their correct spelling would be produced by application of such a system. Thus, if the orthographic representation corresponding to /dæn/ were inaccessible for whatever reason, application of phoneme–grapheme rules would most likely arrive at the correct spelling DAN; however, if the orthographic representation of /jat/ were inaccessible, application of the same rules is most unlikely to result in the correct spelling YACHT. This contrast is often described by saying that English spellings differ in terms of the regularity or irregularity of the relationship between their pronunciation and their spelling. We refer to this as the "probability of correct phoneme–grapheme conversion" (see Hanna, Hanna, Hodges, & Rudorf, 1966, for the PCG probabilities in English). Words such as /dɪd/ would be said to have a high phoneme–

grapheme conversion probability, whereas words such as *doubt* (which could be spelled as DOWT, DOUTE, DOUGHT, etc.) would have a low probability of being correctly produced by application of phoneme–grapheme correspondence rules.

Given these assumptions, we can make specific predictions regarding JG's performance in spelling tasks; specifically we would expect that (a) most high-frequency words, regardless of their probability of correct phoneme–grapheme conversion, should be spelled correctly because orthographic representations should not be damaged for these items, but that (b) low-frequency items, being less accessible, will be more often spelled through the PGC system, and we should, therefore, expect that the spelling of low-frequency items should differ depending on the phoneme–grapheme conversion probabilities of the items: low-probability/low-frequency words should be spelled incorrectly more often according to PGC system than high-probability/low-frequency words. Table 6.4 shows the results obtained by JG. High-frequency words showed no effect on phoneme–grapheme probability ($\chi^2 = .37$, ns), whereas low-frequency words could be distinguished according to grapheme–phoneme conversion probabilities ($\chi^2 = 4.42$, $p < .05$).

Another means of determining whether JG had intact knowledge of PGC rules was to ask her to spell unfamiliar or invented nonwords such as /klejk/, which we could expect to be spelled KLAKE, KLAIK, or KLAICK. Based on her performance with familiar words, we would expect her to produce phonologically plausible renditions of unfamiliar or invented items, just as normal subjects do (Campbell, 1983). In fact, JG was able to produce plausible spellings for 100% of the nonwords she was asked to write and for 98% of those she was asked to spell orally. The evidence thus converges on an explanation of JG's performance that indicates that

TABLE 6.4

JG's Written and Oral Spelling Performance with Words of High and Low Frequency and High and Low Phoneme–Grapheme (PGC) Probabilities

Frequency	PGC probability	
	High	Low
High frequency		
Written spelling	100%	90%
Oral spelling	100%	98%
Low frequency		
Written spelling	80%	50%
Oral spelling	93%	65%

the OOL was damaged and that the responses observed when she was asked to write were the result of the functioning of an undamaged PGC system.

The case of ML would appear to be different. Good comprehension and the fact that both written and oral spelling were equally affected suggested a deficit to a component beyond the semantic system, yet shared by oral and written spelling processes. The absence of a frequency effect was an indication, however, that the OOL might not be the locus of impairment in this patient. Phonologically plausible errors were not observed and, additionally, words of both high and low PGC probability were equally affected: high, 37% correct; low, 30% correct. When asked to spell nonwords, ML performed as she had with words: 38% correct in written spelling and 45% correct in oral spelling of nonwords. In fact, errors with nonwords took the same form as those with words: substitutions, deletions, transpositions, and additions of letters (e.g., /mʃræm/ as RUSHRAM; /dansɛpt/ as DNCEPT; /fɔjt/ as FIOT; and /riʃ/ as RRECECH).

It has been assumed that a postlexical memory component or buffer is necessarily involved in written and oral spelling (Caramazza, Miceli, Villa, & Romani, 1987; Wing & Baddeley, 1980). The location of this component in relation to the lexical processing system is shown in Figure 6.3. The purpose of this memory component, referred to as the GRAPHEMIC BUFFER, is to store orthographic representations while allographic conversion and letter-name conversion processes take place. Allographic and letter-name conversion processes take abstract letter identities and assign them a particular form: name, case, and font as needed. These processes are thought to act serially, processing one letter at a time. The graphemic buffer maintains the whole letter string available while the sequential conversion processes take place. Thus, an impairment to the graphemic buffer would be expected to produce comparable error rates in both oral and written spelling of both words and nonwords.

It would appear that, in the case of ML, the results described thus far are consistent with damage to the graphemic buffer:

1. Absence of a frequency effect: We would not expect lexical factors such as frequency to be reflected in damage to such a component because it is postlexical; that is, it should not matter whether a word is of high or low frequency in the lexicon, because to the graphemic buffer it is simply a string of letters to be temporarily stored.

2. Similar performance in oral and written spelling: Because of the location of the graphemic buffer within the processing system, we

would expect oral and written spelling to be affected equally by damage to the graphemic buffer.

3. Similar performance with words and nonwords: Because the buffer stores orthographic information regardless of its origin, word and nonword spelling should be similarly affected.

4. Effects of representation length: Memory components are typically restricted in the number of elements that can be held simultaneously active, and disorders of memory are often characterized by a reduction in the capacity of the component. Damage to the graphemic buffer is thought to result in more errors when longer sequences are stored. If we examine ML's performance in written and oral spelling according to the length of the response, we find that, whereas performance is as good as 61% (60/99) with three-and four-letter words, accuracy falls to 4% (2/50) with seven- and eight-letter words (see Table 6.5).

All the evidence gathered suggests that ML, although impaired in the processing of words, did not have damage to the orthographic output lexicon (i.e., to the stored information regarding the orthographic representation of words), but rather to a postlexical memory component referred to as the graphemic buffer (for other cases with hypothesized damage to the graphemic buffer, see Caramazza et al., 1987; Miceli, Silveri, & Caramazza, 1987; Posteraro, Zinelli, & Mazzucchi, 1988).

In this section we have described the impaired spelling of two patients who made apparently superficially similar errors in both oral and written spelling. As a result of testing predictions motivated by the architecture of the lexical processing system, however, we have concluded that one suffered from a lexical deficit to the OOL, whereas the other had damage to the nonlexical component referred to as the graphemic buffer. This example illustrates how apparently similar patterns of impaired performance may stem from damage to different underlying mechanisms.

TABLE 6.5

ML's Spelling Accuracy in Three Tasks According to Stimulus Length

Letter length	Writing to dictation	Written naming: pictures	Oral spelling
3–4	55% (41/75)	76% (13/17)	86% (6/7)
5	33% (27/123)	45% (10/22)	63% (12/19)
6	20% (17/86)	8% (1/12)	36% (10/28)
7–8	5% (2/42)	N/A	0% (0/8)

Similar to the PGC system in writing, for reading a system of rules mapping letters or letter clusters into their possible pronunciations is proposed and referred to as a system of grapheme–phoneme correspondences (GPC) (see Figure 6.3) (for a discussion of this topic, see Coltheart, 1978; Venezky, 1970; but see Humphreys & Evett, 1985, for opposing views). In normal subjects such a system would be used in attempting to produce pronunciations for words that are not represented in the OIL, words we have never or seldom encountered in their written form. Consistent with this hypothesis is the performance of patients such as MP (Bub, Cancelliere, & Kertesz, 1985), who had no trouble reading nonwords but was significantly impaired in word reading. MP's performance in reading resembled the pattern of impairment described above for patient JG in writing: significant effects of frequency (high-frequency words, 88% correct; low frequency words, 79%) and regularity (regular, 96%; irregular, 41%). Furthermore, the majority of reading errors consisted of phonologically plausible PRONUNCIATIONS of the written form (e.g., AISLE → /ejzəl/), often referred to as regularization errors. It was concluded that MP's performance pattern was, at least in part, the result of an impairment to the OIL in the context of an intact GPC system. This resulted in phonologically plausible readings of items for which a pronunciation could not be computed normally[1] (for other cases whose reading performance reflects the use of the GPC system, see Hillis & Caramazza, in press, and papers in Patterson, Marshall, & Coltheart, 1985).

These examples suggest that the patterns of performance we observe subsequent to brain damage are the result of the operation of the damaged components in concert with all available intact components. Thus, damage to the OOL in the presence of an intact PGC system will result in phonologically plausible responses in spelling, whereas damage to the OIL may result in phonologically plausible readings or regularization errors.

Patients who exhibit certain error patterns subsequent to brain damage are often described as using "compensatory strategies" (e.g., see Kolk & Grunsven, 1985). Thus JG might be said to produce phonologically plausible spellings as the result of a strategy induced by the presence of damaged components. What is meant by such a statement is not entirely clear. One possibility is precisely what has been suggested

---

1. A deficit to one of the systems that represents relationships between phonology and orthography does not necessarily result in damage to the other. For example, Beauvois and Derouesne, (1979) described a patient who, like JG, had difficulty writing words but not nonwords. In reading, however, the patient apparently had a deficit to the GPC system as evidenced by a difficulty only in the reading of nonwords.

in the preceding paragraph. We argued there that, subsequent to brain damage, a person will produce an output on the basis of whatever damaged and intact components are available. On this account, phonologically plausible spellings simply reflect the functioning of the PGC system available to the person before brain damage, although this system is not used for familiar words because these, in an undamaged system, are represented in the OOL. Brain damage, therefore, simply reflects the output of a system given that certain components have been damaged (see Caramazza, 1984, 1986, for a discussion of the transparency principle). This view allows one to use brain-damaged performance as a window into the cognitive system and, as a consequence, as a tool that can be used to make inferences about what the system must have been like before brain damage—the work of cognitive neuropsychology.

The other possible interpretation of compensatory strategies is that, subsequent to brain damage, the cognitive system undergoes a transformation such that previously unrelated components establish links to one another and new, previously nonexisting, components are developed. Although such a view is, of course, a logical possibility, it is important to realize the implications of this position. It would mean that we have no theory of the cognitive system to use as a basis for interpreting observed patterns of impaired performance. This would be the case because the system would have been transformed, presumably differently for different patients according to individual needs, as well as the form and extent of the damage. We would have no way of knowing the shape of the transformation since data from one patient to another would be irrelevant, given that each would be functioning with a differently configured cognitive system. Thus, not only would we have no basis for interpreting patient data, but we also would be unable to use patterns of brain-damaged performance to provide information concerning the structure of the normal cognitive system.

Although it is possible that neurological damage results in a reorganization of the cognitive system, because of the paralyzing implications of such a possibility, in the absence of positive evidence regarding reorganization, we should be willing to accept such a·view only to the extent to which we are unsuccessful in accounting for patterns of brain damage in terms of a theory of the structure of the normal cognitive system.

SEMANTIC ERRORS

Naming typically refers to the act of producing, in written or spoken form, the name that corresponds to an item. Thus, one might pronounce or write the name of an object, a picture, an item, or an action that one has in mind. In terms of the model we have been discussing, object or picture naming would require an object recognition component for input, semantic processing, and the use of the POL or OOL to produce spoken or written output, respectively (see Figure 6.2). Naming an item one has in mind would originate in the semantic system and involve one of the output lexicons.

In analyzing data produced by two neurologically impaired patients with comparable error rates in the oral naming of objects presented visually and tactilely, we found that performance on a number of other tasks needed to be considered before we could draw conclusions regarding the nature of the patients' underlying deficits. In Table 6.6 are examples of some of the actual errors produced by RGB in naming tasks. The responses (e.g. "pineapple" for banana) clearly show a semantic similarity to the target and are, therefore, commonly referred to as semantic errors. In fact, as shown in Table 6.6, 80/81 of RGB's errors on these tasks can be classified as being semantically related to the stimulus item. Also in Table 6.6 are examples of errors produced by patient KE on the same tasks (Hillis, Rapp, Romani, & Caramazza, in press). These errors also bear a semantic relationship to the target. Like RGB, when KE made an error (see Table 6.6), he responded almost exclusively (86%; 147/171 with a word that was semantically related to the target.

On the basis of these data, one might conclude that the two patients had similar impairments. Consequently, given that earlier in this chapter, RGB's deficit was attributed to the phonological output lexicon, we might be tempted to conclude that KE also suffered from an impairment to the same functional component of the lexical system. However, recall that the model of lexical processing that we are using as the basis for the interpretation of our data makes a number of predictions regarding

TABLE 6.6

Examples of Semanitic Errors in Oral Naming with Object and Tactile Input for KE and RGB as well as the Proportion of Semantic Errors/Total Errors

Task	RGB	KE
	lemon→sour	lemon→orange
	clam→octopus	clam→crab
	kangaroo→racoon	racoon→rabbit
	mittens→socks	shirt→sock
	banana→pineapple	peach→banana
Object naming	98% (63/64)	85% (126/149)
Tactile naming	100% 17/17)	95% (21/22)

performance on other tasks given a hypothesized impairment in the POL. Specifically, we should observe relatively good performance and an absence of semantic errors on all tasks that do not involve the POL. On the basis of the data presented thus far, however, we are not in a position to determine if KE's performance is consistent with these predictions.

Table 6.7 presents the results obtained by RGB and KE on a number of the critical tasks. RGB, as seen earlier, was relatively unimpaired in tasks not involving the POL. KE, on the other hand, showed comparable semantic error rates on all of the tasks. A possible conclusion is that KE had a number of deficits in addition to a POL deficit similar to the one exhibited by RGB. If we return to our model of lexical processing, however, we find that the one component of the system that is involved in all tasks of lexical processing is the semantic system. Given its central, mediating role between input and output systems, we would expect that damage to such a system would have comparable impact on all tasks that involve lexical processing, regardless of input–output or orthographic–phonological status. This is precisely what we observe in the case of KE: he made semantic errors in all production tasks, as well as in comprehension tasks where he was simply required to say whether a word and picture matched (e.g., whether the word /lajǝn/ and the picture of a tiger corresponded to the same item) (Table 6.7). These results yield the conclusion that KE, unlike RGB, had a deficit to the semantic system.

Given that the deficit for RGB presumably involved an output lexicon, whereas for KE it did not, we would expect that for RGB, but not for KE, performance should have been affected by the frequency of occurrence of the words that serve as stimuli. The data support this prediction. RGB showed a significant frequency effect such that, in

TABLE 6.7

Semantic Error Rate (Semantic Errors/Total Errors) for KE and RGB on Six Tasks

Task	RGB	KE
Oral reading	98% (59/60)	82% (116/142)
Oral naming: pictures	98% (62/63)	85% (126/149)
Oral naming: tactile	100% (17/17)	95% (21/22)
Written naming: pictures	0% (0/12)	71% (107/150)
Writing to dictation	0% 0/12)	60% (84/139)
Auditory word/picture matching	— (0/0)	96% (77/80)
Written word/picture matching	— (0/0)	79 (54/68)

reading, low-frequency words resulted in significantly fewer correct responses (60% correct) than did high-frequency words (71% correct) (χ^2 = 4.68, $p < .03$). KE's performance did not appear to be affected by this parameter; he accurately read equal numbers of low- and high-frequency words.

An interesting question is raised by these results: Why should the same type of error—a semantic error—result from damage to different components—the POL and the semantic system? Damage to the semantic component may take different forms. It is believed that in some cases the semantic representations can be damaged in such a way that it is difficult to distinguish between items that are similar. For example, it is probably the case that APPLE [fruit, edible, round, sweet, smooth skinned, red, yellow, green] and PEACH [fruit, edible, round, sweet, fuzzy skinned, yellow] have more shared semantic features than they have differentiating features. A loss of some of the differentiating features would render the two items almost indistinguishable. The patient should, as a consequence of such damage, have difficulty not only in discriminating between the two in comprehension tasks, but also in producing the correct name in a naming task (for reviews, see Caramazza & Berndt, 1978; Lesser, 1978).

Damage to either of the output lexicons, on the other hand, should not affect a patient's ability to understand the meaning of words, and good comprehension should be observed. In the case of damage to one output component, semantic errors are explained by assuming that, in a naming task, the presentation of a peach for example, necessarily results in the activation of some of the features of semantically related items (e.g., of apple). If the semantic representation of peach does not result in the activation of the damaged output form /pitʃ/ in the POL, another, accessible phonological representation that is normally activated by the semantic representation because it shares semantic features with peach (e.g., /æpl/) could be produced instead (for discussion, see Caramazza & Hillis, in press; Gordon, Goodman-Schulman, & Caramazza, 1987; Nolan & Caramazza, 1982; Patterson, 1978).

In summary, we have described the performance of two patients with basically very similar errors in picture and tactile naming. By considering their performance in the context of a model of lexical processing, we have shown, however, that these patients have deficits affecting different lexical components. This example illustrates the point that questions such as the following serve only to create confusion: What is THE source of semantic errors in aphasic patients? There apparently is no reason to assume that patients who make similar errors have similar deficits or damage to different underlying components must necessarily result in different error types.[2]

Semantic errors have also played a prominent role in the discussion of a syndrome observed in reading and referred to as DEEP DYSLEXIA (Marshall & Newcombe, 1966, 1973; see also papers in Coltheart, Patterson, & Marshall, 1980). Deep dyslexia is typically described in the following manner (Morton & Patterson, 1980): (a) semantic (e.g., "table" for CHAIR), derivational (e.g., "walked" for WALKING), and visual (e.g., "chair" for CHAIN) paralexias in reading single words aloud; also omissions; (b) severe if not total impairment in reading nonsense words; (c) part-of-speech effects in word reading with nouns read better than adjectives which, in turn, are read better than verbs or function words; and (4) abstractness effects in word reading such that imageable, concrete words are read better than abstract words. These symptoms are considered to represent a category of disorder or a syndrome because a number of patients have been observed in whom these symptoms cooccur; the semantic error is believed to be the central or defining feature of the syndrome.

The fact that a quite specific constellation of behaviors should be observed across a number of patients is commonly taken as an indication that the observed performance pattern results from damage to a common mechanism. Consequently, reports of syndromes typically lead to attempts to understand what the mechanism underlying the symptoms might be. The example of deep dyslexia provides us with the opportunity to explore the notion that the observation of symptom cooccurrence necessarily reflects damage to a single functional component.

We can turn to the model with which we have been working to determine the location of a functional deficit that would result in only the constellation of symptoms that serve to define deep dyslexia. An impairment to nonword reading suggests a deficit to GPC mechanisms, but such damage does not predict the observed pattern of performance with words. Although the production of semantic, derivational, and

---

2. We have not, of course, described a number of other patterns of impaired performance that can be observed in naming tasks; clearly, however, if the theory of lexical processing is correct, these also should be explainable as the result of damage to one of the underlying components. For example, a commonly observed behavior occurs when a patient is apparently unable to produce any response when asked to provide the name of an item. (This deficit is referred to as ANOMIA.) Within this model, such responses can be considered to occur when the POL is damaged to such a large extent that neither the correct response nor any semantically similar responses become active enough to serve as the basis of a spoken response.

visual paralexias, as well as word class and abstractness–concreteness effects, might be consistent with a semantic deficit, many of these patients show good comprehension for many of the words that result in semantic errors, and certainly the nonword difficulties cannot be explained by a semantic deficit. No single lexical component, when damaged, would produce this performance pattern. In fact, no one has yet been successful in accounting for the syndrome in terms of a single underlying deficit.[3]

In addition, if one claims that this constellation of symptoms can result ONLY from damage to a single component, then the expectation is that the occurrence of one of the symptoms should be predictive of the other symptoms. This expectation certainly does not hold for deep dyslexia. Patients have been described who exhibit one or more of the symptoms of deep dyslexia, but no others. For example, of the symptoms of deep dyslexia, RGB (Caramazza & Hillis, 1990b) and KE (Hillis et al., 1990a) exhibited only semantic errors and difficulty in nonword reading; patients LB (Caramazza, Miceli, Silveri, & Laudanna, 1985) and WB (Funnell, 1983) had difficulty only with nonwords. These findings are consistent with the conclusion, at least within the lexical processing framework we have described, that deep dyslexia can be understood only as the result of multiple deficits (Nolan & Caramazza, 1982; Shallice & Warrington, 1975).

We have seen, therefore, that the cooccurrence of symptoms does not necessarily implicate a common deficit to the functional architecture of a cognitive system. Nonetheless, the question remains: Why should this coincidence of symptoms be repeatedly observed? This question has two possible answers: (a) The symptoms may reflect damage to a number of different mechanisms that are anatomically adjacent in the brain. According to this view, damage to a particular brain region, unless very selective, may be expected to affect a number of functional components. (b) The theory we are using as the basis for the interpretation of patient performance is wrong. This alternative is entirely possible, of course, but if a new theory is developed that would predict that this particular constellation of symptoms should result from damage to a single underlying mechanism, the theory must also be able to account for all the other patterns of observed impairment that are accounted for by the current theory. This has not yet been done for the case of deep dyslexia.

Just as the cooccurence or association of symptoms need not be an

---

3. At a neuroanatomical level an explanation has been proposed which is referred to as the Right Hemisphere Hypothesis. This suggestion, however, has been widely criticized. (For a review of the RHH, see Coltheart et al., 1980; Patterson & Besner, 1984; Saffran, Bogyo, Schwartz, & Marin, 1980; Zaidel & Schweigher, 1984.)

indication of a common functional deficit, the dissociation of performance on different tasks does not necessarily indicate that different components are required to perform the various tasks. An example of a dissociation leading to the claim of multiple components has resulted from the observation of what has been termed MODALITY-SPECIFIC APHASIA. Patients have been described who demonstrated an inability to name objects presented in one modality, despite correct naming of the items in other modalities. For example, Lhermitte and Beauvois (1973) described the patient JF who made numerous errors (primarily semantic) in naming objects and pictures whose function he was able to mime, but many fewer errors in naming objects or pictures upon presentation of their characteristic sound, their definition or their tactile presentation (for other relevant cases, see Beauvois, 1982; Beauvois, Saillant, Meininger, & Lhermitte, 1978; Denes & Semenza, 1975; Hillis, 1988; Riddoch & Humphreys, 1987; Silveri & Gainotti, 1988). This pattern of performance involves a possible paradox: Adequate miming of the functions of visually presented objects, as well as good naming to definition, sound, or tactile input, would appear to require an intact semantic system, whereas the presence of semantic errors in object and picture naming suggests a damaged semantic system. One means of reconciling this discrepancy is to suggest that there are multiple semantic systems and that, in the case of JF, the connection between the system of "visual semantics" and the system of "verbal semantics" required for correct naming was damaged (see Shallice, 1987, for discussion). This would result in poor naming, despite adequate comprehension (as demonstrated by miming) of visually presented items, as well as in good naming and comprehension in all other modalities.

The claim of modality-specific semantic systems, therefore, raises the possibility that the specific functional architecture with which we are working and which specifies a single amodal semantic system might be incorrect. Specifically, it has been suggested that in contrast to the single semantic system represented in Figure 6.2, there are numerous semantic systems differentiated according to modality (Beauvois et al., 1978; Lhermitte & Beauvois, 1973; Warrington & Shallice, 1984; see Shallice, 1987, 1988, for discussion). Thus, there would be a semantic system for visual information which is addressed when a person is presented with an object or picture, a verbal semantic system to represent the meaning of words, perhaps an auditory system to represent the meaning of sounds, and so forth (for a discussion of what might be meant by the term modality-specific semantics, see Caramazza, Hillis, Rapp, & Romani, 1990; Hillis, et al., 1990; Riddoch, Humphreys, Coltheart, & Funnel 1988).

Caramazza et al. (1990) and Hillis et al. (1990) have argued, however, that the data regarding modality-specific aphasia do not require such conclusions since they can naturally be accounted for within a theory that posits a single central semantic component. For example, in the case of JF, it can be shown how damage to those processes that address the semantic system from an object recognition component (Figure 6.2) could result in the observed performance pattern. The authors argued that such damage could often result in the activation of semantic representations that would be inadequate for naming but sufficient for correct miming. They further pointed out that proponents of the modality-specific semantics proposal have failed to articulate the content of the various semantic systems: What is represented in visual semantics? How is it similar to or different from the information represented in the other semantic systems? For example, how is the meaning of DOG different in visual and verbal semantic systems?

It is not enough, therefore, to observe a dissociation in order to conclude that the dissociation must reflect a distinction among underlying functional components, just as, in the case of deep dyslexia, it was not enough to observe an association in order to conclude that a common component must be implicated. A common component can be inferred if, within some theory, there is a component whose function is such that, when damaged, the observed association should occur. Likewise a distinction among components will be motivated only if, within some theory, a pattern of performance cannot be accounted for without postulating additional components. Thus, although the functional architecture of the lexical processing system proposed in this chapter may very well be incorrect, it has not been shown to be incorrect with these examples.

MORPHOLOGICAL ERRORS

We have seen, in previous sections, that similarity of performance levels and error types does not guarantee similarity of underlying impairment. Nonetheless, it is common practice to group patients by error type, assign a name to this grouping, and assume that patients categorized in this manner form a homogeneous group that will be similar in all other relevant respects. A common example of such a practice is the classification of AGRAMMATISM (for a review, see Berndt & Caramazza, 1980; and papers in Kean, 1985). Patients are typically classified as agrammatic according to the following characteristics of speech production: omission and/or substitution of function words and inflections, and reduced phrase length. (Some would include as part of the classification criteria the symptom of "asyntactic" comprehension; (for a critical evaluation of this position, see Zurif, Gardner, & Brownell, 1989; but also see Berndt, 1987; Caramazza & Badecker, 1989). Patients categorized according to these criteria are then treated as a group; for example, common rehabilitation programs are applied and test results are averaged across patients. Note that these practices are necessarily based on the assumption that patients similarly classified are fundamentally homogeneous with regard to the nature of their underlying deficit; otherwise, why average across their performance and apply common treatment programs?

Even a very simplistic consideration of what might be involved in producing correct sentences, however, might distinguish between mechanisms that determine an appropriate syntactic structure for the sentence to be uttered and mechanisms that select and represent the individual words to be used. A deficit to either of these levels of processing would be expected to result in an impairment in sentence production. We examined this possibility by considering the performance of two patients who, according to the above criteria, are aggrammatic; however, we found them to have fundamentally different underlying deficits.

Table 6.8 contains samples of spontaneous speech of both patients,

TABLE 6.8

Spontaneous Speech Samples and Error Rates for ML and FS

ML

Cleaning . . . Annie Thompson . . . Boston . . . got up four
dollars . . . taken for little children . . . eaten . . . not eaten three
days . . . touch by the story . . . made up purse her . . . for her

couple having picnic . . . boy flying kite . . . playing in the
water . . . a sailboat, flagpole, dog . . . the boat is down
water . . . dog watch boy

FS

Then returns my house   Then I listen to the television
Pio ritorna la mia casa   Pio io ascolto il televisione

or then make lunch because, dear doctor, I live alone!
o poi fare il pranzo perche', caro dottore, vive solo!

then I telephone, receives, make because the days long
Pio telefono, riceve, fare, perche' il giornate lungo

	ML	FS
Omission of function words	62% (108/173)	22% (54/242)
Function word substitution	2% (4/173)	20% (48/242)
Inflection/derivation errors	15% (5/33)	27% (75/275)

with translations provided for FS (Miceli & Caramazza, 1988), an Italian patient. Both patients omitted function words; FS in particular made numerous inflectional substitution errors (e.g., *leggeva* [he was reading] → *leggere* [to read]). If a lexical deficit involving an output component were to be the source of the observed omissions and substitutions, we would expect errors in other tasks involving that lexical component.

The performance patterns of the two patients can be directly compared on their ability to repeat single words: prefixed, suffixed, and function words (see Table 6.9). ML (Caramazza & Hillis, 1989a) made no errors on this task, whereas FS was similarly impaired across all word types. In addition, ML did not make errors of the sort observed in her spontaneous speech in any other task involving single word production: reading, repetition, or writing. This indicated that ML did not have a lexical deficit affecting function words and morphological affixes. In fact, we concluded that ML's deficit in sentence production could be attributed to an impairment at the level of the sentence planning mechanisms that specify the morphemes and function words to be selected from the output lexicons for production.

On the other hand, an analysis of FS's error types indicated a close resemblance between the errors observed in sentence production and those observed in repetition of single words. Consequently, in the case of FS, the role of a lexical deficit in sentence production could not be ruled out. We see once again that patients with apparently similar performance patterns may differ in terms of their underlying impairments: FS with a lexical deficit affecting sentence production and ML with apparently no deficit at the level of single words.

A more detailed analysis of the errors produced by FS in repetition of single words revealed aspects of the internal structure of the POL. We noticed that the majority of the errors (84.5%) were morphological in nature. Most of the morphologically based errors consisted of correct repetition of the stem of the stimulus word and the substitution of the affix (e.g., *vestire* [to wear] → *vestivi* [you were wearing]). Only 15.5% of

TABLE 6.9

Accuracy of Repetition Performance for ML and FS with Prefixed, Suffixed and Function Words

	ML	FS
Function words	100%	31%
Prefixed words	100%	48%
Suffixed words	100%	33%

the errors were phonemic paraphasias (e.g., *pagata* [paid] → *pagara* [nonword]). This distribution of errors suggests that, although FS had some impairment affecting the selection and/or the production of individual sounds, as evidenced by the phonemic paraphasias, such a deficit cannot account for the massive presence of morphological errors. It would appear, instead, that a deficit specifically affecting morphological structure played a major role in this FS's impairment.

Additionally, a striking feature of these morphologically based errors is that they were essentially all (615/637 or 96.7%) inflectional errors. This result suggested a selective deficit to mechanisms in the lexicon dedicated to inflectional processing. Comparable proportions of errors were made on derived and inflected words: 33.4% accuracy for each type in a specially designed list of derived and inflected words matched for length and frequency. Nonetheless, errors for both inflected and derived words consisted predominantly of inflectional errors. For example, the inflected word *leggeva* (he was reading) → *leggere* (to read) and the derived word *regionale* (regional, singular) → *regionali* (regional, plural).

Within the model of lexical processing proposed here, the deficit suffered by FS can best be described as an impairment to those processes that select specific affixes within the inflectional component of the lexicon. That is, the stems or root forms and derivational affixes are correctly selected, whereas inflectional affixes are often misselected. Such a deficit should give rise to the frequent inflectional substitutions observed in the course of sentence production and repetition.

This example illustrates the difficulties involved in attempts to develop legitimate categories of impairment (for detailed discussions of problems of classification and categorization, see Badecker & Caramazza, 1985; Caramazza, 1984, 1986; Ellis, 1987; McCloskey & Caramazza, 1988; but see also Shallice, 1988; Zurif et al., 1989; Caplan, 1986). The classification of a patient is based on the assumption that similar performance on one or more particular tasks—sentence production in this case—is the result of one or more similar deficits. Clearly then, classification is only warranted (a) to the extent to which one can motivate the assumption of similarity of underlying deficits or, alternatively, (b) to the extent to which it would not matter that patients similarly classified might differ in this fundamental respect.

Important in a consideration of alternative (a) is the nature of neurological impairment. The extent and location(s) of impairment will differ from patient to patient. Because of this, different cognitive functions may be affected in patients who otherwise share certain deficits. Thus, although two patients may have damage to the same underlying component, one of the two patients may have damage to additional components as well. Thus, similar performance on Tasks 1–5, suggesting an impairment to mechanism X, does not guarantee similar performance on Tasks 6–10. If performance on Tasks 1–5 is the classification or grouping criterion, then very heterogeneous groups may result. Within the common practices of research or treatment, group heterogeneity is extremely problematic. One cannot expect a positive outcome if patients grouped according to the criterion of agrammatism, for example, receive a common treatment. Similarly, research attempts to further our understanding of the cognitive system and its impairments will yield incorrect conclusions if such patients are grouped and conclusions are drawn based on average group results. For data and discussion of the heterogeneity of performance in aggrammatic production, see Miceli, Silveri, Romani, and Caramazza (1989) and Saffran, Berndt, and Schwartz (1989).

Although there may be purposes for which group heterogeneity with respect to underlying disfunction is unimportant, it is not obvious what these might be.

In this section, by examining two cases of apparently agrammatic aphasia, we illustrated the difficulties involved in attempts to classify and group patients, and found evidence that supports the notion that certain sentence production deficits can be understood, at least in part, as deficits to the morphological aspects of lexical processing, whereas others are best understood as impairments to processes specific to sentence planning.

Conclusion

With these examples, we hoped to show how patterns of impaired performance cannot be understood simply upon consideration of performance levels, error types, or the observation of dissociations or associations of symptoms. These overt manifestations of damage to the functional components of processing can be interpreted only within a theoretical framework that provides a basis for their interpretation. A detailed description of the possible underlying mechanisms and their functions is clearly necessary.

The level of detail at which theories need to be specified will become apparent when we evaluate the issue of whether impaired performance can be considered to result from damage to a representation itself— resulting in loss of the representation—or from damage to those mechanisms that access the representation—making the representation difficult to recover. Shallice (1987) discussed this issue and proposed a number of criteria which, he argued, can be used to distinguish deficits of storage from deficits of access. One criterion mentioned is consistency. Shallice argued that loss of a representation should result in the consistent inability to identify a given item across test sessions, whereas an access difficulty should result in inconsistent performance across repeated testing. We argue that this issue, like all others raised in this chapter, cannot be decided without making reference to a specific theory of lexical processing at the level of interest; in this case, a description of the structure of representations and access mechanisms will be required.

We have shown earlier that, without making reference to a theory indicating the possible processing components and their interrelationships, it could not be determined if a particular pattern of performance (e.g., the production of semantic errors) has only a single possible source. Likewise, it is impossible, without making reference to a description of mechanisms of access and storage, to determine if a particular pattern—in this case, inconsistent performance—can result only from damage to an access mechanism, while consistent performance results only from damage to a stored representation.

For example, one might imagine that the mechanism that accesses the POL from the semantic system works in the following manner. A semantic representation consisting of a set of features, such as <animal, mammal, domestic, four legged, hairy, barks, canine>, serves as input to the POL. Phonological representations in the POL are activated by the semantic input in proportion to the degree to which they share semantic features in their access specification. In this example, the phonological units /dag/, /bigl/, /kæt/, /lajən/, and so forth, are all activated to some degree, and the representation that receives the most activation, /dag/, may reach threshold for output and subsequent production. As discussed in an earlier section of this chapter, the ease (measured by accuracy or speed) with which a lexical representation reaches threshold is a function of at least two parameters: the degree of fit between the input and the access code for a representation, and the activation threshold of the representation (as indexed by frequency of usage). Thus where two or more phonological representations are equally activated by a semantic input, the lexical entry with the lowest threshold (most frequent) will be the one produced as a response (Caramazza & Hillis, 1990b).

Let us consider whether the consistency criterion proposed by Shallice (1987) distinguishes between access and storage deficits for this type of model of lexical access and representation. What are the expectations of damage to the access procedure? It depends on the assumptions we are willing to make about the consequences of damage to the hypothesized access procedure. Thus, for example, we might imagine that ONE consequence of brain damage is that semantic representations would activate phonological representations to a lesser extent than normal. In this case, the phonological representation for the correct response would still receive the most activation, but not necessarily enough to reach threshold. If, however, there is a semantically related lexical representation with a lower threshold of activation, it could be the one to reach threshold and to be produced CONSISTENTLY as a response. In such a situation, one would observe consistently incorrect responses to the target.[4]

Consider the case of damage to the stored semantic representations themselves. One type of damage could take the form of the "loss" of some of the features that comprise the meaning of words. One consequence of this situation would be that the semantic representation computed for an object would now be underspecified in such a way that it activates equally a number of phonological representations in the POL, including the correct one. For example, considering only the semantic category of animal terms, if damage were to result in the loss of all features except <animal, domestic, and hairy>, the residual information would activate equally *cat, dog, Pekingese,* and so forth. Assuming that the semantic information computed under the hypothesized conditions of damage is too impoverished to activate any one phonological representation to threshold, a response may be selected at random from the set of phonological representations that have the highest levels of activation, leading to inconsistent errors and error responses and, by chance, correct responses as well.

Thus, it is possible to articulate plausible models of lexical processing which, when damaged at the level of access procedures or stored representations, lead to expectations about the consistency of performance that are opposite those derived by Shallice (1987). Obviously, then, it is not possible to say, independently of a specific theory of lexical processing, that a particular pattern of consistency in performance signals a deficit to access mechanisms and another pattern of consistency of performance signals a deficit to stored representations. In other words, it is not possible to establish general criteria for determining when representations/access mechanisms are impaired without a description of the structure and function of the relevant mechanisms. More importantly for present purposes, we see that the kinds of expectations that we may derive from a model depend crucially on increasingly detailed claims

---

4. In the particular instantiation considered here, whether an item is consistently misnamed and whether a consistent error response is produced depends entirely on the distribution of thresholds of semantically related cohorts.

about the processing structure of the components that comprise a particular functional architecture.

We hope that we showed with this chapter how a theory is an enormously powerful and useful tool for the interpretation of human behavior—normal or impaired. Furthermore, we hope that it has become apparent that it is not the case that the need for theory can be dispensed with. All interpretation is based on some theory we have of cognitive structure; the theories simply differ in terms of the degree to which we are aware of them and of our use of them, and in terms of the level of detail at which they are described. If that is the case, then the progress we make in understanding language and cognitive disorders will depend to a large extent on our willingness and ability to develop theories that are both explicit and detailed.

Acknowledgments

The work on this chapter was supported by NIH grants NS22201 and 23836 to The Johns Hopkins University. We would like to thank Lisa Benzing, Argye Hillis, and Michael McCloskey for helpful comments.

References

Badecker, W., & Caramazza, A. (1985). On considerations of method and theory governing the use of clinical categories in neurolinguistics and cognitive neuropsychology: The case against agrammatism. *Cognition, 20,* 97–125.

Badecker, W., & Caramazza, A. (1989). Neurolinguistic studies of morphological processing: Toward a theory based assessment of language deficit. In E. Perecman (Ed.), *Integrating theory and practice in clinical neurology.* New York: IRBN Press.

Basso, A., Capitani, E., & Laiacona, M. (1988). Progressive language impairment without dementia: A case with isolated category specific naming defect. *Journal of Neurology, Neurosurgery and Psychiatry, 51,* 1201–1207.

Basso, A., Taborelli, A., & Vignolo, L. A. (1978). Dissociated disorders of speaking and writing in aphasia. *Journal of Neurology, Neurosurgery and Psychiatry, 41*(6), 556.

Baxter, D. M., & Warrington, K. E. (1987). Transcoding sound to spelling: Single or multiple sound unit correspondences. *Cortex, 23,* 653–666.

Baxter, D. M., & Warrington, K. E. (1985). Category-specific phonological dysgraphia. *Neuropsychologia, 23,* 11–28.

Beauvois, M. F. (1982). Optic aphasia: A process of interaction between vision and language. *Philosophical Transactions of the Royal Society of London,* Series B 298, 35–47.

Beauvois, M. F., & Derouesne, J. (1979). Phonological alexia: Three dissociations. *Journal of Neurology, Neurosurgery and Psychiatry, 42,* 1115–1124.

Beauvois, M. F., & Derouesne, J. (1981). Lexical or orthographic agraphia. *Brain, 104,* 21–49.

Beauvois, M. F., Saillant, B., Meininger, V., & Lhermitte, F. (1978). Bilateral tactile aphasia: A tacto-verbal dysfunction. *Brain, 101,* 381–401.

Behrmann, M., Moscovitch, M., Black, S. E., & Mozer, M. C. (in press). Perceptual and conceptual factors in neglect: Two contrasting case studies. *Brain.*

Berndt, R. S. (1987). Symptom co-occurrence and dissociation in the interpretation of agrammatism. In M. Coltheart, G. Sartori, & R. Job (Eds.), *The cognitive neuropsychology of language.* Hillsdale, NJ: Erlbaum.

Berndt, R. S. (1988). Category-specific deficits in aphasia. *Aphasiology, 3/4,* 237–240.

Berndt, R. S., & Caramazza, A. (1980). A redefinition of the syndrome of Broca's aphasia: Implications for a neuropsychological model of language. *Applied Psycholinguistics, 1,* 225–278.

Bub, D., Cancelliere, A., & Kertesz, A. (1985). Whole-word and analytic translation of spelling to sound in a non-semantic reader. In K. E. Patterson, J. C. Marshall, & M. Coltheart (Eds.), *Surface dyslexia.* London: Erlbaum.

Butterworth, B. (1983). Lexical representation. In B. Butterworth (Ed.), *Language production* (Vol. 2). London: Academic Press.

Campbell, R. (1983). Writing non-words to dictation. *Brain and Language, 19,* 153–178.

Caplan, D. (1986). In defense of agrammatism. *Cognition, 24,* 263–276.

Caramazza, A. (1984). The logic of neuropsychological research and the problem of patient classification in aphasia. *Brain and Language, 21,* 9–20.

Caramazza, A. (1986). On drawing inferences about the structure of normal cognitive systems from the analysis of patterns of impaired performance: The case for single patient studies. *Brain and Cognition, 5,* 41–66.

Caramazza, A. (1988). Some aspects of language processing revealed through the analysis of acquired aphasia: The lexical system. *Annual Review of Neuroscience, 11,* 395–421.

Caramazza, A., & Badecker, W. (1989). Patient classification in neuropsychological research. *Brain and Cognition, 16,* 256–295.

Caramazza, A., & Berndt, R. S. (1978). Semantic and syntactic processes in aphasia: A review of the literature. *Psychological Bulletin, 85,* 898–918.

Caramazza, A., & Hillis, A. E. (1989). The disruption of sentence production: Some dissociations. *Brain and Language, 36,* 625–650.

Caramazza, A., & Hillis, A. E. (1990a). Levels of representation, coordinate frames and unilateral neglect. *Cognitive Neuropsychology.*

Caramazza, A., & Hillis, A. E. (1990b). Where do semantic errors come from? *Cortex, 26,* 95–122.

Caramazza, A., Hillis, A. E., Rapp, B. C., & Romani, C. (1990). Multiple semantics or multiple confusions? *Cognitive Neuropsychology, 7(3),* 161–189.

Caramazza, A., Miceli, G., Silveri, M. C., & Laudanna, A. (1985). Reading mechanisms and the organization of the lexicon: Evidence from acquired dyslexia. *Cognitive Neuropsychology, 2,* 81–114.

Caramazza, A., Miceli, G., Villa, G., & Romani, C. (1987). The role of the graphemic buffer in spelling: Evidence from a case of acquired dysgraphia. *Cognition, 26,* 59–85.

Coltheart, M. (1978). Lexical access in simple reading tasks. In G. Underwood (Ed.), *Strategies of information processing.* London: Academic Press.

Coltheart, M., Patterson, K. E., & Marshall, J. C. (Eds.). (1980). *Deep dyslexia.* London: Routledge & Kegan Paul.

Costello, A. de L., & Warrington, E. K. (1987). Dissociation of visuo-spatial neglect and neglect dyslexia. *Journal of Neurology, Neurosurgery and Psychiatry, 50,* 1110–1116.

Cummings, D. W. (1988). *American English spelling.* Baltimore, MD: The Johns Hopkins University Press.

Denes, G., & Semenza, C. (1975). Auditory modality-specific anomia: Evidence from a case of pure word deafness. *Cortex, 11,* 401–411.

Dennis, M. (1976). Dissociated naming and locating of body parts after left anterior temporal lobe resection: An experimental case study. *Brain and Language, 3,* 147–163.

Ellis, A. (1987). Intimations of modularity, or, the modularity of mind. In M. Coltheart, G. Sartori, & R. Job (Eds.), *The cognitive neuropsychology of language.* London: Erlbaum.

Ellis, A., Flude, B. M., & Young, A. W. (1987). 'Neglect dyslexia' and the early visual processing of letters in words and nonwords. *Cognitive Neuropsychology, 4,* 439–464.

Funnell, E. (1983). Phonological processing reading: New evidence from acquired dyslexia. *British Journal of Psychology, 74,* 159–180.

Goodglass, H., & Budin, C. (1988). Category and modality specific dissociations in word comprehension and concurrent phonological dyslexia. *Neuropsychologia, 26,* 67–78.

Goodglass, H., & Kaplan, E. (1972). *The Boston Diagnostic Aphasia Examination.* Philadelphia, PA: Lea Febiger.

Goodglass, H., Klein, B., Carey, P., & Jones, K. J. (1966). Specific semantic word categories in aphasia. *Cortex, 2,* 74–89.

Goodman, R. A., & Caramazza, A. (1986a). Aspects of the spelling process: Evidence from a case of acquired dysgraphia. *Language and Cognitive Processes, 1*(4), 263–296.

Goodman, R. A., & Caramazza, A. (1986b). Dissociation of spelling errors in written and oral spelling: The role of allographic conversion in writing. *Cognitive Neuropsychology, 3* (2), 179–206.

Gordon, B. (1983). Lexical access and lexical decision: Mechanisms of frequency sensitivity. *Journal of Verbal Learning and Verbal Behavior, 22,* 146–160.

Gordon, B., Goodman-Schulman, R. A., & Caramazza, A. (1987). *Separating the stages of reading errors.* (Reports of the Cognitive Neuropsychology Laboratory, No. 28). Baltimore, MD: The Johns Hopkins University.

Hanna, R. R., Hanna, J. S., Hodges, R. E., & Rudorf, E. H. (1966). *Phoneme-grapheme correspondences as cues to spelling improvement.* U.S. Department of Health, Education and Welfare, Office of Education, Washington, DC: U.S. Government Printing Office.

Hart, J., Berndt, R., & Caramazza, A. (1985). Category-specific naming deficit following cerebral infarction. *Nature (London), 316,* 439–440.

Henderson, L. (1989). On mental representation of morphology and its diagnosis by measures of visual access speed. In W. Marslen-Wilson (Ed.), *Lexical representation and process.* Cambridge, MA: MIT Press.

Hillis, A. (1988). *"Optic aphasia": A breakdown between visual recognition and semantic interpretation?* Paper presented at the annual convention of the American Speech-Language-Hearing Association, Boston, MA.

Hillis, A. E., & Caramazza, A. (1989). The graphemic buffer and attentional mechanisms. *Brain and Language, 36,* 208–235.

Hillis, A. E., & Caramazza, A. (in press). *Category-specific naming and comprehension impairment: A double dissociation. Brain.*

Hillis, A. E., & Caramazza, A. (in press). The reading process and its disorders. In D. Margolin (Ed.), *Cognitive neuropsychology in clinical practice.* New York: Oxford University Press.

Hillis, A. E., Rapp, B. C., Romani, C., & Caramazza, A. (1990). Selective impairment of semantics in lexical processing. *Cognitive Neuropsychology, 7(3),* 191–243.

Howes, D., & Solomon, R. L. (1951). Visual duration thresholds as a function of word probability. *Journal of Verbal Learning and Verbal Behavior, 20,* 417–430.

Humphreys, G., & Evett, L. (1985). Are there independent lexical and nonlexical routes in word processing? An evaluation of the dual-route theory of reading. *Behavioral and Brain Sciences, 8*(4), 689–739.

Jackendoff, R. (1983). *Semantics and cognition*. Cambridge, MA: MIT Press.

Kean, M.-L. (Ed.). (1985). *Agrammatism*. Orlando, FL: Academic Press.

Kinsbourne, M., & Rosenfeld, D. B. (1974). Agraphia selective for written spelling. *Brain and Language, 1*, 215–225.

Kinsbourne, M., & Warrington, E. K. (1962). A variety of reading disability associated with right hemisphere lesions. *Journal of Neurology, Neurosurgery and Psychiatry, 28*, 563–567.

Kinsbourne, M., & Warrington, E. K. (1965). A case showing selectively impaired oral spelling. *Journal of Neurology, Neurosurgery and Psychiatry, 28*, 563–566.

Kolk, H. H. J., & Van Grunsven, M. J. F. (1985). Agrammatism as a variable phenomenon. *Cognitive Neuropsychology, 2*, 347–384.

Lesser, R. (1978). *Linguistic investigation of aphasia*. London: Arnold.

Lhermitte, E., & Beauvois, M. F. (1973). A visual-speech disconnexion syndrome: Report of a case with optic aphasia, agnosic alexia and colour agnosia. *Brain, 96*, 695–714.

Marshall, J. C., & Newcombe, F. (1966). Syntactic and semantic errors in paralexia. *Neuropsychologia, 4*, 169–176.

Marshall, J. C., & Newcombe, F. (1973). Patterns of paralexia: A psycholinguistic approach. *Journal of Psycholinguistic Research, 2*, 175–199.

McCarthy, R., & Warrington, E. K. (1985). Category specificity in an agrammatic patient: The relative impairment of verb retrieval and comprehension. *Neuropsychologia, 23*, 709–727.

McCarthy, R. A., & Warrington, E. K. (1988). Evidence for modality-specific meaning systems in the brain. *Nature (London), 334*(4), 428–430.

McCloskey, M., & Caramazza, A. (1988). Theory and methodology in cognitive neuropsychology: A response to our critics. *Cognitive Neuropsychology, 5*(5), 583–623.

McKenna, P., & Warrington, E. K. (1978). Category-specific naming preservation: A single case study. *Journal of Neurology, Neurosurgery and Psychiatry, 41*, 571–574.

Meyer, D. E., & Schvaneveldt, R. W. (1971). Facilitation in recognizing pairs of words: Evidence of a dependence between retrieval operations. *Journal of Experimental Psychology, 90*, 227–334.

Miceli, G, & Caramazza, A. (1988). Dissociation of inflectional and derivational morphology. *Brain and Language, 35*, 24–65.

Miceli, G., Silveri, C., & Caramazza, A. (1987). The role of the phoneme-to-grapheme system and of the graphemic output buffer in writing: Evidence from an Italian case of pure dysgraphia. In M. Coltheart, G. Sartori, & R. Job (Eds.), *Cognitive neuropsychology of language*. London: Erlbaum.

Miceli, G., Silveri, C., Nocentini, U., & Caramazza, A. (1988). Patterns of dissociation in comprehension and production of nouns and verbs. *Aphasiology, 2*, 351–358.

Miceli, G., Silveri, C., Romani, C., & Caramazza, A. (1989). Variations in the pattern of omissions and substitutions of grammatical morphemes in the spontaneous speech of so-called agrammatic patients. *Brain and Language, 36*, 447–492.

Miceli, G., Silveri, C., Villa, G., & Caramazza, A. (1984). On the basis for the agrammatic's difficulty in producing main verbs. *Cortex, 20*, 207–220.

Michel, F. (1979). Preservation du langage écrit malgré un déficit majeur du language oral. *Lyon Medical, 241*, 141–149.

Miller, G. A., & Johnson-Laird, P. N. (1976). *Language and perception*. Cambridge, MA: Harvard University Press.

Morton, J. (1969). The interaction of information in word recognition. *Psychological Review, 76*, 165–178.

Morton, J. (1981). The status of information processing models of language. *Philosophical Transactions of the Royal Society of London, 295*, 387–396.

Morton, J., & Patterson, K. (1980). A new attempt at an interpretation, or, an attempt at a new interpretation. In M. Coltheart, K. Patterson, & J. Marshall (Eds.), *Deep dyslexia*. London: Routledge & Kegan Paul.

Nolan, K., & Caramazza, A. (1982). Modality-independent impairments in word processing in a deep dyslexic patient. *Brain and Language, 16*, 237–264.

Patterson, K. E. (1978). Phonemic dyslexia: Errors of meaning and the meaning of errors. *Quarterly Journal of Experimental Psychology, 30*, 587–601.

Patterson, K. E., & Besner, D. (1984). Is the right hemisphere literate? *Cognitive Neuropsychology, 1*(4), 315–341.

Patterson, K. E., & Marcel, A. d. (1977). Aphasia, dyslexia and the phonological coding of written words. *Quarterly Journal of Experimental Psychology, 29*, 307–318.

Patterson, K. E., Marshall, J. C., & Coltheart, M. (Eds.). (1985). *Surface dyslexia*. London: Erlbaum.

Posteraro, L., Zinelli, P., & Mazzucchi, A. (1988). Selective impairment of the graphemic buffer in acquired dysgraphia: A case study. *Brain and Language, 35*, 274–286.

Rabinowicz, B., & Moscovitch, M. (1984). Right hemisphere literacy: A critique of some recent approaches. *Cognitive Neuropsychology, 1*(4), 343–350.

Riddoch, M. J., & Humphreys, G. (1987). Visual object processing in optic aphasia: A case of semantic access agnosia. *Cognitive Neuropsychology, 4*, 131–185.

Riddoch, M. J., Humphreys, G., Coltheart, M., & Funnell, E. (1988). Semantic systems or system? Neuropsychological evidence re-examined. *Cognitive Neuropsychology, 5*, 3–25.

Saffran, E. M., Berndt, R. S., & Schwartz, M. (1989). The quantitative analysis of agrammatic production: Procedure and data. *Brain and Language, 37*, 440–479.

Saffran, E. M., Bogyo, L. C., Schwartz, M., & Marin, O. S. M. (1980). Does deep dyslexia reflect right-hemisphere reading? In M. Coltheart, K. E. Patterson, & J. Marshall (Eds.), *Deep dyslexia*. London: Routledge & Kegan Paul.

Saffran, E. M., & Marin, O. S. M. (1977). Reading without phonology. *Quarterly Journal of Experimental Psychology, 29*, 515–525.

Sanders, R., & Caramazza, A. (1990). Operation of the phoneme-to-grapheme conversion mechanism in a brain injured patient. *Journal of Reading and Writing, 2*(1), 61–82.

Sartori, G., & Job, R. (1988). The oyster with four legs: A neuropsychological study on the interaction of visual and semantic information. *Cognitive Neuropsychology, 5*, 105–133.

Semenza, C., & Zettin, M. (1989). Evidence from aphasia for the role of proper names as pure referring expressions. *Nature (London), 342*, 678–679.

Shallice, T. (1981). Neurological impairment of cognitive processes. *British Medical Bulletin, 37*, 187–192.

Shallice, T. (1987). Impairments of semantic processing: multiple dissociations. In M. Coltheart, G. Sartori, & R. Job (Eds.), *The cognitive neuropsychology of language*. London: Erlbaum.

Shallice, T. (1988). *From neuropsychology to mental structure*. Cambridge: Cambridge University Press.

Shallice, T., & Warrington, E. K. (1975). Word recognition in a phonemic dyslexic patient. *Quarterly Journal of Experimental Psychology, 27*, 187–199.

Silveri, M. C., & Gainotti, G. (1988). Interaction between vision and language in category specific semantic impairment for living things. *Cognitive Neuropsychology, 5*, 677–709.

Taft, M. (1985). The decoding of words in lexical access: A review of the morphographic approach. In D. Besner, T. G. Waller, & G. E. Mackinnon (Eds.), *Reading research: Advances in theory and practice* (Vol. 5). Orlando, FL: Academic Press.

Venezky, R. (1970). *The structure of english orthography*. The Hague: Mouton.

Warrington, E. K. (1975). The selective impairment of semantic memory. *Quarterly Journal of Experimental Psychology, 27*, 635–657.

Warrington, E. K. (1981a). Neuropsychological studies of verbal semantic systems. *Philosophical Transactions of the Royal Society of London, Series* B 295, 411–423.

Warrington, E. K. (1981b). Concrete word dyslexia. *British Journal of Psychology, 72*, 175–196.

Warrington, E. K., & McCarthy, R. A. (1983). Category specific access dysphasia. *Brain, 106*, 859–878.

Warrington, E. K., & McCarthy, R. A. (1987). Categories of knowledge: Further fractionation and an attempted integration. *Brain, 110*, 1273–1296.

Warrington, E. K., & McCarthy, R. A. (1988). Evidence for modality-specific meaning systems in the brain. *Nature (London), 334*, 428–430.

Warrington, E. K., & Shallice, T. (1984). Category specific semantic impairments. *Brain, 197*, 829–854.

Wing, A. M., & Baddeley, A. D. (1980). Spelling errors in handwriting: A corpus and a distributional analysis. In U. Frith (Ed.), *Cognitive processes in spelling*. London: Academic Press.

Zaidel, E., & Schweiger, A. (1984). On wrong hypotheses about the right hemisphere: Commentary on K. E. Patterson and D. Besner, "Is the right hemisphere literate?" *Cognitive Neuropsychology, 1*(4), 351–364.

Zingeser, L. B., & Berndt, R. S. (1988). Grammatical class and context effects in a case of pure anomia: Implications for models of language production. *Cognitive Neuropsychology, 5*(4), 473–516.

Zurif, E., Gardner, H., & Brownell, H. (1989). The case against the case against agrammatism. *Brain and Cognition, 10*, 237–255.

7

Sentence Processing in Aphasia

RITA SLOAN BERNDT

The capacity for producing and comprehending sentences is the feature of human language that most clearly distinguishes it from other systems of communication. All known languages provide some means for combining a finite number of words to create an infinite number of well-formed and interpretable sentences. This "generative" capacity of language appears to be unique to humans, and it emerges consistently (and early) in the communicative attempts of normal children. Although they have been studied and described from many different perspectives in the 30 years since the publication of Chomsky's (1957) *Syntactic Structures*, the syntactic representations and processes that underlie sentence formulation and interpretation are still debated (Bock, 1987b; Frazier, 1988).

A widely held and long-standing belief is that studies of aphasia can contribute to our understanding not only of how the brain carries out this unique human activity (DeBleser, 1987), but of how syntactic processes function in the normal speaker–listener (Caramazza & Berndt, 1987; Lesser, 1978; Saffran, 1982). In 1981, when the first edition of *Acquired Aphasia* was published, there was considerable optimism that studies of aphasia could indeed place strong constraints on the form that candidate models of sentence processing could take. In a chapter of that volume entitled "Syntactic Aspects of Aphasia," Berndt and Caramazza set out the testable (and, as it turned out, quite easily falsifiable) hypothesis that a form of aphasia (AGRAMMATISM) existed with a set of symptoms that reflected a central syntactic impairment that affected performance (in all modalities) in all tasks that require syntactic processing, that is, in the production and comprehension of written or spoken sentences.

ACQUIRED APHASIA, SECOND EDITION

Had this thesis been upheld, it would have indicated that the same set of syntactic representations are exploited in comprehension and production. Although intuitively appealing, this view remains largely unsupported (see Shallice, 1988, for a recent review). Moreover, the selective impairment of syntactic capacities in agrammatism would have provided an extraordinary opportunity for the investigation of other aspects of language (phonology, semantics, pragmatics) in relative isolation from syntax. Unfortunately (perhaps), this strong version of the syntactic deficit hypothesis (see Schwartz, Linebarger, & Saffran, 1985, for other possible versions) was not supported by subsequent investigations of individual cases. These studies uncovered multiple dissociations among the set of symptoms that had been argued to arise from a single, syntactic deficit (for reviews, see Caramazza & Berndt, 1985; Howard, 1985; Goodglass & Menn, 1985).

Contemporary research on sentence processing in aphasia, to be reviewed here, presents a much more complicated, but in some ways more optimistic, picture. Although it now seems unlikely that studies of sentence processing in aphasia will uncover a deficient set of syntactic representations or operations that can be interpreted in linguistic terms, the processes that now appear to be most affected in many patients may prove to be more amenable to remediation than had they actually reflected a "loss" of syntactic representations (Saffran & Schwartz, 1988). At least preliminary indications are that some sentence processing impairments can be improved by focusing attention on a theoretically defined element within a general model of sentence processing. These possibilities will be reviewed in the conclusion of this chapter.

The Syntactic Deficit Hypothesis (Circa 1980)

The notion that brain damage could selectively affect individual components of the normal language system was based on long-standing distinctions among aphasic symptoms that were associated with different sites of focal left-hemisphere lesions. Foremost among these distinctions for accounts of sentence processing is the difference between agrammatism and paragrammatism (Kleist, 1916). More recent summaries of this dichotomy (Goodglass, 1968) have emphasized the following characteristics: Agrammatic speakers produce halting, effortful attempts at communication that frequently result in incomplete, fragmented sentences in which syntactic complexity is reduced from normal levels and content words (especially nouns) are produced much more frequently than are grammatical words (articles, pronouns, auxiliary verbs, and some prepositions). Bound grammatical elements (especially verb inflections) are frequently omitted, and auditory comprehension is relatively spared. The following is an excerpt of a patient classified as agrammatic recounting the fairy tale, "Cinderella":

> Cinderella (5 sec) mother and one two sisters (9 sec) two sisters is (4 sec) pants shoes (5 sec) "what's wrong? you stay home Cinderella" [spoken with character voice] (2 sec) two sisters at a ball (3 sec) a magic wand (2 sec) nice lady (2 sec) her godmother (2 sec) "what's wrong?" [character voice] (3 sec) at the ball no money

Paragrammatic speakers produce sentences, including grammatical elements, fluently and with apparent ease, although often incorrectly. Content words (especially nouns) are frequently the source of phonemic error, and grammatical words and inflections may be inappropriately substituted for one another. Comprehension even of isolated content words is impaired. The following is a partial transcription of "Cinderella" from a patient whose speech demonstrates characteristics of paragrammatism:

> Cinderella /rotərəf/ grandmother and two /mɪf/ sisters . . . her /smʌf/ mother was mad was mad to her sisters . . . and she came hoping to be that she could've been chosen as the for the /s/ /s/ /s/ /prɪrz/ and had to go the but she had to leave before they /faɪned/ nine o'seven o'clock . . . and then . . . the one that was listen to find the whole whole kingdom . . .

Although it was clear even 10 years ago that the range of syntactic structures produced by paragrammatic speakers was subnormal (Gleason et al., 1980), virtually all discussion of syntactic impairment in aphasia focused on agrammatism.

The psychologically and linguistically motivated accounts of agrammatism (as opposed to more neuroanatomically oriented accounts) can be divided, roughly, into three types. One approach attempted to explain the omission of grammatical elements in sentence production through the operation of phonological principles (Goodglass, 1976; Kean, 1978). These accounts differed importantly, however, in terms of the database they attempted to explain. Goodglass and colleagues focused on actual data from patients in a variety of contexts (Goodglass & Berko, 1960; Goodglass, Fodor, & Schulhoff, 1967), and Kean focused on an "idealized agrammatism" that has never been reported in pure form.

Other approaches were motivated by the occurrence among agrammatic speakers of an auditory comprehension disorder that could be demonstrated only in tasks that were especially designed to REQUIRE the patient to process the structure, as well as the word meanings, in sentences, (Caramazza & Zurif, 1976; Heilman & Scholes, 1976). These arguments can be distinguished further into those in which impaired processing of grammatical morphemes was believed to be the primary deficit (Bradley, Garrett, & Zurif, 1980; Zurif, 1982), and those in which an impairment in the processing of grammatical morphemes was thought to reflect a more basic deficit to syntactic processing that also compromised the interpretation and production of word order (Berndt & Caramazza, 1980; Saffran, Schwartz, & Marin, 1980a; Schwartz, Saffran, & Marin, 1980).

All of these attempts to explain the sentence processing deficits of agrammatism have been undermined (albeit to somewhat differing degrees) by three major findings that have emerged from recent research.

Overlap Among the Symptoms of Agrammatism and Paragrammatism

The emphasis on agrammatism that has characterized recent research in sentence processing in aphasia gained a major impetus from the double dissociation of that "syndrome" from paragrammatism. This double dissociation was an effective and persuasive rebuttal to the argument that structural elements of sentences are particularly susceptible to any sort of processing disruption, perhaps because of their relative lack of "content." Moreover, the agrammatism/paragrammatism distinction fueled speculation that the neuroanatomical site subserving syntactic processes was discrete enough to be discoverable (Caramazza & Zurif, 1976).

Several findings have blurred the sharp distinction between agrammatism and paragrammatism. First, when differences in fluency are ignored (these differences are, after all, not necessary to the syntactic arguments), the sentence production patterns of the two types of patients show considerable overlap. Agrammatic speakers frequently substitute among, rather than omit, grammatical morphemes, and this is especially (but not only) true for the bound grammatical morphemes of languages in which the omission of an inflection yields a nonlexical stem (Grodzinsky, 1984; Miceli & Mazzucchi, 1990). Furthermore, paragrammatic patients sometimes omit, rather than substitute, grammatical markers and produce other structurally aberrant sentences that are not easily interpretable as resulting from lexical substitutions or semantic error (Butterworth & Howard, 1987). Finally, the syntactic comprehension impairment that has been found among agrammatic aphasics also has been found among some patients whose speech is best characterized as paragrammatic (Caramazza, Berndt, & Basili, 1983; Martin & Blossom-Stach, 1986). The agrammatism/paragrammatism distinction has been criticized on a variety of other grounds (Heeschen, 1985; Heeschen & Kolk, 1988), including even its historical adequacy. DeBleser (1987) has translated a number of papers from the early German aphasia literature demonstrating clear appreciation for the considerable overlap of omission and substitution symptoms even within the same patient.

Thus, there is some basis for the belief that sentence processing deficits may take a variety of forms, may co-occur with many other symptoms of aphasia, and may be associated with lesions to a number of different neuroanatomical regions.

Dissociation of Sentence Production from Comprehension

The strongest version of the syntactic deficit hypothesis of agrammatism emphasized the similar nature of the comprehension and production symptoms that were found among agrammatic speakers. Although such co-occurrence continues to be the rule rather than the exception, a number of patients have been described with the agrammatic pattern of omission of grammatical morphemes who demonstrate normal comprehension (Caramazza & Hillis, 1989; Kolk, Van Grunsven, & Keyser, 1985; Miceli, Mazzucchi, Menn, & Goodglass, 1983; Nespoulos et al., 1988). The problem presented by this dissociation for the syntactic deficit hypothesis is that it suggests that BOTH comprehension and production symptoms do not arise from a single functional impairment. It is possible that more detailed study of the production pattern of agrammatic speakers will uncover symptoms that are necessarily related to the comprehension patterns (Berndt, 1987). Nonetheless, it is clear that the omission of grammatical morphemes in spontaneous speech is not necessarily related to a sentence comprehension impairment.

Dissociations Among the Symptoms of Agrammatic Production

The "idealized agrammatism" that was the focus of much early attention is not a very good description of the sentences produced by most patients. Dissociations have been found in individual patients (a) between grammatical morpheme omission and other sentence structural abnormalities (Berndt, 1987; Kolk & Van Grunsven, 1985; Miceli et al., 1983; Saffran, Schwartz, & Marin, 1980b); (b) between bound and freestanding grammatical morphemes (Miceli & Mazzucchi, 1990; Saffran, Berndt, & Schwartz, 1989); and (c) among specific elements WITHIN the classes of freestanding and bound grammatical morphemes (Miceli, Silveri, Romani, & Caramazza, 1989). Some of these patterns were described some years ago by Tissot, Mounin, and Lhermitte (1973), who distinguished among three types of grammatical disturbance: (a) fragmented, halting, and limited speech output, but without major structural errors; (b) a primarily morphological impairment in which bound and freestanding grammatical markers are omitted but word order is intact; and (c) a primarily constructional impairment in which sentences are virtually nonexistent but morphological elements are produced. More recent descriptions have uncovered an even more complex set of patterns; it is unlikely that a linguistically motivated framework can be offered that would predict all of them.

Other approaches can be adopted to the problem of symptom variability, however. Kolk and colleagues have developed a model of sentence processing in aphasia that readily accommodates (even predicts) all of the above-described types of variability (Kolk & Van Grunsven, 1985; Kolk et al., 1985). Within this framework, several possible deficits are described that could undermine patients' attempts to comprehend and/or to produce sentences. None of these postulates a loss of syntactic representations or processing mechanisms; instead, they constitute a possible set of performance limitations. For example, some aspects of patient performance might be interpreted as a result of short-term memory limitation. Alternatively, performance might be undermined by changes in the thresholds of word activation or an increase in noise in the system (Stemberger, 1984), or to an exacerbated decay rate caused by pathological delays in patients' processing.

The patients' methods of adapting to these limitations is the important aspect of Kolk's model. Faced with the likelihood of failing to articulate a well-formed sentence, patients will adopt a number of positive and negative adaptations: they might choose simple sentence forms with predictable structures and/or they might omit unessential items. In fact, they might adopt any of the characteristics of the "simplified speech register" of normal speakers trying to make themselves understood to a foreigner. This adaptation theory differs qualitatively from other models to be reviewed herein, all of which assume that the observable behavior is the result of the patient's deficit, accompanied, perhaps, by a limited number of specified heuristics that might be adopted for specific tasks. Both the advantages and the disadvantages of Kolk's model stem from the same fact: the theory is unaffected by demonstration of dissociations among symptoms. Since symptom dissociations are at present the major evidentiary base that constrains neuropsychological modeling, Kolk's model is difficult to test. It would appear, however, that the model predicts that the precise form that a patient's symptoms take (substitutions, omissions, etc.) should be subject to change through therapeutic intervention. To date there have been no reports of attempts to change patients' adaptive responses, but it is possible that some aspects of the model might be tested in this way.

The listing of symptom dissociations summarized above has left us with few obvious candidates for a unitary account of sentence processing deficits in aphasia. In fact, the seemingly limitless possibilities for symptom patterns have stimulated a call for abandonment of the syndrome-driven approach to aphasia research (Caramazza, 1986), an attack on the theoretical utility of the concept of agrammatism (Badecker & Caramazza, 1985), and a lively debate on these issues (see, e.g., *Brain and Cognition, 10*(2), 1989; *Cognitive Neuropsychology, 5*(5), 1988).

These methodological discussions should not be allowed to overshadow the valuable contribution that recent work on agrammatism has made to our appreciation of the variety of sentence processing deficits that can occur in aphasia, and to the methods used to study them. First, the time appears to be past when theories of aphasia were offered based on "idealized" syndromes. The standard currently requires real data from patients who are described in some detail. Second, several studies are now available that include systematic analysis of sentence production (Butterworth & Howard, 1987; Miceli et al., 1989), at least one of which was designed to be replicable (Saffran et al., 1989). It is not inconceivable that some reasonably objective set of sentence production symptoms may be uncovered that will prove to be theoretically defensible as a grouping criterion. Third, a rich source of information about sentence processing in aphasia is now available (in English) for patients speaking a variety of different languages. Studies of Dutch-speaking patients by Kolk and colleagues and of Italian-speaking patients by Miceli and colleagues have proven to be important sources of information about the variety of ways that sentence processing symptoms can dissociate. Large multilanguage studies are currently under way (e.g., Menn & Obler, 1990) which will allow detailed consideration of the potential for impairment of sentence structural elements in a range of languages along the continuum from highly configurational to highly inflectional. Studies of aphasic speakers of languages other than English are needed to address issues such as the relative vulnerability to brain damage of the different means available in human languages for encoding sentence structural information. We are only now beginning to reap the benefits of these analyses.

The remainder of this chapter will review recent findings on sentence processing in aphasia against the background of patient variability reviewed above. To limit the complexity (and length) of this review, the focus is on auditory-verbal language. Thus, dissociations of verbal from written language will not be considered.[1]

Sentence Production

A Model of Normal Production

The ease with which normal speakers produce complex and well-formed sentences should not be taken as evidence that sentence production is a simple matter. The problem that must be explained by models of normal sentence production is formidable: How does the human speaker constrain what may be a complex, multidimensional conceptual "message" into a linear string of correctly chosen words that conveys to a listener the basic information about "who does what to whom," as well as other information such as when, how, and why they did it? For English speakers, the linguistic devices that must be considered in structuring an utterance to convey such information include the order in which words are produced, as well as a relatively small number of bound and freestanding grammatical morphemes (e.g., verb inflections, auxiliary verbs, determiners). One critical issue is how lexical information is coordinated with these different structural devices during the act of speaking (Bock, 1987b).

The model of normal sentence production that has dominated attempts to explain sentences produced by aphasic patients is built upon a database of speech errors produced by normal speakers (Fromkin, 1973; Garrett, 1975, 1980). Regularities in the occurrence of particular error types suggest that there are two separate steps in the structural formulation of a sentence that take place after the conceptual message has been generated and before the relevant phonetic representation specifies the identity of the sounds that will need to be articulated.

---

1. This limitation to auditory-verbal language also means that this text does not consider other types of communication systems that might involve sentence processing. For example, Weinrich et al. (1989) demonstrated remarkable sparing of comprehension of some aspects of syntax in a globally aphasic patient trained with a computerized, iconographic visual communication system (C-VIC). The extent to which C-VIC exploits the same lexical and syntactic representations that are used in auditory-verbal processing is a question of considerable theoretical interest that is currently under investigation.

The first of these two (labeled the FUNCTIONAL level) is a level of representation that serves to guide the coordination problem: based on conceptual information in the intended message, clause-size units of semantically specified lexical items are assigned roles in a predicate–argument-type structure. At this level only the semantic–syntactic identity of the words to be spoken is available (not pronunciation), and this representation is marked in some fashion as to the roles they will play in the ultimate sentence (e.g., a noun might be marked as agent of the action, or as logical subject of the predicate).[2] This abstract, unordered representation of marked lexical information serves as input to the "positional level": phrase-size units of ordered words are created through the insertion of phonologically specified lexical elements into a syntactic frame made up of bound and freestanding grammatical elements. This representation, which also includes some information about phrasal stress assignment, provides a basis for the elaboration of phonetic form and the creation of the next (PHONETIC) level of representation.

One important aspect of the processing that is presumably carried out between the functional and positional levels is that the creation of the structural frame at the positional level, as well as the ultimate insertion of words into that frame, is only partly conditioned by the assignment of logical roles at the functional level. For example, the functional level representation of the two sentences

$$\text{The boy kisses the girl} \tag{1}$$

and

$$\text{The girl is kissed by the boy} \tag{2}$$

2. Garrett (1975, 1980) did not state explicitly the type of formal representation that is available at the functional level, because the speech error data do not provide evidence that allows an unambiguous characterization. Moreover, it appears that the original model adopted representational assumptions that were closely tied to the currently prevailing model of transformational grammar; thus, the tendency is to align the functional level with "deep structures" and the positional level with "surface structures." As the linguistic theories changed to grant more importance to lexically specified information (see Wasow, 1985), the characterization of the levels themselves changed somewhat. For example, Garrett (1982) described the functional level of representation as involving predicate–argument structures, which he characterizes as "more abstract" than deep structures. Other interpretations of the functional level representation characterize the information represented at this level more semantically, that is, as thematic roles such as AGENT (the one causing the action), PATIENT (the one who is acted upon), and so forth. For present purposes, the important point is that the roles that semantic entities play in the message to be conveyed are represented at the functional level in a form that is very abstract, devoid of the information about word pronunciation and order that is represented at the positional level.

is essentially the same; different surface manifestations occur because the syntactic frame available at the positional level assigns the role of grammatical subject to the logical subject (or thematic agent) in Sentence 1, but assigns the role of grammatical subject to the logical object (or thematic patient) in Sentence 2. The factors that determine which syntactic frame will emerge at the positional level were not spelled out in Garrett's model, nor were the processes that support the "mapping" from logical to grammatical roles in the creation of the positional level.

In fact, attention to these kinds of issues requires consideration of an information base other than the occurrence of normal speech errors. For example, the formulation of a sentence in the passive rather than active voice (such as in the examples above) appears to be motivated by a variety of pragmatic and contextual constraints that prevail as messages are being formulated (Levelt, 1989). In addition, a number of factors that affect the relative accessibility of words during sentence formulation can have predictable effects on the syntactic frames chosen (Bock, 1982, 1987a).

Several lines of experimental investigation have converged in recent years on variants of Garrett's model that allow for considerably more interaction between lexical retrieval and the formulation of a syntactic structure than is allowed in the strictly one-directional model sketched above (Bock, 1987b; Dell, 1986). In part, these modifications of the model have been motivated by a reconsideration of the normal speech error corpora that suggests considerable influence of phonological factors on the commission of functional level errors (Dell & Reich, 1981; Stemberger, 1985). These data, along with experimental results demonstrating small but consistent effects of phonological priming on the selection of syntactic structures such as active and passive voice (Bock, 1987a), indicate that some phonologically specified lexical information (from the positional level) must be available to influence the assignment of logical roles at the functional level. Because retrieval of the phonological forms of words is a problem experienced by many aphasic patients, this modification to the model may allow consideration of a possibly systematic relationship between lexical retrieval problems and the production of syntactically deviant sentences. This possibility will be considered below.

Another type of modification of Garrett's model relevant to interpretation of aphasic deficits has been made explicit by Bock (1987b), but was alluded to by Garrett himself as a possibility that was not precluded by the available data (1980, p. 217). This change involves the specification of the roles assigned to lexical items at the functional level, with Bock arguing that words are assigned directly to grammatical functions corresponding to roles in the surface structure (Bock, 1987b, p.

372). Bock made two assertions within this formulation to account for the speech error data and for a series of experimental results: first, variations in the "conceptual accessibility" of words will greatly influence assignment of words to grammatical functions such as subject and object, and second, the grammatical subject of the sentence will be assigned first, unless there are strong contraindications.

In Bock's model, much that determines the ultimate form a sentence will take occurs prior to this level of "functional integration": words become differentially active because of previously occurring sentences, other conversational or environmental influences, or experimental semantic priming. Some of these words are verbs that carry with them inherent information about functional relations, that is, about the mappings between thematic roles and grammatical roles. Different forms of the same verb (e.g., active and passive forms) become available, and these different forms have different "base" strengths, with the active form more likely to prevail. Functional integration involves linking together these activated elements according to the functional relations specified by the verb, beginning with the assignment of a word to the role of grammatical subject.

Thus, the most activated or accessible nominal concepts are linked to the sentence subject role, and most often linked to the active verb form that has a higher base level of activation, producing an active voice sentence. However, if the noun with the thematic role of patient rather than that of agent in an event is for some reason more accessible, the verb form will be overridden and the (thematic) patient/(grammatical) subject will be linked to a passive verb form. The functional representation created initiates two further processes: the generation of constituent structures and the retrieval of lexical–phonological representations. Bock (1987b) reviewed evidence indicating that differential activation levels of phonological representations exert an influence on the order in which words are produced within constituents. Thus, there are two separate points in Bock's formulation at which disruption in the retrieval of lexical information could interfere with the successful formulation of a syntactic structure.

One of the most important differences between Garrett's and Bock's models for purposes of interpreting data from aphasia concerns the different approaches they take to the mapping between thematic or logical roles (who is doing what to whom) and grammatical roles (sentence subject, object). While supplying no details about the processes that might be involved, Garrett's model identifies separate representational levels for the two types of information (functional level for logical roles, positional level for grammatical roles), suggesting that some processes that link nouns at the two levels must be carried out. In contrast, Bock assigned this mapping function to the lexical representations of verbs. For example, part of what is activated with a concept involving a transfer of goods between two persons is that (at least) two verbs could pertain, one mapping the thematic role of agent onto the grammatical subject ("give"), the other mapping the thematic role of goal onto the grammatical subject ("receive"). The implications of these differences in accounting for patients' production deficits, and for approaching remediation of those deficits, are discussed below.

Interpreting Sentence Production Deficits from the Normal Model

Garrett (1982) interpreted the description of agrammatism (i.e., deficient grammatical morpheme production with spared lexical production) and jargonaphasia (i.e., spared grammatical morpheme production with impaired lexical production) as evidence in support of the distinction within his model between open class (content) words and closed class (grammatical) elements. Garrett goes on to consider a possible account of agrammatism as a deficit at the positional level within his model. Adopting an explicit interpretation of the positional level as representing phonologically statable elements within a formal grammar, Garrett interpreted the omissions produced by idealized agrammatic patients as a phonological deficit (cf. Kean, 1978).

Other accounts of sentence production deficits have invoked quite different types of impairments at the positional level (or to the processes that must be carried out to create the positional level representation). Schwartz (1987) elaborated a linguistic model offered by Lapointe (1983) that concerns the processes that construct the planning frames at the positional level. According to Lapointe, planning frames are constructed from a store of prepackaged fragments of morphosyntactic structures consisting of lexical items and various grammatical markers. To explain agrammatic patients' omission of grammatical markers, Lapointe argued that more complex fragments would be more difficult to gain access to for output purposes. Schwartz's modification of this proposal assumes that this restriction within the morphosyntactic fragment store to simpler elements results in a bias toward unexpanded phrases and a limitation in the number of ways that phrases can be combined. Such limitation could explain the tendency of agrammatic patients to omit content words (such as adjectives), and to otherwise simplify their utterances in terms of clause and phrase structures.

In another attempt to implicate the positional level in sentence construction impairments, Caramazza and Hillis (1989) focused on the performance of a single patient who omits some grammatical morphemes and also commits word order errors in spoken and written sentences. Caramazza and Hillis attempted to elaborate somewhat on the nature of the processes that might go into generating a positional level representation. They noted, for example, that the construction of a phrasal frame does not determine the precise form that specific grammatical morphemes need take. For example, the specification that a particular noun phrase (NP) occurs in a phrasal frame does not help to select the form of the determiner that will occur with the NP. Presumably, information specified at the functional level would be required to delimit the choice of definite or indefinite article. These sorts of considerations led Caramazza and Hillis to suggest that there are different levels of information specified at the functional level that interact with different subprocesses in the formation of a fully specified positional level. Assuming that all or any of these subprocesses could be selectively impaired in aphasia, such an elaborated model (if one could be articulated) might provide a means of accommodating the variety of forms that sentence production deficits can take.

Accounting for Symptom Dissociations from the Model

Although no such elaborated model has emerged, several attempts have been made to modify the basic model in ways that allow some attribution of particular types of symptom dissociations to a breakdown in one or more describable functions or representations.

OVERLAP OF OMISSION/SUBSTITUTION OF GRAMMATICAL MORPHEMES

The occurrence of grammatical morpheme substitutions among the speech errors of agrammatic patients, and the omission of grammatical morphemes by paragrammatic speakers, reviewed above, has been invoked as a major problem for unitary accounts of sentence production disorder. In considering the model that has been sketched here, it is not at all clear why this should be so. If a functional deficit is postulated in the processes that generate a specific representation within the model, then that representation should be disrupted. There is nothing within the model, or in the simple postulation that there is a "deficit," that predicts what form that disruption should take (see also Caramazza & Hillis, 1989). Perhaps a more cogent question to consider is why there is so little co-occurrence of omission and substitution errors within the same patient given this lack of apparent constraint to one or the other type of error. Some of the accounts that have been developed, however, do offer a principled reason that omissions rather than substitutions should occur (e.g., Schwartz, 1987), but this specificity has been more the exception than the rule.

Butterworth and Howard (1987) have argued that a different type of model is necessary to accommodate the variability of omission–substitution patterns in a patient's sentence productions. These authors analyzed sentences produced by five paragrammatic patients; as noted above, they uncovered a plethora of omission—substitution errors, as well as a variety of constructional problems, in the patients' productions.[3] Butterworth and Howard proposed a model with six independent systems (semantic, syntactic, lexical, etc.), each of which is subject to a control system that initiates and terminates operation of its system and that checks its input and output. The presence of all varieties of error types in the patients' data, which might be hard to accommodate as a disruption to any one (or even to more than one) of the systems themselves, can thus be attributed to a transient malfunction of one or more of the control operations. The authors go on to consider how each error type (omission, substitution, etc.) might result from a failure of one of these control operations. Although some examples are given, it remains difficult to say precisely how a deficit to one of the control operations can be distinguished from a deficit to the system that it controls.

---

3. It must be noted here that demonstrations of dissociations among types of words omitted and substituted by a patient rest entirely on the methods used to score their speech. The systematic quantification of aphasic speech (especially spontaneous speech rather than elicited productions) is made difficult by uncertainty about the precise form of the patient's target (see Saffran et al., 1989, pp. 444–445, for discussion). Several recent production analyses have been reported that fail to state the criteria that were used to reconstruct patients' utterances, and that fail to demonstrate either (a) that these criteria can be reliably applied to the same patient's sentences by different investigators, or (b) that the same patient will produce the same pattern on different occasions. When the data are to be subjected to statistical analysis such as analysis of variance (Bates et al., 1988), information about scoring reliability is essential for the proper interpretation of significance levels. Likewise, if the point of the paper is that enormous variability is exhibited in the patient data (Miceli et al., 1989), it would seem to be important to demonstrate unequivocally that the scoring techniques did not contribute to the variability. Providing examples of sentences scored in particular ways (e.g., Butterworth & Howard, 1987) is helpful in that it makes the scope of the classification–decision problem clear to the reader, but it would be more interesting to know the extent to which two skilled analysts (e.g., Butterworth & Howard) made the same classification decisions.

DISSOCIATIONS AMONG THE GRAMMATICAL MORPHEMES

In the model outlined above, the grammatical morphemes, both bound and free, are not retrieved through the lexical selection processes that effect the production of content words. Based on evidence from normal speech errors, all syntactically relevant closed class elements are viewed as a homogeneous set from which the syntactic frame represented at the positional level is created. Dissociations within these elements, such that one type of element is omitted while another is retained, requires some modification of the model. Lapointe (1985) offered a linguistically motivated modification to the processes responsible for the creation of the positional level representation that accounts for some of the dissociations among the omission patterns of agrammatic patients. Lapointe's data showed that patients tended to produce verb forms in which inflections were present, but obligatory auxiliaries were either omitted or incorrect (i.e., they were substitutions rather than omissions). This type of pattern motivated the proposal that verb affixes and auxiliaries are retrieved in two separate operations: First, a structural frame is created that includes the verb affix as well as slots for the auxiliary and the main verb. Next, the auxiliary is retrieved from a store of function words. Lapointe's formulation includes a formal hierarchy of complexity for various verb forms that roughly predicts the likelihood that specific verbal elements will be produced.

This modification accounts for only a subset of the available data. First, it cannot accommodate more general dissociations between freestanding and bound grammatical morphemes that affect other than verbal elements (Miceli et al., 1989; Saffran et al., 1989), nor can it explain some of the dissociations WITHIN each of the two classes of grammatical morphemes (Miceli et al., 1989). To date, no modification of the model and no new linguistic–psycholinguistic model has been offered that can explain the enormous variability in omission–substitution symptoms that has been reported for the morphologically rich Italian language (Miceli & Mazzucchi, 1990; Miceli et al., 1989). It may well be that these patterns are conditioned, not only by multiple deficits to specific linguistic operations or representations, but also by individual "strategic" responses that patients might adopt to compensate for their deficits (cf. discussion of Kolk et al., 1985, above).

DISSOCIATION OF GRAMMATICAL MORPHEME
PRODUCTION FROM SENTENCE CONSTRUCTION

Two aspects of sentence constructional capacities have been identified that can dissociate from the omission of grammatical morphemes. A double dissociation has been reported of the omission of grammatical morphemes from STRUCTURAL SIMPLIFICATION, as defined by a variety of measures of phrase length, phrasal elaboration, and so forth (Berndt, 1987; Parisi, 1987). Patients have been reported who omit grammatical morphemes but produce relatively long and complex sentences (Kolk et al., 1985; Miceli et al., 1983); other patients have been described who produce normal grammatical morphemes but abnormally simple and foreshortened utterances (Saffran et al., 1989). As noted immediately above, the production model (and its modifications) provides several possible sources of deficiency in grammatical morpheme production. What about the symptom of structural simplification? Little attention has been given to this symptom, and it would appear that a failure to elaborate structures that are otherwise produced relatively normally (i.e., without omission of grammatical elements) could arise from a number of levels within the model. For example, Levelt (1989) recently described some of the important (and complex) conceptual operations that might constitute the message level. There appears to be considerable potential for pathologically induced limitation at this level that would result in impoverished sentence structures.

The possibility that is being considered here is that structural simplification might result from a DEFICIT at the message level; that is, patients might not be able to use the environmental or discourse information that is available to constrain their conceptual acts (perceptions, feelings, thoughts, etc.) into statable propositions. This possibility differs substantially from a proposal by Kolk et al. (1985), who attributed patients' simplified utterances and agrammatic speech to decisions that may or may not be made at the message level. Within the adaptation model (discussed above), a "telegraphic" speech register, which is argued to be part of the normal repertoire, may be adopted by the patient in anticipation of difficulty he or she expects to have in formulating a complex sentence. Once the simplified form of the proposition is chosen, it is automatically executed by the "sentence structure system" (functional, positional, and phonetic levels within Garrett's model.) Thus, unlike the other proposals to be considered here, Kolk's model does not postulate a deficit at a specific level of the production model, but an anticipatory, compensatory mechanism that applies before syntactic operations are executed.

The modification of the production model offered by Bock (1987b) presents another possible source of structural simplification that might be dissociable from grammatical morpheme omissions. Most aphasic patients suffer some degree of lexical, or lexical–phonological, impairment—deficits that have been considered to be largely independent of sentence structural problems. Bock's formulation (reviewed above) identifies several points in the sentence production process at which the factors influencing selection of a lexical item can affect the form that a syntactic structure will take.

The "influences" that Bock has considered are relatively subtle ones operating within a limited time frame in the speech of fluent speakers; she does not consider what might happen to syntactic structures in conditions of serious (and chronic) lexical inaccessibility. One possibility, frequently described in the aphasia literature but true for normal speakers as well, is that a more accessible word will be substituted for a less accessible word; for example, *thing* will be substituted for *astrolobe*. However, if word retrieval deficits are more pervasive, or if retrieval latencies are simply slowed in general, the important lexical influences that have been shown to affect the construction of a syntactic frame may not be available when they are needed. Bock's demonstration of an influence on syntactic structure of the phonological priming of candidate words (a "backwards" influence in terms of the original serial model) suggests that even phonologically based word retrieval deficits could result in syntactic disruption without a frank syntactic deficit. Precisely why such an influence would take the form of structural simplification remains to be determined; however, with intact processes for creation of a positional level representation, and some residual word retrieval ability, some type of sentence construction should be possible.

The second type of grammatical morpheme–sentence construction dissociation that has been reported involves the symptom of INCORRECT WORD ORDER FOR SUBJECT AND OBJECT NOUNS. Saffran et al. (1980a) reported that a group of agrammatic speakers had great difficulty starting with the subject noun in transitive and locative sentences when asked to describe pictures showing two nouns that were semantically reversible in terms of possible logical roles, and also alike in animacy (girl carrying boy; book on pillow). This finding has important theoretical implications, because word order is the primary syntactic device used in English to distinguish grammatical subject from object. Since it also contradicts a long-standing assertion that agrammatic patients do not experience difficulty with word order (Goodglass, 1968), and has been declared to be incorrect on the basis of at least one study (Bates, Friederici, Wulfeck, & Juarez, 1988),[4] some clarification of the word order deficit claim, and its methodological basis, is in order.

---

4. An additional study that is interpreted as a failure to replicate Saffran et al. (1980a) was reported by Kolk and Van Grunsven (1985). These authors employed a written "sentence order test" as their sole production task, which was similar to one of the tests

The disruption of word order in agrammatism has not been postulated to undermine basic noun–verb–noun (N-V-N) order (see below); thus, an analysis that compares patient performance with random ordering (Bates et al., 1988), or with what might be expected if the patient had "no syntax" (Kolk & Van Grunsven, 1985), is not relevant to the argument. Moreover, the argument is that some patients cannot effectively assign sentence subject status to a noun strictly on the basis of that noun's thematic role, but appear to use nonlinguistic characteristics of the message, such as animacy, to select a noun with which to begin. (This strategy will work very frequently in spontaneous speech.) Thus, experimental tests of the word order claim need to control noun animacy, as well as other variables that might influence noun accessibility. Finally, in keeping with the spirit of this review, it must be noted that it is quite possible that not all patients who omit grammatical morphemes will be found to have difficulty with word order, and that such dissociation in no way diminishes the importance of accounting for the occurrence of a word order deficit when it does occur.

In fact, there is some indication that dissociation of word order errors and grammatical morpheme omission can be found in both directions. Caramazza and Berndt (1985) described results of a picture description task administered to five patients. The intended roles of the nouns produced by two agrammatic patients could not be unambiguously interpreted as word order errors because of the patients' difficulty producing the morphological elements of the verb that would distinguish active and passive voice; in contrast, three fluent aphasic patients (without agrammatism) produced clear word order errors. Another example of this latter dissociation is discussed at the end of this section.

Saffran and colleagues have offered an explanation of the production problems found in agrammatism that can accommodate dissociations between these symptoms, as well as the dissociation of grammatical morphology from structural simplification (Saffran, 1982; Saffran et al., 1980a, 1980b). "Idealized agrammatism" (i.e., all three symptoms occur-

---

used by Saffran and colleagues. It is unclear to what extent these sentence anagram tests exploit the representations and processes employed in verbal sentence production. In terms of the model discussed here, it would seem that the phonetic level is obviously not relevant, and that the message and functional levels are severely constrained in that the lexical items have been chosen. The positional level syntactic frame information (i.e., the grammatical morphemes) would seem to be of great importance to support the mapping from the functional level to assure correct word order, but the processing requirement vis-à-vis the positional level in the sentence order task has changed from a phonologically constrained production task to a reading comprehension task.

ring together) is postulated as resulting from two separate deficits in Garrett's model. Grammatical morpheme omission, which is assumed to be functionally linked to agrammatic patients' articulation disturbance, is attributed within the model to a deficit very close to the processes of motor coding. That is, the grammatical morphemes are assumed to be adequately specified at the positional level; thus, patients' apparent awareness of their omissions can be explained. Saffran and colleagues argued that the positional level representation is not adequately translated through the operation of phonological and phonetic processes into articulatory commands. This aspect of the argument has not fared well against the backdrop of patient variability; several patients have been reported who have no articulation disturbance but who omit grammatical morphemes (Kolk et al., 1985; Miceli et al., 1983).

The second deficit postulated by Saffran and coworkers was offered to account for the constructional deficits often found in agrammatism: the structural simplification and the word order problem. This argument places a deficit at the functional level of Garrett's model. The problem was argued to reside in the creation of functional argument structures: in the encoding of relations among the semantic elements that will ultimately comprise the sentences. Faced with such a deficit, the patient produces an utterance by directly mapping from conceptual information at the message level to lexical retrieval to surface N-V-N form without benefit of the predicate–argument structures, or thematic relations, that distinguish agents from patients, themes, goals, and so forth.

At least part of this deficit at the functional level was believed to involve a difficulty with main verbs. Saffran et al. (1980b) noted that many agrammatic patients have considerable difficulty producing main verbs, and often produce nouns in place of verbs in their attempts at sentences (e.g., one of their patients described a picture of a woman photographing a flower as "the girl is Polaroid the flower"; Saffran et al., 1980a, p. 279.) Since verbs determine the arguments that will be filled by sentence nouns, a problem realizing verbs for production could be an important component of this failure to encode functional relations. Saffran and colleagues stopped short of claiming that a problem with the retrieval or representation of verbs was responsible for the functional level disturbance.

Verb Deficits and Sentence Formulation

Saffran and colleagues emphasized the importance of the verb as a repository of information about the form that a sentence will ultimately take. This information is essential in determining the order in which nouns will be produced around the verb or other predicate, as well as in specifying the grammatical morphemes (auxiliary and inflection) that will constitute the form of the verb. Several group studies have indicated that poor verb retrieval is a characteristic of agrammatic aphasics even in naming tasks, whereas other types of patients (anomic aphasics) are BETTER able to produce verbs than nouns (Miceli, Silveri, Villa, & Caramazza, 1984; Zingeser & Berndt, 1990). This double dissociation is important, since the syntactic and conceptual complexity of verbs might be argued to make them particularly vulnerable to the effects of brain damage (see Berndt, 1988; Zingeser & Berndt, 1988, for arguments). Several logical possibilities exist as to how a selective verb deficit might be related to sentence production (see Berndt, 1988; Miceli et al., 1984); it is not an easy matter to sort them out.

To address the direction of the relationship between verb retrieval and sentence formulation, as well as to probe the extent to which the symptoms of agrammatism could dissociate, we carried out several investigations of a fluent aphasic patient who showed some of the characteristics of agrammatism (Mitchum & Berndt, 1989). The patient (ML) is a former attorney who suffered a left-hemisphere CVA approximately 6 years prior to the initiation of this study. In most ways, ML's clinical profile resembles that of a Wernicke's aphasic: speech is fluent, sometimes paragrammatic, and his comprehension is moderately impaired. The following is a portion of ML's version of "Cinderella":

> In ancient times we go through Cinderella upstairs in the attic . . . we have the mopping and the baking and the but all these dresses were very rags . . . Cinderella said no because she real sad in the attic . . . two girls go to horses and carriage . . . suddenly fairy godmother comes.

When his spontaneous speech was subjected to the quantitative analysis proposed by Saffran et al. (1989), several symptoms of agrammatism emerged. Despite normal production of a variety of freestanding grammatical morphemes (e.g., determiners, pronouns), the elements of verb morphology (auxiliary verbs and inflections) were frequently omitted. In addition, the variety of verbs produced was very limited, consisting for the most part of high-frequency and quite general verbs. Moreover, ML had considerable difficulty producing well-formed sentences, and those he did produce were very simple. Finally, he showed a significant decrement in verb production in naming tasks, compared with frequency-matched nouns.

In an attempt to determine the relationship between verb retrieval and sentence formulation, we elicited sentences from ML in a variety of conditions in which aspects of the message, as well as specific verbs and nouns, were made differentially accessible. First, we provided pictured (or videotaped) scenarios that showed a simple transitive action occurring between two people (e.g., a man hugging a woman). ML described these scenes in three conditions: without any cues, with a constraint to begin the sentence with a particular noun (half the time constraining him to produce a passive voice sentence), and with a constraint to begin with a particular noun and use a particular verb. Thus, we provided him with at least the phonological forms of nouns and verbs to aid his sentence construction, while we constrained the proposition to be expressed. Results were clear: regardless of condition, ML produced errors in ordering nouns around the verb. These word order errors occurred even in the unconstrained condition (in the half of trials in which either noun could plausibly be the subject), as well as in sentences that were morphologically correct actives as well as passives. Thus, ML had great difficulty mapping logical roles onto grammatical roles, despite intact ability to produce the surface forms of active and passive voice.

In another task without a specified message to be conveyed, ML was asked to create a sentence using a specific (unambiguous) noun or verb. When given a target noun to embed in a sentence, ML produced very simple sentences with very high-frequency ("empty") verbs, but used the nouns appropriately:

> *we have the <u>kitchen</u>*
> *I love the <u>hat</u>*
> *we have a <u>jug</u> of wine*
> *please get the <u>ketchup</u>*

Target verbs were very often used in sentences with these same empty verbs, with the targets most often in a context that required no overtly realized subject:

> *I love to <u>read</u>*
> *we go to <u>dig</u>*
> *the beggar said please <u>give</u> the beggar*
> *take it to the room and <u>follow</u> the road*

Almost half of the verb target sentences used these infinitival or imperative constructions; in addition, many of ML's responses were unclear as to the form class of the verb target:

> *I get my tea and she have and <u>spill</u>*
> *he get the bucket where the <u>pour</u>*
> *go to the store and my get <u>sells</u>*

To preclude the strategy of using subjectless verb forms, and thus to probe ML's ability to embed verbs in a predicate–argument structure, we presented him with the verb targets again, but with their present progressive (*–ing*) forms. ML was unable to use this form appropriately in verb position, or even to demonstrate a minimal appreciation of grammatical class (although he seemed to understand something about their meanings):

> *get an <u>eating</u> sandwich*
> *in the den we have a <u>reading</u>* (self-correction):
>   *we have the book and <u>reading</u>*
> *can I have a large <u>drinking</u> of water*
> *the <u>spilling</u> was water in the glass*

It seems clear in this case that the problem with verb retrieval goes beyond gaining access to the phonological form of the verb. Rather, the crucial information regarding sentence structure—information about what sorts of noun arguments go with the verb, or even that there ARE noun arguments—appears to be unavailable. Although this patient did not demonstrate the halting, dysprosodic, and morphologically impoverished speech that has been regarded as the hallmark of agrammatism, he did demonstrate other agrammatic symptoms. In his case, poor sentence construction seemed to be intimately related to impoverished verb representations. Only the highest frequency and least specific verbs were used consistently with appropriate arguments.

These results seem to be most easily accommodated on the sentence production model by referring to Bock's modification along the lines of lexical–functional grammar (Bresnan & Kaplan, 1982). Within that formulation, all information concerning the mapping between logical roles (or predicate–argument structures) and grammatical roles (subject, object) is carried as part of the verb representation; a deficit that is selective for verbs would undermine this mapping operation without the necessity to postulate additional processing deficits. This possibility is considered further in the discussion, given below, of sentence comprehension deficits in aphasia.

Sentence Comprehension

A Framework for Normal Comprehension

As noted above, the ease with which normal speakers appear to construct sentences belies the complexity of the operations that must be carried out to accomplish the fluent production of well-formed sen-

tences. This mismatch between the apparent simplicity of the phe-
nomenological experience and the apparent complexity of the actual
processes is, if anything, even more striking for sentence comprehension. In most conditions, normal speakers are not aware of much "processing" between the sensory experience of hearing someone speak and
the interpretation of that speech. It feels as if sound is mapped directly
onto meaning, and that this mapping happens continuously even while
the speech is ongoing. For those concerned with aphasic disorders, however, it is clear that much can go wrong between hearing someone speak
and understanding what they have said. The goal here is to sketch a
model of some of the operations that need to be carried out on a spoken
sentence in order to arrive at a correct interpretation of its meaning, and
then to attempt an interpretation of some patterns of aphasic sentence
comprehension disorders in light of that model.

It might be possible, for the sake of reducing the complexity of this
review, simply to "reverse" the production model and continue to refer
to the same levels of representation. To some extent this is possible,
since sentence production was not described within that model at a level
of detail that invoked very many processes or representations that could
not also apply to comprehension. Nonetheless, some important differences must be emphasized between the tasks of producing and of
understanding sentences. The first involves the time course within
which processing must be completed, which is not under the control of
the listener. Sentence comprehension requires the interpretation of a
fleeting, sequential auditory stimulus, with (presumably) the necessity
of backtracking over a memory representation of that input if elements
are missed or misinterpreted. There is considerable evidence that auditory comprehension normally involves immediate interpretation of
semantic and syntactic elements as the sentence is being processed
(Marslen-Wilson & Tyler, 1980). Thus, disruption in the temporal aspects of processing, or a limitation of memory capacity, might be expected to have important effects on patients' abilities to understand
sentences.

Another difference between comprehension and production models
involves the relative lack of restrictions on interaction among components of processing that characterizes some comprehension models. As
noted above, recent revisions to the production model have focused,
among other things, on modifying its serial processing requirement to
allow an influence from lower levels onto higher levels; this is true to an
even greater extent for models of sentence comprehension, some of
which have placed virtually no limitations on how information from
different levels might interact (see Frazier, 1988, for review). Thus, it is
important to emphasize that any working framework with distinct levels

of processing may lead to the mistaken impression that these processes must be carried out in succession.

Finally, the "linearization" problem is quite different for production, (where the linear sequence is the GOAL and everything must work toward it) and comprehension (where the linear sequence is the STARTING POINT, and can be abandoned as soon as it is no longer needed.) Little attention has been given, however, to aphasic deficits that might implicate these processing characteristics that are specific to comprehension; in fact, as with production, the actual processes that are carried out to generate structural representations are largely undescribed. For our purposes, then, it seems best to emphasize the comparability of operations in comprehension and production, and to use a framework that encourages this comparison.

We will assume, then, that auditory comprehension of sentences begins with analysis of a complex and ongoing acoustic event into linguistic (phonetic and lexical) elements. The details of acoustic–phonetic conversion are themselves controversial (see Pisoni & Luce, 1987; Blumstein's chapter 5), and are not considered here. This exclusion is not to be taken as an argument that these early aspects of processing have no bearing on sentence comprehension, but only that the details of this level of the system, as well as the methods used to study them, have not focused on specifically sentence-level processes. Thus, our framework begins after the acoustic waveform has been phonetically interpreted. From this information, the listener needs to construct a structural representation that, despite different linguistic formulations, at least characterizes the phrasal organization of the sentence into hierarchically interpretable constituents (subject NP, object NP, etc.). In some ways this representation must be similar to the more "syntactic" interpretations of the positional level in Garrett's model: lexical elements are ordered into syntactic frames made up of appropriate grammatical morphemes. Arriving at this type of representation must be quite different for comprehension and production, however. In comprehension the representation must be parsed from the spoken input as the sentence continues to be spoken. Moreover, unlike the situation for production, in which (presumably) the speaker could regenerate the intended message if needed and start over, in most comprehension situations there is a single opportunity to extract the information needed to build this representation.

The grammatically interpretable constituent structure available in this type of representation yields to a semantic interpretation of the lexical and structural information available in the constituent representations; that is, the listener must comprehend the meanings of the major lexical items and interpret their roles in a functional argument structure. The representation generated by the processes needed to accomplish this is the same type of information described at the functional level of the production model. (The issue of whether representational elements within these levels constitute THE SAME representations for production and comprehension is considered below.) Thus, the important aspects of the model again focus on the mapping processes that connect the constituent and functional levels. In this case, they take as input a structural representation of sentence constituents and give as output a semantically interpreted proposition. Also again, we can distinguish two ways of approaching these mapping processes. From a perspective based on transformational grammar (a Garrett-type approach), some set of procedures is needed to align the two levels of representation. From a perspective based on lexical-functional grammar (a Bock-type approach), the information about how functional roles map onto grammatical roles is available as part of the lexical representation of the verb. This distinction may seem to be unnecessarily subtle, but it becomes important in interpreting aphasic patients' sentence comprehension performance.

Sentence Comprehension in Aphasia: Assigning Thematic Roles to Sentence Nouns

The type of comprehension disorder at issue here is one that emerges in patients with relatively good comprehension of single words. These patients fail in sentence–picture matching tasks in which (a) the sentence to be understood cannot be interpreted simply by mapping knowledge of content word meaning onto knowledge of the real world, and (b) the distractor items depict plausible interpretations that might be given to the sentence if the patient failed to comprehend the structural information in the sentence.

Although syntactic complexity of the sentence may be a predictor of performance in some patients, it is not the essential element. For example, the sentence "the boy that the bee stung cried and ran home" is a complex sentence, but one in which the content word meanings alone yield a highly predictable interpretation. When paired with distractors showing, for example, a girl victim, a dog biting, or a child laughing, such a sentence could be easily associated with the correct picture if the patient understood the meanings of the nouns and verbs. In contrast, the sentence "the girl kisses the boy" is less complex, but when paired with a distractor showing a boy kissing a girl would be impossible to interpret based on word meanings alone. In addition, the listener would need to "know" that the subject of "kisses" maps onto the thematic role of agent of the action. It is this recovery of the functional (thematic) roles of the nouns in semantically reversible sentences that has been most at issue in studies of sentence comprehension in aphasia.

The most recent wave of interest in this issue (see Howard, 1985, for a historical discussion) can be traced to a paper by Caramazza and Zurif (1976), who demonstrated that patients classified as Broca's and conduction aphasics had difficulty in a sentence–picture matching task when presented with center-embedded relative clause sentences such as "the cat that the dog is biting is black" and a distractor showing a cat biting a dog. Since that time, numerous studies have reported various degrees of replication of that result with groups of Broca's aphasics. Some of these studies have included sentences that are simpler than those employed by Caramazza and Zurif, such as simple active voice sentences with transitive verbs (Gallaher & Canter, 1982; Jones, 1984), and sentences with locative prepositions that do not require interpretation of the morphological elements of the verb that signal active and passive voice (Schwartz, Saffran, & Marin, 1980). Virtually all of the studies of sentence comprehension reported in recent years have focused on groups of patients, usually characterized as agrammatic speakers.

Various explanations have been given for the pattern of comprehension impairment described. Some have focused on the creation of the constituent level or on the intactness of constituent level representations (Berndt & Caramazza, 1980; Bradley et al., 1980); others have attributed the problem to an inability to extract from sentence word order the information about the relations in force between sentence nouns (available at the constituent level) that is needed to construct the functional level (Schwartz et al., 1980), or to a deficit in the interpretation of all relational information such as that carried by prepositions and some verbs (Jones, 1984; Saffran et al., 1980b). This possibility is considered in the conclusion of this chapter.

Another explanation for this type of comprehension disorder was not motivated by the comprehension model, but by the assumed requirement that information be stored in memory while sentences are being interpreted (Clark & Clark, 1977). The type of sentence comprehension disorder described above is often demonstrated by patients with clear limitations of short-term memory, and this co-occurrence of deficits has led to the hypothesis that the two symptoms are functionally related in those patients (see Saffran, 1990, for review).

Kolk and Van Grunsven (1985) suggested that memory limitations, in the form of diminished capacity or an exacerbated decay rate, might also undermine sentence comprehension in agrammatic aphasics. This notion was developed in an attempt to account for the variability found across patients on a task, and within patients on a variety of tasks. Patients could easily differ in terms of the degrees of their memory limitations; tasks clearly differ in terms of memory demands. Martin and coworkers tested this hypothesis using passive voice sentences that were either truncated passives ("John was applauded") or full passives ("John was applauded by Kathy") (Martin, Wetzel, Blossom-Stach, & Feher, 1989). If comprehension failure results either from a capacity limitation or from premature decay of the representation formed from the speech signal, then patients should perform better on the truncated passives, because those sentences place less burden on memory than do the full passives. The hypothesis was not upheld, as the patients performed very similarly on the two sentence types.

Martin (1987) also demonstrated the dissociability of sentence comprehension performance from the ability to "rehearse" information in memory using subvocal articulation. An "articulatory loop" is postulated to be a central component of working memory, and might reasonably be expected to be at risk in agrammatic aphasics who typically suffer from a disorder of articulation. Nonetheless, nonfluent patients with articulation disorders but without agrammatism, who were limited in their ability to carry out articulation-based rehearsal, performed well on Martin's tests of sentence comprehension.

The final word on the issue of a memory contribution to sentence comprehension disorders has probably not been heard, however. One problem hindering serious consideration of this issue has been the lack of a coherent model of the memory requirements of sentence processing; the available memory model was designed to account for list repetition (Baddeley, 1986), and fails to consider the different forms in which sentence-level information might be stored (e.g., auditory, lexical, syntactic, semantic). Saffran (1990) recently proposed that several distinct memory records may exist to support different aspects of sentence processing, any one of which might be subject to selective disruption by brain damage. Several attempts have been made to account for the performance of patients within this account (Berndt & Mitchum, 1990; Berndt, Mitchum, & Price, in press; Saffran & Martin, 1990), but none of these concerns the performance of patients with agrammatic speech output. The possibility that the comprehension problems experienced by some types of aphasic patients might be secondary to a memory limitation is thus still viable; however, it is unlikely that any sort of general memory account of the comprehension pattern at issue here will be tenable.

Another piece of evidence that memory limitations do not underlie all sentence comprehension disorders emerged from a study reported by

Schwartz, Linebarger, Saffran, and Pate (1987). This study did not employ the sentence–picture matching task described above, but required patients to judge the semantic coherence of sentences. For example, patients were asked to judge whether the following types of sentences were "good" or "silly":

(structure based)	*"the puppy dropped the little boy"*
	"the little boy was dropped by the puppy"
(lexically based)	*"the spoon ate the table"*
	"the table was eaten by the spoon"

In addition, all of the sentence types were "padded" into quite lengthy versions of the same basic structures, often with multiple clauses:

"the puppy ran around excitedly and accidentally dropped the little boy onto the wet grass, which upset Louise"
"yesterday morning, the spoon which I bought years ago ate the table in the front room"

In the structure based condition, the stimuli were semantically reversible sentences much like those employed in the sentence–picture matching tasks described above. (There were, in addition, a variety of more complex sentences involving relative clauses, all of which were represented in both structure based and lexically based conditions.) Thus, although relieved in this task of interpreting pictures, the patient still performed the same linguistic operations as required by sentence–picture matching; that is, he or she had to assign the thematic roles (agent, patient) to nouns based on an appreciation of the grammatical roles (subject, object) indicated by the surface structure of the sentence.

The stimulus sentences were further characterized in terms of the relation between the positions of the nouns in the surface form of the sentence, and their interpretation in a functional argument structure. Based on a recent version of Chomsky's theory (1981), in which noun phrases in passive voice and other types of sentences are represented as having been "moved" from their D(eep)-structure position (preceding the verb) to their S(urface)-structure position (following the verb), passive voice and other sentences involving such hypothesized movements were characterized as having "moved arguments." (Note that this linguistic theory is intended as a formal characterization of the relation between levels of representation, not as a performance model of how the speaker or listener accomplishes the translation from one level to the other.)

Agrammatic patients performed well in the lexically based conditions, although significantly poorer in the moved arguments and padded conditions than in the base conditions. Nonetheless, their performance in all of the lexical conditions was quite good (mean error rate around 10%). In the structure based condition, patients showed considerable ability to assign thematic roles on the basis of grammatical roles, even in the padded condition, although their performance was below that of nonaphasic brain-damaged controls. Only in the moved arguments condition of the structure based set did performance approach chance levels.

These results indicate that the patients have some difficulties interpreting thematic roles that correspond to surface-structure elements even in active voice and other base sentences. Nonetheless, they have retained considerable ability to do so even when the surface structure is complex, which suggests that their appreciation of basic constituent structures of sentences is largely intact; they were apparently able to parse the padded sentences (containing relative clauses and other complexities) into a structure that could be correctly interpreted most of the time. Performance could not have been based on a default strategy such as assuming the first noun encountered is the subject. The padded versions contained too many candidate nouns which, interpreted as agent, would have rendered the sentences anomalous. Memory load also apparently was not a significant factor; the padded sentences were very long, yet performance was quite comparable to performance on the base sentences.

In the moved arguments conditions, however, patients had serious problems assigning thematic roles correctly (i.e., in rejecting sentences such as "the bird was eaten by the worm"). The explanation of this finding offered by Schwartz et al. (1987) is that the set of procedures for mapping between thematic roles and grammatical roles (already something of a problem for these patients) is made more difficult when the relationship between a D-structure ordering and an S-structure ordering is not "transparent." Although virtually nothing is known about how these mapping procedures are carried out, formal linguistic theories postulate complex and quite indirect linkings between these two levels. The idea, then, is that an impaired mapping process is most likely to fail when the roles to be mapped are only indirectly and nontransparently linked, such as in passive voice sentences.

Grodzinsky (1984, 1986) offered a structural account of agrammatic comprehension, also motivated by Chomsky (1981), which reaches a conclusion that differs markedly from that of Schwartz et al. (1987), although it also emphasizes the issue of moved arguments. Grodzinsky (1984) argued that the agrammatic condition is one in which some types of information are unspecified at the level of S-structure, a level of representation argued by Schwartz and colleagues to be intact. Grammatical elements that enter into particular types of structural relations, as well as the "empty elements" ("trace" and "PRO") that mark lexical positions when they are moved from their original positions, are left unspecified. Thus, in the S-structure representation of a passive voice sentence, the initial noun is linked to its D-structure object position by a trace, which is not specified in the agrammatic patient's S-structure representation.

In this case, the initial noun phrase is not assigned a thematic role in the usual way, but instead the patient adopts a heuristic based on the linear order of the nouns in the sentence. The first noun is assigned the role of agent; however, the prepositional phrase after the verb (which phrase the patient can interpret, according to Grodzinsky) also assigns the thematic role of agent to its nouns. Thus, two sentence nouns have been assigned the role of agent. The strategy of the patient will be to guess between the two, resulting in chance performance on passive sentences. Active voice sentences (with no moved arguments) do not present these problems, because they do not require an interpretation of a trace; they should be comprehended well.[5]

One problem with this account is that it does not correspond well to the available data. The 10 agrammatic patients tested by Jones (1984) performed quite poorly on active voice sentences. Friederici and Graetz (1987) reported a high level of comprehension among German-speaking Broca's aphasics of three variants of passive voice sentences. Other studies have shown considerable variability in performance that fails to adhere to the pattern predicted (see, e.g., Table 1 of Shankweiler, Crain, Gorrell, & Tuller, 1989; or Table 1 of Linebarger, Schwartz, & Saffran, 1983a). In addition, Martin et al. (1989) tested Grodzinsky's hypothesis concerning thematic assignment in passive voice sentences with the truncated and full passive sentence comprehension test described above. Since the truncated passives contain no by-phrase to provide conflicting assignment of agent status to the second noun, patients should consistently interpret the first noun as agent; that is, they should perform worse on the truncated than on the full passives. This prediction was not upheld, however, as patients performed equivalently on the two types of sentences.

Another attempt to account for sentence comprehension deficits in aphasia from syntactic theory has gone through significant changes in

5. Considerable controversy has surrounded the linguistic analysis that forms the basis for Grodzinsky's hypothesis (Caplan & Hildebrandt, 1986; Sproat, 1986). An evaluation of the theoretical adequacy of Grodzinsky's account is outside the scope of this review, which is concerned with the adequacy of the data offered to support it.

the last few years (Caplan, Baker, & DeHaut, 1985; Caplan & Futter, 1986; Caplan & Hildebrandt, 1988; Hildebrandt, Caplan, & Evans, 1987). Caplan and colleagues have relied on an experimental paradigm that requires the patient to manipulate doll-like objects in response to sentences. A range of syntactic structures is tested in addition to the active–passive transitive types that have been discussed thus far. Patients are asked to act out "who is doing what to whom" in response to the sentences, after their comprehension of the names of the dolls is established. Some of the sentences are quite complex and utilize two verbs, for example,

> *Patrick was believed by Joe to be eating*
> *The bear was given by the donkey to the goat*

In these cases, the patient is taught to respond only to the latter part of the sentences, and to show who is doing the action stated in the second verb.[6] The data are scored only with regard to the identity of the noun objects chosen; patients' interpretations of the action verbs is not assessed.

Based on this paradigm, Caplan et al. (1985) listed the factors that contribute to increased difficulty for aphasic patients in general: deviations from subject–verb–object word order, an increased number of arguments per verb, and more than one verb per sentence. The sentence types were grouped (and ranked) as to their difficulty. In addition, specific patterns of deficit have been argued to characterize the performance of individual patients, and are said to represent two primary kinds of deficit: a disruption of a specific parsing operation (which yields a syntactic representation), or a disruption to some aspect of the syntactic representation itself (Caplan & Hildebrandt, 1988). Either of these deficits might represent an actual loss of information, in which case it should always be manifested, or a problem of utilization, in which case

---

6. A number of methodological problems with this paradigm can be mentioned. It is not clear, for example, how patients are to understand which part of the sentence is the "last part" when correct performance requires choosing the first noun as the actor (e.g., "John promised Joe that he would kneel"). This is an important problem, since in general patients performed poorly when required to choose as agent of second verb a noun from the beginning of the sentence. A second question can be raised concerning what the patient is supposed to do when a sentence does not explicitly demand an action in the second part of the sentence. In the example above, it is not stated that any kneeling took place. Should John then be designated, since he is the agent of the only action described by this particular sentence? Note that if such an interpretation is applied, the response will be correct. The point is that there are even more potential reasons for a patient to act in a particular way when performing this task than the numerous possibilities listed by Caplan and colleagues.

performance will be variable. To account for the data from groups of patients, as well as from several individual patients, however, it was necessary to invoke two additional factors. The patients' deficits interacted, it was argued, with the overall processing requirements demanded by the sentence; thus, a particular parsing operation might be available to a patient in a simple sentence, and impossible in a more complex one. Also, the actual performance that the patient might exhibit reflects not only the deficit and its interaction with processing load, but the heuristics that might be used to solve the problem in the face of the deficit.

The problem with the attempts of Caplan and colleagues to account for their patients' deficits is that, despite a sophisticated linguistic analysis and data from a large number of patients, the account does not explain anything because it can explain everything. That is, although some interesting descriptive facts are provided about patient performance with complex sentences, the number of unconstrained factors that can be invoked to accommodate failed predictions renders the account unfalsifiable.

One thing to be noted about the accounts of Grodzinsky and of Caplan and colleagues is that the linguistic level of representation that is at issue is the S-structure in Chomsky's (1981) model. Although obviously much more elaborated, this representation corresponds roughly to the syntactic frame and ordered lexical terms that we have been calling the constituent level. Thus, the deficit postulated by both groups of researchers is to the syntactic representation that allows constituents to be interpreted as filling grammatical roles such as subject, object, and so forth, or to the parsing operations required to recover this representation from the phonetic analysis of the speech signal. In contrast, Schwartz and coworkers (1987) argued that this syntactic level is adequate; the problem is attributed to an inability to interpret available grammatical roles as representing positions in a functional argument structure. The next section reviews evidence concerning the adequacy of the syntactic structures patients can recover from spoken sentences, obtained from tasks that do not require assignment of thematic roles to sentence nouns.

Parsing Operations and Syntactic Representations

A variety of methods can be used to assess directly the form of the syntactic representations that patients construct from spoken sentences. The primary paradigm used is one in which subjects are asked to judge the syntactic well-formedness of sentences; they are not asked to interpret their meanings. In an important study, Linebarger et al. (1983a) demonstrated that a group of four agrammatic aphasics who failed on sentence–picture matching tasks with semantically reversible sentences was nonetheless quite good at judging the syntactic acceptability of sentences. The subjects showed an appreciation for a range of syntactic facts, including knowledge about the subcategorization requirements of specific lexical items (i.e., restrictions on the kinds of complements that can apply to verbs), and an ability to interpret discontinuous elements in sentence structures. For example, the patients were able to detect the subtle differences in the following pairs of sentences that renders one grammatical and the other ungrammatical:

> *I want you to go to the store now*
> *I hope you to go to the store now*
>
> *Did the old man enjoy the view?*
> *Did the old man enjoying the view?*

Perhaps most importantly, such performance demonstrates remarkable sensitivity to the structure-marking role of a range of grammatical function words. Since these elements are often omitted from agrammatic speech, and since they are important elements indicating syntactic structure, it has been hypothesized (as noted above) that the agrammatic deficit reflects a primary impairment in processing this category of words (e.g., Bradley et al., 1980; Zurif, 1982). Even proposals of more selective involvement of grammatical morphology (e.g., Grodzinsky, 1984; Zurif & Grodzinsky, 1983) have difficulty with the high level of sensitivity to grammatical morphology demonstrated in this task (Linebarger, Schwartz, & Saffran, 1983b).

The sensitivity of agrammatic aphasics to these grammatical morpheme elements was also demonstrated for speakers of the highly inflected language of Serbo-Croatian. Lukatela, Crain, and Shankweiler (1988) tested six agrammatic patients on a grammaticality judgment task that focused particularly on appreciation of the subcategorization requirements of verbs. For example, in English the requirement that the verb "to sleep" cannot take a direct object but can take a prepositional phrase produces the difference in grammaticality between "he slept the car" and "he slept in the car"; in Serbo-Croatian, the difference between a direct object and the object of a preposition is signaled by an inflection on the noun. Agrammatic subjects proved to be remarkably sensitive to these types of distinctions.

Several methodological concerns have been raised about the grammaticality judgment task. Since interpretation of the meaning of the sentence is not measured, and since patients are not asked to say what is wrong with the ungrammatical sentences, ANY clue to ungrammaticality could be used to achieve a high level of performance. Linebarger and coworkers reported the measures they used to avoid such cues, including a procedure for matching ungrammatical sentences to grammatical sentences that served as a model for intonation contour. Nonetheless, the possibility remained that some subtle prosodic abnormality could signal the ungrammaticality of sentences with an unusual sequence of open and closed class words. This possibility was essentially ruled out by Berndt, Salasoo, Mitchum, and Blumstein (1988), who showed that very little decrement in performance occurred on the task when the sentence stimuli were signal-processed to remove the intonation contour.

Another type of methodological concern was raised by Zurif and Grodzinsky (1983) and echoed by Wulfeck (1988). Their concern was that the grammaticality judgment task is somehow unnatural when compared with more traditional sentence comprehension tasks. According to Wulfeck, the two types of tasks "involve different kinds of processing" (p. 81). Zurif and Grodzinsky were concerned that the grammaticality judgment task requires only "off-line" processing, and that syntactic parsing may be possible in an off-line task, and not possible in an "on-line" comprehension task where interpretation is carried out immediately. Both of these concerns seem to beg the question: What is different about the two tasks? Linebarger et al. (1983a) seem to have answered this question in terms of a model of sentence comprehension: that is, the grammaticality judgment task measures only the construction of a syntactic representation, whereas sentence–picture matching and anomaly judgment tasks (Schwartz et al., 1987) assess the ability to generate a semantic interpretation of the syntactic representation.

Zurif and Grodzinsky (1983) appear to equate their distinction between on-line and off-line tasks to one between comprehension tasks and metalinguistic tasks, respectively. On-line sentence comprehension is usually taken to refer to the time course of processing as it is being carried out; on line tasks provide some (reaction time) measurement of the chronology of that processing. Under this definition, grammaticality judgment and sentence–picture matching are both off-line tasks.

Recently, however, the grammaticality judgment task was rendered on-line by Shankweiler et al. (1989), who presented patients with a grammaticality judgment task in a reaction time context. The types of sentences employed differed somewhat from those used by Linebarger et al. (1983a) in that they focused on substitutions within and between the distinct classes of grammatical morphemes. The on-line nature of the procedures employed allowed Shankweiler et al. to address additional questions about patients' abilities to construct a syntactic representation. The words within the ungrammatical sentences that caused the ungrammaticality were systematically placed either early, middle, or late in the sentence. Normal subjects would be expected to show word position effects in their reaction times (i.e., faster response times to incorrect words detected later in the sentence). Word position effects in other types of tasks have been interpreted as an indication that subjects have generated a syntactic representation of the sentence (Marslen-Wilson & Tyler, 1980). In this experiment, significant word position effects would suggest that the constructed syntactic representation in some way speeded subjects' judgments that the ungrammatical element did not fit the structure. Shankweiler et al. also varied the size of the gap between the ungrammatical element and another word in the sentence that entered into that ungrammaticality. For example, in the sentence,

"The baker told the helper that the bread were rising,"

the within-category substitution of "were" occurs late in the sentence, and it is close to the word "bread" that renders it ungrammatical.

Again, agrammatic subjects demonstrated considerable sensitivity to surface-structure elements in the sentences, and also showed the normal pattern of word position effects. This latter result, in addition to the fact that both the normal controls and the agrammatic subjects showed significant effects of the distance between elements of the ungrammaticality, suggests that the patients retained the ability to construct a relatively normal representation of the structure of the sentence as they were hearing it. It should be noted that four of the six patients tested performed poorly on sentence–picture matching with reversible sentences.

Studies using the grammaticality judgment task have uncovered impressive residual ability to construct syntactic representations among agrammatic aphasics. Nonetheless, criticisms of the methodology can still be marshaled that emphasize putatively different requirements for "noticing an error" and for generating a syntactic structure. Although no one has succeeded in explaining how one might notice a structural error if one had not successfully generated a structural representation, it is reassuring that other evidence of retained structural capacities in aphasia has been obtained using on-line tasks that do not depend on patients' judgments of well-formedness. These studies have also uncovered ways in which the structural representations generated may not be entirely intact.

The task that has been employed is word monitoring: Subjects listen to a sentence and press a reaction time key when a particular target word is recognized. This task has been widely employed in studies of normal sentence comprehension, specifically to address questions regarding the time course of activation of specific types of information during processing (Marslen-Wilson, 1989). Some of the word monitoring experiments carried out with aphasic patients have required them to monitor directly for the target word that is of interest. In an early application of this method to aphasic performance, Swinney, Zurif, and Cutler (1980) found that agrammatic aphasics (unlike controls) were slower to respond when monitoring for grammatical function words than for content words. Friederici (1983, 1985) also found slower responses to function words than to content words in the monitoring times of German agrammatic patients, which was a reversal of the effect shown by normal subjects. In addition, however, Friederici noted differences in response times within the function word category of prepositions that seemed to relate to the role played by the preposition in the sentence context. The same differences among patients' responses to prepositions based on their grammatical function have also been demonstrated in an off-line grammaticality judgment task (Friederici, 1982).

These studies suggest that the agrammatic patients' ability to process grammatical function words is not entirely normal. Nor is it abolished: Patients were quite accurate at detecting the presence of the grammatical elements. The central question, of course, is the effect that this non-normal processing of grammatical elements might have on patients' ability to construct a syntactic representation. Several other word monitoring studies have begun to address questions regarding the types of structural representations that patients construct, and these have employed the word monitoring study in a somewhat different way. In the work to be reviewed next, subjects monitor for a target word that is not particularly at issue, but which occurs in the sentence immediately following some important structural manipulation. Often this manipulation involves an ungrammatical element. In general, normal response times are slowed by the occurrence of irregularities in the sentences, often to different degrees for different types of violations.

Tyler (1985) was the first to apply this type of approach to an analysis of aphasia. In one type of manipulation, the focus was on the semantic and syntactic restrictions on elements that can follow specified verbs. A base sentence was constructed in which an acceptable noun followed the verb; this was then varied to produce several types of violations. In pragmatically implausible violations, the noun following the verb was not grammatically precluded, but was not a likely completion of the sentence given knowledge of the real world. In the selection restriction violations, the noun following the verb was not concordant with the semantic specification of the verb. In the strict subcategorization trials, the noun following the verb violated the restrictions on permissible verb arguments. The following are sample sentence fragments for the target word *guitar:*

(base)	*the young man grabbed the guitar and . . .*
(pragmatic)	*the young man buried the guitar and . . .*
(selection restriction)	*the young man drank the guitar and . . .*
(subcategorization)	*the young man slept the guitar and . . .*

Normal subjects were slower to respond to all of these violations than to the base sentence, but the SMALLEST reaction time cost occurred to the pragmatic violations. An agrammatic patient tested by Tyler also showed slower response times in all conditions, but for him the LARGEST reaction time cost occurred in the pragmatic condition. In another study (Tyler, 1989), this same patient showed the normal word position effects (i.e., a reaction time advantage for targets occurring later in the sentence) only when sentences were semantically interpretable; unlike normal subjects, he failed to show word position effects in semantically anomalous, but syntatically well-formed, sentences. Nonetheless, because his monitoring latencies in the anomalous condition were faster than in a scrambled word condition with no syntactic structure, it appears that he was able to extract some syntactic information even from the anomalous prose.

Using a new set of word monitoring studies, Tyler (1989) attempted to delineate more precisely the type of syntactic structures this patient generated in anomalous sentences (i.e., without benefit of coherent semantic information). In work with normal subjects, Tyler and Warren (1987) had shown that the processing of anomalous sentences depends on the organization of the speech input into "local" phrases that are syntactically and prosodically well formed. These local phrases appear to be integrated into a larger prosodic structure. Results with the aphasic patient indicated that his use of different types of information differed depending on whether semantic information was available. In anomalous sentences, he appeared to structure the input into phrases using local syntactic information (either word order or grammatical markers). In normal sentences, local syntactic information seemed to be less important, as local syntactic violations were not disruptive. Thus, at least one agrammatic patient is quite sensitive to some types of syntactic information. In light of the discussion above regarding the interpretation of thematic roles from syntactic structures, it is particularly important to note that this patient is very sensitive to the structural consequences of verbs. Nonetheless, it is also clear that this patient is overly reliant on semantic and pragmatic information, possibly to the point of ignoring the information that he can extract from syntactic structure if semantic information is available as well.

In another attempt to distinguish local from more global structures, Baum (1989) tested a group of Broca's aphasics on a word monitoring task with materials representing three types of "local" violations (i.e., those occurring within a clause) and three types of "long distance" violations (i.e., those occurring across a clause boundary). In addition, each violation type was also padded with extraneous words and phrases so that the distance between the elements making up the ungrammaticality could be assessed. Normal subjects' monitoring times were more affected by an ungrammaticality occurring in the local than in the long distance conditions, but they did show sensitivity to grammaticality even in the long distance condition. The agrammatic group, however, was sensitive to grammaticality only in the local condition. This result cannot be easily attributed to a memory limitation, since the effect was obtained with the longer padded sentences in the local violation conditions. This study, together with Tyler's (1989) results, suggests that agrammatic patients are sensitive to some kinds of structural facts but not to others. Interestingly, Baum's results also indicate a retained appreciation for subcategorization restrictions on the verb (one of her local conditions). Beyond this converging evidence that these patients may have retained important facts about the structural implications of verb representations, it is still unclear precisely what syntactic information remains available and what information does not.

Comprehension, Production, and Remediation of the Mapping Deficit

This review was initiated with a litany of the dissociations that have been obtained among the symptoms that had been interpreted as reflections of a single underlying deficit. One of these, the dissociation of the production symptoms of agrammatism from comprehension failure, has been interpreted as an indication that common structural mechanisms are not exploited in comprehension and production (Shallice, 1988). Because this is an important claim, the nature of the reported dissociation deserves more careful scrutiny. Intact comprehension occurring with structurally impoverished sentences has been reported relatively rarely; comprehension failure with intact sentence production is more common.

Most of the studies of sentence comprehension reported above were studies of groups of patients whose production deficits were not characterized aside from noting that they were agrammatic or, sometimes, that they were classified as Broca's aphasics. An exception is provided by the study of Martin et al. (1989), who analyzed the sentences produced by four patients using the quantitative analysis system developed by Saffran et al. (1989). This system allows some assessment of structural simplification in measures that express the degree to which words are used in propositional structures, and the extent to which they are elaborated, but it is concerned primarily with production of bound and free-standing grammatical morphemes. Martin et al.'s patients demonstrated little correlation between the severity of these aspects of their sentence production and the degree of their apparent sentence comprehension impairment. As suggested by Martin et al., however, what is really needed to assess the relationship between comprehension and production is detailed study of a specific aspect of sentence processing in a single patient, using tasks especially designed to separate that aspect of processing from others.

Although many such studies have been directed at patients' single word processing (especially of written words; see Shallice, 1988, for review), few investigations of sentence processing have taken this approach. Moreover, the outcome of such a study would still beg the question of the NECESSITY of any symptom co-occurrence that is uncovered. Even very similar impairments in comprehension and production could represent two parallel deficits in completely separate systems. A new approach has been taken to this question that appears to hold much promise for theoretical as well as clinical progress. The argument is as follows: If similar impairments of comprehension and production result from the same processing impairment (i.e., to a single component that is shared), then treatment focused on that component that succeeds in improving the symptom in comprehension should be accompanied by a change in production, even if production processes were not targeted in the treatment (see Byng & Coltheart, 1986; Mitchum & Berndt, 1988, for discussion). Such "targeted intervention" studies necessarily require a model of the system that is under investigation, as well as careful and detailed diagnosis of the nature of a patient's deficits.

Results of this type of intervention study have been reported for two patients with differing degrees of sentence processing impairment. Both patients had been aphasic for years before the initiation of this treatment, and had completed years of speech therapy. Byng (1988) carried out a series of diagnostic tests with an agrammatic patient (BRB) which suggested that the functional locus of his deficits in both comprehension and production was the set of procedures for mapping between logical (thematic) and grammatical roles. The patient had difficulty producing verbs in spontaneous speech, and demonstrated problems comprehending thematic and grammatical relations in a verb comprehension test in which "reverse role" distractors were available (e.g., distinguishing between "give" and "take" portrayed in a videotaped segment).

Thus it might be assumed that the nature of the patients' deficits involved loss of the specific information encoded in verbs about the functional relations between thematic roles and the verb's required arguments. (In some models, as emphasized throughout this review, verb representations carry information not only about their own argument restrictions, but also about the relationships between their arguments and possible thematic roles.) However, the therapy program directed at the patient's impairments did not involve verbs at all, but focused on mapping logical and grammatical roles from prepositions in reversible contexts. Not only did this intervention (carried out with written words) reestablish the patient's comprehension of reversible locative sentences, but it was also followed by an improvement in his comprehension of reversible active and passive sentences. Moreover, significant gains were found in sentence production, in the form of a significant increase in the number of arguments included with the verb in spontaneous speech. The mapping process that was reinstated in this patient was apparently very abstract, presumably granting to him not only an appreciation of the necessity of word order in the expression of relationships, but also the important information that those word orders are dictated by a single sentence element (i.e., the preposition or the verb).

A similar study was carried out by Jones (1986) with a very severely nonfluent man, essentially a holophrastic speaker who produced virtually no verbs. The patient also had great difficulty interpreting reversible sentences. This intervention was also conceived of as focused on mapping (in this case, explicitly between the positional and functional levels of Garrett's model). Jones went to some lengths to prevent the patient from attempting to produce the sentences during the therapy, which focused on identifying elements such as action, agent, and theme, in written sentences. Posttreatment assessments demonstrated considerable change in comprehension of reversible sentences, but also showed improvement in sentence production: Verbs began to appear, and utterances showed a propositional quality that had been absent prior to treatment. Eventually, following a new treatment directed explicitly at production, the patient showed remarkably improved (though still agrammatic) sentence production.

These studies allow a number of interesting conclusions in addition to the obvious but important one that apparently long-standing sentence processing disorders can yield to treatment under the right conditions. Moreover, the roughly described level of the system that was the focus of these interventions—the "mapping operations" that link thematic and grammatical roles—is precisely the processing level that appears to be the most egregiously underspecified in the models. Thus it is possible that detailed studies such as these that even more closely control the information made available to the patient might contribute in important ways to specifying what these operations involve. For example, it is conceivable that some of the treatment techniques that were used in the studies reviewed here contributed to an improved constituent structure representation, and that this was responsible for the post-treatment gains. Future studies might employ some of the on-line methods described above to assess the integrity of this level of representation before and after treatment in order to assess the effect of mapping therapy on that level.

Most importantly, however, the remarkable carryover to sentence production demonstrated in these studies suggests that it is premature to abandon attempts to find processing or representational commonalities in sentence comprehension and production. The experimental methods available to address this issue with normal subjects are few and complex (see Monsell, 1987); careful study of the sentence processing capabilities of patients in both domains could contribute substantially to our understanding of the processing resources that are exploited both for comprehension and for production.

Conclusions

Research conducted in the past 10 years has uncovered considerable variability in the forms that sentence processing disorders can take in aphasia. Symptoms that once appeared to be quite similar across patients and consistent within a patient have been shown to be dauntingly variable when performance is carefully scrutinized. This variability may indicate that most if not all of these symptoms can arise from several distinct functional disorders.

Nonetheless, some patterns have emerged that require an account, even if that account will not work for all similar patients. This review has emphasized the constructional problems that have been shown to characterize the sentences produced by aphasic patients (both agrammatic patients and others), in addition to symptoms relating to the use of grammatical morphemes. One possibility that was raised concerning production is that poor access to verbs (or to some aspect of verb representations) might underlie at least some patients' constructional deficits. In our discussion of the case ML, poor verb retrieval, constructional deficits, and omission of the morphological elements of the verb were shown to co-occur in the context of relatively intact ability to produce nouns and other freestanding grammatical morphemes. This co-occurrence of deficits does not indicate that any one of them is causal; a targeted therapy study is under way to address that issue.

With regard to comprehension, recent research has succeeded in separating two aspects of sentence comprehension that appear to be distinct. The ability to recover a structural representation of sentence constituents in simple sentences appears to be largely intact in most patients studied, although parsing operations needed to support more complex syntactic analysis may be more frequently impaired. Even when constituent structures appear to be intact, however, patients often fail to interpret correctly the thematic relations conveyed by the sentence. One possible explanation is that the grammatical-to-thematic mapping information carried by the verb is no longer available. If this is so, an impairment of verb-specific thematic information may co-occur with intact appreciation of required verb arguments, since this letter information appeared to be spared in a variety of on-line studies. An alternative possibility that must be explored in future work is that a set of procedures needs to be carried out to link the roles of sentence nouns at what we have called the functional and constituent levels of representation. Although much has been done to describe the types of misalignments of these representations that can make this mapping difficult, little information is available to suggest the nature of these mapping procedures. Finally, it has been suggested here that some of the processes and representations involved in sentence processing might prove to be common to comprehension and production; this issue may need at least another 10 years for resolution.

Acknowledgments

The preparation of this chapter was supported by NIH (Deafness and Communicative Disorders) grant RO1-DC00262 to the University of Maryland School of Medicine. The author is grateful to Maryne C. Glowacki for assistance in the preparation of the manuscript.

References

Baddeley, A. D. (1986). *Working memory.* Oxford: Oxford University Press.

Badecker, W., & Caramazza, A. (1985). On consideration of method and theory governing the use of clinical categories in neurolinguistics and cognitive neuropsychology: The case against agrammatism. *Cognition, 20,* 97–126.

Bates, E. A., Friederici, A. D., Wulfeck, B. B., & Juarez, L. A. (1988). On the preservation of word order in aphasia: Cross-linguistic evidence. *Brain and Language, 33,* 323–364.

Baum, S. R. (1989). On-line sensitivity to local and long-distance syntactic dependencies in Broca's aphasia. *Brain and Language, 37,* 327–338.

Berndt, R. S. (1987). Symptom co-occurrence and dissociation in the interpretation of agrammatism. In M. Coltheart, G. Sartori, & R. Job (Eds.), *The Cognitive neuropsychology of language.* Hillsdale, NJ: Erlbaum.

Berndt, R. S. (1988). Category-specific deficits in aphasia. *Aphasiology, 2*(3/4), 237–240.

Berndt, R. S., & Caramazza, A. (1980). A redefinition of the syndrome of Broca's aphasia: Implications for a neuropsychological model of language. *Applied Psycholinguistics, 1,* 225–278.

Berndt, R. S., & Mitchum, C. C. (1990). Auditory and lexical information sources in immediate recall: Evidence from a patient with deficit to the phonological short-term store. In G. Vallar & T. Shallice (Eds.), *Neuropsychological impairments of short-term memory.* Cambridge: Cambridge University Press.

Berndt, R. S., Mitchum, C. C., & Price, T. R. (in press). Short-term memory and sentence comprehension: An investigation of a patient with crossed aphasia. *Brain.*

Berndt, R. S., Salasoo, A., Mitchum, C. C., & Blumstein, S. E. (1988). The role of intonation cues in aphasic patients' performance of the grammaticality judgment task. *Brain and Language, 34,* 65–97.

Bock, J. K. (1982). Toward a cognitive psychology of syntax: Information processing contributions to sentence formulation. *Psychological Review, 89,* 1–47.

Bock, J. K. (1987a). An effect of the accessibility of word forms on sentence structures. *Journal of Memory and Language, 26,* 119–137.

Bock, J. K. (1987b). Co-ordinating words and syntax in speech plans. In A. W. Ellis (Ed.), *Progress in the psychology of language.* (Vol. 3). London: Erlbaum.

Bradley, D., Garrett, M., & Zurif, E. (1980). Syntactic deficits in Broca's aphasia. In D. Caplan (Ed.), *Biological studies of mental processes.* Cambridge, MA: MIT Press.

Bresnan, J., & Kaplan, R. M. (1982). Introduction: Grammars as mental representations of language. In J. Bresnan (Ed.), *The mental representation of grammatical relations.* Cambridge, MA: MIT Press.

Butterworth, B., & Howard, D. (1987). Paragrammatisms. *Cognition, 26,* 1–37.

Byng, S. (1988). Sentence processing deficits: Theory and therapy. *Cognitive Neuropsychology, 5*(6), 629–676.

Byng, S., & Coltheart, M. (1986). Aphasia therapy research: Methodological requirements and illustrative results. In E. Hjelmquist & L. G. Nilsson (Eds.), *Communication and handicap: Aspects of psychological compensation and technical aids.* Amsterdam: Elsevier/North-Holland.

Caplan, D., Baker, C., & DeHaut, F. (1985). Syntactic determinants of sentence comprehension in aphasia. *Cognition, 21,* 117–175.

Caplan, D., & Futter, C. (1986). Assignment of thematic roles to nouns in sentence comprehension by an agrammatic patient. *Brain and Language, 27,* 117–134.

Caplan, D., & Hildebrandt, N. (1986). Language deficits and the theory of syntax: A reply to Grodzinsky. *Brain and Language, 27,* 168–177.

Caplan, D., & Hildebrandt, N. (1988). *Disorders of syntactic comprehension.* Cambridge, MA: MIT Press.

Caramazza, A. (1986). On drawing inferences about the structure of normal cognitive systems from the analysis of impaired performance: The case for single-patient studies. *Brain and Cognition, 5,* 41–66.

Caramazza, A., & Berndt, R. S. (1978). Semantic and syntactic processes in aphasia: A review of the literature. *Psychological Bulletin, 85*(4), 898–918.

Caramazza, A., & Berndt, R. S. (1981). Syntactic aspects of aphasia. In M. T. Sarno (Ed.), *Acquired aphasia* (pp. 157–182). New York: Academic Press.

Caramazza, A., & Berndt, R. S. (1985). A multicomponent deficit view of agrammatic Broca's aphasia. In M.-L. Kean (Ed.), *Agrammatism.* Orlando, FL: Academic Press.

Caramazza, A., & Hillis, A. E. (1989). The disruption of sentence production: Some dissociations. *Brain and Language, 36,* 625–650.

Caramazza, A., & Zurif, E. B. (1976). Dissociation of algorithmic and heuristic processes in language comprehension: Evidence from aphasia. *Brain and Language, 3,* 572–582.

Chomsky, N. (1957). *Syntactic structures.* The Hague: Mouton.

Chomsky, N. (1981). *Lectures on government and binding.* Dordrecht: Foris.

Clark, H. H., & Clark, E. V. (1977). *Psychology and language.* New York: Harcourt Brace Jovanovich.

DeBleser, R. (1987). From agrammatism to paragrammatism: German aphasiological traditions and grammatical disturbances. *Cognitive Neuropsychology, 4*(2), 187–256.

Dell, G. S. (1986). A spreading activation theory of retrieval in sentence production. *Psychological Review, 93,* 283–321.

Dell, G. S., & Reich, P. A. (1981). Stages in sentence production: An analysis of speech error data. *Journal of Verbal Learning and Verbal Behavior, 20,* 611–629.

Frazier, L. (1988). Grammar and language processing. In F. J. Newmeyer (Ed.), *Linguistics: The Cambridge survey.* Cambridge: Cambridge University Press.

Friederici, A. D. (1982). Syntactic and semantic processes in aphasic deficits: The availability of prepositions. *Brain and Language, 15,* 249–258.

Friederici, A. D. (1983). Aphasics' perception of words in sentential context: Some real-time processing evidence. *Neuropsychologia, 21,* 351–358.

Friederici, A. D. (1985). Levels of processing and vocabulary types: Evidence from on-line comprehension in normals and agrammatics. *Cognition, 19,* 133–166.

Friederici, A. D., & Graetz, P. A. M. (1987). Processing passive sentences in aphasia: Deficits and strategies. *Brain and Language, 30,* 93–105.

Fromkin, V. A. (1973). *Speech errors as linguistic evidence.* Mouton: The Hague.

Gallaher, A. J., & Canter, G. J. (1982). Reading and listening comprehension in Broca's aphasia: Lexical versus syntactical errors. *Brain and Language, 17,* 183–192.

Garrett, M. F. (1975). The analysis of sentence production. In G. Bower (Ed.), *Psychology of learning and motivation* (Vol. 9). New York: Academic Press.

Garrett, M. F. (1980). Levels of processing in sentence production. In B. Butterworth (Ed.), *Language production* (Vol. 1). New York: Academic Press.

Garrett, M. F. (1982). The organization of processing structure for language production: Applications to aphasic speech. In D. Caplan, A. R. Lecours, & A. Smith (Eds.), *Biological perspectives on language.* Cambridge, MA: MIT Press.

Gleason, J. B., Goodglass, H., Obler, L., Green, E., Hyde, M., & Weintraub, S. (1980). Narrative strategies of aphasic and normal-speaking subjects. *Journal of Speech and Hearing Research, 23,* 370–382.

Goodglass, H. (1968). Studies on the grammar of aphasics. In S. Rosenberg & K. Joplin (Eds.), *Developments in applied psycholinguistics research.* New York: Macmillan.

Goodglass, H. (1976). Agrammatism. In H. Whitaker & H. A. Whitaker (Eds.), *Studies in neurolinguistics* (Vol. 1). New York: Academic Press.

Goodglass, H., & Berko, J. (1960). Agrammatism and inflectional morphology in English. *Journal of Speech and Hearing Research, 3,* 257–267.

Goodglass, H., Fodor, I. G., & Schulhoff, C. (1967). Prosodic factors in grammar—evidence from aphasia. *Journal of Speech and Hearing Research, 10*(1), 5–20.

Goodglass, H., & Menn, L. (1985). Is agrammatism a unitary phenomenon? In M.-L. Kean (Ed.), *Agrammatism.* Orlando, FL: Academic Press.

Grodzinsky, Y. (1984). The syntactic characterization of agrammatism. *Cognition, 16,* 99–120.

Grodzinsky, Y. (1986). Language deficits and the theory of syntax. *Brain and Language, 27,* 135–159.

Heeschen, C. (1985). Agrammatism versus paragrammatism: A fictitious opposition. In M.-L. Kean (Ed.), *Agrammatism.* Orlando, FL: Academic Press.

Heeschen, C., & Kolk, H. (1988). Agrammatism and paragrammatism. *Aphasiology, 2*(3/4), 299–302.

Heilman, K. M., & Scholes, R. J. (1976). The nature of comprehension errors in Broca's conduction and Wernicke's aphasics. *Cortex, 12*(3), 258–265.

Hildebrandt, N., Caplan, D., & Evans, K. (1987). The man left$_t$ without a trace: A case study of aphasic processing categories. *Cognitive Neuropsychology, 4*(3), 257–302.

Howard, D. (1985). Agrammatism. In S. Newman & R. Epstein (Eds.), *Current perspectives in dysphasia.* London and New York: Churchill-Livingstone.

Jones, E. V. (1984). Word order processing in aphasia: Effect of verb semantics. *Advances in Neurology, 42.*

Jones, E. V. (1986). Building the foundations for sentence production in a non-fluent aphasic. *British Journal of Disorders of Communication, 21,* 63–82.

Kean, M.-L. (1978). The linguistic interpretation of aphasic syndromes. In E. Walker (Ed.), *Explorations in the biology language.* Montgomery, VT: Bradford Books.

Kleist, K. (1916). Uber Leitungsaphasia und grammatische storungen. *Montasshrift fur Psychiatrie und Neurologie, 40,* 118–199.

Kolk, H. H., & Van Grunsven, M. (1985). Agrammatism as a variable phenomenon. *Cognitive Neuropsychology, 2*(4), 347–384.

Kolk, H. H., Van Grunsven, M., & Keyser, A. (1985). On parallelism between production and comprehension in agrammatism. In M.-L. Kean (Ed.), *Agrammatism.* Orlando, FL: Academic Press.

Lapointe, S. G. (1983). Some issues in the linguistic description of agrammatism. *Cognition, 14,* 1–39.

Lapointe, S. G. (1985). A theory of verb form use in the speech of agrammatic aphasics. *Brain and Language, 28,* 196–234.

Lesser, R. (1978). *Linguistic investigations of aphasia.* New York: Elsevier/North-Holland.

Levelt, W. J. M. (1989). *Speaking: From intention to articulation.* Cambridge, MA: MIT Press.

Linebarger, M. C., Schwartz, M. F., & Saffran, E. M. (1983a). Sensitivity to grammatical structure in so-called agrammatic aphasics. *Cognition, 13,* 361–392.

Linebarger, M. C., Schwartz, M. F., & Saffran, E. M. (1983b). Syntactic processing in agrammatism: A reply to Zurif and Grodzinsky. *Cognition, 15,* 215–225.

Lukatela, K., Crain, S., & Shankweiler, D. (1988). Sensitivity to inflectional morphology in agrammatism: Investigation of a highly inflected language. *Brain and Language, 33,* 1–15.

Marslen-Wilson, W. (Ed.). (1989). *Lexical representation and process.* Cambridge, MA: MIT Press.

Marslen-Wilson, W., & Tyler, L. K. (1980). The temporal structure of spoken language understanding. *Cognition, 8,* 1–71.

Martin, R. C. (1987). Articulatory and phonological deficits in short-term memory and their relation to syntactic processing. *Brain and Language, 32,* 159–192.

Martin, R. C., & Blossom-Stach, C. (1986). Evidence of syntactic deficits in a fluent aphasic. *Brain and Language, 28,* 196–234.

Martin, R. C., Wetzel, W. F., Blossom-Stach, C., & Feher, E. (1989). Syntactic loss versus processing deficits: An assessment of two theories of agrammatism and syntactic comprehension deficits. *Cognition, 32,* 157–191.

Menn, L., & Obler, L. K. (1990). *Agrammatic aphasia: Cross-language narrative source book.* Baltimore, MD: John Benjamins.

Miceli, G., & Mazzucchi, A. (1990). The nature of speech production deficits in so-called agrammatic aphasia: Evidence from two Italian patients. In L. Menn, & L. K. Obler (Eds.), *Agrammatic aphasia: Cross-language narrative source book.* Baltimore, MD: John Benjamins.

Miceli, G., Mazzucchi, A., Menn, L., & Goodglass, H. (1983). Contrasting cases of Italian agrammatic aphasia without comprehension disorder. *Brain and Language, 19,* 65–97.

Miceli, G., Silveri, M. C., Romani, C., & Caramazza, A. (1989). Variation in the pattern of omissions and substitutions of grammatical morphemes in the spontaneous speech of so-called agrammatic patients. *Brain and Language, 36,* 447–492.

Miceli, G., Silveri, M. C., Villa, G., & Caramazza, A. (1984). On the basis for the agrammatics' difficulty in producing main verbs. *Cortex, 20,* 207–220.

Mitchum, C. C., & Berndt, R. S. (1988). Aphasia rehabilitation: An approach to diagnosis and treatment of disorders of language production. In M. G. Eisenberg (Ed.), *Advances in clinical rehabilitation. II.* New York: Springer.

Mitchum, C. C., & Berndt, R. S. (1989). *Verb retrieval and sentence production.* Paper presented at the Academy of Aphasia, Santa Fe, NM.

Monsell, S. (1987). On the relation between lexical input and output pathways for speech. In A. Allport, D. G. MacKay, W. Prinz, & E. Scheerer (Eds.), *Language perception and production: Relationships between listening, speaking, reading and writing.* Orlando, FL: Academic Press.

Nespoulous, J.-L., Dordain, M., Perron, C., Ska, B., Bub, D., Caplan, D., Mehler, J., & Lecours, A. R. (1988). Agrammatism in sentence production without comprehension deficits: Reduced availability of syntactic structures and/or of grammatical morphemes? A case study. *Brain and Language, 33,* 273–295.

Parisi, D. (1987). Grammatical disturbances of speech production. In M. Coltheart, G. Sartori, & R. Job (Eds.), *The cognitive neuropsychology of language.* Hillsdale, NJ: Erlbaum.

Pisoni, D. B., & Luce, P. A. (1987). Acoustic-phonetic representations in word recognition. *Cognition, 25,* 21–52.

Saffran, E. M. (1982). Neuropsychological approaches to the study of language. *British Journal of Psychology, 73,* 317–337.

Saffran, E. M. (1990). Short-term memory impairment and language processing. In A. Caramazza (Ed.), *Advances in cognitive neuropsychology and neurolinguistics.*

Saffran, E. M., Berndt, R. S., & Schwartz, M. F. (1989). The quantitative analysis of agrammatic production: Procedure and data. *Brain and Language, 37,* 440–479.

Saffran, E. M., & Martin, N. (1990). Short-term memory impairment and sentence processing: A case study. In G. Vallar & T. Shallice (Eds.), *Neuropsychological impairments of short-term memory.* Cambridge: Cambridge University Press.

Saffran, E. M., & Schwartz, M. F. (1988). 'Agrammatic' comprehension it's not: Alternatives and implications. *Aphasiology, 2*(3/4), 389–394.

Saffran, E. M., Schwartz, M. F., & Marin, O. S. M. (1980a). The word order problem in agrammatism: production. *Brain and Language, 10,* 263–280.

Saffran, E. M., Schwartz, M. F., & Marin, O. S. M. (1980b). Evidence from aphasia: Isolating the components of a production model. In B. Butterworth (Ed.), *Language production* (Vol. 1). London: Academic Press.

Schwartz, M. F. (1987). Patterns of speech production deficit within and across aphasia syndromes: Application of a psycholinguistic model. In M. Coltheart, G. Sartori, & R. Job (Eds.), *The cognitive neuropsychology of language.* Hillsdale, NJ: Erlbaum.

Schwartz, M. F., Linebarger, M. C., & Saffran, E. M. (1985). The status of the syntactic deficit theory of agrammatism. In M.-L. Kean (Ed.), *Agrammatism.* Orlando, FL: Academic Press.

Schwartz, M. F., Saffran, E. M., & Marin, O. S. M. (1980). The word order problem in agrammatism: comprehension. *Brain and Language, 10,* 249–262.

Schwartz, M. F., Linebarger, M. C., Saffran, E. M., & Pate, D. S. (1987). Syntactic transparency and sentence interpretation in aphasia. *Language and Cognitive Processes, 2,* 85–113.

Shallice, T. (1988). *From neuropsychology to mental structure.* New York: Cambridge University Press.

Shankweiler, D., Crain, S., Gorrell, P., & Tuller, B. (1989). Reception of language in Broca's aphasia. *Language and Cognitive Processes, 4*(1), 1–33.

Sproat, R. (1986). Competence, performance and agrammatism: A reply to Grodzinsky. *Brain and Language, 27,* 160–167.

Stemberger, J. P. (1984). Structural errors in normal and agrammatic speech. *Cognitive Neuropsychology, 1*(4), 281–313.

Stemberger, J. P. (1985). An interactive activation model of language production. In A. Ellis (Ed.), *Progress in the psychology of language* (Vol. 1). London: Erlbaum.

Swinney, D. A., Zurif, E. B., & Cutler, A. (1980). Effects of sentential stress and word class upon comprehension in Broca's aphasics. *Brain and Language, 10,* 132–144.

Tissot, R. J., Mounin, G., & Lhermitte, F. (1973). *L'agrammatisme.* Brussels: Dessart.

Tyler, L. K. (1985). Real-time comprehension processes in agrammatism: A case study. *Brain and Language, 26,* 259–275.

Tyler, L. K. (1989). Syntactic deficits and construction of local phrases in spoken language comprehension. *Cognitive Neuropsychology, 3*(6), 333–356.

Tyler, L. K., & Warren, P. (1987). Local and global structure in spoken language comprehension. *Journal of Memory and Language, 26,* 638–657.

Wasow, T. (1985). Postscript. In P. Sells, *Lectures on contemporary syntactic theories: An introduction to government-binding theory, generalized phrase structure grammar, and lexical-functional grammar.* Stanford, CA: Center for Study of Language and Information.

Weinrich, M., Steele, R. D., Carlson, G. S., Kleczewska, M., Wertz, R. T., & Baker, E. (1989). Processing of visual syntax in a globally aphasic patient. *Brain and Language, 36* (3), 391–405.

Wulfeck, B. B. (1988). Grammaticality judgments and sentence comprehension in agrammatic aphasia. *Journal of Speech and Hearing Research, 31,* 72–81.

Zingeser, L., & Berndt, R. S. (1988). Grammatical class and context effects in a case of pure anomia: Implications for models of language production. *Cognitive Neuropsychology, 5* (64), 473–516.

Zingeser, L., & Berndt, R. S. (1990). Retrieval of nouns and verbs in agrammatism and anomia. *Brain and Language, 39,* 14–32.

Zurif, E. (1982). The use of data from aphasia in constructing a performance model of language. In M. A. Arbib, D. Caplan, & J. C. Marshall (Eds.), *Neural models of language processes*. New York: Academic Press.

Zurif, E., & Blumstein, S. (1978). Language and the brain. In M. Halle, J. Bresnan, & G. Miller (Eds.), *Linguistic theory and psychological reality*. Cambridge, MA: MIT Press.

Zurif, E., & Grodzinsky, Y. (1983). Sensitivity of grammatical structure in agrammatic aphasics: A reply to Linebarger, Schwartz, and Saffran. *Cognition, 15*, 207–213.

8

Explanations for the Concept of Apraxia of Speech

HUGH W. BUCKINGHAM, JR.

The term APRAXIA OF SPEECH has had an extremely variable history and has been used to describe different types of behaviors, in different types of patients, and under different stimulus conditions. The term has been used, often with qualifying modifiers, to describe syndromes or parts of syndromes. Since there is, and has been, so much variability in the way the term has been used, it becomes very confusing when it is simply incorporated to label a specific patient. Because there have been different conceptualizations of "apraxia," it stands to reason that apraxia of speech may also not be completely well defined throughout the literature on the topic. The purpose of this chapter is to outline the various ways in which apraxia has been explained so that the reader will have a proper appreciation of the complexities involved. In this chapter I propose that under certain interpretations there are additional forms of apraxia of speech that differ from the frontal speech apraxias. Frontal lobe apraxia of speech has been referred to as aphemia, Broca's aphasia, motor aphasia, anarthria, verbal aphasia, phonetic disintegration of speech, apraxia, apraxic dysarthria, cortical dysarthria, and oral verbal apraxia.

I propose further that certain phonological functions as understood by linguists operate IN PARALLEL WITH and at a distinct level from the hierarchically organized sensorimotor practic functions of the brain. The phonological functions involve selecting and sequencing of phoneme-like units that speakers BELIEVE themselves to be uttering. In actuality, they are uttering sounds, or PHONES, which may then be considered as being produced by nervous firings giving rise to complex and synchronous muscular contractions resulting in acoustic impingements on the air. Practic brain function is involved at the neurological level throughout the whole process from ideation to production. However, these processes must be worded carefully so as not to imply that phonemes are articulated. The nature of the phoneme is such that it cannot be uttered. It is a "psychologically real" abstract unit for which no invariant factor, articulatory or acoustic, has yet been found. Consequently, an anomaly results when it is maintained that phonemes are uttered, produced, articulated, distorted, and so forth. Phonological functions of selecting and sequencing phonemes are much too abstract and ideational in nature to be considered "motoric."

Another claim made in this chapter is that the subphonemic errors made by Broca's aphasics typically involve disturbed limb–praxic function for the vocal tract musculature involving motor commands for outputting speech sounds (phones)—the units for which, together with their serial order, being "fed forward" from the ideational level.[1] The result is an effortful, groping speech output, usually seen when the left frontal lobe is damaged in the region of the third convolution. This syndrome has also been referred to as an apraxia of speech, which leads to the principal thesis of this chapter. One can plausibly argue, given the historical development of the notion of apraxia, that the apraxias in general admit of alternate explanations: one that involves disconnection

---

1. I am aware that as this sentence reads I am dangerously close to the fallacy that John Hughlings Jackson (1878/1931b) warned against. He believed that a "psychical state" (an "idea of a word" or simply "a word") cannot produce an articulatory movement, which is clearly a physical phenomenon. Rather, it was "discharge of the cells and fibers of the anatomical substratum of a word [which] produces the articulatory movement" (p. 156). In general, Jackson stated, "In our studies of diseases of the nervous system we must be on our guard against the fallacy that what are physical states in lower centers fine away into psychical states in higher centers; that, for example, vibrations of sensory nerves become sensations, or that somehow or another an idea produces a movement" (p. 156). Phonemes, like words, are abstractions and like the "psychical" elements of Jackson do not "fine away" into physical articulatory production. I believe that this dualism of Jackson is appropriate and should be carefully considered when dealing with phonemes and neurological theories of speech production; that is, the problems are precisely what Jackson was defining last century (also see Engelhardt, 1975). Phonemes are mentalistic constructs of the mind; they have psychological not physical reality. Fromkin and Rodman (1988) write, "A phoneme is an abstract unit. We do not utter phonemes; we produce phones" (p. 78); that is, we produce phonetic segments. They quote the early twentieth century linguist Edward Sapir: "In the physical world the naive speaker and hearer actualize and are sensitive to sounds, but what they feel themselves to be pronouncing and hearing are 'phonemes' " (p. 70).

lesions and another that involves cortical lesions of centers. The explanatory mechanisms for both are different. This state of affairs has resulted in much confusion over the issue of apraxia and the consequent notion of apraxia of speech. The problems have been recalcitrant principally because the arguments are at the level of explanation and not at the level of data.

Historical Background

Prior to the work of John Hughlings Jackson and Hugo Liepmann, who are usually credited with developing the notion of apraxia (e.g., Harrington 1985, 1987; Brown, 1988b), Paul Broca (1861/1960) considered two alternative views for explaining the speech problem of his patient, Leborgne (Tan) (also see Schiller, 1979). The first, which he eventually adopted, was that the patient had lost his "faculty of articulate speech."[2] This was an intellectual faculty and consisted of the "memory for the procedure one has to follow in order to articulate the words" (p. 54). This was not a general faculty of speech, but rather one aspect dealing with "the faculty to coordinate the movements which belong to the articulate language" (pp. 54–55). Broca also considered the possibility that aphemia might "be a kind of locomotor ataxia, limited to the articulation of sounds" (p. 54). Were this to be the case, Broca reasoned, the disorder would not be the loss of an intellectual faculty "which belongs to the thinking part of the brain" (p. 54) but rather "it would only be a special case of the general coordination of actions, a faculty which depends on the motor centers of the central nervous system" (p. 54). At the time of Broca's paper, the "Bell-Magendie" sensorimotor dichotomy had not reached the cerebral cortex (Young, 1970); consequently, it was difficult to conceive of a CORTICAL motor (nonintellectual) system, and therefore damage to the cortex should only disrupt "intellectual faculties"; motor organization and function were not considered to be intellectual. Broca states quite succinctly, "Everyone knows that the cerebral convolutions are not motor organs" (p. 70). Subsequent to Broca's presentation, the stage was set for the arguments as to whether Broca's aphasia involves

2. The preponderance of the word FACULTY at the time Broca was writing is due to the development of the so-called faculty psychology of the eighteenth-century Scottish philosophers Thomas Reid and Dugald Stewart. Franz Gall drew heavily from the Scottish school when developing his theories of phrenological faculties. These theories subsequently influenced Bouillaud, who passed them on to Auburtin and Broca. Thirty-five years before Broca, Bouillaud (1825) argued (in support of Gall) that the "faculty of articulate language" is mediated in the anterior lobes of the brain (Young, 1970).

language or speech, although in 1861 the discussion was whether it was an intellectual impairment or a nonintellectual problem with locomotion. This quandary parallels the present-day disputes over whether lesions in areas 44 and 45 of the dominant left hemisphere cause an aphasia or an apraxia. It is claimed that the second option focuses on the motor system rather than on the language system.

Benton and Joynt (1960) showed that speech-specific lingual paralysis secondary to brain damage is a long-observed phenomenon, having been reported by Soranus of Ephesus (A.D. 98–135), Paracelsus (1493–1541), and Johann Schenck von Grafenberg (1530–1598). The same observation of speech-specific lingual paralysis was made by Auburtin and Bouillaud (Stookey, 1963), both of whom were precursors of Broca. In addition to noting simply that the patient could swallow, masticate, and so forth, but could not utter words normally, Baillarger (Alajouanine, 1960) and Auburtin (as reported in Broca, 1861/1960, p. 52) observed that the patient could quite fluently produce speech automatisms. Still, a third observation of the Broca's aphasic was made. Broca wrote "that they can immediately WHEN BEING ASKED bring their tongue up, down, right, etc. But, however precise these movements may appear to us they are infinitely less so than the excessively delicate movements which the language demands" (p. 54, emphasis added). From this description provided by Broca, we have apraxia of speech without oral–facial apraxia (at least no involvement of the tongue).

A fourth description was also provided: a "nonprotrusion" of the tongue upon VERBAL request. Jackson (1866/1931a) wrote,

> In some cases of defect of speech the patient seems to have lost much of his power to do anything HE IS TOLD TO DO, even with those muscles that are not paralyzed. Thus, a patient will be unable to put out his tongue when we ask him, although he will use it well in semi-involuntary actions, e.g., eating and swallowing. (p. 121, emphasis added).

He added, "He will not make the particular grimace he is told to, even when we make one for him to imitate" (p. 121). Twelve years later, in an article appropriately entitled "Remarks on Non-Protrusion of the Tongue in Some Cases of Aphasia," Jackson (1878/1931d) again wrote, "It will have been noticed by every medical man that some patients who have loss or defect of speech do not put out the tongue WHEN THEY ARE ASKED" (p. 153, emphasis added). Jackson, unlike Broca, was describing an apraxia of speech WITH oral–facial apraxia. Jackson was the first to stress that the disorder was one of volitional movement; he considered that encoding a propositional message was highly volitional as was the protrusion of the tongue upon verbal–acoustic command. Incorporating volition, as an explanatory device for certain movement disorders goes back at least to Jackson (1874/1931c), who described the "three degrees of the use of the word 'no.' " Uttering *no* when requested to do so is more volitional than uttering *no* in the normal course of conversation. Its production was considered most automatic (and consequently less volitional) when used emotionally as a negative command. It is important to point out that Jackson had to rule out any paralysis in order to account for the less volitional movements. In his explanations, he also had to rule out comprehension loss. A failure to perform on verbal command is not a significant observation if it can be shown that the patient simply does not understand the command.

This historical development is well known now, especially with von Bonin's (1960) publication and the selected writings of Jackson (edited by J. Taylor, 1931). Several investigators of apraxia of speech have referred to the pioneering work of Jackson (De Renzi, Pieczuro, & Vignolo, 1966, p. 50; Head, 1926, p. 94; Johns & LaPointe, 1976, p. 185; Mateer & Kimura, 1977, p. 262).

It is necessary, however, to mention that at this point in history an intriguing ambiguity was developing. The results of this ambiguity are evident today. The patient who, to the verbal command, was unable to grimace or to protrude the tongue for Jackson might have had a lesion disconnecting the area for comprehending language and the area for outputting the motor commands. He would not necessarily have had any lesions in the motor zones of the frontal lobes. On the other hand, the lesion could have been in the frontal cortical motor zones. In this case, disconnection would not serve as the crucial element of explanation, but rather the explanation would rest at the motor level. The disconnection hypothesis crucially involved LANGUAGE as a stimulus condition; the other did not. Therefore, the mechanisms would be quite distinct. The nondisconnection hypothesis would emphasize the mechanism as breakdown in motor planning and sequencing, whereas the other would emphasize disconnection of motor zones and language comprehension zones. Geschwind (1975) stated, "The explanation . . . tries to account for all the apraxias on the basis of disconnection of the areas in which the command is comprehended from those areas where the command is carried out" (p. 190). The nondisconnection proponents require that their "apraxia" be caused by some lesion in an important cortical area. The disconnection position does not require this. Again, I am making the claim that once the phrase "when they are asked" comes up in the history of aphasia, the interpretive ambiguity arises. I further claim that the ambiguity has led to the two distinct views of apraxia; the issues became crystalized when aphasiologists began trying to characterize an "apraxia of speech."

Nowadays, however, much of the zeal and furor with which the anatomical connectionist accounts were proposed has subsided. There is growing evidence from the neurosciences that a strict anatomical connectionist explanatory paradigm is seriously flawed and needs radical rethinking and resynthesis (e.g., Deacon, 1989; but also see the recent connectionist account for interhemisphere information transfer in Gazzaniga's, 1989, essay). The recent death of Norman Geschwind has no doubt taken some of the wind out of the sails of cerebral connectionism, since he was such a vigorous, productive, and articulate proponent of this view. Furthermore, it should be emphasized that the anatomical connectionism of Meynert and Wernicke that was rekindled by Geschwind has little if anything to do with the so-called "connectionist" arguments of parallel distributed processing models. The only link between the two is their shared affinity with the basic tenets of the decades-old association psychology (see Buckingham, 1984, for a discussion of the associationist roots of anatomical connectionism).

The work of Hugo Liepmann shows that he utilized both types of explanation. His "limb-kinetic" apraxia was caused by lesions in the frontal motor association areas, and his "ideational" apraxia stemmed from damage to the sensory association zones in the posterior temporoparietal regions (Brown, 1972, 1988; Head, 1926). Liepmann felt that motor aphasia was a particular form of limb-kinetic apraxia of the "glossolabiopharyngeal" apparatus; subsequently, he added the larynx to this string of anatomical modifiers (Head, 1926, p. 99). According to Liepmann, a limb–kinetic apraxia was characterized by a "loss of kinaesthetic memories of a definite part of the body" (Head, 1926, p. 97). The patient had "lost the power to execute certain combinations of acquired movements" and "delicate movements" were impossible (Head, 1926, p. 98). Accordingly, Liepmann, when speaking of motor aphasia as a type of limb-kinetic apraxia, was extending the notion of "limb" to the speech articulators as well as to the arms. In a sense, this is not unreasonable. When Liepmann discussed this type of apraxia, he did not make reference to the stimulus-specific language command, but rather invoked the Jacksonian notion of volition as the key explanatory device. That is, the patient could be said to be apraxic in his speech behavior, even though no one had provided a verbal command to behave linguistically, that is, to speak. Clearly, except for repetition, speakers articulate of their own accord—something quite different from performing some behavior upon verbal command from a second party. Again, disconnection apraxia principally involves motor isolation from auditory zones for language comprehension or from posterior visual zones. The historical oddity in all this is that Liepmann also introduced the first in-depth description of ideomotor types of apraxia, which were clearly connectionistic in nature.[3] Here, the ideational and motor-kinesthetic processes are separated from one another rather than lesioned themselves. By postulating an internal initiating ideational component, Liepmann could explain this type of apraxia without restricting the output disturbances to those elicited by linguistic verbal commands. (See Paillard, 1982, for an excellent integration of recent neurophysiological research into the overall framework of Liepmann.) Once again, the "will" was incorporated as the command generator, so to speak. These confusions no doubt led Geschwind (1965) to state that "the designation 'apraxia' is an inadequate one unless the stimulus conditions are specified" (p. 606). For this reason, it has always been strange to me, at least, that researchers who describe nonconnectionistic apraxias of speech elicit so much of their data by asking patients to REPEAT (Johns & Darley, 1970). Disconnection explanations are classic for repetition deficits (Kinsbourne, 1972; Wernicke, 1874/1977). Aside from a supramarginal gyrus ideokinetic apraxia, Liepmann (1900) also described the "sympathetic" ideokinetic apraxia of the left limbs arising from callosal disconnections in the anterior regions or from left prefrontal lesions, both of which disconnect the dominant language zones from the right hemisphere motor areas.

Before leaving the earlier studies of apraxia, it is instructive to look at how Henry Head's discussion of the issue served to extend the interpretive ambiguity. When writing about Liepmann and apraxia in his chapter entitled "Chaos," Head provided some more chaos by beginning the section with the clear implication that the apraxic behavior is secondary to a linguistic command, such as "told to protrude his tongue," "show his teeth to command," and "execute such movements to order" (Head,

---

3. A disconnection theory will, of course, admit of a lesion to some center if that center is anatomically connected to (and between) Wernicke's area and a primary motor area. Consequently, the ensuing explanation will still be connectionistic. I have in mind the lesions in the prefrontal motor association cortex, which still, according to Geschwind's model, disconnect the primary cortical motor area from Wernicke's area rather than destroy "programmed memories for movement," and so on. In addition, there is Geschwind's (1969) description of lesions which simply disconnect the angular gyrus from Wernicke's area, and lesions that actually damage the gyrus itself. The resulting syndromes are different, but in both cases, the essential mechanism is disconnection of Wernicke's area from the occipital visual cortex. Certainly, Geschwind uses center explanations in dealing with certain failures to respond on imitation, but these failures are not apraxic-like, rather they are due to motor weakness. We will see later that Geschwind has another explanation for certain other failures on imitation.

1926, p. 93). Up to this point in Head's treatment, the label APRAXIA is directly linked with the language stimulus condition as an essential component. It would therefore be subject to a connectionist explanation. However, by page 95 in Head's discussion, we are told that an apraxia of speech is a disorder with the "higher mechanics of verbal formulation" (p. 95). Since formulation is involved, it is now possible to consider the stimulus condition as self-induced on the part of the speaker. It is this point at which the "will" is usually invoked. Once the concept of volitional or purposive behavior comes to the foreground, the will may serve as the stimulus condition. Consequently, the disconnection explanation would no longer be necessary. As we shall see, this is exactly what happened in the further developments in apraxia of speech and the concomitant nonconnectionistic explanation, and this persists to the present (e.g., Katz, 1988a, Tuller & Story, 1987, 1988; Ziegler & von Cramon, 1985, 1986).

It would appear, then, that ample historical precedent exists for two quite distinct explanations for movement disorders, which are both referred to as "apraxia." One explanation leads to the acceptance of an apraxia of SPEECH; the other does not. Consequently, one's position as to what constitutes an apraxia in general has largely determined one's stand on whether it makes sense to talk about an apraxia of speech. Several current stands are discussed next against this historical backdrop.[4]

Current Stands

One current position regarding apraxia of speech is often referred to as the "Mayo School" position. The influence of F. L. Darley, Arnold Aronson, and J. R. Brown is obvious, and many researchers (with clinical and theoretical goals alike) have, in one way or another, been extending their views (See Wertz, LaPointe, & Rosenbek, 1984). The list of publications is long indeed; much of the work has appeared since the late 1960s. The excellent summaries provided by Johns and LaPointe (1976), Rosenbek, Kent, and LaPointe (1984), and Rosenbek (1984) are written from the point of view of the Mayo tradition of a center lesion apraxia of speech. Their claim is that this is what others have called Broca's aphasia. Furthermore, the apraxia of speech is caused by lesions

4. Table I in Johns and LaPointe (1976) contains an illuminating collection of clinical descriptions of limb-kinetic speech deficits from Auburtin (1861) to Shankweiler, Harris, and Taylor (1968).

in the frontal motor association areas, although this school, in the early stages of its formulations, seemed to feel that any articulatory disturbance was apraxic in nature, that is, essentially motoric. As it turns out, recent thinking has shown this to be more likely than originally thought (Buckingham & Yule, 1987). I return to this issue later in the chapter. The further important claim of this school is that an apraxia of speech is not a language problem at all. Two clear historical points are made by this school. First, it adopts Broca's postulated (but ultimately not chosen) explanations that the "aphemic" disorder is primarily motoric, not a higher level linguistic problem. Second, the school would agree with Liepmann that what is involved is a type of limb-kinetic apraxia of the glossolabiopharyngeal musculature. Consequently, the mechanism involved need not be connectionistic. In addition, the Mayo position separates apraxia of speech from oral–facial apraxia, although like most others (e.g., De Renzi et al., 1966), the proponents are well aware that the two most often occur together.

Another proposal may be regarded as the result of a reaction to the early positions of the Mayo School that every nondysarthric articulation problem was an apraxia of speech. This second proposal makes a clear distinction between frontal articulatory disorders and posterior articulatory disorders. The work reported in Canter (1973), Trost and Canter (1974), and Burns and Canter (1977) shows that the nature of the articulation parameters in anterior versus posterior patients is quite distinguishable. An apraxic, nonfluent character is seen in the frontal lobe subjects, whereas the temporoparietal lesion patients show a fluent and well-articulated phonemic disorder where, for instance, all allophones of substituted phonemes have their predicted phonetic shapes. This second current proposal brings to bear not only neuroanatomical questions, but also LINGUISTIC questions. Much argumentation now involves determining exactly what is and what is not phonemic. As we shall see, the interpretations are often quite inconsistent, the reason being twofold: The abstract nature of the phoneme has not been fully appreciated, nor has the possibility of a subtle motor deficit in the posterior aphasias.

Luria (1973) has been surprisingly reminiscent of Liepmann in his views of apraxia. He equated Broca's aphasia (efferent motor aphasia) with a kinetic apraxia, and afferent motor aphasia with kinesthetic apraxia of speech. He correlated the phonological paraphasias of sensory aphasics with an ideational apraxia. It turns out, however, that Luria had admitted of only center-lesion explanations for apraxic behavior. An excellent example is taken from Luria's (1973) description of the speech problems secondary to lesions in the inferior postrolandic zones of the parietal lobe, that is, the cortical sensory area for the speech musculature. He wrote,

> If a lesion of the secondary (kinaesthetic) zones of the post-central region
> affects the LOWER ZONES OF THIS REGION OF THE LEFT (DOMINANT) HEMISPHERE,
> i.e., the region of secondary organization of kinaesthetic sensation in the face,
> lips and tongue, the kinaesthetic apraxia may manifest itself in a special
> manner in the organization of movements of the speech apparatus, leading to
> the distinctive disorder of speech which has been called AFFERENT MOTOR
> APHASIA. (p. 174)

Luria, in the same manner as Liepmann, has viewed any voluntary movement as mediated by a "complex functional system" involving ideation, kinesthetic afferentiation, and kinetic organization. Each of these organizational levels has its anatomical substrate, and one or another type of apraxia will arise secondary to lesions in the respective areas. Movement parameters for speech will be disturbed in various ways depending upon the localization of damage along the posterior to frontal axis. The articulatory aspect, therefore, of the different types of aphasia will be characterized as one or another type of "apraxia of speech," from ideational to kinetic.[5] The ideational level of apraxic behavior is much closer to the level at which we characterize the more abstract aspects of sound systems of human language, which has given rise to the notion of an "apraxia of language" as far as the phonology of language is concerned (e.g., Buckingham, 1983). In sum, Luria (1972) criticized the notion of conduction aphasia and in general has been critical of disconnectionism. It is clear, therefore, that he would emphasize center-lesion theories of apraxia rather than disconnectionist theories. Consequently, it has not been at all difficult for Luria to conceive of apraxia of speech, in fact, he has considered several possible forms for it.

   Brown (1972) has agreed with Luria to the extent that there is "interference at comparable stages in microgenesis of speech and movement" (p. 198). Brown wrote that "disorders of movement, like those of speech, are disturbed in a posterior–anterior fashion" (p. 195). Worded differently, "the movement complex passes from a conceptual to a motoric form [see footnotes 1 and 5], undergoing a progressive differentiation comparable to that which occurs in the speech system" (p. 195). More recently, Brown (1975a, 1975b, 1977, 1988a) has refined his notion of

---

5. One could certainly argue that "ideation-to-kinetic" feedforward microgenesis schemes come dangerously close to Jackson's (1878/1931b) edict against the direct mind–brain leap taken in models that allow psychic states to fine away into physical states. This parallels the problem alluded to in footnote 2 of going from phoneme to articulation (see also Kelso & Tuller, 1981, p. 227).

microgenesis of action. For Brown (1975a) "the term microgenesis has been proposed for the continuous formative activity which underlies cognition" (p. 26). For instance, he wrote (1977), "Both facial and limb apraxia can occur with frontal and temporoparietal lesions. In this respect, they are comparable to phonemic paraphasia, which also occurs with anterior and posterior pathology" (p. 72). Blumstein (1973) supported this; in fact, she found MORE phonemic paraphasia with anterior-lesioned patients. At the phonemic level, the anterior versus posterior differences appeared to be quantitative, not qualitative, just as Poeck and Kerschensteiner (1975) found for oral apraxia. Similarly, De Renzi et al. (1966) wrote, "Oral apraxia characterizes patients whose speech productions may be very different from one another" (p. 68). For aphasic speech errors in anterior versus posterior populations, the qualitative distinctions do not reside in the phonemics of the errors but rather in the allophonics. There seems to be more incorrect allophonic production by frontal patients, who nevertheless at other times also produce correct allophones of incorrectly selected phonemes, as do the posterior patients. I return to this question later. In any event, for Brown, the more anterior the lesion is, the more "maladroit" the action.

Brown (1975a) more recently wrote,

> There is little evidence for the view that language is formed posteriorly and somehow conveyed, by way of thalamus, insula or an association bundle, to Broca's area for motor speech. Rather, there appears to be simultaneous realization out of a common deep structure into the final perceptual and motoric forms of the language act. (p. 26)

(Also see Deacon, 1989, for more on the failure of "feedforward" theories.) This means that damage along the posterior–anterior plane of the cortex at one or another location will NOT give rise to qualitatively different types of disturbed action. This is quite a different position from his earlier view (Brown, 1972, chap. 17, p. 195), that the microgenesis of action took the route of the posterior–anterior axis over the cortical mantle along which distinct apraxic syndromes could be placed (i.e., more or less Liepmann's conception). In any event, Brown acknowledged center lesion apraxias rather than disconnecting lesion apraxias. One other important distinction has been made by Brown (1975a) when he wrote, "The 'centers' of traditional neuropsychology are rather to be considered as LEVELS by means of which cognition is carried one stage further" (p. 29). Pathways, for Brown, "do not serve to associate ideas, perceptions of movements, written words to spoken words, etc., but rather link up temporally transformations occurring at different points in the microgenetic sequence" (p. 29). In addition, his model incorporates distinct levels of speech apraxias. I mentioned earlier that in many cases of nonconnectionistic explanations of apraxia, the concepts of volition and will play important roles. This is the case with Brown as well. For instance, "object facilitation" for transitive movements is said to bring "about a more concrete (i.e., less volitional) setting for the desired movement. In this sense, movements with objects are comparable to performance in conversational speech" (Brown, 1972, p. 197). The clear implication is that spontaneous conversational speech is less volitional than being requested to do something such as provide linguistic labels for objects, repeat a linguistic form, describe some scene, or imitate a transitive movement (without the object).

Brown proposed his dynamic microgenesis model as an alternative to disconnection theory. We witness this in his discussion of conduction aphasia (Brown, 1975b). The speech paraphasia and the movement apraxia represent disturbances at comparable levels in the actualization of speech and movement. Since speech is a form of movement, the two collapse into one and thus we have (for conduction aphasia) an "ideomotor apraxia of speech." Brown avoided reference to an interruption of pathways and instead claimed that the patient shows apraxic behavior because the language input stimulus (the request) presses the volitional system, not because the language area is cut off from the motor zones. J. W. Brown (personal communication, 1978) would actually state this somewhat differently. Instead of a language input stimulus pressing a volitional system, he would prefer to say that it is the level of representation of an act that determines whether it has a volitional or automatic character. Therefore, in Brown's model the linguistic command does not play the essential role that it does in the disconnection model. A spontaneous act for Brown would represent a developing crystalization of that act at a more "preliminary" level. That act is therefore more automatic. The act executed secondary to a command to do it exists at a "higher" representational level and consequently determines the increased volitional nature of the performance. The various forms of apraxia, according to Brown, reflect or point to stages in the ontogeny of a motor act, and he has paralleled this with the view that the distinct forms of aphasia characterize stages in the development of a linguistic production. According to Brown (1977), facial apraxia is a "disorder of VOLITIONAL facial action appearing in performances initiated in the test situation with no alteration of spontaneous facial motility. The more automatically elicited performances are better preserved, whereas actions elicited by written or spoken commands are impaired" (p. 72, emphasis added).

Much has been said about apraxia from supramarginal gyrus lesions

(Brown, 1972; Denny-Brown, 1958; Geschwind, 1965; Mateer & Kimura, 1977). Predictably, those who admit of center-lesion explanations have considered supramarginal gyrus apraxia of speech. The supramarginal gyrus is a crucial zone for the discussion of apraxia in general AND of apraxia of speech. Although it is a cortical area of the parietal lobe strategically located for the language zones, it is also anatomically quite near the arcuate fasciculus fibers traveling through opercular regions (Galaburda, 1982). Some have preferred to call the repetition disturbance of conduction aphasia an "ideokinetic apraxia for the formation of sounds" (Kleist, 1916). Center-lesion theories of apraxia, of course, are premised on such statements as "memory for movement is stored in this area." If the area is damaged, the patient will be apraxic whether or not be is TOLD TO DO anything. Denny-Brown (1958) seems to be representative of those investigators who emphasize posterior center-lesion theories of apraxia of speech. He wrote,

> Although the complex movements of lips, tongue and larynx show disturbances that are apractic in nature, these occur in isolation from other types of body apraxia, as if the praxis of speech had developed independently in the dominant insula and parietal operculum, more removed from the parietal-occipital region concerned in other types of ideation apraxia. Thus apraxia of the tongue is a special and particular variant of motor apraxia, associated most commonly with executive aphasia, and usually dissociated from apraxia of facial expression. (pp. 12–13)

Denny-Brown made no mention here of a relevant stimulus (the linguistic command), a characteristic of center-lesion theories of apraxia. It should be pointed out, however, that by 1965 he had shifted his focus to frontal lesions (Broca's aphasia) and consequent speech disturbances. He (Denny-Brown, 1965) described a Broca's aphasic with lesions in the left third and part of the second frontal convolution. The patient (a) had difficulty initiating words, (b) had occasional substitution and anticipation of segments and syllables, (c) had a "slowing of rhythm," and (d) showed great variability. Denny-Brown concluded, "This particular difficulty is associated with varying degrees of apraxia of the tongue, lips, face, and respiratory control" (p. 462). Denny-Brown still admits of center-lesion apraxias, but now the region involved for apraxia of speech is in the dominant frontal lobe instead of the insular and parietal opercular zones described in the 1958 paper.

In a series of articles (Kimura, 1976, 1977a; Kimura & Archibald, 1974; Mateer & Kimura, 1977), Kimura has suggested that, "lesions of the left hemisphere impair the performance of complex motor sequences, regardless of whether the sequences are meaningful or not" (Kimura &

Archibald, 1974, p. 346). Her belief has been that speech disturbances and apraxia are simply distinct manifestations of a breakdown in the control of the action of motoric sequencing. The actual sequential control system is in the parietal lobe according to Kimura (1976; Kimura & Watson, 1989). Kimura's theory is that the movements need only be complexly coordinated, not necessarily meaningful (i.e., symbolic). The reasoning has been extended to her hypothesis that "the left hemisphere is particularly well adapted, not for symbolic function per se, but for the execution of some categories of motor activity which happen to lend themselves readily to communication" (Kimura, 1976, p. 154).[6] The problem here, of course, is to determine just what is complex and what is not. In a sense, the issue may reduce simply to the fact that multiple or sequential movements are more difficult to produce than single isolated ones. It should be pointed out that Kimura has begun to think that the problem is "a failure to achieve target motor responses when more than one is required rather than just an improper ordering of those targets" (Mateer & Kimura, 1977, p. 274). Similarly, Kimura (1977b) has stated that her analysis of apraxic errors (due to left posterior lesions) reveals that the principal difficulty rests, not with ordering the movements, but rather with selecting and/or executing new postures, whether of brachial or oral musculature (also see Kimura, 1982; Kimura & Watson, 1989).

More germane to this chapter, however, are Kimura's assumptions and explanations for apraxia. She clearly has admitted center-lesion explanations of apraxia and not supported disconnection theories. Kimura's views of apraxia seem to have clouded her understanding of the disconnection view, which always stipulates the linguistic command stimulus. By failing to isolate the "relevant stimulus" in Geschwind's model, she missed the point when examining his work. The following quotation from Kimura and Archibald (1974) is indicative of misunderstanding at the explanatory level. They wrote, "Section of the corpus callosum drastically diminishes the control of the left hemisphere over the left hand, . . . which would seem to support Geschwind's suggestion that cortico-cortical pathways are involved in the left hemisphere's bilateral control of movement" (p. 347). Left-handed "sympathetic" apraxias arise from left frontal or anterior callosal lesions that disconnect left Wernicke's area from right hemisphere motor zones. The disconnection theory is NOT that "memory for movements" and so forth

6. Kimura's position is that human language articulation is an overlaid function that developed over ancient neural architectures of early man, architectures that no doubt were involved early on with the control and timing of sequential movement (Calvin, 1983; Deacon, 1989).

is located, say, in the supramarginal gyrus. In fact, Geschwind (1965, pp. 612–613) argued against this view. Kimura and Archibald (1974) continued, "However, the inadequacy of the left hemisphere control over the left hand in callosally sectioned patients has been demonstrated largely via verbal instruction" (p. 347). This quotation more than anything else demonstrates their misunderstanding of the connectionistic theory of apraxia, because it implies that nonverbal instructions should have been used. Again, for Geschwind, in order to demonstrate an apraxia in the split-brain cases, the input command should be via verbal instruction. Thus, it is rather pointless for Kimura and Archibald to proceed. They wrote, "It is quite possible that non-verbal instruction, of the kind involved in imitating movement sequences, could proceed via extra-callosal pathways" (p. 347). Geschwind would certainly agree that the movement could be produced with a nonverbal input command, but largely because the right hemisphere could get the command information from, for instance, the right visual cortex.

Geschwind's connection model certainly holds for those patients who can nevertheless perform to imitation. There are problems, however, in explaining those patients who are apraxic to imitation also, since, as Geschwind (1975) admitted, "We are led to expect that the patient[s] will respond correctly to non-verbal stimuli, which can reach motor regions without going through the speech areas" (pp. 190–191). Geschwind (1975) wrote, "Clearly some factor other than disconnection between language and motor areas seems to be necessary to account for these findings" (p. 191). The other factor invoked by Geschwind (1975) is that of cerebral dominance for limb (arm, hand) movement that (contrary to Kimura's theory) may or may not be in the same hemisphere for speech (Heilman, Coyle, Gonyea, & Geschwind, 1973; also see Heilman, 1979; Heilman & Gonzalez-Rothi, 1985, for excellent summaries of the apraxias in general). This addition to Geschwind's disconnectionism does not necessarily compromise his model, since the dominant hemisphere can be said to "lead" or "drive" the nondominant hemisphere in many instances. Heilman et al. (1973) and Rubens, Geschwind, Mahowald, and Mastri (1977) supported the model that incorporates dominance theory AND disconnectionism. Of course, in the instances of lack of improvement on imitation, the issue of a verbal language input does not play a role. Nevertheless, disconnection theory still offers the most plausible explanation for the sympathetic apraxias.

Kimura and Archibald (1974) discussed purported counterevidence for the pathway involved in sympathetic apraxia. From the outset, Liepmann (1900) and Bonhoeffer (1914) predicted the possibility of a left-handed apraxia from right frontal lobe damage, where the hemiplegia was not serious enough to render apraxia testing worthless. Geschwind has repeatedly made similar predictions. Kimura and Archibald (1974) wrote, "The difficulty with this view is that one would occasionally expect apraxia to appear only in the left hand, from a right hemisphere lesion . . . because the control from the left cortex to left hand had been disrupted in its passage through the right hemisphere" (p. 347). It is somewhat strange to see this wording; this is precisely what the prediction has been from the beginning! It would appear that Kimura and Archibald were unaware of the prediction. They further stated that in their "own series of patients, the hypothesis was testable only in three patients who had right hemisphere damage without hemiplegia, and in these patients both hands performed equally well on movement copying" (p. 347). There are two serious problems with this statement. In the first place, all we are told is that Kimura and Archibald's patients had right-hemisphere damage with no hemiplegia. In these cases it is crucial to state WHERE in the right hemisphere. For all we know, these three patients could have had postrolandic involvement, in which case the purported counterevidence collapses. Geschwind (1975) commented on right-hemisphere sympathetic apraxia. He wrote,

> Such cases are rare; in most instances the area of destruction is large enough to affect the actual precentral motor regions on the right, and the resulting left-sided paralysis makes it impossible to assess the presence of apraxia. I have, however, seen one patient with a left-sided apraxia in whom radioisotope-brain-scanning showed a lesion deep in the right frontal lobe. (p. 190)

In these rare cases, it is essential that the site of the right-hemisphere lesion be specified. It must be frontal, small enough so as not to occasion paralysis, and strategically located so as to disrupt the anterior callosal fibers coming from the left. The second error, which is more to the point of the present chapter, is that Kimura and Archibald's three patients were tested on MOVEMENT COPYING. There is much tactile and visual information in the movement-copying task that can get to the right hemisphere for left-hand movement. This is not counterevidence for the connectionistic theory, since the stimulus input command is not spoken language. In fact, Geschwind (1965) stressed that "'apraxia' is not a unitary disturbance, since under appropriate conditions these patients could carry out complex motor tasks" (p. 612). Again, it appears that the essential aspects of a connectionistic explanation of apraxia have not been appreciated by Kimura and Archibald. I should also reiterate that Kimura's center-lesion theories of apraxia quite predictably have led her to admit of apraxias of speech. In fact, as I showed, the speech apraxias for her are simply one manifestation of complex nonsymbolic movement disorders that arise secondary to posterior left-hemisphere damage.

It should be clear to the reader at this juncture that all the center-lesion theories of apraxia usually admit of at least one distinct "apraxia of speech": Kleist—ideomotor apraxia of speech; Denny-Brown—ideomotor (insular–parietal operculum) and frontal lobe apraxia of speech; Luria and J. Brown—Kinetic, ideomotor, and ideational apraxias of speech;[7] Kimura—posterior (supramarginal gyrus) apraxia of speech; Canter and Darley (Mayo School)—frontal lobe (around central sulcus) apraxia of speech. I would emphasize that this enumeration of different types of apraxia of speech has more serious consequences for the concept "apraxia of speech" as a whole than does the enumeration of different terminological classifications of ONE form of apraxia of speech (the limb-kinetic).

Johns and LaPointe's (1976) theoretical assumption is that there IS an apraxia of speech, and it is a type of limb-kinetic apraxia for the speech musculature; it is essentially Liepmann's view of that type of apraxia. Their literature survey and in-depth discussion of terminological confusion almost entirely deals with limb-kinetic center-lesion apraxia of speech and the plethora of nomenclature it has had throughout the history of aphasia. Table 1 in their article comes from the work initiated by Johns in his doctoral dissertation research on this form of apraxia of speech. Again, it is based on center-lesion theory, obviously not connection theory. Throughout history (they begin with Auburtin, 1861), this frontal lobe apraxia of speech has been referred to as "aphemia, Broca's aphasia, motor aphasia, anarthria, verbal aphasia, phonetic disintegration of speech, apraxia, apraxic dysarthria, cortical dysarthria, and oral

---

7. Brown (1972, chap. 10) drew a strong correlation between ideational apraxia posterior fluent paraphasic speech. He wrote,

> We may almost speak of ideational apraxia as a 'fluent' apraxia, contrasting it with 'non-fluent' apraxias of anterior origin. In ideational apraxia there is an abundance of partial movements, each normal in itself, and the overall movement sequence, though disorganized, has an ease and an effortless quality as is seen in the speech of posterior aphasia. (p. 170)

Again, this is essentially Luria's view as well; consequently, I have grouped them together here, although as J. W. Brown pointed out to me (personal communication, 1978) he never actually made the correlation complete by specifically referring to an ideational apraxia of SPEECH. From the above quotation, however, it would not have been very far fetched had he done so. Again, as mentioned earlier, this close relation between ideational apraxia and the speech in posterior aphasia led me to suggest an "apraxia of language" (Buckingham, 1983), where the *phonology* of language was implicated.

verbal apraxia" (Johns & LaPointe, 1976, p. 163). The context of the actual descriptions, however, reveals that "generally good clinical agreement has existed" (p. 163). There is never much argument with the actual descriptions; I would imagine that the connectionist would give similar descriptive details of the typical Broca patient.[8]

There are, however, a few places in Johns and LaPointe's (1976, pp. 186, 191) review where they mentioned disconnection phenomena and where they referred to another center-lesion type of apraxia of speech. When discussing the De Renzi et al. (1966) findings concerning the possible (but not often obtaining) separation of limb-kinetic apraxia of speech and oral–facial apraxia, they compared the two possible anatomical explanations suggested in that paper. One is that oral nonverbal movements and oral verbal (speech) movements could be mediated by two distinct frontal cortical association areas. Note that this view would NOT be in accord with Kimura's model discussed earlier, although it is clearly a center-lesion hypothesis. The second consideration of De Renzi et al. (1966), however, as Johns and LaPointe (1976) wrote, is "that apraxia from commands can result from lesions to pathways connecting frontal and temporal lobes; and apraxia from imitation can result from lesions disrupting occipital and frontal fasciculi" (p. 186). Later in their review, they outlined speech disturbances that may stem from lack of cortical sensory feedback information, and they noted that perhaps there could be another type of apraxia of speech. In fact, they pointed out that Jay Rosenbek, one of the most influential clinicians and researchers of the Mayo tradition, "revised the concept of apraxia of speech to include sensory-perceptual influences rather than the traditional view of it as strictly a motor, or output, speech disorder" (pp. 191–192). The various peripheral oral sensation studies in limb-kinetic apraxias of speech have shown sensory deficits. These deficits could presumably occur from lesions that extend to the lower postrolandic region, and therefore what Rosenbek discovered was that Luria's "afferent apraxia" could be an added component to limb-kinetic apraxia.

It is unfortunate that Johns and LaPointe (1976) did not include discussion of Kimura's work on posterior apraxia of speech or of the whole question of disconnection explanation in apraxia. Kimura denied that frontal lesions result in anything more than weakness, slowness, and incoordination of movement. In addition, Geschwind (1965) wrote that "'limb-kinetic' apraxia has not been defined clearly enough to separate it

8. It is usually noted that a large percentage of Broca's aphasics have more extensive lesions of "the operculum from anterior frontal through Broca's area to anterior parietal regions, the insula, both banks of the central (Rolandic) fissure . . . usually extending deep into the hemisphere" (Mohr, 1976, p. 228).

from mild pyramidal disturbance" (p. 617). Certainly, there is no frontal apraxia of speech for Geschwind (or any apraxia OF SPEECH, for that matter) because of his connectionistic paradigm. Geschwind has explained Broca's aphasia as due to a disconnection between Broca's area and the motor face area on the motor strip anterior to the rolandic fissure, but he denies that anything is gained by using the term apraxia of speech, since patients are seen with Broca's aphasia who do not have an oral–facial apraxia and others are seen with Wernicke's aphasia who do have an oral–facial apraxia. Furthermore, as mentioned above, patients with distinct aphasic outputs may have qualitatively similar oral–facial apraxias, and patients with no speech problems at all may have an oral–facial apraxia. There is no frontal apraxia of speech for Kimura either, since for her complex praxis for movement is a dominant POSTERIOR function of the brain. These theories have challenged the theoretical position of the Mayo tradition as to apraxia of speech. Nevertheless, what I am arguing for in this chapter is that it is hopelessly ambiguous to simply say that this or that is an apraxia of speech without further specifying the neuroanatomical explanation being used, the location of the lesion, the stimulus conditions that evoked the behavior said to be apraxic, and the actual phonetic disorder itself.

General Characteristics of Limb-Kinetic Apraxia of Speech

Patients with a limb-kinetic apraxia of speech have at least five typically observable behaviors. In attempting to articulate, these patients often show a groping behavior, which indicates that they have the underlying phonological form in mind. Although there are difficulties with initiating the articulated sequence, articulatory preposturing quite often reveals the vocal tract configuration for the initial segments of the word to be uttered. This initial preposturing may also include some noncontiguous coarticulatory information (see Katz, 1987, 1988a, for experimental confirmation of this brute force observation), so that, for example, the lips may be rounded for the preposturing of /k/ when a patient is groping for the word /klu/ (*clue*). In light of the fact that these patients often manifest sequencing impairments, the coarticulated /k/, rounded by the influence of the noncontiguous high-back vowel /u/, is easier to produce than the sequential transition to the /l/, which is contiguous to the /k/. This demonstrates that coarticulation and transitionalizing are separate processes, and that coarticulated information is often coded within syllable units. Limb-kinetic apraxics' disturbances often are exacerbated on elicitation, which, of course, relates to the issue of volitional level and confrontation testing.

I would now like to mention some of the difficulties I have interpreting various of the supposed linguistic and nonlinguistic diagnostic characteristics of the limb-kinetic type of apraxia of speech, that is, the frontal Broca's patient. PROGRAMMING, INCOORDINATION, and VARIABILITY are three terms that, to my way of thinking, have led to many inconsistencies and have in general not served to differentiate syndromes very well. INITIATION, SELECTION, and SEQUENCE have not been sharply enough defined, and the term PHONEME itself has caused no little confusion because of its abstract nature.

When we are told that an apraxia of speech involves disorders in the "programming" of motor speech, we need to know immediately what the units of speech are that are involved and precisely where in the encoding process we are. It is not clear that the phonemic level is motoric in any sense whatsoever. Is the motor level allophonic? Are the allophones specified within broadly defined syllabic units that may straddle lexical boundaries? One should not lose sight of the fact that PROGRAM is a metaphor and may be used as a descriptor at any level of abstraction whatsoever and therefore may be used at the earliest ideational levels or at the latest output levels (see footnotes 1 and 5).

It is important to distinguish between an "incoordination" of the musculature used for speech and an "incoordination" of the set of synchronous nerve impulses that eventually impinge on different muscle groups for properly timed articulatory events. Disturbed laryngeal control is certainly a type of incoordination that is seen in frontal lobe patients; it is not muscular, but rather neural (see Marshall, Gandour, & Windsor, 1988).

VARIABILITY OF BEHAVIOR is another open-ended term that not only is somewhat confusing but also can define practically any aphasic or apraxic. Presumably, this term came into use as a way to differentiate the apraxic from the dysarthric. Using the term to distinguish an apraxic from an aphasic, however, would be disastrous. Not only do all types of aphasics exhibit variability in their language behavior, but so do apraxics. The variability, however, is explained in two quite different ways. The connectionist, like Geschwind, as I pointed out earlier, attributes the variability to the different stimulus conditions under which the patient is requested to do something. If the request is nonverbal, the patient often is able to carry out the movement pattern despite the fact that it could not be performed to verbal request. On the other hand, center-lesion explanation must invoke volition, will, and so forth; limb-kinetic speech apraxias are characterized by the "islands of error-free productions" that are often thought to be more automatic, less propositional, and therefore less volitional. Recall, however, the different interpretation of center-lesion apraxic disturbances in Brown's theory to which I alluded earlier. The term VARIABILITY, therefore, does not even distinguish between theories of apraxia, rather what distinguishes them is their explanatory mechanisms.

Canter, Burns, and Trost (1975) suggested a useful distinction for getting around the problems with the vague term SEQUENCING. They differentiated between "transitionalizing" from phoneme to phoneme (it would have been more proper to say from phone to phone) and the sequential ordering of phonemes. Therefore, we could say that the essential problem with posterior patients is with sequential ordering, whereas the problem with the Broca patient is with "sequential flow." Note that the "syntagmatic" disorder of the motor aphasic described by Luria (and linguistically characterized by Jakobson) is that of Canter's sequential flow, although, until it is disambiguated in this way, SYNTAGMATIC as a descriptive term will not work, since the posterior "paradigmatic" aphasics will exhibit the sequential ordering disturbances that are clearly "syntagmatic" in nature (Buckingham, 1977, 1986).

The qualitative aspect of phonemic paraphasia in terms of substitution, deletion, addition, and linear switch is no different for ANY aphasic, including any patient with limb-kinetic apraxia of speech. The cortical system for selecting and sequencing phonemic units will show disruption at times for frontal patients as well as for posterior patients. For instance, it confuses the issue when we try to distinguish frontal from posterior syndromes by stating that only posterior cases show selection difficulties; the frontal patient does also. I have seen many posterior cases where there are addition, deletion, and linear types of phonemic paraphasia. It is not diagnostic of any group to show that substitution errors, for example, are more frequent than other error types. Buckingham and Kertesz (1976, p. 52) showed that, of the analyzable phonemic paraphasias of a neologistic jargonaphasic, there were far more substitution errors. Earlier, Blumstein (1973, pp. 46–47) demonstrated that (using her classification of aphasia), when one analyzes the phonemic errors of Broca's conduction, and Wernicke's aphasics in terms of substitution, simplification, linear switch ("environment" in Blumstein's terms), and addition, one finds that all the groups have the same relative difficulty. Each group had more substitution errors, followed by simplifications (deletions), and next by linear switches. Least in number for all groups were addition paraphasias. Evidently, as Blumstein (1973) stated, "the phonological errors characteristic of aphasic speech reflect a systematic disorganization of phonology independent of a particular lesion site" (p. 47). In addition, the fact that error sounds are usually off target by only one dimension (feature) as opposed to two or three is not diagnostic either for any one group, since, again, Blumstein's study (1973, p. 49) showed that ALL aphasics will exhibit substitutive paraphasias that in the majority of cases differ from the target phonemic unit by one distinctive feature. The distinctions that would be diagnostic for each group would be quantitative in nature, not qualitative—at least at the phonemic level. Furthermore, there is increasing evidence to believe that many of the so-called strictly paradigmatic phonemic substitutions involve phonemic false evaluation on the part of hearers (e.g., Buckingham & Yule, 1987).

Experimental Studies

The actual situation with substitution errors is more complex, however, and we must make some finer SUBPHONEMIC distinctions. In this way we might come up with a better diagnostic for differentiating patients with limb-kinetic apraxias of speech from the posterior patients. Let us assume that there may be two possible disturbances, one at a nonmotoric phonemic level and the other at some lower stage of speech production (see Ziegler, 1987). Breakdown at either level may result in a substitutive error. The problem was well stated by De Renzi et al. (1966): "It is hard to decide if the substitution of voiced consonantal sounds (e.g., b, v, g), by the corresponding voiceless consonants (p, f, k, respectively) is due to wrong choice of phonemes . . . or to lack of synergy of the vocal cords with the muscles of articulation" (p. 55).

The phonetic counterpart for the linguistic distinctive feature [voice] for syllable initial stop consonants involves the time interval between the release of the consonantal closure and the onset of vocal fold vibration of the larynx for the following vowel; this is the VOICE-ONSET TIME (VOT). Generally speaking, the closer the voice onset occurs to the time of release, the more likely the consonant will be filtered through the linguistic system as [+voice], for a language such as English. The parameters are language dependent, and there will always be a range of values of onset times where variation within the range causes no perceptual differences for hearers. For instance, the VOT value of syllable initial /d/ in English may range from −180 to +25 msec, but most adult values range from 0 to +20 msec. Time of stop release is always zero with respect to VOT, so that a VOT of −180 msec means that the folds start vibrating 180 msec BEFORE stop release. For /t/, the VOT values range from +40 to +120 msec. The consonants /b/–/p/ /g/–/k/ have different ranges, the bilabials ranging to the left of the alveolars and the velars ranging to the right. Therefore, for example, the /k/ will have the longest VOT lag of the stops. The phonetic counterpart of the linguistic nondistinctive feature [aspiration] is the VOT lag subsequent to closure release; the longer the voicing lag, the more aspiration. Aspiration is a characteristic of English syllable initial /p/, /t/, and /k/, except when these segments follow /s/, in which case their VOT lags shorten considerably. The shortened lag places them perceptually closer to their [+voice] counterparts.

A study by Blumstein, Cooper, Zurif, and Caramazza (1977) comparing anterior subjects with posterior subjects on voice-onset timing[9] parameters showed a "lack of synergy" for the former group. Although at times they will produce phonemic substitutions (certainly to be expected, given Blumstein, 1973), this group produces asynergic phonetic substitutions that in several instances turn out to be unexpected, incorrect ALLOPHONIC productions. In the case of /t/, for instance, the anterior patient is likely to substitute the allophone of /t/ that normally occurs after /s/, as in [stap], in syllable initial position (see Blumstein, Cooper, Goodglass, Statlender, & Gottlieb, 1980, for the addition of conduction aphasics and of a dysarthric speaker with brain stem damage in comparative VOT studies). To a native speaker of English with a "good phonetic ear" or with, for example, a knowledge of a language such as Spanish (Abramson & Lisker, 1973), this will be recognized (perceived) as a voiceless initial unaspirated stop. By many (probably most), however, it will be perceived as belonging to /d/ and not as an incorrect allophone belonging to /t/. Accordingly, the patient will be credited with a phonemic error, when in fact a phonetic error had been produced! That is, the phonemic target of the speaker will be falsely evaluated by the hearer.

Sands, Freeman, and Harris (1978) followed the improvement over a 10-year period of a patient with a limb-kinetic apraxia of speech. They found that, at the end of this period, errors of place and manner of articulation as well as deletion errors were greatly reduced. What persisted were essentially errors in voicing, and thus it was concluded that the remaining apraxic disturbance was one of temporal coordination of the abductory (spreading) and adductory (bringing together) laryngeal processes with upper articulatory events.

9. Experimental analysis with such parameters as VOT has provided a far superior account of phonemic versus phonetic error and will no doubt help clarify the nature of "phonetic disintegration." This is an extremely important issue, since many have claimed that apraxia of speech (or verbal apraxia) is phonetic disintegration (Alajouanine, Ombredane, & Durand, 1939, Shankweiler & Harris, 1966; Shankweiler et al., 1968).

Freeman, Sands, and Harris (1978) followed up with a more detailed study of VOT in apraxia and found that it differed markedly from productions in non–brain-damaged normals. They noted that apraxic articulations did not include voicing lead for voiced stops and that lag times for voiced stops were longer than normal. On the other hand, the lag times for voiceless stops were shorter than normal. All of these apraxic changes resulted in more closely compact VOT ranges around the point of stop release. Consequently, there was a clear overlapping of [+voice] or [−voice] perceptual categories. Apraxics produced little or no prevoicing leads or long lags. Since VOT is the acoustic cue for perceiving the [±voice] distinction for syllable initial consonants, apraxic incoordinations will trigger perceptual categorial switches in HEARERS. Finally, the authors noted that the apraxics' VOT range constriction to the short lag area (+20 to +30 msec) mirrors VOT ranges in young children, but they offered no explanation for this.

Kewley-Port and Preston (1974), as discussed in Cooper (1977), offered an account of VOT acquisition in children in terms of complexity of neural control. In the first place, vocal fold vibration is brought about by three factors: (a) folds must be adducted, (b) they must be relatively relaxed, and (c) a sufficient drop in pressure across the larynx must be maintained in order to permit an accelerated airflow. The neural control for these three factors is different for the three VOT types: prevoicing, short lag, and long lag. It turns out that the short-lag VOT is neuromuscularly less complex, because, unlike with prevoicing and long lag, factor (c) is mechanically produced. For short-lag VOTs, the speaker need only adduct the folds prior to release of stop closure and keep them relatively lax. Upon release of closure, a sufficient drop in transglottal pressure takes place automatically due to the equalization of mouth pressure. This enables initiation of glottal vibration shortly after the release. For prevoicing or long-delay VOT, the maintenance or delay of cross-glottal pressure drop requires more complexly timed and controlled neural commands. Eventually, the child comes to master the more complex neuromuscular coordination. It appears that the apraxic has lost it. As I discuss later, however, dysarthric speech is characterized by abnormally long voice lags for voiceless consonants, and, consequently, one must be cautious when interpreting neuromuscular complexity explanations for voice-onset lag times.

Incorrect allophonic production may, in some cases, even sound like a foreign accent to some listeners. In fact, one characterization of a foreign accent is precisely that the nonnative speaker often produces some inappropriate phonetic variant of the target phoneme for the language he or she is speaking (Ardila, Rosselli, & Ardila, 1988; Blumstein,

Alexander, Ryalls, Katz, & Dworetzky, 1987). Whitaker (1975) described a patient with left frontal damage whose speech output gave the partial impression of being Spanish in origin. (Ardila et al.'s (1988) patient was a Spanish speaker whose speech gave the impression of being English in origin.) Whitaker wrote that the patient had characteristics of Broca's aphasia with apraxia of speech. This patient was from central Michigan, had not been outside the area, and had never studied a foreign language. Whitaker wrote, "There were striking problems with aspiration; initial voiceless stops were often unaspirated" (p. 27). One suspects that the patient was having difficulties with temporal coordination, although no acoustic measurements were taken. Other phonetic characteristics of this syndrome were clearly not phonemic in nature and gave the impression of being ataxic. This type of subphonemic foreign accent output secondary to frontal rolandic area lesions has been described by several others as a cortical dysarthria (Whitaker, 1975, pp. 23–25). This does not mean that the cortical frontal lobe patient is impossible to distinguish from the patient with upper or lower motor neuron damage, who also produces phonetic errors.

The phonetic distortions are less variable in the motor neuron group than in the cortical group, and, unlike the motor neuron dysarthrias, the limb-kinetic patients quite often produce phonemic errors with proper allophonic realization. Blumstein et al. (1980) and Itoh, Sasanuma, Hirose, Yoshioka, and Ushijima (1980) have been able to distinguish dysarthric speech from limb-kinetic apraxic speech. Blumstein et al. showed that, unlike Broca's aphasics, whose VOT range was quite restricted, the dysarthric patients productions for consonants were distributed over a wider VOT range. Broca's VOT values for voiceless consonants rarely surpassed +150 msec, whereas the predominant voiceless productions for the dysarthrics were abnormally long. This is why dysarthric speech at times seems overly aspirated. Furthermore, unlike the Broca productions, the dysarthric productions showed no phonetic overlap between voiced and voiceless categories. This would explain why hearers rarely attribute phonemic errors to dysarthrics, but often do so to apraxics. Itoh et al. (1980) clearly demonstrated that the pattern and velocity of dysarthric (one patient with ataxia and the other with amyotrophic lateral sclerosis) articulations are distinct from those of limb-kinetic apraxia of speech. For the most part, VOT studies have concentrated on syllable-initial stops.

Still another type of substitutive phonetic error can be seen. It represents a phonetic problem, but unlike the $[p^h] \rightarrow [p]$ in English, where the incorrectly substituted phone may be assigned to the same phonemic unit to which the target phone belongs, the error MUST be assigned to a different phonemic unit from that of the target, even though the phonetic error may not imply a phonemic selection error. Itoh, Sasanuma, and Ushijima (1979) studied velar movements in the speech of a limb-kinetic type of patient by fiber-optic techniques. The patient's lesion involved "the cortical surface near the anterior tip of the Sylvian fissure of the left hemisphere and immediately subjacent subcortical white matter" (p. 229). Due to asynchronous velar movement, a phonetic change of [n] → [d] (i.e., improper lowering of the velum) was demonstrated. The phonetic error, however, is assigned to a phonemic unit distinct from that of the target phone. The phoneme /n/ does not have [d] as a possible allophonic alternation in Japanese; consequently, the phonetic error [d] must be assigned to /d/. However, as the authors pointed out, the fiber optic measurements showed that, despite variation in the slope of velar lowering, the pattern of anticipatory lowering was constantly preserved. This was interpreted by the authors as indicating that "the observed variation of the pattern of velar movements and the resultant phonetic change do not stem from a selection or retrieval error of a target phoneme in the process of speech production, namely, an error of phonological processing" (p. 235). Obviously, then, the error is primarily [n] → [d], not /n/ → /d/, although the target phone and the error phone must be assigned to /n/ and /d/, respectively.

Itoh et al. (1980) again measured temporal asynchronies among articulators in apraxia; this time, however, they used a different technique. By placing radioactive pellets upon the lower lip, the lower incisor (for tracking jaw movement), the dorsum of the tongue, and the nasal surface of the velum, a computer-controlled X-ray microbeam system could track the simultaneous movements of these structures during articulation. This procedure further demonstrated the variability and temporal disorganization in the speech of limb-kinetic apraxics.

It is certainly true that the patient with limb-kinetic apraxia of speech may or may not have a concomitant oral–facial apraxia AND may or may not have a concomitant aphasia. That is, some sort of "pure" apraxia of speech may be seen. Therefore, it would be best not to claim that Broca's aphasia equals apraxia of speech. The typical Broca's aphasic clearly has more than the articulatory asynchronies we have been discussing; the apraxia is usually but one component and is most often accompanied by agrammatic production and comprehension[10] (see Berndt's chapter in this volume).

Lecours and Lhermitte (1976) demonstrated that an apraxic (for them,

10. Recall the arguments of A. Damien Martin (1974). See also the papers in Kean (1985) and more recent polemics, such as Grodzinsky (1989).

"anarthric") phonetic disintegration can exist in isolation from aphasia and from dysarthria. Their patient had cortico-subcortical softening of the inferior half of the left precentral gyrus, with Broca's area nevertheless intact. Although Lecours and Lhermitte called this "pure" form of phonetic disintegration "a relatively infrequent form of aphasia" (p. 109), the patient had no other aphasic symptomatology. Although some of the errors in this case were at the phonemic level, the vast majority were subphonemic.

More recently there has been a spate of acoustic-perceptual studies of the speech apraxias. Kent and Rosenbek (1983), for example, published an in-depth study of the acoustic patterns produced by apraxic speakers. Like most of the studies before this, the exemplars were elicited under different stimulus–response parameters. In this investigation, the patients: (a) repeated monosyllabic words, polysyllabic words, phrases, and short sentences; (b) produced conversational speech; (c) described pictures; and (d) read paragraphs aloud. Again, nondisconnectionist studies tend to collapse speech production data gathered across quite different stimulus–response settings. The major conclusions from this study were the following: (a) slow speaking rates with prolongations of transitions and steady states and intersyllabic pauses; (b) a tendency to equalize stress on vowels, which resulted in reduced vocalic centralizing and enhanced maintenance of full vowel quality; (c) articulatory movements toward spatial targets that were often slow and inaccurate for both vowels and consonants; (d) frequent asynchrony between laryngeal and supralaryngeal mechanisms; (e) frequent initiation difficulties; (f) overly complex sound sequences that were often produced as a result of the articulatory struggle itself. The authors also observed that these patients produced occasional errors of segment selection; however, one must be very careful, since "segment selection" errors may not result from motoric difficulties at all. As mentioned above, the segment selection error may simply be in the mind of the hearer, and in that case, the production may very well be apraxic rather than selectional. If the selection error is actually encoded by the patient, then it is unlikely that the error is apraxic in nature. The authors also noted that their patients occasionally produced intrusions, metatheses, and omissions. These kinds of errors also are unlikely to stem necessarily from the motoric–phonetic disruption (see Buckingham, 1986, p. 204, footnote 2, for further remarks on this point).

There has also been a welcome increase in the examination of anticipatory coarticulation in apraxia of speech. Ziegler and von Cramon (1985), using a gated speech stimuli paradigm, assessed the temporal extent of anticipatory vocalic speech gestures. The language was

German, and the vowels examined were /i:/, /y:/, and /u:/. These German vowels made it possible to separate out the feature [+round] from the [front] versus [back] parameter, since German has front rounded and unrounded vowel phonemes. The actual lexical forms that were elicited, recorded, digitized, and gated were /gə tí:tə /, /gə tý:tə /, and /gə tú:tə /. The vowels in question received the tonic accent, and the forms themselves were placed into the carrier phrase, "Ich habe /—/ gehört (I have heard /—/). The single apraxic subject was to repeat the carrier phrase with the form in it. The forms were then gated and subsequently played to groups of hearers for vowel identification. One dysarthric and three normal subjects also produced these forms, the productions being similarly gated for subsequent presentation to hearers. The gated (G) portions for /gə tý:tə /, for example, were as follows: G1— the initial /gə-/ portion; G2–4—$\frac{1}{10}$, $\frac{2}{10}$, and $\frac{3}{10}$ of the /-tVt-/ period (i.e. increasing portions of the burst spectrum of the first /t/); and G5—$\frac{1}{2}$ of the /-tVt-/ period, which would then, obviously, include the actual vowel in question. Relative millisecond values rather then strict millisecond values for the gated units were necessary to control for the variation in productions, such as abnormal prolongations.

For each gated stimulus, the listeners were asked to judge whether the gated stimulus was the beginning of /gə tí:tə /, /gə tý:tə /, or /gə tú:tə /. They had to mark the vowel /i/, /y/, or /u/ on a response sheet, and they were instructed to guess when unsure. Other details aside, the normal speaker productions showed correct vowel identification by hearers significantly ($p < .001$) above chance as soon as plosion was perceivable (i.e., from G2 on) for the initial /t/. For the apraxic speaker productions, hearers were not consistent, especially for /i:/ versus /y:/ until G5. Thus, the rounding for the front rounded vowel /y:/ was not apparent with any regularity in the burst. Also, with the first gated stimulus /gə-/ of the form /gə tú:tə/ as produced by the apraxic, hearers revealed high rates of confusions between /i:/ and /u:/ rather than between /y:/ and /u:/. Lack of anticipatory lip rounding could have caused these confusions. Other apraxic productions showed some anticipatory coarticulation, but only later on, say at G3 or G4. These results, then, suggested to the authors that in apraxia of speech, rather than being totally absent, anticipatory coarticulation is simply DELAYED.

In a follow-up study, Ziegler and von Cramon (1986) more closely examined the acoustic waveform of the exemplars produced by the normals and by the apraxic subject in the 1985 study by examining the formant frequencies and the linear prediction reflection coefficients in the burst spectra that preceded the vowels in question. For the normal productions, vocalic formant information appeared in outline form as early as the vowel portion of the schwa in /gə-/, and actually crossed the initial /t/ of the /-tVt-/ portion. Anticipatory vocalic information for the apraxic exemplars, however, did not uniformly appear until later in the waveform. Thus, the 1986 acoustic study provided strong support for the "delay" in anticipatory coarticulation found in the 1985 perceptual study.

Tuller and Story (1987) were in essential agreement with the delay account of anticipatory coarticulation of Ziegler and von Cramon (1985, 1986), but at the same time Tuller and Story stressed that not all nonfluent patients show a delay and that delay in general is a relative phenomenon depending upon factors such as unit length of items being uttered, the specific vowel in question, and the choice of measurement points. Also, it is certainly reasonable that listeners would make use of a very complex combination of spectral cues for extracting vocalic anticipatory coarticulatory information in consonantal portions of the waveform, and that these cues would not necessarily be restricted to what was focused upon in these studies: formant frequencies (for vowel quality) and characteristic spectral prominence (for rounding) (Katz, 1987). Furthermore, Tuller and Story (1987) pointed out that time-locked points established for the appearence of anticipatory coarticulation information in the waveform is based on collapsed figures based on multiple speakers, and that there is substantial temporal variation across speakers. Therefore, since, "no current time-based theory of anticipatory co-articulation suggests that the absolute temporal extent of anticipation is the same across speakers" (Tuller & Story, 1987, p. 256), it is difficult to know precisely how much of the observed delay in the speech of apraxics is truly abnormal and how much is simply indicative of the variation found in normal speakers.

The interesting point in all this is, of course, that Tuller and Story's (1987) results can agree both with Ziegler and von Cramon and with Katz (1987, 1988a; Katz, Machetanz, Orth & Schönle, 1990), who essentially found no significant differences. Katz compared normal subjects with both anterior and posterior aphasics and found that hearers could perceive vocalic information in the speech of all groups at roughly the same early points. As would be expected, however, Ziegler's and Katz's studies used different stimuli. Ziegler's German language work used trisyllabic forms that were embedded in carrier phrases, all of which were to be uttered by the apraxics. Katz, on the other hand, worked only with English syllables and, unlike Ziegler's study where subjects REPEATED, Katz's subjects READ aloud monosyllabic words and nonwords. These design differences alone would make direct comparisons between the two studies difficult. Katz's syllables were the following:

[si], [su], [ti], [tu], [ki], [ku], [sti], [stu], [ski], and [sku]. These stimuli were digitized, and the stops and fricatives were located. Fourier analysis and linear predictive coding were employed to obtain the spectral picture of the aperiodic segments of the prevocalic consonants, and for each stimulus, 24-msec windows were placed over early and late portions of the consonantal waveforms. The late window was the final 20 msec of the consonant, and the early window differed for the stops and the fricative. For [s], the early window included a full 70 msec prior to vocalic transition onset, whereas for the stops [t] and [k], the early windows included the initial 20 msec of the waveform, in other words, the release portion.

Katz's acoustic analysis demonstrated that the apraxic subjects as well as the fluent and normal subjects had "robust" coarticulatory anticipation of the vowels in [ki] and [ku]. Coarticulatory vowel information was equally apparent in the [s] and [t] of [su] and [tu] across subjects for both [round] and [place]. With the CCV stimuli, all groups produced early acoustic correlates of anticipatory coarticulation of the vowel in the [s] spectrum, the information traveling across the intervening stop. The 10 listeners in Katz's study performed above chance in recognizing the upcoming vowel from the spectral information in the early portions of the consonantal waveforms of all speakers. Although, as a group, the apraxic exemplars were identified above chance, these exemplars received lower identification scores than did those produced by the fluent and normal speakers. In addition, it is interesting to observe the performance of three of the five apraxic speakers who were able motorically to produce the CCV stimuli. One actually showed GREATER than normal degrees of spectral shift in the fricative portions of the [stV] and the [skV]. Another revealed normal shifts for [stV] but not for [skV]. The third showed normal anticipatory shifts for both CCV types. Tuller and Story (1987, p. 257) considered the differences in Ziegler's and Katz's stimuli, and suggested that the early appearance of vocalic anticipatory information in the consonantal spectra in Katz's study is likely due to the use of monosyllabic (and presumably, therefore, stressed) forms. These isolated stressed monosyllabic forms would naturally allow for more extensive articulatory PREPOSTURING during the initial fricatives (for the [s] in both CV and the CCV forms). Although Ziegler did not use fricatives, his stimuli were embedded within larger ranges of phonological material, and, therefore, as Tuller and Story suggested, the articulations in Ziegler study may very well have been subject to greater temporal and spatial constraints, inhibiting exaggerated preposturing.

In a later study, Tuller and Story (1988) looked at normal, fluent, and nonfluent (apraxic) subjects not only on anticipatory coarticulation, but also on "carryover" (left-to-right coarticulation). Both aphasic groups performed somewhat worse than normals for carryover phenomena, but essentially similarly among themselves. However, for anticipatory coarticulation, the two aphasic groups were clearly different. The apraxics, as opposed to the fluents and the normals, demonstrated a delay in coarticulatory shifts in prevocalic fricatives. Although this study did not use such lengthy stimuli as did Ziegler, bisyllabic word pairs were used. Length of stimuli, therefore, seems to be a crucial factor determining whether an apraxic speaker will exhibit anticipatory coarticulation. It is also probably advisable to place the articulatory material to be analyzed within a larger span of material, rather than using forms in isolation or placing them at initial positions. Exaggerated preposturing by patients with apraxia of speech may also be more likely to be produced at the initiation of words or phrases. Heightened or exaggerated initial preposturing is most likely what Buckingham (p. 288) observed informally 10 years ago in the first edition of the present book, and which led to his brute force claim there (see above, p. 289).

As alluded to above, the phenomenon of "phonemic false evaluation" (e.g., Buckingham & Yule, 1987) has obscured many earlier studies of apraxia of speech and has made the interpretation of many of those studies difficult indeed. In those early studies of segmental production in apraxia of speech, many of the presumed phonemic substitutions where in fact only category substitutions in the minds of those who were listening to the apraxics. More refined technological instrumentation finally demonstrated that many of what were initially felt to be phonemic substitutions, were in actuality phonetic asynchronies that shifted acoustic cues in one way or another such that hearers encoded phonemic category shifts in their minds. The problem was that those hearers subsequently credited what they themselves encoded as phonemic substitutions to the speakers. Indeed, much confusion naturally ensued. In the first edition of the present chapter, this point was discussed against the background of the early studies (e.g., Blumstein et al., 1977) that revealed the actual motoric underpinnings of these falsely evaluated phonemic substitutions.

Since then, another study of ostensive phonemic substitutions in anterior aphasia (Keller, 1978) has been scrutinized in Buckingham (1982) in an attempt to suggest that there was a motoric underpinning for the phonemic substitutions, and that in reality the phonemic substitutions were encoded by the hearer, while the motor disruption was encoded by the speaker. Keller observed what he felt to be phonemic level vowel substitution in apraxia of speech, whereby patients would select mid vowels for high vowels and low vowels for mid vowels. In other words, the phonemic vowel substitutions were in the direction of lower vowels for higher vowels. He explored four hypotheses to account for these vowel lowerings: (a) loss of fine-grained control for the selective contraction of a few single muscles for higher vowels, resulting in a strong simultaneous contraction of the genioglossus and hyoglossus (the two principal intrinsic tongue muscle groups); (b) paradigmatic selection disorders that seem to favor lower vowel counterparts; (c) inaccurate proprioceptive feedback; and (d) incomplete auditory feedback. Each of these hypotheses is problematic. The first would account only for the increased productions of [a] and would not account for errors such as /i/ to /e/. The second appears to be constructed in accordance with the data it seeks to explain. The third and fourth hypotheses do not explain the DIRECTIONALITY of the errors. Keller did not consider a much more likely scenario: auditory impression of vowel lowering due to abnormal nasalization of the vowels in question resulting from faulty velar control.

Speech apraxic patients such as those studied by Keller (1978) often have, "a marked variability in terms of the pattern of velar movements" (Itoh et al., 1979, p. 227). Recently, Katz et al. (1988; Katz et al., 1990), in a kinematic analysis of an anterior aphasic (patient EG) using electromagnetic articulography, noted that their patient's velum was relatively low throughout his speech production, although the patient "did not sound overly nasal." Nevertheless, my claim would be that it is quite possible that enough nasality was coming through to affect the formant structure of the vowels so produced. There is experimental evidence that, "vowel nasalization is accompanied by an auditory lowering of the vowel" (Wright, 1975, p. 382). In this study, Wright demonstrated that subjects consistently perceived nasalized high and mid vowels as lower. Wright's claim is that nasalization of high and mid vowels will cause their first formants to rise, thereby imparting an auditory lowering.

More recently, Beddor, Krakow, and Goldstein (1986) examined listener misperceptions of the height of nasalized vowels, and their findings are extremely illuminating for the point I am trying to make. They found that listeners misperceive vowel height of nasalized vowels only in those cases where nasalization is motorically inappropriate and where there is no conditioning nasal consonant in the phonological structure of some target word. Although Beddor et al. were seeking listener-oriented explanations for diachronic sound changes, their findings strengthen my contention that the apraxic vowel lowering phonemic substitutions could very well have been in the minds of the hearers, that is, phonemic false evaluation. The crucial factor is that the nasalization would be abnormal and inappropriate in the case of the brain-damaged apraxic with disrupted velopharyngeal control. The majority of the "lowerings" would be expected to be in words where there was no nasal consonant in the underlying form. In addition, Krakow, Beddor, and Goldstein (1988) observed that hearers' perception of the height of nasal vowels is influenced not only by degree of nasalization and by whether a nasal consonant is in the phonological representation of the word, but also by the LENGTH of the vowel. More perceptions of lowering occurred when the vowels were longer in duration. Consequently, for the preception of motor aphasic speech, one would expect an even greater tendency to perceive vowel lowering, since these same patients very often produce abnormally lengthened vowels as well (e.g., Kent & Rosenbek, 1983).

Beddor et al. (1986) disagreed with Wright (1975) that the important acoustic phenomenon is a raising formant one. Rather, they pointed out that what is happening with nasalized vowels occurs in the region or vicinity of the first formant, rather than that something is affecting the first formant exclusively. For P. S. Beddor (personal communication, 1988), the perceptual lowering of high and mid nasalized vowels is due to the additional nasal formant, which raises what she calls the "center of gravity" of high and mid vowels relative to their oral counterparts. As opposed to Wright's first formant raising theory, Beddor's account also explains the observation that low nasalized vowels will perceptually raise, since the "center of gravity" of low vowels is lowered by the added nasal formant. Low nasalized vowels should actually lower further, if Wright is correct. Nevertheless, the perceptual consequences of both studies lend credence to my suggestion that phonemic false evaluation is a likely candidate for explaining why certain patients with apraxia of speech from anterior lesions seem to be substituting high and mid vowel phonemes for their lower counterparts. Again, the phonemic selection characterization may only be in the minds of the hearers, whereas the apraxic's problem would be more properly characterized as faulty ve-lopharyngeal control. See Krakow et al. (1988) for further remarks on the issue of nasal vowels and perceived height.

Up to this point, phonetic–apraxic errors have been discussed with reference to patients with typical anterior left cerebral lesions (i.e. non-fluent patients) who are said to have apraxia of speech and who are often labeled as Broca's aphasics. The phonemic false evaluation claims are marshaled in to demonstrate that motor–phonetic disruptions are behind many of the so-called phonemic substitutions in apraxia of speech. Could there be, as well, a subtle apraxic component in the fluent left posterior lesion aphasias that might also be leading to phonemic false evaluation? That is, could any of the often observed phonemic substitutions in Wernicke's aphasia, or in conduction aphasia, be in the minds of the listeners as well?

In several publications, beginning with Blumstein et al. (1980), motor–phonetic abnormalities have, in fact, been charted in the speech of otherwise fluent, posterior aphasics. Subsequent to this publication, there have been several others: MacNeilage, Hutchinson, and Lasater (1981); MacNeilage (1982); Shinn and Blumstein (1983); Tuller (1984); Duffy and Gawle (1984); Ryalls (1986); Kent and McNeil (1987) and Baum, Blumstein, Naeser & Palumbo. Different types of phonetic asynchronies (e.g., fricative elongation, abnormal vowel lengthening, abnormal prevoicing for VOT) have been found in these studies, some of which would have only phonetic consequences but others of which could very likely have phonological consequences—for hearers, that is. It goes without saying that an unambiguous phonemic selection error adumbrates a phonemic level problem for the aphasic. The fact is, however, that not all so-called phonemic selection errors are encoded at the level of phonemic selection by the aphasic. These subtle phonetic disruptions in fluent aphasia are phonetic nonetheless, and, again, some may have phonological consequences and some may not. The picture does not seem to be as clear-cut as Ziegler (1987) would have it. In that study, Ziegler claimed that, "Aberrations in the sound pattern of Wernicke's aphasics reflect a dysfunction affecting the discrete structure in the inventory of phonetic plans, whereas patients with apraxia of speech exhibit problems of realizing properly selected phonological units" (p. 177).

Not only may many apraxic patients produce phonemic substitutions (although far fewer than we originally thought), but many of the phonetic control problems now seen in fluent aphasics do not necessarily have phonological consequences, and therefore do not necessarily affect the discrete structure in the inventory of phonetic plans (which is simply another way of talking at the level of phonology). For example, the abnormal prevoicing of Wernicke's aphasics reported in Blumstein et al. (1980) would not affect the phonological structure of English, and therefore would not indicate a selection problem. Slight abnormalities in a production of the spectral portion of a stop may be due to a phonetic control problem involving laryngeal manipulation, but it may give rise to phonemic category shifts in the feature [place] for perceivers. Abnormally lengthened voiceless fricatives may lead a hearer to perceive the voiced counterpart, and one would certainly expect abnormal vowel length control before final obstruents to at least occasionally lead to misperceptions of the [± voice] phonemic category of those obstruents. It appears now that one can no longer simply assume that the only production errors of the posterior aphasic are phonemically based paraphasias. Moreover, Dogil (1989) recently demonstrated a startling amount of motor disruption in the early phase of jargonaphasia in a Wernicke's aphasic.

Clearly much more instrumental research is needed to understand the nature of these motor problems in the speech of anterior and posterior fluent aphasics. Perceptual studies must also be run on the exemplars exhibiting the phonetic abnormalities to better understand the perceptual consequences these apraxic abnormalities have for hearers. A study such as Tuller's (1984) must take the fluent exemplars of abnormal vowel length in those words that had final obstruents and play those exemplars to have listeners judge [± voice] for those final consonants. Fine-tuned instrumental studies must be carried out on the speech of anterior patients to find those instances of abnormal nasalization around vowel productions. Those exemplars then need to be played to groups of listeners for judgment of vowel height.

It should be clear to the reader that the experimental studies of apraxia outlined above are directed not at studying what patients do on linguistic command, but rather at measuring articulatory, acoustic, and perceptual parameters. Thus, they tacitly accept the nonconnectionistic, center-lesion view of apraxia. Disconnection explanations play no role whatsoever in the accounts of the apraxic productions in these studies. Rather, they focus upon subphonemic errors, variability, and nonfluency.

VARIABILITY is often used to distinguish the dysarthric from the cortically damaged patient, but it is a nonlinguistic descriptor and need not be specifically linked to speech behavior. Furthermore, variability can be used only to distinguish apraxic distortions from dysarthric distortions. It will not serve to differentiate apraxia from aphasia, since aphasic behavior itself is quite variable. FLUENCY, in terms of struggle, may certainly be used to distinguish (within reason) between frontal and posterior cases, as long as we can be sure it is a motoric struggle and not a word-finding block, which can also cause struggling and groping behavior in the patient. Furthermore, we are now aware of a subtle apraxic component in posterior fluent aphasia.

More crucially, I would argue that the actual descriptions of apraxic speech errors are valid only if they are made at the allophonic, post-phoneme selection level. Consequently, any theory that states that apraxia of speech is a motoric disturbance composed of "substitutions, addition, and repetitions of phonemes" (Mayo Clinic and Mayo Foundation, 1976, p. 232) will have to demonstrate how the substitutions, additions, and repetitions of phonemes are different from posterior aphasic errors that can be characterized in the same way. More importantly, theories that are worded in terms of phonemes will have to show what it means for the switch (at the selection level) of /m/ to /p/, for instance, to be motoric. As mentioned earlier, it is impossible to conceive of a motor disorder at the phonemic level; no invariant articulatory (as measured by cineradiography or by electromyography) or acoustic (as measured spectrographically) pattern has ever been found that uniquely specifies some phonemic unit. Yet, the psychological reality of those units is unquestionable. Therefore, phonemes cannot be submitted to physical scrutiny, and, by the same token, it is anomalous to describe motor disorders of speech in terms of them.

Conclusion

In conclusion, it is safe to say that ample historical precedent exists for two different neuroanatomical explanations for apraxia: center lesion and disconnection. Whether one or a combination of these explanations will ultimately come to be accepted, only time will tell. It does appear, however, that experimental studies of phonetic parameters in apraxia of speech no longer focus on anatomical disconnection. This is especially obvious in those cases where the speech output that is measured is not strictly elicited by linguistic command (i.e. by repetition). The studies on the center-lesion limb-kinetic apraxias of speech predictably claim that the cortical regions damaged are those that (somehow) contain the information for proper articulatory timing, whether single or multiple gestures are involved. Disconnection accounts for the apraxia postulate blocks in the information passage from Wernicke's area to cortical motor centers. Center-lesion theories, on the other hand, do not eliminate from analysis speech samples collected from stimulus conditions other than those that involve relays between language comprehension and motor execution. In fact, as this chapter has shown, many exemplars analyzed in recent studies of apraxia of speech have not been elicited through repetition. Often, as experimental design will be set up to allow subjects to repeat a word that they cannot read, where the general procedure is to have the subjects read. All the exemplars are nevertheless grouped together for analysis. Rarely is it asked any more whether, for instance, an apraxic would demonstrate delays in anticipatory coarticulation when repeating, but not when reading. Nevertheless, once we fully understand the phonetics of the errors, we will be in a better position to truly distinguish apraxia, dysarthria, and true phonemic paraphasia. The technology of the day is allowing us to do precisely this with increasing sophistication and clarity. The emphasis is clearly on the micro-phonetic details and their acoustic and perceptual consequences, rather than on the nature of the elicitation of the speech itself. Consequently, cerebral connectionist accounts of apraxia of speech are, for all intents and purposes, practically nonexistent today.

Acknowledgments

In the first edition of this book, I expressed my appreciation to Norman Geschwind who sadly died several years ago. This revised version is dedicated to him. I would also like to express my appreciation to Jason W. Brown and Leonard LaPointe for their helpful remarks on earlier drafts of this chapter. Naturally, they are not to be held responsible for any of my interpretations. This chapter is an updating of the author's paper, which originally appeared in *Brain and Language*, 1979, *8*, 202–226.

References

Abramson, S., & Lisker, L. (1973). Voice-timing perception in Spanish word-initial stops. *Journal of Phonetics, 1*, 1–8.

Alajouanine, T. (1960). Baillarger and Jackson: The principle of Baillarger-Jackson in aphasia. *Journal of Neurology, Neurosurgery and Psychiatry, 23*, 191–193.

Alajouanine, T., Ombredane, A., & Durand, M. (1939). *Le syndrome de la désintegration phonétique dans l' aphasie.* Paris: Masson.

Ardila, A., Rosselli, M., & Ardila, O. (1988). Foreign accent: An aphasic epiphenomenon? *Aphasiology, 2*, 493–499.

Auburtin, E. (1861). Sur la forme et le volume du cerveau: Sur le siége de la faculté du language. *Bulltein de la Société d'Anthropologie (Paris) 2*, 214–233.

Baum, S. R., Blumstein, S. E., Naeser, M. A., & Palumbo, C. L. (1990). Temporal dimensions of consonant and vowel production: An acoustic and CT scan analysis of aphasic speech. *Brain and Language, 39*, 33–56.

Beddor, P. S., Krakow, R. A., & Goldstein, L. M. (1986). Perceptual constraints and phonological change: A study of nasal vowel height. *Phonology Yearbook, 3*, 197–217.

Benton, A. L., & Joynt, R. J. (1960). Early descriptions of aphasia. *Archives of Neurology, 3*, 205–222.

Blumstein, S. E. (1973). *A phonological investigation of aphasic speech.* The Hague: Mouton.

Blumstein, S. E., Alexander, M. P., Ryalls, J. H., Katz, W., & Dworetsky, B. (1987). On the nature of the foreign accent syndrome: A case study. *Brain and Language, 31*, 215–244.

Blumstein, S. E., Cooper, W. E., Goodglass, H., Statlender, S., & Gottlieb, J. (1980). Production deficits in aphasia: A voice-onset time analysis. *Brain and Language, 9*, 153–170.

Blumstein, S. E., Cooper, W. E., Zurif, E. B., & Caramazza, A. (1977). The perception and production of voice-onset time in aphasia. *Neuropsychologia, 15*, 371–383.

Bonhoeffer K. (1914). Klinischer und anatomischer befund zur lehre von der apraxie und der "motorischen sprachbehn." *Monatsschrift für Psychiatrie und Neurologie, 35*, 113–28.

Bouillaud, J. B. (1825). Recherches cliniques propres à démonstrer que la perte de la parole correspond à la lésion des lobules antérieurs du cerveau. Et à confirmer l'opinion de M.

Gall sur le siège de l'organe du language articulé. *Archives Generales de Medecine, 8,* 25–45.

Broca, P. (1960). Remarks on the seat of the faculty of articulate language, followed by an observation of aphemia. In G. von Bonin (Ed.), *Some papers on the cerebral cortex.* Springfield, IL: Thomas. (Original work published 1861)

Brown, J. W. (1972). *Aphasia, apraxia and agnosia.* Springfield, IL: Thomas.

Brown, J. W. (1975a). On the neural organization of language: Thalamic and cortical relationships. *Brain and Language, 2,* 18–30.

Brown, J. W. (1975b). The problem of repetition: A study of "conduction" aphasia and the "isolation" syndrome. *Cortex, 11,* 37–52.

Brown, J. W. (1977). *Mind, brain and consciousness: The neuropsychology of cognition.* New York: Academic Press.

Brown, J. W. (1988a). *The life of the mind: Selected papers.* Hillsdale, NJ: Erlbaum.

Brown, J. W. (Ed.). (1988b). *Agnosia and apraxia: Selected papers of Liepmann, Lange, and Potzl.* Hillsdale, NJ: Erlbaum.

Buckingham, H. W. (1977). A critique of A. R. Luria's neurodynamic explanation of paraphasia. *Brain and Language, 4,* 580–587.

Buckingham, H. W. (1982). Critical issues in the study of aphasia. In N. J. Lass (Ed.), *Speech and language: Advances in basic research and practice* (Vol. 8). New York: Academic Press.

Buckingham, H. W. (1983). Apraxia of language vs. apraxia of speech. In R. A. Magill (ed.), *Memory and control of action.* Amsterdam: North-Holland.

Buckingham, H. W. (1984). Early development of association theory in psychology as a forerunner to connection theory. *Brain and Cognition, 3,* 19–34.

Buckingham, H. W. (1986). The scan-copier mechanism and the positional level of language production: Evidence from phonemic paraphasia. *Cognitive Science, 10,* 195–217.

Buckingham, H. W., & Kertesz, A. (1976). *Neologistic jargon aphasia.* Amsterdam: Swets & Zeitlinger, B. V.

Buckingham, H. W., & Yule, G. (1987). Phonemic false evaluation: Theoretical and clinical aspects. *Clinical Linguistics and Phonetics, 1,* 113–125.

Burns, M. S., & Canter, G. (1977). Phonemic behavior of aphasic patients with posterior cerebral lesions. *Brain and Language, 4,* 492–507.

Calvin, W. H. (1983). *The throwing madonna: Essays on the brain.* New York: McGraw-Hill.

Canter, G. (1973, October). *Dysarthria, apraxia of speech, and literal paraphasia: Three distinct varieties of articulatory behavior in the adult with brain damage.* Paper presented at the meeting of the American Speech and Hearing Association, Detroit, MI.

Canter, G., Burns, M., & Trost, J. (1975). Differential phonemic behavior in anterior and posterior aphasic syndromes. Paper presented at the 13th annual meeting of the Academy of Aphasia, Victoria, B.C.

Cooper, W. E. (1977). The development of speech timing. In S. J. Segalowitz & F. A. Gruber (Eds.), *Language development and neurological theory.* New York: Academic Press.

Deacon, T. (1989). Holism and associationism in neuropsychology: An anatomical synthesis. In E. Perecman (Ed.), *Integrating theory and practice in clinical neuropsychology.* Hillsdale, NJ: Erlbaum.

Denny-Brown, D. (1958). The nature of apraxia. *Journal of Nervous and Mental Disease, 126,* 9–32.

Denny-Brown, D. (1965). Physiological aspects of disturbances of speech. *Australian Journal of Experimental Biology and Medical Science, 43,* 455–474.

De Renzi, E., Pieczuro, A., & Vignolo, L. A. (1966). Oral apraxia and aphasia. *Cortex, 2,* 50–73.

Dogil, G. (1989). The phonological and acoustic form of neologistic jargon aphasia. *Clinical Linguistics and Phonetics, 3,* 265–279.

Duffy, J. R., & Gawle, C. A. (1984). Apraxic speakers' vowel duration in consonant-vowel-consonant syllables. In J. C. Rosenbek, M. R. McNeil, & A. E. Aronson (Eds.), *Apraxia of speech: Physiology, acoustics, linguistics, management.* San Diego, CA: College-Hill Press.

Engelhardt, H. T. (1975). John Hughlings Jackson and the mind-body relation. *Bulletin of the History of Medicine, 49,* 137–151.

Freeman, F. J., Sands, E. S., & Harris, K. S. (1978). Temporal coordination of phonation and articulation in a case of verbal apraxia: A voice onset time study. *Brain and Language, 6,* 106–111.

Fromkin, V., & Rodman, R. (1988). *An introduction to language* (4th ed.). New York: Holt, Rinehart & Winston.

Galaburda, A. (1982). Histology, architectonics, and asymmetry of language areas. In M. A. Arbib, D. Caplan, & J. C. Marshall (Eds.), *Neural models of language processes.* New York: Academic Press.

Gazzaniga, M. (1989). Organization of the human brain. *Science, 245,* 947–952.

Geschwind, N. (1965). Disconnexion syndromes in animals and man. *Brain, 88,* 237–294, 585–644.

Geschwind, N. (1969). Anatomy of the higher functions of the brain. In R. S. Cohen & M. Wartofsky (Eds.). *Boston studies in the philosophy of science* (Vol. 4). Dordrecht: Reidel.

Geschwind, N. (1975). The apraxias: Neural mechanisms of disorders of learned movement. *American Scientist, 63,* 188–195.

Grodzinsky, Y. (1989). Agrammatic comprehension of relative clauses. *Brain and Language, 37,* 480–499.

Harrington, A. (1985). Nineteenth century ideas on hemispheric differences and "duality of mind." *Behavioral and Brain Sciences, 8,* 617–660.

Harrington, A. (1987). *Medicine, mind, and the double brain: A study in nineteenth-century thought.* Princeton, NJ: Princeton University Press.

Head, H. (1926). *Aphasia and kindred disorders of speech* (Vols. 1 and 2). London: Cambridge University Press.

Heilman, K. M. (1979). The neuropsychological basis of skilled movement in man. In M. S. Gazzaniga (Ed.). *Handbook of behavioral neurology: Vol. 2. Neuropsychology.* New York: Plenum.

Heilman, K. M., Coyle, J. M., Gonyea, E. F., & Geschwind, N. (1973). Apraxia and agraphia in the left-hander. *Brain, 96,* 21–28.

Heilman, K. M., & Gonzalez-Rothi, L. J. (1985). Apraxia. In K. M. Heilman & E. Valenstein (Eds.), *Clinical neuropsychology* (2nd ed.). New York: Oxford University Press.

Itoh, M., Sasanuma, S., Hirose, H., Yoshioka, H., & Ushijima, T. (1980). Abnormal articulatory dynamics in a patient with apraxia of speech: X-ray microbeam observation. *Brain and Language, 11,* 66–75.

Itoh, M., Sasanuma, S., & Ushijima, T. (1979). Velar movements during speech in a patient with apraxia of speech. *Brain and Language, 7,* 227–239.

Jackson, J. (1931a). Notes on the physiology and pathology of language. In J. Taylor (Ed.). *Selected writings of John Hughlings Jackson* (Vol. 2). London: Hodder & Stoughton. (Original work published 1866)

Jackson, J. (1931b). On affections of speech from disease of the brain. In J. Taylor (Ed.), *Selected writings of John Hughlings Jackson* (Vol. 2). London: Hodder & Stoughton. (Original work published 1878)

Jackson, J. (1931c). On the nature of the duality of the brain. In J. Taylor (Ed.). *Selected writings of John Hughlings Jackson* (Vol. 2). London: Hodder & Stoughton. (Original work published 1874)

Jackson, J. (1931d). Remarks on the non-protrusion of the tongue in some cases of aphasia.

In J. Taylor (Ed.). *Selected writings of John Hughlings Jackson* (Vol. 2). London: Hodder & Stoughton. (Original work published 1878)

Johns, D. F., & Darley, F. L. (1970). Phonemic variability in apraxia of speech. *Journal of Speech and Hearing Research, 13*, 556–583.

Johns, D. F., & LaPointe, L. L. (1976). Neurogenic disorders of output processing: Apraxia of speech. In H. Whitaker & H. A. Whitaker (Eds.), *Studies in neurolinguistics* (Vol. 1). New York: Academic Press.

Katz, W. F. (1987). Anticipatory labial and lingual coarticulation in aphasia. In J. Ryalls (Ed.), *Phonetic approaches to speech production in aphasia and related disorders*. Boston, MA: Little, Brown.

Katz, W. F. (1988a). Anticipatory coarticulation in aphasia: Acoustic and perceptual data. *Brain and Language, 35*, 340–368.

Katz, W. F. (1988b). "Methodological considerations" reconsidered: Reply to Sussman et al. (1988). *Brain and Language, 35*, 380–385.

Katz, W. F., Schonle, P. W., Machetanz, J., Hong, G., Hohne, J., Wenig, P., & Veldscholten, H. (1988, October). *A kinematic analysis of anticipatory coarticulation in an anterior aphasic subject using electromagnetic articulography*. Paper presented at the 26th annual meeting of the Academy of Aphasia, Montreal.

Katz, W., Machetanz, J., Orth, U., & Schönle, P. (1990). A kinematic analysis of anticipatory coarticulation in the speech of anterior aphasic subjects using eletromagnetic articulography. *Brain and Language, 38*, 555–575.

Kean, M.-L. (Ed.). (1985). *Agrammatism*. Orlando, FL: Academic Press.

Keller, E. (1978). Parameters for vowel substitutions in Broca's aphasia. *Brain and Language, 5*, 265–285.

Kelso, J. A. S., & Tuller, B. (1981). Toward a theory of apractic syndromes. *Brain and Language, 12*, 224–245.

Kent, R. D., & McNeil, M. R. (1987). Relative timing of sentence repetition in apraxia of speech and conduction aphasia. In J. Ryalls (Ed.), *Phonetic approaches to speech production in aphasia and related disorders*. Boston, MA: Little, Brown.

Kent, R. D., & Rosenbek, J. C. (1983). Acoustic patterns of apraxia of speech. *Journal of Speech and Hearing Research, 26*, 231–249.

Kewley-Port, D., & Preston, M. S. (1974). Early apical stop production: A voice onset time analysis. *Journal of Phonetics, 2*, 195–210.

Kimura, D. (1976). The neural basis of language qua gesture. In H. Whitaker & H. A. Whitaker (Eds.), *Studies in neurolinguistics* (Vol. 2). New York: Academic Press.

Kimura, D. (1977a). Acquisition of a motor skill after left-hemisphere damage. *Brain, 100*, 527–542.

Kimura, D. (1977b). *Studies in apraxia*. Paper presented at the 15th annual meeting of the Academy of Aphasia, Montreal.

Kimura, D. (1982). Left-hemisphere control of oral and brachial movements and their relation to communication. *Philosophical Transactions of the Royal Society of London, Series B, 298*, 135–149.

Kimura, D., & Archibald, Y. (1974). Motor functions of the left hemisphere. *Brain, 97*, 337–350.

Kimura, D., & Watson, N. (1989). The relation between oral movement control and speech. *Brain and Language, 37*, 565–590.

Kinsbourne, M. (1972). Behavioral analysis of the repetition deficit in conduction aphasia. *Neurology, 22*, 1126–1132.

Kleist, K. (1916). Ueber Leitungsaphasie und grammatische Störungen. *Monatsschrift für Psychiatrie und Neurologie, 40*, 118–199.

Krakow, R. A., Beddor, P. S., & Goldstein, L. M. (1988). Coarticulatory influences on the perceived height of nasal vowels. *Journal of the Acoustical Society of America, 83,* 1146–1158.

Lecours, A. R., & Lhermitte, F. (1976). The "pure form" of the phonetic disintegration syndrome (pure anarthria); Anatomo-clinical report of a historical case. *Brain and Language, 3,* 88–113.

Liepmann, H. (1900). Das krankheitsbild der Apraxie (motorischen asymbolie) auf grund eines falles von einseitiger apraxie. *Monatsschrft für Psychiatrie und Neurologie, 8,* 15–40, 102–32, 182–97. (English translation in D. A. Rottenberg & F. H. Hochberg [Eds.], *Neurological classics in modern translation.* New York: Hafner, 1977.)

Luria, A. R. (1972). Aphasia reconsidered. *Cortex, 8,* 34–40.

Luria, A. R. (1973). *The working brain: An introduction to neuropsychology.* New York: Basic Books.

MacNeilage, P. F. (1982). Speech production mechanisms in aphasia. In S. Grillner, B. Lindblom, J. Lubker, & A. Persson (Eds.), *Speech motor control.* Oxford: Pergamon.

MacNeilage, P. F., Hutchinson, J. A., & Lasater, S. A. (1981). The production of speech: Development and dissolution of motoric and premotoric processes. In J. Long & A. Baddeley (Eds.), *Attention and performance IX.* Hillsdale, NJ: Erlbaum.

Marshall, R. C., Gandour, J., & Windsor, J. (1988). Selective impairment of phonation: A case study. *Brain and Language, 35,* 313–339.

Martin, A. D. (1974). Some objections to the term apraxia of speech. *Journal of Speech and Hearing Disorders, 39,* 53–64.

Mateer, C., & Kimura, D. (1977). Impairment of non-verbal oral movements in aphasia. *Brain and Language, 4,* 262–276.

Mayo Clinic and Mayo Foundation. (1976). *Clinical examinations in neurology* (4th ed.). Philadelphia, PA: Saunders.

Mohr, J. P. (1976). Broca's area and Broca's aphasia. In H. Whitaker & H. A. Whitaker (Eds.), *Studies in neurolinguistics* (Vol. 1). New York: Academic Press.

Paillard, J. (1982). Apraxia and the neurophysiology of motor control. *Philosophical Transactions of the Royal Society of London, Series B, 298,* 111–134.

Poeck, K., & Kerschensteiner, M. (1975). Analysis of the sequential motor events in oral apraxia. In K. J. Zülch, O. Creutzfeldt, & G. C. Galbraith (Eds.), *Cerebral localization.* New York: Springer-Verlag.

Rosenbek, J. C. (1984). Advances in the evaluation and treatment of speech apraxia. In F. C. Rose (Ed.), *Advances in Neurology, 42: Progress in aphasiology.* NY: Raven Press.

Rosenbek, J. C., Kent, R. D., & LaPointe, L. L. (1984). Apraxia of speech: An overview and some perspectives. In J. C. Rosenbek, M. R. McNeil, & A. E. Aronson (Eds.), *Apraxia of speech: Physiology, acoustics, linguistics, management.* San Diego, CA: College-Hill Press.

Rosenbek, J. C., McNeil, M. R., & Aronson, A. E. (Eds.), (1984). *Apraxia of speech: Physiology, acoustics, linguistics, management.* San Diego, CA: College-Hill Press.

Rubens, A. B., Geschwind, N., Mahowald, M. W., & Mastri, A. (1977). Posttraumatic cerebral hemispheric disconnection syndrome. *Archives of Neurology (Chicago), 34,* 750–755.

Ryalls, J. (1986). An acoustic study of vowel production in aphasia. *Brain and Language, 29,* 48–67.

Sands, E. S., Freeman, F. J., & Harris, K. S. (1978). Progressive changes in articulatory patterns in verbal apraxia: A longitudinal case study. *Brain and Language, 6,* 97–105.

Schiller, F. (1979). *Paul Broca: Founder of French anthropology, explorer of the brain.* Berkeley: University of California Press.

Shankweiler, D., & Harris, K. S. (1966). An experimental approach to the problem of articulation in aphasia. *Cortex, 2,* 277–292.

Shankweiler, D., Harris, K. S., & Taylor, M. L. (1968). Electromyographic studies of articulation in aphasia. *Archives of Physical Medicine and Rehabilitation, 48,* 1–8.

Shinn, P., & Blumstein, S. E. (1983). Phonemic disintegration in aphasia: Acoustic analysis of spectral characteristics for place of articulation. *Brain and Language, 20,* 90–114.

Stookey, B. (1963). Jean-Baptiste Bouillaud and Ernest Auburtin: Early studies on cerebral localization and the speech center. *JAMA, Journal of the American Medical Association, 184,* 1024–1029.

Sussman, H. M., Marquardt, T. P., MacNeilage, P. F., & Hutchinson, J. A. (1988). Anticipatory coarticulation in aphasia: Some methodological considerations. *Brain and Language, 35,* 369–379.

Taylor, J. (Ed.). (1931). *Selected writings of John Hughlings Jackson* (Vols. 1 and 2). London: Hodder & Stoughton.

Trost, J., & Canter, G. (1974). Apraxia of speech in patients with Broca's aphasia: A study of phoneme production accuracy and error patterns. *Brain and Language, I,* 63–80.

Tuller, B. (1984). On categorizing speech errors. *Neuropsychologia, 22,* 547–558.

Tuller, B., & Story, R. S. (1987). Anticipatory coarticulation in aphasia. In J. Ryalls (Ed.), *Phonetic approaches to speech production in aphasia and related disorders.* Boston, MA: Little, Brown.

Tuller, B., & Story, R. S. (1988). Anticipatory and carryover coarticulation in aphasia: An acoustic study. *Cognitive Neuropsychology, 5,* 747–771.

von Bonin, G., (Ed.). (1960). *Some papers on the cerebral cortex.* Springfield, IL: Thomas.

Wernicke, C. (1977). [The aphasia symptom-complex: A psychological study on an anatomical basis.] In G. Eggert (Ed. and Trans.), *Wernicke's works on aphasia: A source-book and review.* The Hague: Mouton. (Original work published 1874)

Wertz, R. T., LaPointe, L. L., & Rosenbek, J. C. (1984). *Apraxia of speech in adults: The disorder and its management.* Orlando, FL: Grune & Stratton.

Whitaker, H. A. (1975). *Levels of impairment in disorders of speech.* Paper presented at the 8th International Congress of Phonetic Sciences, Leeds, England.

Wright, J. (1975). Effects of vowel nasalization on the perception of vowel height. In C. A. Ferguson, L. M. Hyman, & J. J. Ohala (Eds.), *Nasalfest: Papers from a symposium on nasals and nasalization.* Stanford, CA: Stanford University, Department of Linguistics.

Young, R. M. (1970). *Mind, brain and adaptation in the nineteenth century.* Oxford: Oxford University Press.

Ziegler, W. (1987). Phonetic realization of phonological contrast in aphasic patients. In J. Ryalls (Ed.), *Phonetic approaches to speech production in aphasia and related disorders.* Boston, MA: Little, Brown.

Ziegler, W. (1989). Anticipatory coarticulation in aphasia: More methodology: A reply to Sussman et al. (1988) and Katz (1988b). *Brain and language, 37,* 172–176.

Ziegler, W., & von Cramon, D. (1985). Anticipatory coarticulation in a patient with apraxia of speech. *Brain and Language, 26,* 117–130.

Ziegler, W., & von Cramon, D. (1986). Disturbed coarticulation in apraxia of speech: Acoustic evidence. *Brain and Language, 29,* 34–47.

9

Aphasia-Related Disorders

EDITH KAPLAN

Aphasic disturbances of production and comprehension of spoken language are usually associated with a disruption in the encoding and decoding of written language (agraphia and alexia). In addition, disorders of gestural representation (apraxia), calculation (acalculia), right–left orientation, finger localization, and visuospatial ability are commonly associated with aphasia. These capacities may be impaired in isolation or in selective clusters as a function of the locus, extent, and etiology of lesion of the dominant hemisphere. The severity of the dysfunction may depend on such variables as the patient's handedness, history of familial sinistrality, and premorbid capacity. Obviously a careful delineation of the nature and extent of these deficits will contribute to diagnosis and to inferences concerning localization. Equally important, such an evaluation will have impact on the choice of appropriate interventions (e.g., language and cognitive therapies) and considerations for vocational rehabilitation.

The following sections of this chapter review each of the disorders listed in the preceding paragraph, their neuroanatomic substrates, and their characteristic presentation in the adult with damage to the left hemisphere.

Reading Disturbances

Reading seldom escapes unscathed in any form of aphasia, except in the relatively rare cases of PURE WORD DEAFNESS and APHEMIA. Although the severity and character of reading disorders show some systematic

313

ACQUIRED APHASIA, SECOND EDITION

relationship to lesion site and to the form of the oral language disorder, this relationship is considerably less predictable than is the case for the speech pattern. For example, although Broca's aphasics characteristically comprehend written language much better than they produce it, some of them are severely impaired in reading. Thus, it appears most profitable to describe reading disturbances in relation to the components of the reading process and refer incidentally to the predominant association of particular features with a standard syndrome. An exception will be made in the case of PARIETAL ALEXIA, AGRAPHIA, and PURE WORD BLINDNESS, disorders in which written language is selectively disturbed.

The reading process is obviously founded on the ability to perceive and discriminate the elementary components of the written code and to recognize their class membership as letters, words, or numerals. Loss of such recognition capacity may be regarded as a prelinguistic disorder, belonging in the category of VISUAL AGNOSIA. Disorders at this level are usually associated with impaired recognition of visual stimuli of other types, including objects and faces, and need not be associated with aphasia.

Assuming the integrity of this basic recognition capacity, a number of elementary processes are probably operating concurrently in the process of word recognition. These are (a) the appreciation of the individual identity of the letters of the alphabet and the appreciation of their equivalent across styles of print and handwriting; (b) the ability to apply graphophonemic conversion rules so that sequences of letters are mapped by their phonological value onto an integrated sound sequence; (c) the association of written letter sequence, as a whole, to the total phonological representation of a word; and (d) the direct association of a concept to a written word, without phonological mediation.

Although there has been considerable controversy among reading theorists as to the relative role of each of these components in normal reading, it is easy to demonstrate that both graphophonemic conversion and direct phonological access must operate exclusively at certain points. The former process is the only means by which nonsense syllables or novel names can be sounded. The latter is the only means by which such forms as *lbs.* and *Mrs.* can be read aloud, and it probably applies as well to irregularly spelled words like *Worcester* and *reign*.

Beyond the one-word level, there is now evidence both from normal readers (Bradley, Garrett, & Zurif, 1980) and aphasics (Saffran, Bogyo, Schwartz, & Marin, 1980) that the reading of lexical words (i.e., those that refer to a semantic concept) uses a different mechanism from the reading of grammatical morphemes, and, as we will see, aphasia may produce a total dissociation between these two mechanisms. The preservation of these two different and parallel reading capacities is probably related to the ability to understand not only isolated lexical terms, but the syntactic relationships among words in a sentence. Here, again, we will see that aphasia may produce dissociations.

Finally, before examining the clinical features of the alexias, it is important to distinguish between oral and silent reading and possibly between both of these and reading comprehension. Certainly, oral reading may be quite dissociated from silent reading either because of impaired articulatory capacity or because of paraphasic intrusions.

Clinical Features

Reading Comprehension

Even global aphasics retain some ability to match letters and short familiar words across various forms of script, for example, upper- and lowercase print and longhand. Global aphasics and severe mixed aphasics who are unable to select individual words on oral request or on matching to pictures are often still able to find the one word in a group of four or five that does not belong to the same category as the remaining words (e.g., a flower name among a list of foods). The ability to match objects and actions to their pictures is usually preserved in Broca's and Wernicke's aphasia, and the completeness of the patients' recognition vocabulary parallels the severity of the aphasia; that is, words of low frequency are missed more often than are common words. Given the opportunity for semantically based errors, Wernicke's aphasics are more vulnerable than Broca's aphasics. Conduction aphasics and most anomic aphasics perform well on the one-word level. Some anomic aphasics, however, having lesions in the angular gyrus, show a profound reading disorder. Transcortical sensory aphasics, who repeat well without comprehending speech, commonly have an equally severe inability to understand writing—even single words.

Differences between aphasic subgroups become more marked for sentence comprehension, particularly where the understanding of the syntax is vital for disambiguating the sentence. Broca's aphasics have been shown (Caramazza & Zurif, 1976; Samuels & Benson, 1979; von Stockert & Bader, 1976) to have difficulty in using the syntactic features effectively, although they understand the content words well. In contrast, Wernicke's aphasics are usually more severely impaired across the board in sentence comprehension. However, some exceptional patients with Wernicke's aphasia perform well in reading at the sentence level. Conduction aphasics and most anomics (with the noted exception) also read sentences with fairly good comprehension.

Reading at the paragraph level and beyond is almost invariably slow and laborious for aphasics of all types, until and unless they attain a high degree of recovery in oral language, probably because of the verbal memory demands of longer sentences and paragraphs.

Reading of Grammatical Words

A frequent finding among Broca's and mixed aphasics is that they have difficulty in both reading aloud and selecting from multiple choice the small grammatical words of the language (i.e., articles, prepositions, pronouns, forms of the copula, and auxiliary and modal verbs). Their difficulty with this group of high-frequency words contrasts with their success in reading content words of much lower frequency. Gardner and Zurif (1975) have documented the interesting fact that patients may correctly select or read aloud noun or verb homonyms of these grammatical words. For example, they may read *bee* but not *be*, *hymn* but not *him*, *buy* but not *by*. This difficulty may or may not be associated with agrammatism in oral language. It is dramatically prominent in the disorder called DEEP DYSLEXIA, described later.

Oral Reading

Oral reading, much more than silent reading, parallels the pattern of spoken language. Thus, Broca's aphasics who are agrammatic in speech are most likely to read nouns and principal verbs correctly but omit or misread the small words of grammar. Their errors on content words usually involve partial application of graphophonemic rules; that is, word substitutions are usually based on similarity of the first portion of the word, whereas semantic substitutions are uncommon.

In contrast, many Wernicke's aphasics may read aloud as paraphasically as they speak, making semantic substitutions for both content and grammatical words.

Similarly, conduction aphasics' oral reading is usually marked by literal paraphasic errors parallel to those of their speech. Anomic aphasics (with the exception of those with PARIETAL ALEXIA) read well orally. Paradoxically, good oral reading is often observed in transcortical sensory aphasics, who may read aloud without comprehension much as they repeat without comprehension.

Literal Alexia

LITERAL ALEXIA was first described by Hinshelwood (1900). This inability to name letters of the alphabet on sight despite successful word reading is most frequently seen in Broca's aphasics (Albert, 1979). One may hypothesize that the contribution of the spared right hemisphere to the processing of contour information (discussed in greater detail in the section below on constructional disorders) permits whole word reading. Helm-Estabrooks and Kaplan (1989) are currently testing this hypothesis. Preliminary results indicate that alexic aphasic patients are more successful in reading words that have contour, that is, words that contain letters that go above and below the line (e.g., *golf, apple, play*), than words that lack contour (e.g., *rice, camera, ear*).

Surface Alexia

This acquired reading disorder is characterized by a preserved ability to read "regular" words and pseudowords, and an inability to read "irregular" words, whose pronunciations do not conform to typical spelling-to-sound correspondence rules (Patterson & Morton, 1985). The paralexic errors seem to be secondary to a misapplication of grapheme–phoneme correspondence rules. Friedman (1988) noted that word frequency, part of speech, and length of word may affect the extent to which there are "regularization" errors.

Patients with SURFACE ALEXIA are primarily fluent aphasics with temporal or temporoparietal lesions. The associated agraphia of these patients reflects the same difficulties present in their reading.

Deep Dyslexia

Marshall and Newcombe (1966) first described a configuration of symptoms in which their patient's oral reading of lexical words was frequently paralexic; for example, *child* was read as *girl*, *wed* as *marry, air* as *fly, listen* as *quiet*. In addition to these semantic substitutions, many derivational errors (*direction* for *directing*) and visual errors (*terror* for *error*) occurred. Grammatical morphemes were either totally omitted or misread with a different and irrelevant function word (e.g., *you* for *an*). Patients who are totally unable to appreciate the phonic values of written letters also cannot detect homonyms (e.g., *pail* and *pale*) or rhymes using different spelling (e.g., *fight* and *kite*), and they cannot select nonsense words. The term DEEP DYSLEXIA was used to characterize patients who went directly to the semantic value of the word from its printed form, without any appreciation of its sound. The same disorder has been described by Shallice and Warrington (1975) with the term PHONEMIC DYSLEXIA and by Andrewsky and Seron (1975), M. F. Schwartz, Saffran, and Marin (1977), and Patterson and Marcel (1977). The two central problems are that these patients can neither use graphophonemic recoding nor access the phonology of a word directly. Their oral reading is not actually reading in the normal sense; that is, they derive a semantic impression from the written form and apply a spoken word to this meaning that may or may not correspond exactly to the written word. Since grammatical morphemes have no semantic referent, they cannot be dealt with at all by this information processing route.

Although the full syndrome of deep dyslexia is relatively uncommon, many of its components are encountered in aphasics of all types, but most frequently in patients with the speech pattern of Broca's aphasia with agrammatism.

Pure Word Blindness (Alexia without Agraphia)

Dejerine (1892) described the syndrome in which the ability to recognize words was lost, while writing and oral language were unaffected. The lesion most commonly responsible for this syndrome has been confirmed repeatedly (Brissaud, 1900; Geschwind & Fusillo, 1966; Poetzl, 1928; Redlich, 1895; Vincent, David, & Puech, 1930). It involves the splenium of the corpus callosum, the left visual cortex, and the lingual gyrus. This lesion, usually produced by occlusion of the posterior cerebral artery, deprives the language zone of the left hemisphere of all visual input, from both the left and the right hemispheres. The ability to recognize words is severely impaired; however, recognition of numbers and letters is sometimes preserved. In these instances, patients can read laboriously through letter-by-letter spelling, either aloud or silently. The more letters in the word, however, and the more time spent in naming the letters, the more likely are errors. The resulting paralexias tend to be orthographically, rather than semantically, related to the target word. Patients with ALEXIA WITHOUT AGRAPHIA have little difficulty writing, but are virtually incapable of reading what they have written. Spared writing together with the preserved ability to comprehend orally spelled words, as well as letters and words traced on their palms, suggests preservation of stored orthographic information that cannot be accessed through the visual modality. In many instances, this disorder is accompanied by difficulty in naming and understanding color names, a short-term memory disorder, and a right homonomous hemianopia.

In the past decade a number of neuropsychological explanations of PURE ALEXIA have been proposed. Warrington and Shallice (1980) attributed letter-by-letter reading to a deficit of the "visual word-form unit," resulting in a compensatory reliance on "reverse spelling." Patterson and Kay (1982) proposed a disconnection between the "letter-form analysis system" and the "visual word-form system." Friedman and Alexander (1984) rejected Patterson and Kay's disconnection hypothesis and suggested instead a problem with the rapid automatic parallel identification system that necessitated employing a slower sequential processing system.

Alexia with Agraphia

ALEXIA WITH AGRAPHIA has also been called PARIETAL ALEXIA (Hermann & Poetzl, 1926; Hoff, Gloning, & Gloning, 1954) and VISUAL ASYMBOLIA (Brain, 1961). Impairment in reading and writing commonly co-occurs with the fluent aphasias (PARIETAL–TEMPORAL APHASIA; Benson, 1979), particularly in Wernicke's aphasia, which has been described earlier. Alexia with agraphia, however, may occur in relative isolation from aphasia. Dejerine (1891) described a patient with a profound alexia and agraphia that persisted to his death despite the clearing of a mild aphasia. A postmortem examination revealed that the responsible deep vascular lesion involved most of the left angular gyrus. Subsequent reports have confirmed this localization (Benson & Geschwind, 1969).

Since the inferior portion of the angular gyrus is located in the posterior temporal region and the inferior portion of the parietal region, it is not surprising to find an associated anomia with inferior angular gyrus involvement and some or all of the components of the Gerstmann syndrome (agraphia, acalculia, right–left disorientation, and finger agnosia), as well as some visuospatial constructional difficulty.

Most patients with alexia and agraphia are incapable of either spelling aloud or comprehending spelled words. A number of cases of alexia with agraphia and preserved ability to spell and comprehend spelling have been reported (Albert, Yamadori, Gardner, & Howes, 1973; Dejerine & Andre-Thomas, 1904; Kinsbourne & Rosenfield, 1974; Mohr, 1976; Rothi & Heilman, 1981). Rothi and Heilman proposed that underlying the alexia and agraphia, at least in their case, was an inability to transcode between the auditory–verbal and visual–graphic codes. The alternative strategy employed by their patient was to name the letters. They argued that there may be at least three reading strategies: (a) a visual code analysis (letter naming), (b) a whole word pattern analysis, and (c) grapheme–phoneme conversion. Identifying the strategy available to the patient could then more effectively direct the therapeutic approach.

Disorders of Writing (Agraphia)

Writing, like reading, is almost always impaired in aphasia, although the specific form of the writing disorder tends to show some parallels with oral language, particularly with respect to the presence of word-finding disorders, paraphasia, and agrammatism. These parallels are most easily seen in Broca's and Wernicke's aphasias.

Writing in Broca's Aphasia

Writing is usually severely impaired in Broca's aphasia. The poor motor control of the nonpreferred hand (in the presence of right hemiplegia) is not sufficient to account for the degree of awkwardness (Heilman, 1975). Block printing is more common than cursive writing. Letters are oversized, letter reversals occur, and words are misspelled through omission and substitution of letters (literal paragraphia). Recovery of writing may parallel that of speech, and in these cases shows the same features of agrammatism, preponderance of substantives, and reduced output (Goodglass & Hunter, 1970). Impaired writing usually persists as the most severe residual (Kertesz, 1979).

Writing in Wernicke's Aphasia

Wernicke's aphasics usually execute the mechanics of writing easily with their dominant hand—in cursive, well-formed letters—showing an analogy to their facile articulation of speech. Moreover, their writing shows the same propensity for semantic paraphasia, neologistic jargon, and paragrammatic sentence forms as does their speech. The writing, however, is reduced in speed and quantity from normal levels. The narrative writing of Wernicke's aphasics has shorter runs of grammatically coherent words than does their speech. At the same time, the repetitious use of low-information verbs and vague nouns is reduced in their writing as compared with their speech (Goodglass & Hunter, 1970).

Parietal Agraphia

The agraphic component of alexia with agraphia may be so severe that it appears to be an apraxic disorder in forming letters (Marcie &

Hécaen, 1979). It is not simply an impairment of motor execution, as these patients are severely impaired in spelling. In milder instances of this disorder, however, it is apparent that these patients can form grammatically correct sentences.

Pure Agraphia

Reports of isolated agraphia are sparse, and there is little consensus as to a lesion site. Exner (1881) postulated a writing center at the foot of the second frontal gyrus, separate from Broca's area. Other reports of pure agraphia (Assal, Chapuis, & Zander, 1970; Henschen, 1922; Mahoudeau, 1950; Mahoudeau, David, & Lecoeur, 1951; Morselli, 1930; Sinico, 1926; Wernicke, 1903) support a frontal localization. Penfield and Roberts (1959) observed transient agraphia following surgical excision of F2 and F3. Other investigators support a parietal locus (Kinsbourne & Rosenfeld, 1974), whereas a number accept a frontal and posterior localization and maintain that there are two forms of the defect, one a grapheme selection disorder and the other a spatiotemporal disorganization specific to writing (Dubois, Hécaen, & Marcie, 1969).

The demonstrated existence of cases of pure agraphia, as well as dissociations between severity of written and spoken language, argues for a functional autonomy between written and oral codes (Marcie & Hécaen, 1979). This is further supported by the less frequent association of writing disorders with deficits in oral language in left handers.

Rosati and De Bastiani (1979) considered the pure agraphia in their patient having a vascular lesion in the language zone (perisylvian region of the left hemisphere) to represent a discrete form of aphasia. Chedru and Geschwind (1972), however, did not accept pure writing disturbances as a specific language encoding disorder, but rather proposed that writing is susceptible to influences from a wide variety of pathophysiological processes. In the absence of other language disorders, they noted writing to deteriorate to senseless scrawls in confusional states.

During the past decade there have been a number of reports of acquired writing disorders that parallel reading disorders. For some patients, the agraphia does not coexist with a dyslexia; for others, the type of agraphia corresponds to their type of dyslexia; and for still others, the type of agraphia is distinctly different from their type of dyslexia. Analysis of the distinctive errors made by these patients has provided a testing ground for theories of the mental processes that mediate writing and spelling. For a comprehensive review of these cases, and the theories, see Bub and Cherkow (1988).

Phonological Agraphia

Patients with PHONOLOGICAL AGRAPHIA have inordinate difficulty spelling or writing nonsense words to dictation, yet have relatively little difficulty writing words varying in picturability, frequency, or regularity of spelling. Some aphasics with PHONOLOGICAL AGRAPHIA can write the word for an object that they cannot say. In fact, for some patients, writing the word then enables them to say it. Reports of phonological agraphia (Baxter & Warrington, 1983, 1985; Bub & Kertesz, 1982a; Hatfield, 1985; Roeltgen & Heilman, 1984) provide evidence for the dissociation between written and spoken naming.

Surface Agraphia

Like surface dyslexia, SURFACE AGRAPHIA (or LEXICAL AGRAPHIA) is characterized by the relative preservation of the correspondence between sound and print. Thus "regular" words can be written correctly, but there is a misapplication of rules for "irregular" words. The resultant errors are characteristic of phonetic spelling (e.g., "goz" for *goes*; "peese" for *peace*). As in SURFACE ALEXIA, dictated pseudowords and high-frequency words are spelled well, whereas homophones and irregularly spelled lower frequency words are not. For well-detailed case descriptions, see Beauvois and Derouesne (1981), Goodman and Caramazza (1986), Hatfield and Patterson (1983), and Newcombe and Marshall (1985).

Deep Agraphia

Bub and Kertesz (1982b) described a patient whose reading was unimpaired but whose writing contained semantic paragraphias analogous to the paralexias noted in deep dyslexia. For example, the patient wrote "boat" for *yacht* and "smile" for *laugh*. This patient again underscores the independence between the mechanisms that account for encoding and decoding the visual form of the word.

Acalculia

In 1919, Henschen introduced the term ACALCULIA to designate an acquired calculation disorder distinct from an aphasic inability to read and write numbers. Prior to Henschen, there had been a number of case reports of acquired impairment of calculation overshadowing other co-occurring impairments. Lewandowsky and Stadelmann (1908) described a patient who could read and write numbers but was severely impaired in the simplest of oral arithmetic problems. In this patient all other language functions were spared except for increased latency in word finding and an inability to write words spelled aloud. The responsible lesion was a hematoma in the left occipital lobe (surgically removed), which led Lewandowsky and Stadelmann to attribute this relatively isolated deficit to a specific disorder in the optic representation of numbers. Peritz (1918) proposed the left angular gyrus as the center for calculation, a localization supported by Henschen.

Berger (1926) described three cases of acalculia with dominant hemisphere lesions that did NOT involve the angular gyrus (two occipital and one temporal). These "pure" cases (PRIMARY ACALCULIA) were distinct from SECONDARY ACALCULIA, that is, calculation disturbances resulting from problems in attention, memory, language (aphasia, alexia, agraphia), or general cognitive functioning. Obviously, secondary acalculia would therefore occur more frequently than pure or primary acalculia.

The co-occurrence of severe constructional difficulties noted in some cases (e.g., Singer & Low, 1933) led some investigators to consider the role of a spatial component (Critchley, 1953).

In 1961, Hécaen, Angelergues, and Houillier proposed the following classification based on a study of 183 acalculic patients with retrorolandic lesions:

1. Digit alexia and agraphia may or may not be accompanied by an aphasia, alexia, and/or agraphia. In this type, the paralexic substitutions for presented numbers (stimuli) and the paragraphic errors during computation (response) preclude a correct answer. Benson and Denckla (1969) demonstrated intact computational ability in two patients with digit alexia and agraphia by presenting multiple-choice solutions for arithmetic problems that had been originally "solved" incorrectly.

2. Spatial acalculia causes incorrect solutions due to misalignment of numbers, misordered numbers, number reversals, directional confusion, visual neglect, or oculomotor disturbances. Here, too, basic computational skills may or may not be demonstrated to be intact.

3. Anarithmetia is a fundamental, primary impairment of calculation. This does not imply an isolated impairment, but rather one that does not have as its source an alexia or agraphia for numbers or a spatial organizational problem.

Of these three types of acalculia, digit alexia and agraphia and anarithmetia were found to occur predominantly with left-hemisphere lesions, whereas spatial acalculia rarely occurred with left-hemisphere lesions (10%) but occurred in 73.3% of patients with right-hemisphere lesions (Hécaen & Angelergues, 1961).

Within each hemisphere, varieties of acalculic disorders have been identified in virtually all regions of the brain (Grewel, 1969). Some of this variability in lesion loci has been attributed to premorbid individual differences in processing mathematical problems (Leonhard, 1979) involving different neural substrates. Conversely, the nature and severity of the calculation disorder is obviously, in good measure, determined by the specific dysfunctions referable to different lesion loci, which in turn have differential impact on various aspects of the complex function of calculation (Benson & Weir, 1972; Cohn, 1961; Gerstmann, 1940; Hécaen et al., 1961). Furthermore, the complexity of calculation may be impaired differentially as a function of the modality of presentation, the modality of response (Benton, 1963), and the nature and number of operations involved. As Boller and Grafman (1980) and Levin (1979) concluded in their reviews of the acalculias, the mechanisms of anarithmetia and its regional localization require further study.

Taking the lead from Benton (1963) and Boller and Hécaen (1979), a calculation test battery could be developed that (a) establishes the integrity of number recognition, number reading, writing, memory span, and spatial organization; (b) evaluates appreciation of number values (e.g., which of two numbers is greater), number concepts, and so forth; (c) permits a detailed analysis of stimulus parameters and modality of presentation and response; (d) involves a qualitative analysis of errors. Helm-Estabrooks and Kaplan (1989) developed an instrument (The Boston Stimulus Board) to evaluate some of the above factors in severely aphasic and nonvocal patients. Stimuli can be presented orally and/or visually and require a simple pointing response to a visual multiple-choice array, with foils selected to permit an error analysis. Sections were designed to assess the integrity of number recognition, number reading, number concepts, digit span, and arithmetic computation, as well as other cognitive functions.

Finally, a profile of spared and impaired aspects of calculation functions on a background of spared and impaired language, visuospatial ability, and general neuropsychological functioning could provide insights for the development of intervention strategies.

Finger Agnosia

The inability to recognize or otherwise identify fingers on both of one's own hands, on those of the examiner, or on model hands was considered by Gerstmann (1924) to be a consequence of a more general disturbance of the body schema and attributable to a lesion in the parieto-occipital junction around the angular gyrus of the dominant hemisphere. It should be noted that the severity of the impairment in finger naming or comprehension overshadows an impairment in body-part identification in general.

As is the case in each of the specific disorders (e.g., alexia, agraphia, and acalculia described earlier), finger agnosia is manifested in a variety of ways. Schilder (1931) distinguished a finger aphasia, an optic finger agnosia, and a constructive finger apraxia. Performance may be impaired as a function of modality of presentation or response, that is, whether the modality of stimulation is auditory, visual, or tactile and the response verbal or nonverbal (Benton, 1959; Critchley, 1966; Ettlinger, 1963). Correlational studies (Matthews, Folk, & Zerfas, 1966; Poeck & Orgass, 1969; Sauguet, Benton, & Hécaen, 1971) indicate that tasks involving verbal aspects of finger identification correlate with verbal IQ and are highly associated with receptive aphasic disorders; tasks involving nonverbal aspects of finger recognition correlate more highly with performance IQ than verbal IQ and were also associated with a receptive aphasia. Though nonverbal finger recognition was found to be impaired in left (18%) and right (16%) hemisphere lesions, most of the left-hemisphere–damaged patients showed evidence of either an aphasia or general mental impairment (Gainotti, Cianchetti, & Tiacci, 1972).

Finger agnosia rarely occurs as an isolated finding. Gerstmann (1924) suggested that finger agnosia is the primary deficit in a cluster of symptoms (agraphia, acalculia, and right-left disorientation). This tetrad of symptoms, known as the Gerstmann syndrome, will be discussed later.

In a study of nine patients with nonverbal impairment in finger identification, Kinsbourne and Warrington (1962) found a high degree of association with visuoconstructive disorders. Schilder (1935) similarly had reported the frequency of co-occurrence of such constructional defects as drawings (especially of face and hands in the human drawings). Gerstmann (1940) as well recognized the frequency of co-occurrence of a CONSTRUCTIONAL APRAXIA. Goodglass and Kaplan (1972) found finger agnosia to correlate best with arithmetic (.58), three-dimensional block constructions (.52), and stick construction (.52) and a general loading of .74 with a parietal lobe factor.

Right–Left Disorientation

The inability to identify the right and left sides of one's own body, as well as those of another person vis-à-vis, or on a schematic figure, has

been long recognized to occur with lesions lateralized to the left hemisphere and in the presence of an aphasia (Bonhoeffer, 1923; Head, 1926).
Like finger agnosia, right–left disorientation may be selectively impaired as a function of the modality of stimulus and the required response. Verbal tasks (e.g., naming, responding to verbal command) and
nonverbal tasks (e.g., imitation) should be studied separately, as should
tasks of varying levels of complexity, such as identifying single lateralized parts on one's own body, executing double uncrossed (e.g.,
touching RIGHT eye with RIGHT hand) and crossed (e.g., touching right
eye with left hand) commands on one's own body and pointing to parts
of the examiner's body (Dennis, 1976; Sauguet et al., 1971).

Head (1926) and McFie and Zangwill (1960) attributed verbal and
nonverbal (imitation) impairment in right–left orientation to a left-hemisphere lesion and an associated aphasia. Sauguet et al. (1971) supported
this lateralization for orientation only to one's own body. They found
imitation of lateral movements to occur in 38% of patients with right-
hemisphere disease as contrasted with 48% of aphasic patients. Luria
(1966) considered the inability of patients with frontal pathology to make
reversals on the examiner—that is to identify the RIGHT side of the
examiner as the LEFT side (especially on tasks of imitation)—as echo-
praxic. Benton (1969) viewed such errors as conceptual, that is, an inability to understand the relativistic nature of the right–left concept.

Tests of right–left discrimination in extrapersonal space, such as the
Road Map Test (Money, 1965), make greater demands on visuospatial
functions and are as demanding for right- as for left-hemisphere–lesioned patients. Increasing the spatial complexity of the task (e.g., presenting a schematic figure in different spatial orientations) demands the
capacity for mental rotation. Ratcliff (1979) found the presentation of an
inverted mannikin (upside down and back to front) especially sensitive
to posterior right-hemisphere involvement. Again, right–left disorientation is immediately related to the demands of the test. As is the case in
acalculia and finger localization (described earlier), the complexity of the
task requires sensitive sorting out of the components that may be selectively impaired as a function of the lesion site.

The Gerstmann Syndrome

The tetrad of symptoms described in the preceding sections—
agraphia, acalculia, finger agnosia, and right–left disorientation—were,
as a complex, assumed to represent a distinct neuropsychological syndrome (Gerstmann, 1930). Gerstmann assumed that finger identification

is central to the development of calculation. Strauss and Werner (1938) demonstrated a definite relationship between the ability to articulate the fingers and the early development of the number concept. Finger localization and calculation are presumed to be precursors of right–left orientation and the ability to write. In addition to the prominence of this cluster of symptoms, Gerstmann noted cases with constructional problems, word-finding difficulty, mild reading difficulty, color naming problems, and/or absence of optokinetic nystagmus. The presence of any or all of these associated problems constitute a secondary syndrome implicating more extensive involvement of the parieto-occipital junction of the left hemisphere. The sudden appearance of either the primary or secondary syndrome has been associated with space-occupying lesions. Kertesz (1979) identified 9 out of 556 aphasics and controls who were observed to have the four components of the syndrome distinct from other deficits. Seven of the 9 cases had a left parieto-occipital lesion, 1 had bilateral lesions, and 1 was a trauma and had a negative scan.

The infrequent occurrence of the specific tetrad of Gerstmann, and the greater frequency of the symptoms occurring separately (Heimburger, Demeyer, & Reitan, 1964), has raised the question of the existence of this syndrome. In 1961, Benton addressed this question in his paper entitled "The Fiction of the 'Gerstmann Syndrome.'" He concluded, as did Poeck and Orgass (1975), that the intercorrelations between the four elements of the Gerstmann syndrome were not any greater than correlations between any one element of the syndrome and defects not included in the syndrome. Strub and Geschwind (1974), on the other hand, argued that the infrequency of occurrence of a specific combination of symptoms is what clinically defines a syndrome. For those who accept the entity of the Gerstmann syndrome, it serves to localize the lesion to the parieto-occipital region of the left hemisphere.

There have been a number of reports of a developmental Gerstmann syndrome. Benson and Geschwind (1970) reported two cases of good readers with the tetrad of symptoms along with constructional difficulties. Rourke and Strang (1978) found children referred to a clinic for deficient calculating ability demonstrated a pattern of deficits analogous to the Gerstmann syndrome—that is, problems in arithmetic, right–left orientation, writing, and finger gnosis—while reading was found to be at or above expected grade level. J. Schwartz, Kaplan, and Schwartz (1981) examined school records of 1438 fifth- and sixth-grade children and identified 22 dyscalculic students (1% of the population). The following seven tests were administered: finger gnosis, right–left orientation, Money Road Map Test, block design subtest of the Wechsler Intelligence Scale for Children–Revised, Rey–Osterrieth Complex Figure, visual reproduction subtest of the Wechsler Memory Scale, and Wide Range Achievement spelling subtest. Ten of the 22 children (45% of the dyscalculic population) were found to have all the components of the Gerstmann syndrome and also (as in Rourke's population) had constructional difficulties. Qualitative analysis of their strategies and errors suggested greater compromise of RIGHT hemispheric functions than was the case in either the 12 dyscalculic children who had no evidence of finger agnosia or the nondyscalculic normal matched peer group. It is of interest that the spelling errors of the Gerstmann group in this study as well as in the Rourke study were predominantly phonetic. It would appear, then, that there is a developmental Gerstmann syndrome, but that, unlike in the adults, it does not indicate left-hemisphere dysfunction.

Constructional Disorders

Impaired performance in producing drawings or geometric configurations is frequently referred to as constructional apraxia. The original conception (Kleist, 1912), however, was reserved for those faulty productions that were NOT the result of either impaired visual or motor executive function, but rather a defect in the TRANSMISSION of the visual information to the motor system. The early descriptions (Kleist, 1912; Poppelreuter, 1914–1917) implied this disconnection mechanism. Current use of the term CONSTRUCTIONAL APRAXIA no longer reflects the original presumed underlying mechanism. For some investigators (e.g., Arrigoni & De Renzi, 1964; Piercy & Smith, 1962), constructional disorders following left- and right-hemisphere lesions reflect the same basic disturbance except that it is more frequent and more severe in right-hemisphere than left-hemisphere lesions. They may reflect larger right-hemisphere lesions, since left-hemisphere lesions probably come to the attention of a physician earlier because of the associated aphasic symptoms.

Benton (1969) demonstrated differences as a function of the nature of the constructional task (e.g., drawing, assembling) and concluded that constructional difficulty does not represent a unitary disorder.

During the last three decades, a number of investigators have observed distinctive lateralized differences in the quality of performance. Warrington, James, and Kinsbourne (1966) and Hécaen and Assal (1970) demonstrated that left-hemisphere–lesioned patients improve with practice, whereas right-hemisphere–lesioned patients worsen with practice. Left-hemisphere–lesioned patients produce more right angles than are given in drawing a cube. Right-hemisphere–lesioned patients underestimate angles in a star; left-hemisphere–lesioned patients overestimate angles. In drawing, right-hemisphere–damaged patients tend to oversketch by producing more lines and more details, whereas left-hemisphere–lesioned patients tend to simplify drawings and delete details. Inattention to the left side of space is far more characteristic of right-hemisphere–lesioned patients.

The Block Design subtest of the Wechsler Adult Intelligence Scales is performed poorly but qualitatively differently by patients with lesions lateralized to opposite hemispheres. A study by Kaplan, Palmer, Weinstein, and Baker (1981) found that patients with focal lesions tend to begin working on a block design in the hemiattentional field contralateral to the noncompromised hemisphere; that is, left-hemisphere–lesioned patients work significantly more often from left to right, whereas right-hemisphere–lesioned patients work significantly more often from right to left. Errors en route to a final solution as well as in the final product are more prevalent in the hemiattentional field contralateral to the lesioned hemisphere; that is, left-hemisphere–lesioned patients make significantly more errors on the right side of the designs, and patients with right-hemisphere lesions make significantly more errors on the left side.

The tendency for right-hemisphere–lesioned patients to use a piecemeal approach (Paterson & Zangwill, 1944) without integrating component parts results in a remarkable inability to maintain the 2×2 or 3×3 matrix (broken configuration). Broken configurations evident in productions of right-hemisphere–damaged patients were virtually absent in the productions of left-hemisphere–lesioned patients. Hemispheric differences were also noted in drawings (e.g., Wechsler Memory Scale Visual Reproductions, Rey–Osterrieth Complex Figure). Patients with left-hemisphere lesions were noted to deal more effectively with contour information than with internal features or details, whereas the reverse obtained for patients with right-hemisphere lesions.

Once again, qualitative analyses of the strategies that patients spontaneously use to compensate for their deficits, along with stimulus parameters that induce or preclude such behaviors, have the potential for contributing to the development of both materials and approaches for therapeutic interventions (Kaplan, 1988).

Apraxia: Disorders of Gestural Behavior

The inability of many aphasics to spontaneously use gesture and pantomime to circumvent their problems in communication has been attributed to an "asymbolia" (Finkelnberg, 1870), a loss of the abstract attitude (Goldstein, 1948), a central communication disorder (Duffy and Duffy, 1981), an intellectual defect (Bastian, 1898; Critchley, 1939), or an apraxic disorder (De Renzi, 1988; Geschwind, 1965, 1975; Goodglass & Kaplan, 1963; Heilman, Rothi, & Valenstein, 1982; Kertesz, Ferro, & Shewan, 1984; Liepmann, 1908). Although controversy remains, the most widely accepted position is that gestural impairment is attributable to an apraxia.

APRAXIA may be defined as a disturbance in the execution of learned purposeful movement to command, out of context, that is not attributable to elementary motor or sensory defects, incoordination, poor comprehension, or intellectual deterioration. The responsible lesion is typically lateralized to the premotor region of the left, or dominant, hemisphere and/or to the corpus callosum.

Geschwind (1965, 1975) described the consequences of a premotor and a callosal lesion as follows: An auditory command to perform a movement, such as "Show me how you would brush your teeth with a toothbrush," is comprehended in Wernicke's area; however, destruction of the premotor area necessary to program and initiate the movement precludes performance with either the right hand or the left hand since the information has no way of getting to the right premotor area. Patients with a midcallosal lesion, as in the case of Geschwind and Kaplan (1962) and Gazzaniga, Bogen, and Sperry (1967), are capable of performing the movement with the right hand (left premotor region is intact) but are incapable of performing it with the left hand since the fiber tract from the left premotor to the right premotor region is destroyed. Another disconnecting lesion occurs in the left arcuate fasciculus. Here the lesion in the fiber tract deep to the parietal lobe connecting Wernicke's area to the premotor area precludes the decoded command from reaching the premotor area (as well as resulting in a conduction aphasia). Liepmann's attribution of motor programming to the dominant hemisphere for handedness, as well as the earlier localization of language to the left hemisphere (in right-handed individuals) by Broca (1861) and Wernicke (1908), explains the frequent co-occurrence of apraxia with an aphasia. Despite this earlier work, Goldstein (1948) argued for a central communication disorder. Patients who could not communicate orally or in writing also could not use the gestural channel. Goodglass and Kaplan (1963) tested the notion of a central communicative disorder. The finding that the severity of aphasia did not correlate with the severity of the gestural disturbance argued against a central communication disorder.[1] Furthermore, the finding of the inability to

---

1. Pickett (1974), using the Porch Index of Communicative Ability (PICA) and 10 com-

imitate the gestures demonstrated by the examiner supported Liepmann's position that the aphasic's gestural deficit represented an apraxic disorder. Body part as object (e.g., the use of a body part to represent an absent implement, such as using the index finger as if it were a toothbrush and then vigorously rubbing teeth with the index finger) was commonly noted in the apraxic aphasic and was later found by Kaplan (1968) to be a characteristic response of 4-year-old normal children. In her developmental study, a distinct developmental progression was noted in the acquisition of gestural representation of absent implements. Using the example of representing brushing teeth with a toothbrush, young children between 2½ and 4 years of age rely on deictic behavior (pointing to the locus of the action, e.g., pointing to the mouth) and manipulation of the object of the action (rubbing the teeth). At age 4, body part as object is the most characteristic mode of representation. By age 8, the children are pretending to hold the absent implement, but the movement is too close to the object of the action (e.g., the teeth) and may degrade into a body part as object. By age 12, children are performing like adults, pretending to hold the implement and utilizing empty space to represent the extent of the implement. It may be inferred that the use of body part as object is employed by apraxic patients to circumvent their difficulty in positioning the hand and reproducing the movement veridically. Gestural representation in dementing patients, in intellectually inferior adults, or in the elderly tends toward more concrete representation and the use of body part as object as in the immature child.

Thus far we have discussed impairment of limb movements to command. Patients with arcuate fasciculus lesions as well as left premotor lesions will have similar difficulty carrying out buccofacial movements.

In all apraxic patients, there is a relatively spared class of movements, axial or whole body movements (e.g., stand up, turn around twice, and sit down). Geschwind (1975) suggested that axial movements are controlled by nonpyramidal systems arising from multiple regions in the cortex, whereas the pyramidal systems controlling unilateral movements arise primarily from the precentral gyrus.

Finally in support of Liepmann's proposition that praxis is localized to the hemisphere dominant for handedness, we may cite a case reported by Heilman, Coyle, Gonyea, and Geschwind (1973). Their patient was left handed and suffered damage to his motor and premotor region of the RIGHT hemisphere. He sustained left-sided hemiparesis WITHOUT an aphasia and a severe apraxia involving the right limb; although this

monly used objects in addition to the 10 items used in the PICA, concluded that gestural ability is related to severity of aphasia rather than to a limb apraxia.

patient's intact left hemisphere was obviously dominant for language, he was apraxic secondary to the lesion of the right hemisphere (dominant for handedness). This case dramatically supports the separate functions of language and praxis and argues for their co-occurrence in aphasia as a result of the proximity of structure affected by one lesion.

Thus far we have focused on the issue of production of gesture and pantomime to verbal command. The role of a general symbolic disturbance underlying COMPREHENSION of symbolic gestures and pantomime has been separately addressed. Duffy, Duffy, and Pearson (1975) found pantomime recognition to be significantly correlated with auditory comprehension, naming ability, and overall linguistic competence and argued for the concept of a central communicative disorder. Opposing this view are the findings of Zangwill (1964) and Alajouanine and Lhermitte (1964), who supported the prevalence of defective pantomime recognition in aphasics but not a correlation with the severity of the aphasia. Gainotti and Lemmo (1976) found a high degree of relationship between the comprehension of symbolic gestures and semantic errors on a verbal comprehension test. Although it was again clear that understanding symbolic gestures was more impaired in aphasics than in other brain-damaged patients, there was a minimal relationship between comprehension and production of symbolic gestures (a finding contrary to Duffy et al., 1975). Finally, Varney (1978) found that deficits in pantomime recognition always co-occurred with reading deficit (but not vice versa). Pantomime recognition was found to be only weakly associated with auditory comprehension and naming ability. Varney concluded along with Vignolo (1969), that the possibility of modality-specific factors may underlie the relationships that have been obtained (in this study, the visual modality).

Despite severe inability to engage in gestural representation to verbal command, apraxic patients perform relatively well in the context of real action with implements. (Heilman, 1975, reported some clumsiness in the use of the nonpreferred limb.) Furthermore, global aphasic, apraxic patients have been demonstrated to have the capacity to use non-orthographic visual stimuli for comprehension as well as for communication (Gardner, Zurif, Berry, & Baker, 1976; Glass, Gazzaniga, & Premack, 1973). Helm-Estabrooks, Fitzpatrick, and Barresi (1982), guided by this body of evidence, developed a therapeutic program (visual action therapy). Beginning with actual utilization of the implement, global aphasics were trained to produce symbolic gestures to represent absent stimuli. On pre–post testing, these patients showed significant improvement on PICA pantomime and auditory comprehension subtests. The results of this study hold promise for therapeutic intervention in apraxic aphasic patients.

Acknowledgment

This work was supported in part by the Medical Research Service of the Veterans Administration and in part by USPH grants NS 07615 and 06209. The author also wishes to thank Anne Foundas and Cheryl Weinstein for their assistance in the preparation of the manuscript.

References

Alajouanine, T., & Lhermitte, F., (1964). Non-verbal communication in aphasia. In A. de Rueck & M. O'Connor (Eds.), *Disorders of language.* Boston, MA: Little, Brown.

Albert, M. L. (1979). Alexia. In K. M. Heilman & E. Valenstein (Eds.), *Clinical neuropsychology.* New York: Oxford University Press.

Albert, M. L., Yamadori, A., Gardner, H., & Howes, D. (1973). Comprehension in alexia. *Brain, 96,* 317–328.

Andrewsky, E., & Seron, S. (1975). Implicit processing of grammatical rules in a case of agrammatism. *Cortex, 11,* 379–390.

Arrigoni, G., & De Renzi, E. (1964). Constructional apraxia and hemispheric locus of lesion. *Cortex, 1,* 170–197.

Assal, G., Chapuis, G., & Zander, E. (1970). Isolated writing disorders in a patient with stenosis of the left internal carotid artery. *Cortex, 6,* 241–248.

Bastian, H. C. (1898). *A treatise on aphasia and other speech defects.* London: H. K. Lewis.

Baxter, D. M., & Warrington, E. K. (1983). Neglect dysgraphia. *Journal of Neurology, Neurosurgery and Psychiatry, 46,* 1073–1078.

Baxter, D. M., & Warrington, E. K. (1985). Category specific phonological agraphia. *Neuropsychologia, 23,* 653–666.

Beauvois, M. F., & Derouesne, J. (1981). Lexical or orthographic agraphia. *Brain, 104,* 21–49.

Benson, D. F. (1979). *Aphasia, alexia, and agraphia.* New York, Churchill-Livingstone.

Benson, D. F., & Denckla, M. B. (1969). Verbal paraphasia as a cause of calculation disturbances. *Archives of Neurology (Chicago), 21,* 96–102.

Benson, D. F., & Geschwind, N. (1969). The alexias. In P. J. Vinken & G. W. Bruyn (Eds.), *Handbook of clinical neurology: Disorders of speech, perception, and symbolic behavior.* New York: American Elsevier.

Benson, D. F., & Geschwind, N. (1970). Developmental Gerstmann syndrome. *Neurology, 20,* 293–298.

Benson, D. F., & Weir, W. F. (1972). Acalculia: Acquired anarithmetia. *Cortex, 8,* 465–472.

Benton, A. L. (1959). *Right-left discrimination and finger localization: Development and pathology.* New York: Harper (Hoeber).

Benton, A. L. (1961). The fiction of the "Gerstmann syndrome." *Journal of Neurology, Neurosurgery and Psychiatry, 24,* 176–181.

Benton, A. L. (1963). *Assessment of number operations.* Iowa City: University of Iowa Hospital, Department of Neurology.

Benton, A. L. (1969). Constructional apraxia: Some unanswered questions. In A. L. Benton (Ed.), *Contributions to clinical neuropsychology.* Chicago, IL: Aldine.

Berger, H. (1926). Ueber Rechenstorungen bei Herderkran Kungen des Grosshirns. *Archiv für Psychiatrie und Nervenkrankheiten, 78,* 238–263.

Boller, F., & Grafman, J. (1980). *Acalculia: Historical development and current significance.* Paper presented at Broca Centennial Conference, Mohonk, NY.

Boller, F., & Hécaen, H. (1979). L'évaluation des fonctions neuropsychologiques: Examen standard de l'unité de recherches neuropsychologiques et neurolinguistiques (Vol. 3). *INSERM. Revue de Psychologie Appliquée, 29,* 247–266.

Bonhoeffer, K. (1923). Zur Klinik und Lokalization des Agrammatismus und der Rechts-links-desorientierung. *Monatsschrift für Psychiatrie und Neurologie, 54,* 11–42.

Bradley, D., Garrett, M., & Zurif, E. B. (1980). Syntactic deficits in Broca's Aphasia. In D. Caplan (Ed.), *Biological studies of mental processes.* Cambridge, MA: MIT Press.

Brain, R. (1961). *Speech disorders.* London: Butterworth.

Brissaud, E. (1900). Cécité verbale sans aphasie ni agraphie. *Revue Neurologique, 8,* 757.

Broca, P. (1861). Perte de la parole. Ramollissement chronique et destruction partielle du lobe antérieur gauche du cerveau. *Bulletin de la Société de l'Anthropologie (Paris), 2,* 219.

Bub, D., & Cherkow, H. (1988). Agraphia. In F. Boller & J. Grafman (Eds.), *Handbook of neuropsychology* (Vol. 1). Amsterdam: Elsevier.

Bub, D., & Kertesz, A. (1982a). Evidence for lexicographic processing in a patient with preserved written over oral single word naming. *Brain, 105,* 697–717.

Bub, D., & Kertesz, (1982b). Deep agraphia. *Brain and Language, 17,* 146–165.

Caramazza, A., & Zurif, D. B. (1976). Dissociation of algorithmic and heuristic processes in language comprehension: Evidence from aphasia. *Brain and Language, 3,* 572–582.

Chedru, F., & Geschwind, N. (1972). Writing disturbances in acute confusional states. *Neuropsychologia, 10,* 343–354.

Cohn, R. (1961). Dyscalculia. *Archives of Neurology (Chicago), 4,* 401–307.

Critchley, M. (1939). *The language of gesture.* London: Arnold.

Critchley, M. (1953). *The parietal lobes.* New York: Hafner.

Critchley, M. (1966). The enigma of Gerstmann's syndrome. *Brain, 89,* 183–198.

Dejerine, J. (1891). Sur un cas de cécité verbal avec agraphie suivi d'autopsie. *Memoires de la Societé de Biologie, 3,* 197–201.

Dejerine, J. (1892). Contribution à l'étude anatomo-pathologique et clinique des différentes variété de cécité verbale. *Memoires de la Société de Biologie, 4,* 61–90.

Dejerine, J., & Andre-Thomas, J. (1904). Un cas de cécité verbale avec agraphie suivi d'autopsie. *Revue Neurologique, 12,* 655–664.

Dennis, M. (1976). Dissociated naming and locating of body parts after left temporal lobe resection. *Brain and Language, 3,* 147–163.

De Renzi, E. (1988). Apraxia. In F. Boller & J. Grafman (Eds.), *Handbook of neuropsychology* (Vol. 2). Amsterdam: Elsevier.

Dubois, J., Hécaen, H., & Marcie, P. (1969). L'agraphie "pure." *Neuropsychologia, 7,* 271–286.

Duffy, R. J., & Duffy, J. R. (1981). Three studies of deficits in pantomimic expression and pantomime recognition in aphasia. *Journal of Speech & Hearing Research, 46,* 70–84.

Duffy, R. J., Duffy, J. R., & Pearson, K. (1975). Pantomime recognition in aphasic patients. *Journal of Speech and Hearing Disorders, 18,* 115–132.

Ettlinger, G. (1963). Defective identification of fingers. *Neuropsychologia, 1,* 39–45.

Exner, S. (1881). *Untersuchungen über die Lokalisation der Funktionen in der Grosshirnrinde des Menschen.* Vienna: Wilhelm Braumuller.

Finkelnberg, F. (1870). Vortrag in der Niedernrheim Gesellschaft der Aerzte, Bonn, Berlin. *Klinische Wochenschrift, 7,* 449.

Friedman, R. B. (1988). Acquired alexia. In F. Boller & J. Grafman (Eds.), *Handbook of neuropsychology* (Vol. 1). Amsterdam: Elsevier.

Friedman, R. B., & Alexander, M. P. (1984). Pictures, images, and pure alexia: A case study. *Cognitive Neuropsychology, 1,* 9–23.

Gainotti, G., Cianchetti, C., & Tiacci, C. (1972). The influence of hemispheric side of lesion on nonverbal tests of finger localization. *Cortex, 8,* 364–381.

Gainotti, G., & Lemmo, M. A. (1976). Comprehension of symbolic gestures in aphasia. *Brain and Language, 3,* 451–460.

Gardner, H., & Zurif, E. B. (1975). Bee but not be: Oral reading of single words in aphasia and alexia. *Neuropsychologia, 13,* 181–190.

Gardner, H., Zurif, E., Berry, T., & Baker, E. (1976). Visual communication in aphasia. *Neuropsychologia, 14,* 275–292.

Gazzaniga, M. S., Bogen, J. E., & Sperry, R. W. (1967). Dyspraxia following division of the cerebral commissures. *Archives of Neurology (Chicago),* 12, 606–612.

Gerstmann, J. (1924). Fingeragnosie: Eine umschriebene Störung der Orientierung am eigenen Korper. *Wiener Klinische Wochenschrift, 37,* 1010–1012.

Gerstmann, J. (1930). Zur Symptomatologie der Hirnläsionen in Ubergangsgebiet der unteren Parietal und mittleren Occipitalwindung. *Nervenartz, 3,* 691–695.

Gerstmann, J. (1940). Syndrome of finger agnosia, disorientation for right and left, agraphia, and acalculia. *Archives of Neurology and Psychiatry, 44,* 398–408.

Geschwind, N. (1965). Disconnexion syndromes in animals and man. *Brain, 88,* 237–294, 585–644.

Geschwind, N. (1975). The apraxias: Neurological mechanisms of disorders of learned movement. *American Scientist, 63,* 188–195.

Geschwind, N., & Fusillo, M. (1966). Color naming defects in association with alexia. *Archives of Neurology (Chicago),* 15, 137–146.

Geschwind, N., & Kaplan, E. (1962). A human deconnection syndrome. *Neurology, 10,* 675–685.

Glass, A. V., Gazzaniga, M. S., & Premack, D. (1973). Artificial language training in aphasia. *Neuropsychologia, 11,* 95–103.

Goldstein, K. (1948). *Language and language disturbances.* New York: Grune & Stratton.

Goodglass, H., & Hunter, M. A. (1970). Linguistic comparison of speech and writing in two types of aphasia. *Journal of Communication Disorders, 3,* 28–35.

Goodglass, H., & Kaplan, E. (1963). Disturbance of gesture and pantomime in aphasia. *Brain, 86,* 703–720.

Goodglass, H., & Kaplan, E. (1972). *Assessment of aphasia and related disorders.* Philadelphia, PA: Lea & Febiger.

Goodman, R. A., & Caramazza, A. (1986). *Aspects of the spelling process: Evidence from a case of acquired dysgraphia* (Reports of the Cognitive Neuropsychology Laboratory, No. 15). Baltimore, MD: John Hopkins University.

Grafman, J. (1988). Acalculia. In F. Boller & J. Grafman (Eds.), *Handbook of neuropsychology* (Vol. 1). Amsterdam: Elsevier.

Grewel, F. (1969). The acalculias. In P. J. Vinken & G. W. Bruyn (Eds.). *Handbook of clinical neurology* (Vol. 4). New York: American Elsevier.

Hatfield, F. M. (1985). Visual and phonological factors in acquired agraphia. *Neuropsychologia, 23,* 13–29.

Hatfield, F. M., & Patterson, K. (1983). Phonological spelling. *Quarterly Journal of Experimental Psychology, 35,* 451–468.

Head, H. (1926). *Aphasia and kindred disorders of speech.* Cambridge: Cambridge University Press.

Hécaen, H., & Angelergues, R. (1961). Etude anatomo-clinique de 280 cas de lésions rétrorolandiques unilatérales des hémiphères cérébraux. *Encéphale, 6,* 533–562.

Hécaen, H., Angelergues, R., & Houillier, S. (1961). Les variétés cliniques des acalculies au cours des lésions retrorolandiques: Approche statistique du problème. *Revue Neurologique, 105,* 85–103.

Hécaen, H., & Assal, G. (1970). A comparison of construction deficits following right and left hemispheric lesions. *Neuropsychologia, 8,* 289–304.

Heilman, K. M. (1975). A tapping test in apraxia. *Cortex, 11,*259–263.

Heilman, K. M., Coyle, J. M., Gonyea, E. F., & Geschwind, N. (1973). Apraxia and agraphia in a left-hander. *Brain, 96,* 21–28.

Heilman, K. M., Rothi, L. J., & Valenstein, E. (1982). Two forms of ideomotor apraxia. *Neurology, 32,* 342–346.

Heimburger, R. F., Demeyer, W., & Reitan, R. M. (1964). Implications of Gerstmann's syndrome. *Journal of Neurology, Neurosurgery and Psychiatry, 27,* 52–57.

Helm-Estabrooks, N., Fitzpatrick, P. M., & Barresi, B. (1982). Visual action therapy for global aphasia. *Journal of Speech and Hearing Disorders, 47,* 385–389.

Helm-Estabrooks, N., & Kaplan, E. (1989). *The Boston Stimulus Board.* San Antonio, TX: Special Press.

Henschen, E. S. (1919). Ueber Sprach, Musik, und Rechenmechanismen und ihre Lokalisationen im Grosshirn. *Zeitschrift für die Gesamte Neurologie und Psychiatrie, 52,* 273–298.

Henschen, E. S. (1922). *Klinische und anatomische Beitrage zur Pathologie des Gehirnes: VII. Uber motorische Aphasie und Agraphie.* Stockholm: E. S. Henschen.

Hermann, G., & Poetzl, O. (1926). *Ueber die Agraphie und ihre Lokaldiagnostischen Beziehungen.* Berlin: Karger.

Hinshelwood, J. (1900). *Letter, word, and mind-blindness.* London: H. K. Lewis.

Hoff, H., Gloning, I., & Gloning, K. (1954). Ueber Alexie. *Wiener Zeitschrift für Nervenheilkunde, 10,* 149–162.

Kaplan, E. (1968). *Gestural representation of implement usage: An organismic-developmental study.* Unpublished doctoral dissertation, Clark University, Worcester, MA.

Kaplan, E. (1988). A process approach to neuropsychological assessment. In T. Boll & B. K. Bryant (Eds.), *Clinical neuropsychology and brain function: Research, measurement, and practice.* Washington, DC: American Psychological Association.

Kaplan, E., Palmer, E. P., Weinstein, C., & Baker, E. (1981). *Block design: A brain behavior based analysis.* Paper presented at the annual European meeting of the International Neuropsychological Society, Bergen, Norway.

Kertesz, A. (1979). *Aphasia and associated disorders.* New York: Grune & Stratton.

Kerteszz, A., Ferro, J. N., & Shewan, C. M. (1984). Apraxia and aphasia: The functional anatomical basis for their dissociation. *Neurology, 30,* 40–47.

Kinsbourne, M., & Rosenfield, D. (1974). Agraphia selective for written spelling. *Brain and Language, 1,* 215–225.

Kinsbourne, M., & Warrington, E. K. (1962). A study of finger agnosia. *Brain, 85,* 47–66.

Kleist, K. (1912). Der gang und der gegenwurtige stand der apraxieforschung. *Zeitschrift für Neurologie und Psychiatrie, 1,* 342–452.

Leonhard, K. (1979). Ideokinetic apraxia and related disorders. In Y. Lebrun & R. Hoops (Eds.), *Problems of aphasia.* Lisse: Swets & Zeitlinger, B. V.

Levin, H. A. (1979). The acalculias. In K. M. Heilman & E. Valenstein (Eds.), *Clinical neuropsychology.* New York: Oxford University Press.

Lewandowsky, M., & Stadelmann, E. (1908). Ueber einen bemerkenswerten Fall von Himblutung und über Rechenströrungen bei Herderkrankung des Gehirns. *Journal für Psychologie und Neurologie, 11,* 249–265.

Liepmann, H. (1908). *Drei Aufsatze aus dem Apraxiegebiet.* Berlin: Karner.

Luria, A. R. (1966). *The higher cortical functions in man.* New York: Basic Books.

Mahoudeau, D. (1950). Considerations sur l'agraphie, à propos d'un cas observé chez un traumatise du crane porteur d'une lesion des deuxième et troisième convolutions frontales gauches. *Semaine des Hopitaux, 26,* 1598–1601.

Mahoudeau, D., David, M., & Lecoeur, J. (1951). Un nouveau, cas d'agraphie sans aphasie révéltrice d'une tumeur métastatique du pied de la deuxième circonvolution frontale gauche. *Revue Neuorologique, 1,* 159–161.

Marcie, P., & Hécaen, H. (1979). Agraphia: Writing disorders associated with unilateral cortical lesions. In K. M. Heilman & E. Valenstein (Eds.), *Clinical neuropsychology.* New York: Oxford University Press.

Marshall, J. C., & Newcombe, F. (1966). Syntactic and semantic errors in apralexia. *Neuropsychologia, 4,* 169–176.

Matthews, C. G., Folk, E. G., & Zerfas, P. G. (1966). Lateralized finger localization deficits and differential Wechsler-Bellevue results in retardates. *American Journal of Mental Deficiency, 70,* 695–702.

McFie, J., & Zangwill, O. L. (1960). Visuo-constructive disabilities associated with lesions of the right cerebral hemisphere. *Brain, 82,* 243–259.

Mohr, J. P. (1976). An unusual case of dyslexia with dysgraphia. *Brain and Language, 3,* 324–334.

Money, J. (1965). *A standardized road-map test of directional sense.* Baltimore, MD: Johns Hopkins Press.

Morselli, G. E. (1930). A proposito di agratia pura. *Rivista Sperimentale di Freniatria, 54,* 500–511.

Newcombe, F., & Marshall, J. C. (1985). Reading and writing by letter sounds. Reading and writing by letter sounds. In K. E. Patterson, J. C. Marshall, & M. Coltheart (Eds.), *Surface dyslexia.* Hillside, NJ: Erlbaum.

Paterson, A., & Zangwill, O. L. (1944). Disorders of visual space perception associated with lesions of the right cerebral hemisphere. *Brain, 67,* 331–358.

Patterson, K. E., & Kay, J. (1982). Letter-by-letter reading: Psychological descriptions of a neurological syndrome. *Quarterly Journal of Experimental Psychology, 34A,* 411–441.

Patterson, K. E., & Marcel, A. J. (1977). Aphasia, dyslexia and phonological coding of written words. *Quarterly Journal of Experimental Psychology, 29,* 307–318.

Patterson, K. E., & Morton, J. (1985). From orthography to phonology: An attempt at an old interpretation. In K. E. Patterson, J. C. Marshall, & M. Coltheart (Eds.), *Surface dyslexia.* London: Erlbaum.

Penfield, W., & Roberts, L. (1959). *Speech and brain mechanisms.* Princeton, NJ: Princeton University Press.

Peritz, G. (1918). Zur Pathopsychologie des Rechnens. *Deutsche Zeitschrift fur Nervenheilkunde, 61,* 234–340.

Pickett, L. W. (1974). An assessment of gestural and pantomimie deficit in aphasic patients. *Acta Symbolica, 5,* 69–88.

Piercy, M., & Smith, V. O. (1962). Right hemisphere dominance for certain nonverbal intellectual skills. *Brain, 85,* 775–790.

Poeck, K., & Orgass, B. (1969). An experimental investigation of finger agnosia. *Neurology, 19,* 801–807.

Poeck, K., & Orgass, B. (1975). Gerstmann syndrome without aphasia: Comments on the paper by Strub and Geschwind. *Cortex, 11,* 291–295.

Poetzl, O. (1928). *Die Optisch-Agnostischen Storungen.* Vienna: Deuticke.

Poppelreuter, W. (1914–1917). *Die psychischen Schadigungen durch Kopfschuss in Kriege.* Leipzig: Voss.

Ratcliff, G. (1979). Spatial thought, mental rotation and the right hemisphere. *Neuropsychologia, 17,* 49–54.

Redlich, E. (1895). Ueber die sogenannte subcorticale Alexie. *Jahrbucher für Psychiatrie und Neurologie, 13,* 1–60.

Roeltgen, D. P., & Heilman, K. M. (1984). Lexical agraphia. *Brain, 107,* 811–827.

Rosati, G., & De Bastiani, P. (1979). Pure agraphia: A discrete form of aphasia. *Journal of Neurology, Neurosurgery and Psychiatry, 42,* 266–269.

Rothi, L. J., & Heilman, K. M. (1981). Alexia and agraphia with letter recognition abilities. *Brain and Language, 12,* 1–13.

Rourke, B. P., & Strang, J. D. (1978). Neuropsychological significance of variations in patterns of academic performance. *Journal of Pediatric Psychology, 3,* 62–68.

Saffran, E. M., Bogyo, L. C., Schwartz, M. F., & Marin, O. S. M. (1980). Does deep dyslexia reflect right hemisphere reading? In M. Coltheart, K. Patterson, & J. C. Marshall (Eds.), *Deep dyslexia.* London: Routledge & Kegan Paul.

Samuels, J. A., & Benson, D. F. (1979). Some aspects of language comprehension in anterior aphasia. *Brain and Language, 8,* 275–286.

Sauguet, J., Benton, A. L., & Hécaen, H. (1971). Disturbances of the body schema in relation to language impairment and hemispheric locus of lesion. *Journal of Neurology, Neurosurgery and Psychiatry, 34,* 496–501.

Schilder, P. (1931). Fingeragnosie, Fingerapraxie, Finger Aphasie. *Nervenarzt, 4,* 625–629.

Schilder, P. (1935). *The image and appearance of the human body.* London: Routledge & Kegan Paul.

Schwartz, J., Kaplan, E., & Schwartz, A. (1981). *Childhood dyscolculia and Gerstmann syndrome.* Paper presented at the American Academy of Neurology, Toronto.

Schwartz, M. F., Saffran, E. M., & Marin, O. S. M. (1977). *An analysis of agrammatic reading in aphasia.* Paper presented at the International Neuropsychological Society, Santa Fe, NM.

Shallice, T., & Warrington, E. K. (1975). Word recognition in a phonemic dyslexic patient. *Quarterly Journal of Experimental Psychology, 27,* 187–199.

Singer, H. D., & Low, A. A. (1933). Acalculia (Henschen): A clinical study. *Archives of Neurology and Psychiatry, 29,* 476–498.

Sinico, S. (1926). Neoplasia della seconda circonvoluzione frontale sinistra: Agratia pura. *Gazzetta degli Ospedali e delle Cliniche, 47,* 627–631.

Strauss, A., & Werner, H. (1938). Deficiency in the finger schema in relation to arithmetic disability. *American Journal of Orthopsychiatry, 8,* 719–725.

Strub, R. L., & Geschwind, N. (1974). Gerstmann syndrome without aphasia. *Cortex, 10,* 378–387.

Varney, N. R. (1978). Linguistic-correlates of pantomime recognition in aphasic patients. *Journal of Neurology, Neurosurgery and Psychiatry, 41,* 564–568.

Vignolo, L. (1969). Auditory agnosia: A review and report of recent evidence. In A. L. Benton (Ed.), *Contributions to modern clinical neuropsychology,* Chicago, IL: Aldine.

Vincent, C., David, M., & Puech, P. (1930). Sur l'aléxie. Production du phénomène à la suite de l'extirpation de la sorne occipitale due ventricule l'atéral gauche. *Revue Neurologique, 1,* 262–272.

von Stockert, T. R., & Bader, L. (1976). Some relations of grammar and lexicon in aphasia. *Cortex, 12,* 49–60.

Warrington, E. K., James, M., & Kinsbourne, M. (1966). Drawing disability in relation to laterality of lesion. *Brain, 89,* 53–92.

Warrington, E. K., & Shallice, T. (1980). Word-form dyslexia. *Brain, 103,* 99–112.

Wernicke, C. (1903). Ein Fall von isolierter Agraphie. *Monatsschrift fur Psychiatrie und Neurologie, 13,* 241–265.

Wernicke, C. (1908). The symptom-complex of aphasia in disease of the nervous system. In E. D. Church (Ed.), *Modern clinical medicine: Diseases of the nervous system.* New York: Appleton.

Zangwill, O. (1964). Intelligence in aphasia. In A. de Rueck & M. O'Conner (Eds.), *Disorders of language.* Boston, MA: Little, Brown.

10

Intelligence and Aphasia

KERRY HAMSHER

Early Controversies

The Discursive Arguments

The purpose of this chapter is to identify and review issues concerning the relation between aphasia and intelligence. The debate that surrounds this topic is far from being concluded and remains a major topic for continuing research in the field of aphasia. This issue has at its heart two underlying themes: First, what is the relation between language and thought; second, to what extent does an aphasic disorder transcend a mere disorder of speech. The first theme has manifold ramifications ranging from contested philosophic debates to questions about vocational rehabilitation for victims of cerebral disease. The second theme is a restatement of the first using the terms and concepts of clinical neurology and neuropsychology. As we shall see, these concepts of "thought" and "language" are much like Siamese twins: At their points of interface, it may not be possible to say where one stops and the other begins; yet each generally operates independently and possesses a unique character.

In Chapter 1, Benton describes the history of concern with the effects of aphasia on intelligent thought, a concern that is deeply rooted in the earliest theories of aphasia. From those early clinical observations of patients with acquired aphasia, two major principles were derived: (a) Aphasia was more than a paralysis of the muscles involved in speech and therefore must involve some mental or cognitive capacity, and (b) the problems manifested by aphasics in the activities of daily living and limitations in communication with others in the environment seemed greater than what could be accounted for by the speech defects alone. In response to the first observation, hypotheses were offered to link a cognitive defect with the consequent disturbances in speech. Bouillaud and Lordat, for example, supposed there was damage to the "organ of memory for words," leading to a concept of aphasia as a specific amnestic defect. Broca, Wernicke, and Lichtheim spoke of defects in association processes that link words with their referent objects or actions. Logically, this concept would allow that both memory for words and a meaningful appreciation of the environment could be preserved but dissociated in aphasia.

The second observation led to questions about the effect of aphasia on thought processes. Trousseau first emphasized the apparent impairment in thought processes in aphasia, followed by J. Hughlings Jackson and Baillarger. Pierre Marie spoke of the necessary impairment of limited but important aspects of intelligence in aphasia. Arnold Pick (1931/1973) declared that "speech symbols represent an important aid to thought" (p. 136). In describing thought processes as cascading events in which the early stages of formulation serve to guide the later stages, Pick suggested that a deficiency in language would degrade the formulation of thought at its earliest stages and thus could give the appearance of intellectual retardation. By this comment one may suppose that Pick felt the real substance of intelligence may remain intact in aphasia but left in waiting for the return of linguistic skills. Findelnburg, Kurt Goldstein, and Head believed aphasia could be conceived as a defect in symbolic thinking. Whether printed or sounded out, words are a convenient way to refer to elements of one's environment and thus are very clearly symbols.

In some senses, these are all appealing concepts of aphasia. It is not clear, however, that any of them can adequately account for either the variety of cognitive deficits that are associated with aphasia or the variability among aphasics in their patterns of cognitive symptomatology. For example, whereas language represents a special use of symbolic thinking—namely, "the use of symbols for purposes of communication" (Benton, 1965, p. 298)—this does not appear to be the only aspect of language that is vulnerable to brain disease. The four major syndromes of aphasia share the symptom of an impairment in naming: In Broca's aphasia, effortful and labored attempts to name result in phonemic paraphasias; in so-called conduction and Wernicke's aphasia, naming is non-effortful and fluent, but there are prominent phonemic and semantic paraphasic errors; in nominal aphasia, paraphasic errors are rare and the defect in naming appears to represent a failure in word retrieval (Goodglass, 1980). Thus, one can see how difficult it would be to explain these various characteristics by one mechanism.

Empirical Formulations

An understanding of the contribution of the right hemisphere to the performance of certain intellectual tasks or functions was largely missing during the early stages of the development of a concept of aphasia. This lack of appreciation for the role of the so-called minor hemisphere persisted despite the contributions of J. Hughlings Jackson, who at the time of Broca's discoveries was suggesting that symptoms of visuospatial impairment, which he called "imperception," could result from right hemisphere lesions, particularly in the posterior zone (Benton, 1977a). Yet, even Jackson lacked a formal theory of intelligence, and none of the early theorists proposed a view of intelligence as an objective and measurable behavioral capacity. The work of Weisenburg and McBride (1935) ushered in both a new approach to the question of the relation between aphasia and intelligence and a new speculation. Their objective assessment of both verbal and nonverbal cognitive performances in aphasic, nonaphasic brain-damaged, and control subjects led them to believe that individual cognitive styles or strategies must play a role. Persons accustomed to solving problems by verbal means might, by this formulation, be the ones most likely to exhibit nonverbal defect in the context of aphasia. Weisenburg and McBride's contribution marked the onset of a new era in which formal conceptualizations of intelligence, and the method of assessment, were brought to bear on the question of the effect of aphasia on intelligence.

Intelligence

The Concept of Intelligence

A definition of the concept of intelligence is at once both controversial and complex. To emphasize here the points of disagreement would be self-defeating, for we cannot realistically evaluate the issues at hand if a consensus definition is circumvented. At the same time, some of the complexity must be preserved if we are going to do justice to the term and meaningfully test the limits of the concept of intelligence in the context of aphasia.

Sir Cyril Burt (1955) ascribed the origin of the concept of intelligence to Plato and Aristotle and credits Cicero with the coinage of the term. The use of tests to assess intelligence, as well as the application of statistics to these data, was introduced by an English scientist, Sir Francis Galton. Galton was interested in supporting the theories of his first cousin, Charles Darwin, by demonstrating that the principles of hereditary descent applied to intellectual as well as physical attributes. To this end he published his study *Hereditary Genius* in 1869 (Galton, 1887). But as Zangwill (1964) pointed out, the real work on the exploration and development of this concept began with the development of intelligence tests for the purpose of addressing socioeducational problems. This work was begun by Alfred Binet, a French lawyer and natural scientist by education, who became a psychologist largely through self-tutoring.

A different conception of the term INTELLIGENCE is sometimes encountered among the general public, where it is taken to mean a state of above-normal thinking capacity. In scientific psychology, intelligence is conceived as a largely but not exclusively biologic characteristic that is expressed in behavior, which varies from one person to the next, and accounts for some individual differences in behavior. Therefore, it is a quantitative concept, as are the concepts of height and weight. At the same time, there appears to be some naturally occurring upper limit to human intelligence, but this limit is not explicitly defined. Unlike height and weight, intelligence cannot be directly observed, touched, or measured in physical terms. It is more well defined and less arbitrary than such concepts as beauty and creativity. Also, the characteristics one looks at to assess intelligence in a subjective fashion are more consistent than, say, the characteristics that might be employed to assess "athleticism" in ping-pong players, football players, gymnasts, and runners.

A distinction is made by most authorities between the application of the concept of intelligence to represent one's ability versus one's actual performance. A highly intelligent individual could on some occasions perform very poorly on an intelligence test for a variety of reasons, such as anxiety or preoccupation. Clearly one could fake a bad performance on an intelligence test, and obviously such an event would not in any real sense lower that person's intellectual competence. Thus, this distinction between capacity and performance is crucial and something to be addressed later in this chapter.

Wechsler (1958) described general intellectual ability as the "global capacity of the individual to act purposefully, to think rationally, and to deal effectively with his environment" (p. 7). Intellectual behavior or functional intelligence, he said, depends on general intellectual ability plus the way in which specific cognitive abilities are combined and such nonintellectual factors as the person's drive and the incentive offered by the situation in which intelligence is being assessed.

Thus, intelligence is a construct that implies an underlying reality, but this reality must be inferred from behavioral observations (Wechsler, 1971). The parallel to this is a working definition of intelligence as a complex trait that is measured by intelligence tests (Wechsler, 1971). Since psychology has developed methods to determine if a particular test is a measure of what we intend to call intelligence, the circularity of the working definition is no longer problematic. These methods derive from our current understanding of the structure of intelligence.

The Structure of Intelligence

Two differing views of the structure of intelligence developed during the first half of the twentieth century. One view, which was articulated by the British psychologist Spearman (1927), holds that intelligence is a unitary trait that is expressed to greater or lesser extent on most any cognitive task. The opposing view is that general intelligence is merely the sum (or average) of a collection of different primary abilities. This point of view was championed by the American psychologist Thurstone (1938). Since Thurstone's primary abilities are not independent of each other and, in fact, are intercorrelated, this position is not fundamentally different from Spearman's position that besides the general factor there are also specific intellectual factors (Piercy, 1969). Modern psychology therefore views intelligence as having both unitary and multiple or factorial aspects. The history that led to this conclusion is described by Matarazzo (1972, pp. 24–62).

Intelligence is generally conceived as being organized in a hierarchial fashion. This notion is borrowed from the facts of evolution, especially with regard to the development of the central nervous system. According to this model, in the normal brain, general ability exerts a downward influence on the next level of organization, which consists of several major or group factors (primary abilities). The group factors, in turn, comprise several specific factors that may be specific to the type of task or method of assessing performance. Whether there are two, three, or more levels of organization within the various spheres of cognitive activity has not been fixed in fact or theory. The question of the number of levels of organization is an arbitrary one, since the answer varies depending upon the number and types of cognitive behaviors sampled, the methods of assessment, and the type of statistical analysis applied.

A concrete example may assist in appreciating the theoretical view of the structure of intelligence. To begin, an extensive battery of cognitive tests would be administered to a cross-section of the general population. The finding that all the test scores correlate positively with each other provides the basis for inferring the presence of a general factor of intelligence, often called g after the manner of Spearman. When the influence of each test's correlation with g is statistically removed, one can determine to what degree two tests are related to each other in a way not accounted for by their shared correlation with g. This leads to the observation that there are clusters of tests that tend to correlate with each other to a high degree and show a low correlation with the remaining clusters of tests. This clustering is how major or group factors are identified. To determine an individual test's correlation with the statistical definition of g, each subject's score on that test would be correlated with the subject's score on the entire battery. Examining these correlations, one will find that some tests correlate with (predict) g better than others. Those tests that correlate most strongly with g are considered the best representatives of measures of general intelligence within the test's group factor. Among verbal tests, vocabulary and general information show this strong relationship with g. Among nonverbal intellectual tasks, Raven's Progressive Matrices and the Block Design subtest from the Wechsler Adult Intelligence Scale-Revised (WAIS-R) are among the best predictors of g.

The Validity of Intelligence

This psychometric framework allows behavioral scientists to develop and validate measures of intelligence within various cultures. Thus, when we speak of measures of general intelligence, we are denoting measures that predict how well a person will likely perform on a wide variety of cognitive tasks. Although eloquently conceived, this view of intelligence would be rather trivial if it were not also true that intelligence, defined and measured by objective means, predicted or coincided with other real-world events and biologic patterns.

When the concept of general intelligence is expressed as a summary score derived from an intelligence test battery, then the technical term INTELLIGENCE QUOTIENT (IQ) may be used. A quotient score is a way of expressing performance level in a standard fashion. By convention, quotient scores have a mean of 100 and a standard deviation of 15 points. The IQ score states a person's standing relative to some reference group. Since performance on intelligence tests progressively increases with age during the developmental years and may progressively decline with age during late life, separate reference groups are needed for various age categories.

Childhood IQs starting from age 7–8 correlate with adult IQ in the range of $r = .70-.85$, suggesting a fair degree of stability. Childhood IQs correlate with adult occupational level ($r = .40-.60$). Similarly, adult IQ scores correlate with adult educational and occupational levels in the same range (approximately $r = .50$) (McCall, 1977). We may infer from these findings that, although performance on an intelligence test battery seems to have an important relationship to adult education and occupational achievements, other factors must also be involved that are not accounted for in the IQ score. Because our concept of intelligence does not require that it account for everything, these summary findings reported by McCall can be considered supportive of the validity of measured intelligence.

Substantial evidence indicates that objective measures of intelligence are in part under hereditary control. For example, the highest correlations in IQs are found among identical twins (about $r = .90$). As expected, there are highly significant but smaller correlations between the IQs of siblings and between parents and children, all of whom share fewer genes than identical twins. There is also evidence that, although these correlations are attenuated when the pairs in these correlations live apart from each other, the pattern of correlations (e.g., identical twins vs. fraternal twins) remains much the same. Moreover, the magnitude of these correlations are similar to those of other complex, multiply-determined traits, such as height and weight. Since the IQ is not a perfectly reliable score, varies within the same individual on different occasions, and is subject to the influence of such personality and environmental factors as drive and incentive, the obtained correlations may be considered minimal correlations. The magnitude of the contributions of heredity and environment is a question that is still at issue; for our purposes, knowing that the IQ is in part under hereditary control is sufficient with regard to the question of the validity of the concept of intelligence expressed as an IQ score (Matarazzo, 1972, pp. 298–317; Vandenberg, 1971).

So far, we have seen that intelligence as a concept has progressed (in a scientific sense) from an abstract concept to a concrete IQ score. This score appears valid in the sense that IQ scores tend to covary with the trappings of the abstract concept of intelligence, such as educational and occupational attainment and performance, and heredity. Further evidence of its validity comes from the observation of its susceptibility to decline with brain damage.

Intelligence and Brain Disease

When speaking of brain disease, one may be tempted to think of something akin to an inflammation, but DISEASE is a broad term that carries no particular implication for the etiology of the diseased or abnormal state. Brain disease may be acquired through such mechanisms as heredity, brain tumors, prenatal trauma or metabolic disorders, postnatal vascular events such as stroke, a shearing of the brain from sudden rotation, and missile wounds such as from a gunshot. Brain disease also can be a secondary consequence of a disease of another organ system, such as renal failure or liver disease. Likewise, the term LESION is not a specific term. A lesion is a site of abnormality. It may be visible radiographically because it alters brain structure or causes a breakdown in the blood–brain barrier, but this is not required. A lesion may also be said to be present as a result of microscopic changes in brain tissue or even changes in intracellular metabolism. For the most part, however, the kinds of lesions referred to in studies of the effects of focal brain lesions on intelligence are ones that have been demonstrated radiographically (on X-ray) or through electrophysiology (i.e., on the electroencephalogram) or have been visualized by a neurosurgeon and occasionally a neuropathologist.

General Intelligence and Brain Disease

Karl S. Lashley, a physiological and behavioral psychologist, brought together psychological and statistical concepts of intelligence, neurological concepts of dementia and mental retardation, and some sparse neuroanatomical observations. From this mixture of data and conjecture, he enunciated two major principles: EQUIPOTENTIALITY and MASS ACTION. Equipotentiality means that the cerebral cortex is considered undifferentiated in its contribution to the performance of intelligent behavior; that is, the contribution of one section of cortex is presumed to be as good as, and equal to, the contribution of some other section. Mass action means that all regions of the equipotential cortex work together, en masse as it were, to produce intelligent behaviors so that a loss in efficiency consequent to brain damage will be proportional to the loss in cortical mass (tissue) regardless of its locus. According to Lashley, these principles applied only to nonlocalized behavioral functions such as learning and intelligence. Lashley (1929) supported these concepts with data on the maze-learning performances of rats in relation to the locus and amount of cortical tissue that was surgically removed. By today's standards, several of his correlations would not be considered statistically significant (reliably greater than zero), so in retrospect his arguments were not as sound as they were thought to be at the time. These principles had value, however, in that they generated research in attempts to defend or refute Lashley's laws.

In a study that was the human analogue of Lashley's classic study, Chapman and Wolf (1959) correlated IQ scores with the neurosurgeon's estimated amount of cerebral tissue removed during operations for the treatment of brain tumors and arteriovenous malformations. Evidence for mass action was found with the stricture that the relationship between intellectual and cerebral tissue loss was much more firm in those patients in whom the cortical excisions were postrolandic (involving the parietal, occipital, and temporal lobes). In an equally monumental study, Blessed, Tomlinson, and Roth (1968) examined the brains of deceased demented patients, most of whom suffered from Alzheimer's disease. A counting was made of the number of senile plaques found in several brain regions. Senile plaques are present in excessive amounts in the brains of demented patients relative to age-matched nondemented controls. Prior to these patients' deaths, they were administered a battery of cognitive tests, and behavioral ratings were obtained from relatives. These investigators found a significant but modest correlation between mean plaque count and scores on the mental test battery, while the plaque count correlated more highly with the ratings of a decline in the patients' personal and social habits. The difference in the magnitude of these correlations may be due to an artifact of assessment, since the behavioral ratings were a direct rating of decline in behavioral status, whereas the mental test scores may have been partially confounded with premorbid ability level. Nevertheless, these and similar findings lend credence to the notion that some summary index of acquired intellectual impairment derived from a battery of cognitive performances provides at least a rough index of the status of the cerebrum (Benton, 1980; Loeb, Gandolfo, & Bino, 1988), particularly the posterior association areas in the parietal and temporal lobes (Duara et al., 1986; Foster et al., 1983).

Focal Brain Lesions and Intellectual Performance

So far we have seen how the concept of intelligence as having both multifactorial and unitary aspects developed from studies of neurologically normal individuals. When a broad array of cognitive abilities are sampled in the investigation of general intelligence, one frequently observes individual patterns of cognitive performance, that is, areas of relative strengths and weaknesses as opposed to equivalent scores across all samples of cognitive performance. Because of what was earlier described as a downward influence of general ability on more specific abilities, we find that if two individuals have broadly separated IQ scores, even in the case where one person's weakness is the other's strength, the person with the lower IQ will seldom surpass the higher IQ individual on any of these more specific intellectual factors. Another way to view this is to say that to some extent particular abilities, such as spatial, verbal, or numerical abilities, are dissociable within the general population. Some evidence suggests that an individual's pattern of specific abilities in the context of their general ability level plays a role in occupational selection. For example, on average, architects may outperform mechanics on measures of general ability, while they share a relative superiority in mechanical and visuoperceptive skills compared with other abilities such as numerical or verbal (see Matarazzo, 1972, pp. 168–174).

Understanding g as a summary statement of intellectual standing in the normal population, the concept of dementia may be viewed as a pathological counterpart to g. In behavioral terms, dementia denotes a generalized decline in all aspects of cognitive functioning which is neurologically represented by widespread cerebral disease or dysfunction (Benton, 1980). In short, dementia implies a significant decline in g from some previous (premorbid) level due to brain disease. Between these two extremes of an intact and devastated cerebrum are the effects of focal brain lesions.

The WAIS, like its predecessor, the Wechsler–Bellevue Intelligence Scale, and its revised version, the Wechsler Adult Intelligence Scale–Revised (WAIS-R), comprises 11 subtests covering a variety of cognitive abilities. Scores from 6 of the subtests are grouped together to yield a verbal IQ score (VIQ), and the remaining 5 subtests are grouped to yield a performance IQ score (PIQ). The full-scale IQ (FSIQ) represents the sum of performances across all the subtests. Several statistical studies using factor analysis (see Matarazzo, 1972, pp. 261–276) suggest that the VIQ is composed of two factors, one of which could be called verbal–conceptual abilities (information, comprehension, similarities, vocabulary) and the other could be called attention–concentration (arithmetic reasoning, digit span). The PIQ is composed of tests assessing perceptual–constructional abilities (block design, picture arrangement, object assembly, picture completion) and psychomotor speed (digit symbol substitution).

The selection and grouping of the WAIS subtests into the verbal and performance scales was largely done on a rational rather than an empirical basis. Although not specifically designed to detect or localize brain disease, this test battery has some usefulness along these lines (Benton, 1977b; Fogel, 1964; McFie, 1976; Wilson, Rosenbaum, & Brown, 1979). For the sake of argument, we will consider the VIQ and PIQ to represent two major intellectual factors. Studies of the WAIS performances of patients with focal or at least largely unilateral brain lesions suggest that the lesions of the left hemisphere often result in a VIQ deficit, whereas lesions of the right hemisphere result in greater impairment of the PIQ. Not all studies are in agreement with this summary statement, but the trend has appeared often enough in many separate clinical settings that it has become accepted with qualifications (G. Goldstein, 1974; Kløve, 1974; Lezak, 1983, pp. 181–224; Smith, 1975; Walsh, 1978, pp. 282–331). Furthermore, McFie (1960, 1969; McFie & Thompson, 1972) reported specific patterns of deficits on the Wechsler subtests that are associated with the intrahemispheric locus of focal brain disease (e.g., frontal vs. temporal vs. parietal lobes). Although these latter findings with the Wechsler tests have not been fully substantiated, the fact that patterns of specific cognitive deficits may be associated with lesions in specific brain areas (foci) is well established (McFie, 1969; Newcombe, 1974; Piercy, 1964; Walsh, 1978).

These illustrative points help to build a conceptual framework for understanding how focal brain lesions may affect intellectual performance. First, depending upon its locus, the lesion may severely compromise a given test performance. Because that test shares some properties with the other tests with which it is factorially grouped—which is the nature of factorial grouping—the effect of that lesion may be seen as partially affecting related test performances. Both the specific test defect and shared deficits on related tests would act to lower the major factor or test group score (e.g., the PIQ). This, in turn, would result in a lowering of the summary or general intellectual score. According to this model, in pathological conditions, specific cognitive defects may exert an upward influence through the structure of intelligence, and its influence would tend to be diminished at higher stages in the hierarchy. To take the analogy one step further, suppose there were a single test that incorporated several of the more specific cognitive abilities, all of which were required for the successful performance of the task. First, in the general population we may expect such a task to have a high correlation with g because of its multifactorial composition. Second, we might expect that focal lesions in different regions of the brain may impair test performance because of impairment of one or several of the more specific abilities incorporated in the test. Studies of the effects of focal brain lesions on cognitive performance may also provide an alternative method to factor analysis to identify the structure and hierarchial organization of intellectual abilities.

It has been asserted that, when g is conceived as the composite sum of various performances that individually may be sensitive to aphasic, apraxic, and agnostic disorders, it may not be possible to assess general intelligence meaningfully in the presence of cerebral disease (Messerli & Tissot, 1974). For instance, a patient with a premorbid IQ of 110 has suffered a stroke resulting in aphasia. After the stroke, this patient obtains a VIQ of 78 and a PIQ of 108 with a resulting FSIQ of 93. Can we say the FSIQ represents a fair and adequate assessment of the patient's general intelligence? It certainly would not reflect the patient's spatial strengths or the severity of the verbal deficits. At this point we reach a theoretical and empirical impasse, for to date we are without an adequate conceptualization of intelligence that can accommodate the findings obtained from normal individuals, demented patients, and patients with focal lesions. As an attempt to arrive at a pragmatic solution, the custom is to use an IQ score derived from nonverbal tests for patients with aphasic disorders and to use a measure of verbal IQ for patients with visuoperceptive or spatial disorders. The supporting reasoning is that specific cognitive defects, such as aphasia or constructional apraxia, are considered to be acquired disabilities much like acquired blindness, deafness, or hemiplegia, which interfere with the usual method of assessing general intelligence.

Language and Intellectual Development

Deafness and Illiteracy

Because of the intimate relationship between language and thought in our everyday experiences, it may take a moment of reflection to disengage the two concepts. True, much of our thought processes are expressed verbally, as in the classroom or when writing an exam or in talking to ourselves to work through solutions to various problems (so-called inner speech). But we can also recall situations and social relations in the form of visual memories, like silent movies, and in this mode we may use visual imagery to replay and rearrange events on our mind. We may find the best route on a map by visual inspection with the aid of spatial judgments, and we may conceive of repairing an automobile engine or an electric appliance without aid of words, but not without thought. To refrain from attempting to put a large square peg through a small round hole surely represents not only perceptual discrimination but also some form of conceptual thought (Piaget, 1936).

Through the use of pantomime, we can communicate nonverbal thoughts to others, although, granted, this may be a tedious and inefficient process compared with oral speech. Infrahuman animals, such as dogs, can be trained to perform many tasks, for example, to fetch a stick and return it to the master in exchange for a pat or some treat. When the same dog spontaneously brings an object in an effort to initiate the game or to receive a reward, we must assume this, too, represents thought as well as learning in the absence of language. Yet those examples do not reveal what level of complexity can be achieved by humans without the aid of words.

Pitner and Lev (1939) compared the intellectual performances of partially deaf children and hearing children in grades 5–8. The mean performance of the hearing-impaired children was 8 IQ points below that of normal children on verbal intellectual measures but only 3 IQ points lower on nonverbal tests. Upon a review of the literature, Furth (1964; Furth & Youniss, 1975) noted that on a variety of tests of reasoning and problem solving, deaf children are often able to perform very closely to the level of hearing children of the same age. Although the retardation in oral and written language acquisition that results from deafness is a formidable obstacle, the many points of intellectual similarity between the deaf and their hearing peers would seem to negate the necessity of language for the development of normal, or near normal, intelligence and conceptual thinking. It has also been noted that environmental circumstances may be pivotal in the degree to which deafness and other forms of sensory deprivation may retard or place limits on learning processes (Kodman, 1963). One must ask to what extent others in the deaf person's environment have tried to communicate using preserved sensory channels, such as the visual, tactile, and proprioceptive modalities. The developmental history of Helen Keller provides strong testimony to the importance of this environmental issue.

The assumption that deaf children, who are without oral or written language, actually lack ANY form of language, however, may not be valid. Since deafness is a peripheral sensory impairment, there is no reason to suppose that the deaf lack or have an impairment of the neural structures that subserve language in the hearing and speaking population. Pilot observations of deaf children between 1.5 and 4 years of age who have not been exposed to a manual sign language suggest they may spontaneously develop their own structured sign system that contains the basic properties of spoken language (Goldin-Meadow & Feldman, 1977). The lack of aural exposure to language with the consequent failure to develop oral speech or its graphic representation may not preclude the development of the fundamental properties of language or the capacity for intelligent thought.

Illiteracy (due to social rather than intellectual restrictions) represent a similar but more limited form of environmental deprivation for an aspect of language in the context of presumably normal neurological mechanisms to acquire it. Despite the incompleteness of the illiterate's language repertoire, thinking, linguistic processing, hemispheric specialization for language, and vulnerability to neurological impairments of language, for the most part, do not appear to differ from those of literate individuals (A. R. Damasio, Castro-Caldas, Grosso, & Ferro, 1976; A. R. Damasio, Hamsher, Castro-Caldas, Ferro, & Grosso, 1976; H. Damasio, Damasio, Castro-Caldas, & Hamsher, 1979).

Developmental Aphasia and Intelligence

DEVELOPMENTAL APHASIA (or CONGENITAL APHASIA) is a term used to describe the condition in which a child shows a relatively specific failure in the acquisition of language functions and manifests abnormalities in either expressive speech alone or in both comprehension and oral speech (Benton, 1964). With rare exceptions—for instance, congenital auditory imperception (Worster-Drought & Allen, 1929)—language functions are similarly affected in the auditory, visual, and tactile modalities. By definition, language abilities must be more severely impaired than other cognitive functions so as to distinguish this specific syndrome from general mental impairment (mental retardation, or amentia). Likewise, other causes for a failure to exhibit normal language for age must be excluded (Benton, 1964; Zangwill, 1978), such as deafness or more pervasive neuropsychiatric disease in which disturbances in verbal communication represent but a subset of core symptoms as in childhood autism (A. R. Damasio & Maurer, 1978).

It is reasonable to query whether the criteria for this behavioral diagnosis begs the question of intellectual deficit in the context of developmental aphasia. To a limited extent it does, since investigators are not likely to argue points of concern to developmental aphasia using data from subjects who are also severely impaired in nonverbal intellectual performance. Also, at very low levels of cognition, numerous technical problems adhere to mental measurements. Inasmuch as the diagnosis requires only a relative disparity between verbal and nonverbal abilities, rather than some absolute level of nonverbal intelligence, the case material reported in the literature can still be informative on this point.

The issue of the status of cognitive functioning in the presence of developmental aphasia is as complex as in the case of adult acquired aphasia. The rarity of the childhood disorder makes it particularly difficult to arrive at statistically reliable empirical formulations. The failure of investigators to describe adequately the symptomatology of the subjects under study makes comparisons across different studies tenuous at best, as does the failure to report or account for demographic variables that influence expected intellectual values, as discussed earlier in the section on the validity of intelligence. The indiscriminate lumping together of children with quite variable patterns of speech and language impairments certainly clouds and may confound experimental findings as well. Two broad classifications are minimally indicated: children with primarily expressive speech defects and children with expressive and receptive language deficits (Benton, 1978).

From the available findings, we may conclude that children with developmental aphasia (or developmental dysphasia), in addition to speech defects, are impaired in verbal intelligence relative to their performance on nonverbal intellectual measures and are more variable than normals in their nonverbal IQs, which tend to be lower than expected given the children's family backgrounds (Benton, 1978). Some of these children do obtain high average to superior nonverbal IQs, but a larger proportion are in the low average to dull normal categories. Although the evidence is insufficient to make a definite statement, generally children in the primarily expressive speech defect category show little impairment in nonverbal intelligence, whereas those in the receptive–expressive group are at much greater risk for these additional deficits.

Benton (1978) reviewed three hypotheses to account for nonverbal intellectual deficits in developmental aphasia. The first view holds that the two types of deficits are fundamentally independent. The extent to which developmental aphasics are impaired in nonverbal intelligence depends upon the extension of the underlying neurological disease to areas beyond the language zone. This places developmental aphasia on a neurological continuum with mental retardation, the latter manifesting cognitive symptoms of bilateral and more symmetric hemispheric dysfunction.

The second hypothesis is similar to that discussed earlier in the section on the concept of intelligence, namely, that developmental aphasia is a handicap that limits and may distort the child's appreciation of his or her environment and his or her communication with others and, in turn, this may have a retarding influence on intellectual development. This implies that through special environmental intervention the handicapping factor may be minimized. On the whole, the evidence does not strongly support this concept. Yet there is a case report by Landau, Goldstein, and Kleffner (1960) of a child with receptive–expressive language impairments who showed a 19-point increment in nonverbal intellectual performance following intensive and protracted language training.

The third hypothesis holds that developmental aphasia represents the expression of an impairment of a more general or higher order cognitive function that is not strictly verbal and may encompass certain nonverbal abilities. Accordingly, the language deficits are not seen as the core disturbance, but rather as a reflection of a disability in a more major cognitive function. This position finds support in the case of the receptive–expressive form of developmental aphasia in which a higher-level auditory–perceptual deficit has been held to be primarily responsible for the failure in language development (Benton, 1964; Tallal & Piercy, 1978; Worster-Drought & Allen, 1929). However, agreement on the specificity of the defect to the auditory modality is controversial (Zangwill, 1978), and others insist that developmental aphasia is specifically a defect in the structure of language (Cromer, 1978).

It is well known that language is acquired on the basis of audition and that the infant must first learn that the mother's spoken language has symbolic significance before the instrumental use of expressive language develops. It is fundamental that we must first be able to perceive something before we can come to know it, let alone make use of it for our own purposes. It must be very frustrating and perhaps confusing to children with expressive developmental aphasia to be able to hear and come to understand language without being able to imitate it faithfully and effortlessly. Considerably more sympathy and understanding must be held out for the child with receptive–expressive developmental aphasia who is deprived of these early experiences demonstrating the symbolic and communicative uses of language. Furthermore, because "communicating with oneself is an important aspect of thinking and that to this extent language is also a tool of thinking" (Benton, 1965, p. 299), it is not surprising that a receptive–expressive disorder will hamper the development of nonverbal problem-solving skills. What is remarkable is how little impairment some of these children show. These observations suggest the tentative conclusion that the neural mechanisms that subserve nonverbal intelligence must be independent of those that subserve language. However, inasmuch as the two cerebral hemispheres and their various lobes work together in concert (Zangwill, 1974)—usually a harmonious one—brain lesions affecting language operations, particularly receptive ones, that have the consequence of disrupting internal communications may also have a disharmonious impact on nonverbal operations. To overcome this, one may have to learn not to attend to faulty "verbal" insights and selectively rely on nonverbal perceptions, reasoning, and innate intuitions. This is likely a far easier task for the deaf child, who has the neurological mechanisms for language, than for the aphasic child, whose apparatus for language is partly nonfunctional or functioning abnormally.

Acquired Aphasia and Cognition

Performance on Tests of Intelligence

Weisenburg and McBride (1935) provided sound evidence that some aphasics show defects in visuoperceptive and spatial abilities and thus seem to have acquired cognitive deficits that exceed the concept of aphasia as strictly a disorder of language. On the other hand, Weinstein and Teuber (1957) reported that the patients who showed the greatest deficit on the Army General Classification Test in their studies of soldiers with missile wounds were those with left temporoparietal lesions, some of whom were aphasic and some of whom were not. Perhaps, then, these extralinguistic symptoms are not so much an expression of aphasia as they are a coincidence of anatomy. If there were areas in the left hemisphere that mediated nonverbal cognitive abilities and if these were situated near the language zone (e.g., Newcombe, 1969, pp. 98–102) or overlapping with it (Basso, De Renzi, Faglioni, Scotti, & Spinnler, 1973; Goodglass, 1974), then it would seem that some aphasics are at risk for extralinguistic cognitive deficits by virtue of the size and locus of their lesions. This formulation would deny that these extralinguistic defects are psychologically (i.e., functionally) related to the aphasic symptoms. Such cognitive symptoms could be as incidental to aphasia as are visual field defects, hemiplegia, or sensory–discriminative impairments. If aphasia, or some forms of it, were psychologically related to nonverbal mental impairment, then language may be viewed as having some paramount role in intelligent thought—perhaps. If not, as suggested by the anatomical explanation, then we could conceive of the cerebrum as composed of several compartments, each of which subserves some different and relatively independent primary mental ability. To try to link aphasic symptoms to nonverbal cognitive deficit would be pure folly if the anatomical hypothesis were correct.

Many investigators have reported that aphasics are more impaired than nonaphasic left-brain–damaged patients on the nonverbal portions of the Wechsler intelligence scales (Orgass, Hartje, Kerschensteiner, & Poeck, 1972). Particularly, it appears to be those aphasics who manifest signs of constructional apraxia who are at greatest risk for nonverbal intellectual impairment (Alajouanine & Lhermitte, 1964; Basso, Capitani, Luzzatti, & Spinnler, 1981; Borod, Carper, & Goodglass, 1982). This association between constructional apraxia and nonverbal intellectual impairment seems to hold, however, for patients with both left- and right-sided lesions (Arrigoni & De Renzi, 1964; Kløve & Reitan, 1958), and therefore is not peculiar to aphasia. Given that the Block Design subtest from the WAIS is often employed to assess constructional praxis (Warrington, 1969), it is not clear how one can separate constructional praxis from nonverbal intelligence. It is also not clear that constructional praxis is as unitary a concept as some clinical investigators would have us believe. The various ways an examiner may test for constructional apraxia, such as by having the patient copy drawings or geometric designs or build forms out of sticks or models out of blocks, are not highly correlated in brain-damaged patients (Benton, 1969). Each one of these tests for apraxia may be tapping one or more specific abilities that belong to a more general spatial factor that may not be fundamentally different from the spatial factor composing the nonverbal intellectual measure. Therefore, there is no compelling reason to attach special significance to the observation that the symptom of constructional apraxia is predictive of impairment in nonverbal intelligence.

Raven's Progressive Matrices (RPM) test has been demonstrated to be a measure of general intelligence obtained through nonverbal means. The test requires subjects to examine a visual array from which a subsection appears to have been cut out. Via either an oral or a pointing response, the subject then indicates which of several multiple-choice alternatives is the correct one. Some items involve the simple completion of a pattern, such as diagonal stripes, and other items incorporate a progression or sequence of figures, such as the systematic rotation or elaboration of figures, which must be discerned and understood in order to make the correct choice. This task calls upon various cognitive abilities, including visuoperception, abstract reasoning, spatial relations, counting, and mental flexibility.

Significant impairment in the performance of the RPM test is seen in patients with both right- and left-hemisphere lesions, particularly in association with constructional apraxia (Arrigoni & De Renzi, 1964; Zangwill, 1975). In right-hemisphere disease, impairment on this task is associated with defects in block building and visual pattern matching, but not in left-hemisphere disease. Among patients with left-hemisphere damage, impairment on the RPM test is associated with the presence of aphasia (Basso et al., 1973), and among aphasics, such defects are primarily restricted to patients with language comprehension impairment (Archibald, Wepman, & Jones, 1967; Costa, Vaughan, Horwitz, & Ritter, 1969; Zangwill, 1969). However, there are patients with severe receptive language deficits who may perform rather well on this task (Kinsbourne & Warrington, 1963; Zangwill, 1964).

Constructional Apraxia

Constructional apraxia was originally viewed as a symptom of cerebral disease in the left posterior quadrant, but numerous studies have since shown that patients with lesions in the right posterior quadrant have the highest incidence and produce the most severe form of this cognitive symptom (see Benton, 1967; Warrington, 1969). When present, it is often associated with general mental impairment (Benton, 1962; Benton & Fogel, 1962). Although general mental impairment may result in the

appearance of constructional apraxia, this is not a consistent consequence, and constructional apraxia may occur as a relatively isolated
cognitive defect, that is, outside the context of general mental impairment. Obviously, there is no relationship between language impairment
and constructional apraxia among patients with right-hemisphere lesions
as there is in patients with left-hemisphere lesions. Specifically, in left-
hemisphere disease, constructional apraxia is associated with the presence of receptive language impairment, and the more severe the receptive disorder, the more likely constructional apraxia will occur (Benton,
1973). The relationship between constructional apraxia and receptive
language disorders with left-hemisphere disease may be described as a
one-way relationship. There is a high probability of receptive impairment
when constructional apraxia is present, but only about one-half of patients with moderate to severe comprehension defects manifest constructional apraxia (Benton, 1973). This probabilistic relation between the
severity of the linguistic defect and the likelihood of constructional apraxia, while consistent with the notion of a functional relation between the
two, does not contradict the anatomical hypothesis described earlier. The
size of the lesion may be another structural factor that relates to both the
locus of the lesion and the severity of the language comprehension defect
(Borod, Carper, Goodglass, & Naeser, 1984).

Visuoperceptive and Visuospatial Performances

Nonverbal intellectual measures, such as the performance scale from
the WAIS or the RPM test, as well as measures of constructional apraxia
are all in part dependent upon visuoperception. Whether on the left or on
the right, brain lesions producing constructional disabilities typically
result in associated visuoperceptive deficits (Dee, 1970). One standardized visuoperceptive task is a facial recognition test that calls for the
matching of photographs of unfamiliar persons taken from different
angles and under different lighting conditions (Benton, Hamsher, Varney, & Spreen, 1983). In patients with focal brain lesions who show no
evidence of general mental impairment, defective performance on this
test is associated with right hemisphere lesions and with lesions of the left
hemisphere, but only in the context of an aphasia syndrome in which
language comprehension is significantly impaired (Hamsher, Levin, &
Benton, 1979). Aphasic patients without significant comprehension deficits as assessed by objective tests (Benton & Hamsher, 1989) and nonaphasic left-hemisphere–damaged patients perform on a par with hospital control subjects who are without history or evidence of neurological
disease. Similarly, a disturbance in perceptual association involving

colors is associated with aphasic impairments in language comprehension and not with "pure" measures of color perception (such as color matching or color discrimination); the opposite pattern is obtained with right-hemisphere lesions (De Renzi, Faglioni, Scotti, & Spinnler, 1972; De Renzi & Spinnler, 1967). The ability to associate colors with objects may be assessed by having patients select colored pencils to shade a drawing of, say, an apple or to point to colors on a multiple-choice array. Interestingly, impairment in this type of performance in the setting of aphasia is correlated with deficits in conceptual performances rather than on tests of facial matching or identifying figures hidden in complex drawings (De Renzi et al., 1972). Among patients with Broca's aphasia, color association correlates with sorting performance on Weigl's Sorting test, whereas among patients with Wernicke's aphasia, color association is correlated with performance on Raven's Coloured Progressive Matrices (Basso, Capitani, Luzzatti, Spinnler, & Zanobio, 1985). Color association defects have been found to be more closely related with language comprehension deficits in the visual than in the auditory modality (Varney, 1982a), even in the very rare instance where such defects occur in the absence of aphasia (Varney & Digre, 1983).

One example of a visuoperceptive performance that is not apparently disrupted in the context of receptive aphasia is global stereopsis. Stereopsis is the ability to appreciate that two objects lie at different distances from the observer based on the fact that each eye receives slightly different retinal images of these objects. If one looks through a stereoscope, which presents separate images to the two eyes, and sees two forms with one eye and the same with the other except with a different horizontal separation, then when both eyes are used one form will appear closer than the other. This is stereopsis. Global stereopsis is similar, except that the two images must be extremely complex, being composed of such things as randomly placed dots. It is impossible to see any forms at all with either eye alone, but when viewed binocularly, part of the background stands out from the rest and the viewer then perceives a form in space. To achieve this visual feat, one must call upon certain higher level visuoperceptive abilities (Hamsher, 1978a). Lesions of the right hemisphere can impair one's capacity to achieve global stereopsis, whereas patients with left-hemisphere lesions perform at the level of hospital control patients (Carmon & Bechtoldt, 1967) even in the context of objectively demonstrated receptive language impairment (Hamsher, 1978b).

Aphasics have been reported to perform more poorly than other brain-damaged groups on a task involving the use of maps, both in the visual and tactile modalities (Semmes, Weinstein, Ghent, & Teuber, 1963). In aphasia this type of apparent spatial deficit is not associated with gener-

alized spatial disorientation as it is in right-hemisphere disease (McFie &
Zangwill, 1960). Yet, on what must be considered a rather pure measure
of "spatial thinking," namely, the Judgment of Line Orientation test
(Benton et al., 1983), which merely calls for matching of lines having the
same spatial orientation, aphasics perform very nearly at the level of non–
brain-damaged control patients, whereas a sizable proportion of patients
with right-hemisphere lesions show severe impairment (Benton, Hannay, & Varney, 1975; Benton, Varney, & Hamsher, 1978). These findings
are in accord with previously described observations suggesting that a-
phasics show little or no impairment on simple and direct measures of
visuoperceptive and spatial capacities, whereas on more complex tasks
that often involve an amalgam of spatial, perceptual, and conceptual
abilities, very severe cognitive disability may emerge in some forms of
aphasia, especially in the context of language comprehension deficits.
Regrettably, as yet, we cannot say why this is so. Perhaps in receptive
forms of aphasia, the victim loses the ability to integrate several specific
mental processes, although individually these processes are retained.
The difficulty levels of the more specific tests do not seem to provide a
useful explanation since, for example, normal persons describe the spatial orientation task as more difficult than the constructional praxis task,
the opposite of the order of difficulty in aphasia.

Conceptual Performances

Conceptual thinking is something of an amorphous concept that has
been applied in such various ways that it is difficult to separate it from
either general intelligence or some specific verbal ability. In fact, some
theorists, for example Bay (1962), would subsume the nonverbal cognitive deficits in aphasia under the rubric of a defect in conceptual or
categorical thinking. It is only when we restrict our usage of the term to its
basic elements that we can employ it in a definable and tractable fashion.
So we shall use CONCEPTIONAL ABILITY to mean the fundamental ability to
generate a concept of a class of things and to discriminate those things
that belong to the class from those that do not. Tasks calling for the sorting
of objects, colors, forms, and so forth, were thought by Kurt Goldstein to
be good representatives of conceptual thinking (K. Goldstein, 1948; Goldstein & Scheerer, 1941). One often-used task is the Weigl Color–Form
Sorting test. The test uses tokens of several colors in the shapes of circles,
squares, and triangles. The subject's task is to form a principle and sort
the tokens accordingly and then form a second principle and re-sort the
tokens to fit it. So the task also involves a conceptual shift.

In an early study using the Weigl sorting task, McFie and Piercy (1952) reported that defective performance was associated with left-hemisphere lesions, based on the observation that failure on this task occurred in 52% of 42 patients with unilateral left-sided lesions and in only 6% of 32 patients with right-sided lesions. Within the left-hemisphere cases, these investigators reported no relationship between conceptual failure and aphasia. A reanalysis of their data, however, suggests that this conclusion may be inaccurate if one considers frontal lobe patients separately. In the left–frontal-lobe group, there were 7 defective performances out of 12, and 6 of the patients with defective performances were nonaphasic. Statistically, there was only a trend for aphasia and defective sorting to be dissociated in left–frontal-lobe disease (the Fisher exact probability of chance association was .14). On the other hand, in patients with lesions outside the frontal lobe, aphasia was positively associated with impaired sorting (Fisher exact probability was .047); that is, only 2 of the 15 defective performances were produced by nonaphasic patients (one of whom had a frontoparietal meningioma). Excluding aphasics, there were 8 cases with left-sided lesions and defective sorting out of 17, and 6 of these patients had frontal or frontoparietal lesions. Thus, in the absence of aphasia, it is likely there exists a positive association between defective performance and frontal lobe involvement (Fisher exact probability was .041).

These analyses highlight an interesting point: Within a single hemisphere, lesions in different loci may result in the same defective cognitive performance but for different reasons. It is now well known that lesions in certain regions of the frontal lobes outside the language zone produce disturbances in sorting behaviors and the ability to perform conceptual shifts (Milner, 1963). These reanalyses also bring McFie and Piercy's (1952) classic study in line with the results of other investigators who have found, on the whole, that defects on sorting tasks are related to the presence of aphasia and, more specifically, aphasia involving receptive language impairment (De Renzi, Faglioni, Savoiardo, & Vignolo, 1966).

Language Comprehension Impairment

Nonverbal Communicative Performances

Up to now we have followed the usual custom of thinking of, or at least referring to, language comprehension impairment and its synonyms as if it were a single entity; however, this may no longer be justified. It is fitting to conclude this chapter on intelligence and aphasia with a discussion of language comprehension impairments since it is primarily in association with such defects that nonverbal intellectual performance is most variable and most vulnerable to impairment. The emphasis here shall be on processes leading to, or occurring with, receptive impairment, with special attention being given to the types of errors made by aphasics. We shall be looking for clues that might help resolve the enigma of nonverbal intellectual impairments in aphasia. If the anatomical hypothesis is correct, then this discussion is largely for naught.

In attempting to explain the basis for the occurrence of nonverbal intellectual deficits in receptive aphasia, both the anatomical hypothesis and the psychological hypothesis suffer from certain inconsistencies. It is often stated that if a symptom of cognitive impairment occurs with equal frequency with lesions of either hemisphere, then it bears no essential relationship with language, which in most individuals resides in the domain of the left hemisphere. That the symptom may have a close association with aphasia in the context of left-sided lesions could be attributed to a coincidence of anatomy. This dictum may not be warranted, however, unless the investigator can demonstrate that the cognitive symptom has the same correlates regardless of whether the lesion is on the right or the left. Of course, because of anatomical coincidence, there may be different additional correlates depending on the side of the lesions, but, at the same time, a core set of related cognitive disabilities should remain invariable. This requirement is derived from the concepts of the structure of intelligence as described earlier, and it is on this point that the anatomical hypothesis is in conflict with the data. The psychological hypothesis stresses the position that behaviors, especially complex cognitive behaviors, have multiple determinants and therefore are subject to distortions for various reasons and from several sources. Exactly what psychological (cognitive, mental) process is the cause of the nonverbal symptoms is the subject of much debate. It may lie in the ability to manipulate symbols or categories. If this were the root cause of both the linguistic and the nonverbal symptoms, however, then it is difficult to explain the substantial proportion of patients with apparently severe receptive deficits and no evidence of a compromise of nonverbal abilities. To postulate the existence of some conceptual center that lies near, or partially overlaps with, the language zone would provide a compromise to the two countervailing hypotheses, but it would also require the assumption of the existence of a set of cognitive abilities that have not previously been shown to have unique properties. For these reasons, the issue of the status of intelligence in aphasia remains unresolved.

Language, as a more or less codified system of symbols used to express or communicate ideas and information, has several forms for expression (e.g., oral speech, written language, gesture). For each mode of expression, a corresponding mode of reception must exist for communication to take place. LANGUAGE is usually used to refer to the use of verbal symbols (words), but we may also think of a nonverbal form of language that allows an individual to communicate with his or her environment.

Spinnler and Vignolo (1966) experimentally demonstrated that defects in the recognition of nonverbal meaningful sounds, such as thunder, the ringing of a door bell, and animal sounds, are associated with aphasia and specifically with impairment in aural comprehension of spoken language. By using a multiple-choice assessment technique, they were also able to show that the types of errors made by aphasics were not random; instead they were predominantly errors involving semantic slippage. For example, if an error were to be made by an aphasic patient in response to a stimulus such as a canary singing, the most likely response choice would be one from the same semantic class, such as a cock crowing, rather than an acoustically similar response, such as a man whistling, or an irrelevant response, such as a train in motion. This impairment is not due to an acquired hearing loss and does not represent a defect in sound discrimination, since receptive aphasics who are impaired on this measure show no defect in the discrimination of meaningless sounds, whereas patients with right-hemisphere lesions may show the opposite pattern (Faglioni, Spinnler, & Vignolo, 1969). Not all aphasics with receptive deficits show a defect in the recognition of meaningful environmental sounds. Those who do, however, have a high frequency of impairment on the Weigl sorting task and the RPM test. These findings have been interpreted as demonstrating the presence of a "cognitive–associative" deficit in comprehension-impaired aphasics (Vignolo, 1969).

Subsequently, Varney (1980) replicated these findings and added three new observations. First, sound recognition impairment is specifically associated with aural comprehension as opposed to the comprehension of written language in the visual modality (reading). Second, sound recognition deficits, when present, appear to represent a primary determinant of aural comprehension impairment rather than an expression of it, because defects in aural comprehension of at least equal severity always accompany sound recognition deficits, whereas there are patients with severe impairments in the understanding of oral speech who are not impaired in recognizing the meaning of environmental sounds. Third, Varney and Benton (1979) demonstrated that a defect in the ability to discriminate phonemes represents another, relatively independent, source of aural comprehension deficits. Thus, the aural comprehension of speech may be impaired for either semantic–

associative or for perceptual–linguistic reasons. The perceptual comprehension defects are most commonly seen in the acute phase of aphasia and tend to recover (Varney, 1984a). On the other hand, defects in the semantic–associative aspects of aural comprehension suggest a much poorer prognosis (Varney, 1984b).

Deficits in the ability to comprehend the meaning of pantomimes represents another form of nonverbal comprehension impairment in aphasia. Goodglass and Kaplan (1963) observed such impairments in the context of aphasia. Because there was not a close association between the severity of aphasia and the severity of the disturbances in gestures and pantomime, they were led to the conclusion that such deficits must in some sense be independent of aphasia. Subsequently, Varney (1978) demonstrated that, although there was no special correlation between pantomime recognition defects and the severity of the disorder in aural comprehension or verbal expression (naming), failure in pantomime recognition was closely allied with disturbances in reading comprehension (i.e., reading for meaning rather than reading aloud). Impairment in the comprehension of pantomimes always occurred in association with defects in reading comprehension of at least equal severity; however, one could be alexic, even severely so, without showing any impairment in the recognition of pantomimes. Thus, in the visual modality, there is likely to be more than one determinant for an acquired impairment in the comprehension of written language. Varney and Benton (1982) also demonstrated that the major error type committed by aphasics was to select from among four response alternatives a response that was semantically associated with the pantomimed stimulus rather than selecting an irrelevant item or one that was visually similar but semantically unrelated to the stimulus. Similar results were found by Duffy and Watkins (1984). These findings suggest a parallel organization of verbal and nonverbal language processing in the visual and auditory modalities.

Nonverbal Intelligence and the Receptive Aphasias

Do these defects in sound and pantomime recognition in association with aphasia tell us anything about the fundamental structure of language, or are they merely instances of a host of findings of nonverbal deficits in comprehension-impaired aphasics? It has been argued that the abilities to comprehend gestural communication and to appreciate the significance of environmental sounds represent the selective advantages that fostered the evolutionary development and refinement of the neural structures in humans that serve these functions. They are considered selective advantages because they may be directly related to one's ability to survive in a primitive and hostile environment. Thus, the human brain may have become preadapted for language through the evolutionary development of these pristine nonverbal communicative abilities (Varney & Vilensky, 1980). Arguments of this sort are necessarily discursive, for when empirical proof cannot be obtained, one must rely on analytic reasoning. Because oral speech arises from audition, it would be natural to expect that mechanisms for understanding sounds as meaningful stimuli must precede the development of speech. Also, it would be difficult to maintain, in view of the very recent and rapid development of reading abilities in human evolution, that the capability for understanding written language in the visual modality was acquired on the basis of a selective advantage that augmented one's probability of surviving.

The final task before us is to relate these recent developments in identifying modality-related subtypes of comprehension impairments to the problem of explaining nonverbal intellectual deficits in aphasia. In our present and limited state of knowledge, it is more reasonable to look for clues rather than solutions to the puzzle. We owe to J. Hughlings Jackson the concept of two classes of behavioral symptoms of brain disease: the negative and the positive. Negative symptoms represent the loss of an ability to produce behaviors that were previously in one's behavioral repertoire. An example would be an inability to recall the name of an object. Positive symptoms represent the emergence of new behaviors that were not previously in the behavioral repertoire. An example of a positive symptom would be misnaming, such as the utterance of semantic or phonemic paraphasias in the attempt to name an object (e.g., calling a knife a fork). Whether the errors described here as semantic (conceptual, associative, symbolic) slippage are negative or positive symptoms may be more an academic argument than a real distinction. If characterized as a loss in the ability to discriminate among members of the same semantic class, they could be considered negative symptoms; if characterized as an active error tendency, perhaps as the result of a derailment in thinking, they could be considered positive symptoms. Since aphasic patients who show these errors of semantic slippage may make their response choices with great conviction and an air of success, it may be convenient to think of these errors as positive symptoms resulting from an active process that causes one to err in a particular direction.

If we were to accept the proposition that some comprehension-impaired aphasics suffer from some form of semantic slippage, we might ask if this error tendency could provide an explanation for the occurrence of nonverbal intellectual deficits in aphasia. Applying this model to the problem at hand, we could conceptualize nonverbal intellectual deficits as the consequence of a newly acquired active error tendency that disrupts performance on complex tasks rather than as the result of a loss in the cognitive abilities the tasks were intended to measure. One convenience of this model is that it does not require the postulation of the bilateral representation of visuoperceptive, spatial, and constructional abilities or other components of nonverbal intelligence. Unfortunately, such a simple model appears inadequate; that is, when Varney (1982b) tested for a relationship between pantomime recognition defects and performance on the WAIS Block Design subtest, none was found. Thus, the hypothesis that a "general asymbolia" could account for both types of nonverbal defects does not appear tenable. At the same time, there is no evidence that the semantic–associative disturbances with regard to either sound recognition defects or pantomime recognition defects in aphasia are dependent upon a specific lesion locus (Varney & Damasio, 1986, 1987). Both types of defects are associated with lesions in a number of cortical and subcortical loci (all of which are associated with aphasia).

The demonstration that there are at least two types of acquired deficits that may result in language comprehension impairment may help to explain the exceptional cases of patients who do not understand oral speech but who show none of the deficiencies in nonverbal intellectual performance that are associated with receptive language impairment. Another dichotomy in subtyping of language comprehension impairment is the distinction between single-word or lexical defects and syntactic processing (Vermeulen, 1982); however, it is not clear that this distinction differs from the perceptual and semantic associative distinctions made above. This is an area that needs further exploration.

Probably, we will need new and more complex hypotheses to explain the high degree of variability in the pattern of nonverbal deficits exhibited by groups of aphasic patients who previously were thought to share the same, unitary symptom of comprehension impairment (Benton, 1982, 1985). The development of brain imaging techniques should help to further refine these hypotheses (H. Damasio & Damasio, 1989). Substantial evidence now shows that both size and locus of lesion affects language comprehension and recovery in aphasia (Kertesz, Harlock, & Coates, 1979; Knopman, Selnes, Niccum, & Rubens, 1984; Lomas & Kertesz, 1978; Selnes, Knopman, Niccum, Rubens, & Larson, 1983; Selnes, Niccum, Knopman, & Rubens, 1984; Tramo, Baynes, & Volpe, 1988; Yarnell, Monroe, & Sobel, 1976). Other, more physiological studies may also be necessary. Another imperative may be to further specify the

syndromes of aphasia to include nonverbal symptomatology that here-
tofore has been omitted in the assessment and classification of aphasic
disorders (Benton, 1982, 1985).

Summary

Intelligence, conceived abstractly, represents one's innate ability to
generate ideas and solve problems of varying complexity and to communicate effectively with others and with one's environment. In an effort to
approximate this abstract concept, psychologists have developed batteries of cognitive tests from which an IQ score can be obtained. Evidence gathered from various sources shows that intelligence, expressed
concretely as an IQ score, meets psychometric criteria and predicts demographic characteristics of individuals that are incorporated in the abstract notion of intelligence.

Neurological disease affecting the cerebrum often results in corresponding impairments in intellectual functioning. In the usual case,
disease of the right hemisphere may be reflected in acquired impairments of nonverbal intelligence, whereas disease of the left hemisphere
may result in verbal intellectual deficits. In a significant proportion of
aphasic patients having receptive language defects, however, nonverbal
intellectual performance appears to be compromised.

The hypotheses offered to account for these incongruous findings fall
into two general classes. One general hypothesis is that some portion of
the cerebral cortex in the left hemisphere, which lies near or overlaps
with the language zone, subserves the same general mental functions as
mediated by the right hemisphere. If lesions resulting in aphasia happen
to invade this region as well, then nonverbal intellectual deficits will
result. This hypothesis denies the existence of a functional relation between nonverbal intelligence and aphasia. The other general hypothesis
suggests the opposite and links disturbances in language with disturbances in thought processes. So far, the evidence brought to bear on this
issue is mixed so, if sampled selectively, allows one to support or refute
either hypothesis.

It is argued that linguistic aspects of language were derived from
pristine nonverbal communicative abilities. Recent investigations of the
capacity of aphasics to comprehend environmental sounds and pantomimes has disclosed the presence of error tendencies, described here as
semantic slippage, in both the auditory and visual modalities. In aphasia,
these error tendencies may disrupt response selections in the performance of nonverbal intellectual tasks, whereas in right-hemisphere dis-

ease, acquired deficits in stimulus processing may be the root causes of nonverbal intellectual impairment. Neural mechanisms to account for these error tendencies have remained elusive.

References

Alajouanine, T., & Lhermitte, F. (1964). Non-verbal communication in aphasia. In A. de Rueck & M. O'Connor (Eds.), *Disorders of language.* Boston, MA: Little, Brown.

Archibald, Y. M., Wepman, J. M., & Jones, L. V. (1967). Nonverbal cognitive performance in aphasic and nonaphasic brain-damaged patients. *Cortex, 3,* 275–294.

Arrigoni, G., & De Renzi, E. (1964). Constructional apraxia and hemispheric locus of lesion. *Cortex, 1,* 170–197.

Basso, A., Capitani, E., Luzzatti, C., & Spinnler, H. (1981). Intelligence and left hemisphere disease: The role of aphasia, apraxia and size of lesion. *Brain, 104,* 721–734.

Basso, A., Capitani, E., Luzzatti, C., Spinnler, H., & Zanobio, M. E. (1985). Different basic components in the performance of Broca's and Wernicke's aphasics on the Colour-Figure Matching Test. *Neuropsychologia, 23,* 51–59.

Basso, A., De Renzi, E., Faglioni, P., Scotti, G., & Spinnler, H. (1973). Neuropsychological evidence for the existence of cerebral areas critical to the performance of intelligence tests. *Brain, 96,* 715–728.

Bay, E. (1962). Aphasia and non-verbal disorders of language. *Brain, 85,* 411–426.

Benton, A. L. (1962). The visual retention test as a constructional praxis task. *Confinia Neurologica, 22,* 141–155.

Benton, A. L. (1964). Developmental aphasia and brain damage. *Cortex, 1,* 40–52.

Benton, A. L. (1965). Language disorders in children. *Canadian Psychologist, 7a,* 298–312.

Benton, A. L. (1967). Constructional apraxia and the minor hemisphere. *Confinia Neurologica, 29,* 1–16.

Benton, A. L. (1969). Constructional apraxia: Some unanswered questions. In A. L. Benton (Ed.), *Contributions to clinical neuropsychology.* Chicago, IL: Aldine.

Benton, A. L. (1973). Visuoconstructive disability in patients with cerebral disease: Its relationship to side of lesion and aphasic disorder. *Documenta Ophthalmologica, 34,* 67–76.

Benton, A. L. (1977a). Historical notes on hemispheric dominance. *Archives of Neurology (Chicago), 34,* 127–129.

Benton, A. L. (1977b). Psychologic testing. In A. B. Baker & L. H. Baker (Eds.), *Clinical neurology* (Vol. 1). Hagerstown, MD: Harper.

Benton, A. L. (1978). The cognitive functioning of children with developmental dysphasia. In M. A. Wyke (Ed.), *Developmental dysphasia.* London: Academic Press.

Benton, A. L. (1980). Psychological testing for brain damage. In H. I. Kaplan, A. M. Freedman, & B. J. Sadock (Eds.), *Comprehensive textbook of psychiatry* (3rd ed., Vol. 1). Baltimore, MD: Williams & Wilkins.

Benton, A. L. (1982). Significance of nonverbal cognitive abilities in aphasic patients. *Japanese Journal of Stroke, 4,* 153–161.

Benton, A. L. (1985). Symbolic thinking and brain disease. *Recherches Sémiotiques/Semiotic Inquiry, 5,* 225–239.

Benton, A. L., & Fogel, M. L. (1962). Three-dimensional constructional praxis. *Archives of Neurology (Chicago), 7,* 347–354.

Benton, A. L., & Hamsher, K. (1989). *Multilingual Aphasia Examination* (2nd ed.). Iowa City, IA: AJA Associates.

Benton, A. L., Hamsher, K., Varney, N. R., & Spreen, O. (1983). *Contributions to neuropsychological assessment*. New York: Oxford University Press.

Benton, A. L., Hannay, H. J., & Varney, N. R. (1975). Visual perception of line direction in patients with unilateral brain disease. *Neurology, 25*, 907–910.

Benton, A. L., & Van Allen, M. W. (1968). Impairment in facial recognition in patients with cerebral disease. *Cortex, 4*, 344–358.

Benton, A. L., Varney, N. R., & Hamsher, K. (1978). Visuospatial judgment: A clinical test. *Archives of Neurology (Chicago), 35*, 364–367.

Blessed, G., Tomlinson, B. E., & Roth, M. (1968). The association between quantitative measures of dementia and of senile change in the cerebral grey matter of elderly subjects. *British Journal of Psychiatry, 114*, 797–811.

Borod, J. C., Carper, M., & Goodglass, H. (1982). WAIS performance IQ in aphasia as a function of auditory comprehension and constructional apraxia. *Cortex, 18*, 199–210.

Borod, J. C., Carper, M., Goodglass, H., & Naeser, M. (1984). Aphasic performance on a battery of constructional, visuo-spatial, and quantitative tasks: Factorial structure and CT scan localization. *Journal of Clinical Neuropsychology, 6*, 189–204.

Burt, C. (1955). The evidence for the concept of intelligence. *British Journal of Educational Psychology, 25*, 158–177.

Carmon, A., & Bechtoldt, H. (1967). Dominance of the right cerebral hemisphere for stereopsis, *Neuropsychologia, 7*, 29–39.

Chapman, L. F., & Wolf, H. G. (1959). The cerebral hemispheres and the highest integrative functions of man. *Archives of Neurology (Chicago), 1*, 357–424.

Costa, L. D., Vaughan, H. G., Jr., Horwitz, M., & Ritter, W. (1969). Patterns of behavioral deficit associated with visual spatial neglect. *Cortex, 5*, 242–263.

Cromer, R. F. (1978). The basis of childhood dysphasia: A linguistic approach. In M. A. Wyke (Ed.), *Developmental dysphasia*. London: Academic Press.

Damasio, A. R., Castro-Caldas, A., Grosso, J. T., & Ferro, J. M. (1976). Brain specialization for language does not depend on literacy. *Archives of Neurology (Chicago), 33*, 300–301.

Damasio, A. R., Hamsher, K., Castro-Caldas, A., Ferro, J., & Grosso, J. T. (1976). Brain specialization for language: Not dependent on literacy. *Archives of Neurology (Chicago), 33*, 662.

Damasio, A. R., & Maurer, R. G. (1978). A neurological model for childhood autism. *Archives of Neurology (Chicago), 35*, 777–786.

Damasio, H., & Damasio, A. R. (1989). *Lesion analysis in neuropsychology*. New York: Oxford University Press.

Damasio, H., Damasio, A. R., Castro-Caldas, A., & Hamsher, K. (1979). Reversal of ear advantage for phonetically similar words in illiterates. *Journal of Clinical Neuropsychology, 1*, 331–338.

Dee, H. L. (1970). Visuoconstructive and visuoperceptive deficits in patients with unilateral cerebral lesions. *Neuropsychologia, 8*, 305–314.

De Renzi, E., Faglioni, P., Savoiardo, M., & Vignolo, L. A. (1966). The influence of aphasia and of hemispheric side of the cerebral lesion on abstract thinking. *Cortex, 2*, 399–420.

De Renzi, E., Faglioni, P., Scotti, G., & Spinnler, H. (1972). Impairment in associating colour to form, concomitant with aphasia. *Brain, 95*, 293–304.

De Renzi, E., & Spinnler, H. (1967). Impaired performance on color tasks in patients with hemispheric damage. *Cortex, 3*, 194–217.

Duara, R., Grady, C., Haxby, J., Sundaram, M., Cutler, N. R., Heston, L., Moore, A., Schlageter, N., Larson, S., & Rapoport, S. I. (1986). Positron emission tomography in Alzheimer's disease. *Neurology, 36*, 879–887.

Duffy, J. R., & Watkins, L. B. (1984). The effect of response choice relatedness on pantomime and verbal recognition ability in aphasic patients. *Brain and Language, 21,* 291–306.

Faglioni, P., Spinnler, H., & Vignolo, L. A. (1969). Contrasting behavior of right and left hemisphere-damaged patients on a discriminative and a semantic task of auditory recognition. *Cortex, 5,* 366–389.

Fogel, M. L. (1964). The intelligence quotient as an index of brain damage. *American Journal of Orthopsychiatry, 34,* 555–562.

Foster, N. L., Chase, T. N., Fedio, P., Patronas, N. J., Brooks, R. A., & Di Chiro, G. (1983). Alzheimer's disease: Focal cortical changes shown by positron emission tomography. *Neurology, 33,* 961–965.

Furth, H. G. (1964). Research with the deaf: Implications for language and cognition. *Psychological Bulletin, 62,* 145–164.

Furth, H. G., & Youniss, J. (1975). Congenital deafness and the development of thinking. In E. H. Lenneberg & E. Lenneberg (Eds.), *Foundations of language development: A multidisciplinary approach* (Vol. 2). New York: Academic Press.

Galton, F. (1887). *Hereditary genius. An inquiry into its laws and consequences* (New and rev. ed., with an American preface). New York: Appleton.

Goldin-Meadow, S., & Feldman, H. (1977). The development of language-like communication without a language model. *Science, 197,* 401–403.

Goldstein, G. (1974). The use of clinical neuropsychological methods in lateralisation of brain lesions. In S. J. Dimond & J. G. Beaumont (Eds.), *Hemisphere function in the human brain.* New York: Halsted Press.

Goldstein, K. (1948). *Language and language disturbances.* New York: Grune & Stratton.

Goldstein, K., & Scheerer, M. (1941). Abstract and concrete behavior: An experimental study with special tests. *Psychological Monographs, 53,* 1–151 (Whole No. 239).

Goodglass, H. (1974). Nonverbal performance. In Y. Lebrun & R. Hoops (Eds.), *Neurolinguistics: Vol. 2. Intelligence and aphasia.* Amsterdam: Swets & Zeitlinger B. V.

Goodglass, H. (1980). Disorders of naming following brain injury. *American Scientist, 68,* 647–655.

Goodglass, H., & Kaplan, E. (1963). Disturbance of gesture and pantomime in aphasia. *Brain, 86,* 703–720.

Hamsher, K. (1978a). Stereopsis and the perception of anomalous contours. *Neuropsychologia, 16,* 453–459.

Hamsher, K. (1978b). Stereopsis and unilateral brain disease. *Investigative Ophthalmology and Visual Science, 17,* 336–343.

Hamsher, K., Levin, H. S., & Benton, A. L. (1979). Facial recognition in patients with focal brain lesions. *Archives of Neurology (Chicago), 36,* 837–839.

Kertesz, A., Harlock, W., & Coates, R. (1979). Computer tomographic localization, lesion size, and prognosis in aphasia and nonverbal impairment. *Brain and Language, 8,* 34–50.

Kinsbourne, M., & Warrington, E. K. (1963). Jargon aphasia. *Neuropsychologia, 1,* 27–37.

Kløve, H. (1974). Validation studies in adult clinical neuropsychology. In R. M. Reitan & L. A. Davison (Eds.), *Clinical neuropsychology: Current status and applications.* Washington, DC: V. H. Winston & Sons.

Kløve, H., & Reitan, R. M. (1958). Effect of dysphasia and spatial distortion on Wechsler-Bellevue results. *Archives of Neurology and Psychiatry, 80,* 708–713.

Knopman, D. S., Selnes, O. A., Niccum, N., & Rubens, A. B. (1984). Recovery of naming in aphasia: relationship to fluency, comprehension and CT findings. *Neurology, 34,* 1461–1470.

Kodman, F., Jr. (1963). Sensory processes and mental deficiency. In N. R. Ellis (Ed.), *Handbook of mental deficiency.* New York: McGraw-Hill.

Landau, W. M., Goldstein, R., & Kleffner, F. R. (1960). Congenital aphasia: A clinico-pathologic study. *Neurology, 10,* 915–921.

Lashley, K. S. (1929). *Brain mechanisms and intelligence. A quantitative study of injuries to the brain.* Chicago, IL: University of Chicago Press.

Lezak, M. D. (1983). *Neuropsychological assessment* (2nd ed.). New York: Oxford University Press.

Loeb, C., Gandolfo, C., & Bino, G. (1988). Intellectual impairment and cerebral lesions in multiple cerebral infarcts: A clinical-computed tomography study. *Stroke, 19,* 560–565.

Lomas, J., & Kertesz, A. (1978). Patterns of spontaneous recovery in aphasic groups: A study of adult stroke patients. *Brain and Language, 5,* 388–401.

Matarazzo, J. D. (1972). *Wechsler's measurement and appraisal of adult intelligence* (5th ed.). Baltimore, MD: Williams & Wilkins.

McCall, R. B. (1977). Childhood IQ's as predictors of adult educational and occupational status. *Science, 197,* 482–843.

McFie, J. (1960). Psychological testing in clinical neurology. *Journal of Nervous and Mental Disease, 131,* 383–393.

McFie, J. (1969). The diagnostic significance of disorders of higher nervous activity: Syndromes related to frontal, temporal, parietal and occipital lesions. In P. J. Vinken & G. W. Bruyn (Eds.), *Handbook of clinical neurology: Vol. 4. Disorders of speech, perception, and symbolic behaviour.* Amsterdam: North-Holland.

McFie, J. (1976). *Assessment of organic intellectual impairment.* New York: Academic Press.

McFie, J., & Piercy, M. F. (1952). The relation of laterality of lesion to performance on Weigl's sorting test. *Journal of Mental Science, 98,* 299–305.

McFie, J., & Thompson, J. A. (1972). Picture arrangement: A measure of frontal lobe function? *British Journal of Psychiatry, 121,* 547–552.

McFie, J., & Zangwill, O. L. (1960). Visual-cognitive disabilities associated with lesions of the left hemisphere. *Brain, 83,* 243–260.

Messerli, P., & Tissot, R. (1974). Operational capacity and aphasia. In Y. Lebrun & R. Hoops (Eds.), *Neurolinguistics: Vol. 2. Intelligence and aphasia.* Amsterdam. Swets & Zeitlinger B. V.

Milner, B. (1963). Effects of different brain lesions on card sorting. *Archives of Neurology (Chicago), 9,* 90–100.

Newcombe, F. (1969). *Missile wounds of the brain: A study of psychological deficits.* London: Oxford University Press.

Newcombe, F. (1974). Selective deficits after focal cerebral injury. In S. J. Dimond & J. G. Beaumont (Eds.), *Hemisphere function in the human brain.* New York: Halsted Press.

Orgass, B., Hartje, W., Kerschensteiner, M., & Poeck, K. (1972). Aphasie und nichtsprachliche intelligenz. *Nervenarzt, 43,* 623–627.

Piaget, J. (1936). *La naissance de l'intelligence chez l'enfant.* Neuchatel: Delachaux & Niestle. (English translation by M. Cook. New York: International Universities Press, 1952.)

Pick, A. (1931). Aphasie. In A. Bethe, G. von Bergman, G. Emblem, & A. Ellinger (Eds.), *Handbuch der normalen und pathologiochen physiologie* (Vol. 15, Pt. 2). Berlin: Springer-Verlag. (English translation by J. Brown. 1973. Springfield, IL: Thomas, 1973.)

Piercy, M. (1964). The effect of cerebral lesions on intellectual function: A review of current research trends. *British Journal of Psychiatry, 110,* 310–352.

Piercy, M. (1969). Neurological aspects of intelligence. In P. J. Vinken & G. W. Bruyn (Eds.), *Handbook of clinical neurology: Vol. 3. Disorders of higher nervous activity.* Amsterdam: North-Holland.

Pitner, R., & Lev, J. (1939). The intelligence of the hard of hearing school child. *Journal of Genetic Psychology, 55,* 31–48.

Selnes, O. A., Knopman, D. S., Niccum, N., Rubens, A. B., & Larson, D. (1983). Computed tomographic scan correlates of auditory comprehension deficits in aphasia: A prospective study. *Annals of Neurology, 13,* 558–566.

Selnes, O. A., Niccum, N., Knopman, D. S., & Rubens, A. B. (1984). Recovery of single word comprehension: CT-scan correlates. *Brain and Language, 21,* 72–84.

Semmes, J., Weinstein, S., Ghent, L., & Teuber, H.-L. (1963). Correlates of impaired orientation in personal and extra-personal space. *Brain, 86,* 747–772.

Smith, A. (1975). Neuropsychological testing in neurological disorders. *Advances in Neurology, 7,* 49–110.

Spearman, C. (1927). *The abilities of man.* New York: Macmillan.

Spinnler, H., & Vignolo, L. A. (1966). Impaired recognition of meaningful sounds in aphasia. *Cortex, 2,* 337–348.

Tallal, P., & Piercy, M. (1978). Defects of auditory perception in children with developmental dysphasia. In M. A. Wyke (Ed.), *Developmental dysphasia.* London: Academic Press.

Thurstone, L. L. (1938). Primary mental abilities. *Psychometric Monographs,* No. 1.

Tramo, M. J., Baynes, K., & Volpe, B. T. (1988). Impaired syntactic comprehension and production in Broca's aphasia: CT lesion localization and recovery patterns. *Neurology, 38,* 95–98.

Vandenberg, S. G. (1971). What do we know today about the inheritance of intelligence and how do we know it? In R. Cancro (Ed.), *Intelligence: Genetic and environmental influences.* New York: Grune & Stratton.

Varney, N. R. (1978). Linguistic correlates of pantomime recognition in aphasic patients. *Journal of Neurology, Neurosurgery and Psychiatry, 41,* 564–568.

Varney, N. R. (1980). Sound recognition in relation to aural comprehension and reading comprehension in aphasic patients. *Journal of Neurology, Neurosurgery and Psychiatry, 43,* 71–75.

Varney, N. R. (1982a). Colour association and "colour amnesia" in aphasia. *Journal of Neurology, Neurosurgery and Psychiatry, 45,* 248–252.

Varney, N. R. (1982b). Pantomime recognition defect in aphasia: Implications for the concept of asymbolia. *Brain and Language, 15,* 32–39.

Varney, N. R. (1984a). Phonemic imperception in aphasia. *Brain and Language, 21,* 85–94.

Varney, N. R. (1984b). The prognostic significance of sound recognition in receptive aphasia. *Archives of Neurology (Chicago), 41,* 181–182.

Varney, N. R., & Benton, A. L. (1979). Phonemic discrimination and auditory comprehension in aphasic patients. *Journal of Clinical Neuropsychology, 1,* 65–74.

Varney, N. R., & Benton, A. L. (1982). Qualitative aspects of pantomime recognition defect in aphasia. *Brain and Cognition, 1,* 132–139.

Varney, N. R., & Damasio, H. (1986). CT scan correlates of sound recognition defect in aphasia. *Cortex, 22,* 483–486.

Varney, N. R., & Damasio, H. (1987). Locus of lesion in impaired pantomime recognition. *Cortex, 23,* 699–703.

Varney, N. R., & Digre, K. (1983). Color "amnesia" without aphasia. *Cortex, 19,* 545–550.

Varney, N. R., & Vilensky, J. A. (1980). Neuropsychological implications for preadaptation and language evolution. *Journal of Human Evolution, 9,* 223–226.

Vermeulen, J. (1982). Auditory language comprehension in aphasia: A factor-analytic study. *Cortex, 18,* 287–300.

Vignolo, L. A. (1969). Auditory agnosia: A review and report of recent evidence. In A. L. Benton (Ed.), *Contributions to clinical neuropsychology.* Chicago, IL: Aldine.

Walsh, K. W. (1978). *Neuropsychology: A clinical approach.* New York: Churchill-Livingstone.

Warrington, E. K. (1969). Constructional apraxia. In P. J. Vinken & G. W. Bruyn (Eds.),

Handbook of clinical neurology: Vol. 4. Disorders of speech, perception, and symbolic behaviour. Amsterdam: North-Holland.

Wechsler, D. (1958). *The measurement and appraisal of adult intelligence* (4th ed.). Baltimore, MD: Williams & Wilkins.

Wechsler, D. (1971). Intelligence: Definition, theory, and the IQ. In R. Cancro (Ed.), *Intelligence: Genetic and environmental influences.* New York: Grune & Stratton.

Weinstein, S., & Teuber, H.-L. (1957). Effects of penetrating brain injury on intelligence test scores. *Science, 125,* 1036–1037.

Weisenburg, T. H., & McBride, K. E. (1935). *Aphasia: A clinical and psychological study.* New York: Commonwealth Fund.

Wilson, R. S., Rosenbaum, G., & Brown, G. (1979). The problem of premorbid intelligence in neuropsychological assessment. *Journal of Clinical Neuropsychology, 1,* 49–53.

Worster-Drought, C., & Allen, I. M. (1929). Congenital auditory imperception (congenital word-deafness): With report of a case. *Journal of Neurology and Psychopathology, 9,* 193–208.

Yarnell, P., Monroe, P., & Sobel, L. (1976). Aphasia outcome in stroke: A clinical neuroradiological correlation. *Stroke, 7,* 516–522.

Zangwill, O. L. (1964). Intelligence in aphasia. In A. V. S. de Rueck & M. O'Connor (Eds.), *Disorders of language.* Boston, MA: Little, Brown.

Zangwill, O. L. (1969). Intellectual status in aphasia. In P. J. Vinken & G. W. Bryun (Eds.), *Handbook of clinical neurology: Vol. 4. Disorders of speech, perception, and symbolic behavior.* Amsterdam: North-Holland.

Zangwill, O. L. (1974). Consciousness and the cerebral hemispheres. In S. J. Dimond & J. G. Beaumont (Eds.), *Hemisphere function in the human brain.* New York: Halsted Press.

Zangwill, O. L. (1975). The relation of nonverbal cognitive functions to aphasia. In E. H. Lenneberg & E. Lenneberg (Eds.), *Foundations of language development: A multidisciplinary approach* (Vol. 2). New York: Academic Press.

Zangwill, O. L. (1978). The concept of developmental dysphasia. In M. A. Wyke (Ed.), *Developmental dysphasia.* London: Academic Press.

11

Artistry and Aphasia

HOWARD GARDNER, ELLEN WINNER, and ALEXANDRA REHAK

Language is our central mode of communication. Accordingly, psychologists interested in the problem of human communication have concentrated on the study of language to the virtual exclusion of other forms of communication. Thus, although the symbol systems of the arts are almost as universal and as well developed among humans as is language, much less is known about the representation of artistic skills in the brain. Moreover, little is known about the relationship of language and artistic modes of communication. For instance, although it is well known that damage to the left hemisphere entails a loss of linguistic capacities, less information is available on whether a breakdown in language entails—or occurs independently of—a breakdown in one or more of the symbol systems of the arts. An understanding of the fate of artistic skills after damage to the brain that has either spared or impaired language should clarify the relationship that obtains between the symbol systems of language and those of the arts.

Any investigation of artistry and aphasia must be built upon a way of thinking about the arts. Work in our laboratory at the Boston University Aphasia Research Center has been guided by a point of view first put forward by the philosopher Nelson Goodman (1968, 1972, 1979) and developed over the past two decades at Harvard Project Zero (Gardner, 1982; Gardner & Perkins, 1989; Winner, 1982). According to this point of view, involvement in the arts entails the ability to "encode" and to "read" symbols, whether they be verbal, pictorial, musical, gestural, or some combination thereof. Rather than simply an arena of entertainment or of emotional gratification, the arts are thus seen as fundamentally cognitive: Mental processes are needed to make sense of artistic symbols, just as they are required to interpret symbols functioning in a scientific, journalistic, or conversational vein. In brief, works of art must be "read," and literacy in the arts proves no less demanding than literacy in the scientific domain.

Such a cognitive approach to the arts (Gardner, 1985) serves here as a point of departure for a psychology (and a neuropsychology) of art, as well as an investigation into the relationship between linguistic and artistic symbols and symbol systems. In what follows, we review certain lines of evidence about the nature of artistry. We consider both music and visual arts, and briefly discuss literary arts; we have chosen to focus on the first two domains because they have been studied more extensively in neuropsychological settings than has literature. We also report a case of visual artistry in a severely aphasic patient who has been treated recently at the Aphasia Research Center.

Three general questions are posed with respect to each art form. What is the relationship between language and the artistic skill in question? What is the predominant mode of information processing in the art form under consideration? What difference exists between those artistic skills that are highly developed and displayed by only a few individuals and those artistic abilities possessed by most normal human beings in our culture?

Music

Preliminary Considerations

Music is a logical candidate for initial consideration in any neuropsychology of the arts. Some form of music is evident in all human cultures, and musical performances and rites date back thousands of years. Music is not only universal; it is also unique among the arts because, unlike literature and nonabstract visual art, it lacks representational content. Representational forms of art have an immediately obvious relation to the "real" world and thereby possess a less "free-standing existence" than music. Indeed, the survival of music in the face of the "triumph" of language poses a riddle for evolutionary theorists: Why has such an apparently "nonadaptive" symbol system continued to figure so importantly in human culture?

Other reasons motivating a neuropsychology of music merit brief mention. Music offers a particularly rich set of roles. In addition to audience member and critic, individuals can participate through singing, playing works produced by others, or creating works of their own, for voice, for instrument, or even for electronic realization by a computer. There are numerous types of music, ranging from folk music to high art, a myriad of styles, and a complex notation that is understood, at least in part, by many literate individuals. This variegated symbolic domain raises a multitude of questions about how competence can be organized in the human brain.

Music proves particularly instructive in relation to aphasia. Despite the fact that it is a nonlinguistic symbol system, music offers striking parallels to language in terms of the symbol manipulation skills necessary to compose and read music. Furthermore, music skills, like language skills, appear to some degree to be lateralized to one cerebral hemisphere (Zatorre, 1984); studying this phenomenon may lead us to a fuller understanding of the relationships both between the two hemispheres of the brain and between the symbol systems they support.

Even to mention the many approaches to music developed over the centuries by musicians, scholars, and, most recently, behavioral scientists would take many pages (for reviews, see Deutsch, 1982; Lerdahl & Jackendoff, 1983; Sloboda, 1985, 1988). Rather than offering a necessarily superficial review of what has been said before, it seems preferable to introduce those organizing principles that have most often emerged in current efforts to study music.

To begin with, one may (following current usage in the cognitive sciences) distinguish two primary approaches in conceptualizing the domain of music. Taking a "bottom–up" approach, one may focus on the elementary components of music—pitch, rhythm, and timbre—and gradually build up from these individual components to that complex interplay that constitutes a musical composition. Adopting the contrasting "top–down" approach, one takes as a point of departure the organized piece of music. According to this approach, it is assumed that musical analysis, like the perception of a musical work, should begin by approaching the organized musical form, or gestalt, with subsequent analysis into components an optional (and possibly advisable) ploy on the part of the analyst or the observer.

Neither approach is wholly adequate. Those researchers who adopt a top–down approach often have difficulty specifying the components of music that contribute to understanding. Those who embrace a bottom–up approach are often unable to effect the bridge from artificial musical stimuli to more naturalistic "whole pieces" of music.

To be sure, a few researchers have exhibited ingenuity in bridging the gap between the building blocks of music and more holistic patterns of perception and production. The most effective methods have utilized a strategy whereby a specific musical fragment is viewed as an instance within a more general musical vocabulary. Thus, Krumhansl (1979) has provided musical contexts to subjects and then asked them to judge the similarity of stimuli presented within these contexts, and Dowling (1978, 1979) has studied the abilities of individuals to discern similarities and differences among musical passages that differ systematically in the kinds of tonal relationships that are featured. Although such efforts still lean heavily on judgments of brief, somewhat contrived stimuli, their incorporation of musical contexts and their focus on musical (as opposed to acoustic) modes of analysis suggest a fruitful way of integrating the two approaches sketched here.

The aforementioned strategies characterize the range of investigations; however, certain issues have proved particularly germane for those researchers working in the neuropsychological tradition. As mentioned, we focus on three organizing issues:

1. *The relationship between linguistic and musical processing.* At least in certain superficial aspects (e.g., the processing of sequential materials over time, the existence of a basic "syntactic component," division into perceptual and productive capacities), music can be analogized to natural language (see Kleist, 1962). But the utility of this comparison remains to be demonstrated.

2. *The predominant mode of musical processing.* Echoing the distinctions raised in the preceding discussion, it is possible to view the apprehension of music primarily in terms of gestalt or holistic processes, primarily in terms of elementary or atomistic factors, or through some amalgam of these two approaches. This issue assumes particular aptness in view of current discussions about processing strategies favored by the two cerebral hemispheres.

3. *Contrasting pattern of skills across levels of talent or accomplishment.* Because of the wide range of competence in the music domain, due to differences in genetic endowment and/or training, it becomes crucial to establish whether superior performances by some individuals are due simply to a greater facility in processing musical elements or whether they reflect qualitatively different strategies.

Components of Music

Most studies in the neuropsychology of music have focused on the extent to which specific musical capacities and skills can be dissociated by brain damage (see Benton, 1977; Marin, 1982; Zatorre, 1984). A pioneering study of this kind was published in 1962 by Milner. Subtests of the Seashore test battery were administered both pre- and postoperatively to epileptic patients who underwent removal of one of their temporal lobes. Following removal of the right temporal lobe, there was a significant drop in scores on subtests measuring sensitivity to timbre, sensitivity to intensity, and tonal memory. Other subtest scores revealed no significant drop. Of greater importance, the performances of patients with left temporal lobe removal were generally comparable to their preoperative levels. Here, then, was early documentation of the relatively greater importance of the right hemisphere in the processing of musical stimuli, as well as a provisional demonstration that musical abilities could be dissociated on a neurological basis.

Subsequent studies utilizing different patient populations and testing techniques have validated the greater importance of the right hemisphere in the processing of musical stimuli and have documented an important division in the organization of musical skills. The left hemisphere has been implicated in the processing of rhythm, a time-dependent sequencing task (Sidtis & Volpe, 1981; Zatorre, 1984). In contrast, the processing of pitch presupposes major participation on the part of the right hemisphere (Gordon, 1970; Kimura, 1973; Shankweiler, 1966; Zattore, 1979). More recent evidence further suggests a decisive role played by the anterior portions of the right frontal lobes in the processing of tonal material (Shapiro, Grossman, & Gardner, 1981). As summarized in a major review by Zatorre (1984), the right temporal lobe takes the primary role in the processing of unfamiliar melodic sequences; the left hemisphere is important for processing familiar melodies.

A recent study by Brownell et al. (submitted) tested both left- and right-hemisphere–damaged patients on a melody completion task and a tone pair task. On the first task, subjects were asked to rate how well a final note completed a simple melody. Right-hemisphere–damaged patients made the least use of tonal goodness in judging the completing note, but both left- and right-hemisphere–damaged patients relied significantly less than normals on tonal goodness. In the tone pair task, subjects judged the similarity of a pair of notes; right-hemisphere–damaged patients relied significantly less than left-hemisphere–damaged patients on tonal goodness. Neither group differed from normal controls in their use of pitch height. Brownell et al. concluded that right-hemisphere damage leads to either a diminished ability to apprehend tonal goodness or an increased attention to pitch height.

Although most experimental research has focused on the perception of musical components, there is some documentation of lateralization in the production of musical entities. Injecting sodium amytal into the carotid arteries of presurgical patients, a number of researchers have been able to mimic (in a reversible manner) the effects of hemispherectomies (see Zatorre, 1984, for a review). The practice of asking patients to sing after such injections has revealed that this skill must be partly controlled by both hemispheres, as at least two researchers found that subjects could not sing after either hemisphere was injected (Borchgrevink, 1980; Gordon, 1970; Bogen & Gordon, 1971). Left-sided injection resulted in both speech and melody impairment, whereas right-sided injection produced a loss in tonal control. Rhythm was left intact in both cases. Zatorre (1984) found that, when played a familiar tune and asked to sing it at a given moment after the injection, patients were evenly split as to which hemisphere enabled them to sing better; 5 of his 12 patients sang equally poorly after either hemisphere was injected.

These findings are consistent with scattered clinical impressions. Many aphasiologists have reported a relative sparing of singing capacities following severe aphasia (Goodglass & Kaplan, 1972), and one promising form of aphasia therapy, in fact, exploits this preserved singing ability as a basis for reconstructing propositional speech (Helm-Estabrooks, 1983). Our own observations indicate that, in left-hemisphere–damaged patients, singing a melody aids in the utterance of articulated words; in contrast, among right-hemisphere–damaged patients, it is the production of the verbal components of music that actually aids in the accurate rendition of melodies (see also Ross & Mesulam, 1979).

Some researchers have asked whether musical capacities may be organized differently in talented or trained individuals. Although the data remain far from conclusive, some intriguing possibilities have been suggested. Bever and Chiarello (1974) devised a task that required the analysis of the internal structure of musical fragments. Individuals with musical training not only performed better on this task, but also displayed a stronger right-ear (left-hemisphere) advantage than musically naive subjects. In a supporting study, Shanon (1980) documented a greater amount of left-hemisphere involvement in tasks requiring complex musical decisions. However, another study, in which patients were required to recognize dichotically presented chords, yielded a contrasting pattern of results (Gordon, 1970): Here musicians demonstrated a right-hemisphere advantage, whereas nonmusicians exhibited no ear preference (see also Gordon, 1980). These latter studies dictate caution in inferring a universal pattern in the performances of musically trained (as opposed to musically naive) subjects: Effects may prove specific to certain stimuli, tasks, or subject groups.

Occasional efforts have been undertaken to examine the "meaning" of musical fragments. In one study, Gardner, Silverman, Denes, Semenza, and Rosenstiel (1977) asked patients to match a simple musical fragment with one or two contrasting geometric patterns. The sets of pictures were varied systematically on a number of graphic dimensions hypothesized to reflect different connotative aspects of musical patterns. Thus, for example, an ascending passage should be paired with an up-pointing line, whereas a descending passage should be paired with a descending line; a continuous tone "matches" an intact circle, whereas a broken tone "matches" a fragmented circle.

Although levels of performance varied considerably across groups of organic patients, a revealing dichotomy emerged: Right-hemisphere–damaged patients proved better able to link a musical passage to a pattern that portrayed the temporal course of the piece (such as regularity–irregularity) than to a pattern that captured gestalt aspects (such as continuity–discontinuity). In contrast, patients with left anterior damage proved better able to match sounds to pictures that captured holistic properties of the piece, and performed less adequately on those stimuli that depicted temporal aspects. Here, then, understanding of the connotative (or expressive) aspects of a piece of music proves consistent with certain hypotheses about preferred modes of information processing in the two hemispheres (Galin, 1974; Kaplan, 1982, Nebes, 1974).

Studies of Larger Musical Fragments

A few investigators have asked subjects to make judgments about actual musical works. For instance, in an effort to document comprehension of the denotative meanings of familiar pieces, Gardner and Denes (1973) asked patients to select which one of four pictures "went with" a familiar piece of music. In half of the instances, the correct answer was based upon the lyrics (not given) of a song; for example, to match the melody of "Row, Row, Row Your Boat" with the correct illustration (a boat), the subject needed to know the lyrics or title. For the other half of the items, knowledge of lyrics was unnecessary: Thus, to match the tune of "Hail to the Chief" with the correct illustration (the president), a subject merely had to know that the piece was usually played at official ceremonies, but did not have to know its unfamiliar title.

Results documented the extent to which musical performance by right-hemisphere–injured patients depends upon verbal information. On those items where correct performance necessitated knowledge of lyrics, right-hemisphere patients outperformed those with left-hemisphere damage. On the other hand, on those items where knowledge of lyrics was irrelevant, and identification could proceed simply on the basis of knowledge of the situation in which such a piece was ordinarily heard, left-hemisphere patients surpassed those with injury to the right hemisphere. Here, then, is further documentation that purely musical components cohere and can be dissociated from verbal aspects of musical stimuli.

Following another line of investigation, Shapiro et al. (1981) asked whether the effects found with atomistic musical stimuli are also in evidence with familiar compositions. Experimenters played familiar pieces and asked subjects merely to judge whether they sounded "right" or "wrong." Groups of subjects proved differentially skilled at this task. Thus, left anterior patients evinced skill at detecting the major kinds of errors, having slight difficulty only with those pieces that were played unusually rapidly or unusually slowly. Left posterior and left central patients performed somewhat more poorly, particularly on items probing sensitivity to tempo. Patients with right anterior damage performed at the lowest level, responding at chance level on every kind of item except the control pieces (pieces that were correctly performed). Counter to the frequently proposed notion that the left hemisphere is dominant for rhythmic processing, it was the right-hemisphere patients who proved poor at detecting rhythmic errors.

This pattern of results may be interpreted as evidence that right-hemisphere patients have a fragile or impaired internal representation of all aspects of the melody. In the absence of such an internal representation, which indicates what the piece is supposed to sound like, it would of necessity prove difficult to determine whether it had been performed correctly. Further evidence for a possible deficit in the overall internal representation (or auditory imagery) of musical material comes from a case study at the Boston University Aphasia Research Center (Judd, Gardner, & Geschwind, 1983). An amateur musician suffering from auditory agnosia secondary to major right-hemisphere involvement proved able to answer challenging theoretical questions about music, yet the same patient could not indicate whether the first note of a familiar piece of music was higher or lower than the second. Such evidence suggests that his internal auditory imagery for known melodies had been severely degraded.

Case Studies

By far the richest and most important information about the organization of musical skills has come from the study of talented individuals who have sustained brain damage. The existence of such a population has made it possible to examine the organization of the highest level of musical skill. Moreover, in cases where examples of premorbid artistry can be examined, it proves possible to make crucial comparisons that may illuminate the effect of brain damage on the organization of music.

In this review, we retain the organizing themes that have guided our presentation of more traditional empirical investigations. We examine the relationship between aphasia and musical achievement, the kinds of strategies used by individuals who have suffered brain disease, and the fate of various discrete and holistic capabilities in light of brain damage. In addition, we comment on the fate of originality, creativeness, and overall sense of form in musical achievements following injury to the brain.

A well-known pair of case studies has highlighted the relationship between the components of linguistic and musical competence. Botez and Wertheim (1959) studied an accordion player who, following removal of a tumor in the second right frontal convolution, suffered several severe amusic disturbances. While able to sing individual pitches, he could not combine them into a song. His repetition of rhythmic and melodic material was poor, and, most importantly, he was unable to play his accordion. Despite these difficulties, the subject had perfectly preserved perceptual and receptive capacities for music. He recognized pieces, spotted deliberate errors introduced in them, and was highly critical of his own performance. Suggesting an analogy to expressive aphasia, Botez and Wertheim spoke of their patient as exhibiting expressive amusia secondary to damage in the right frontal lobe.

Wertheim and Botez (1961) also reported a case of receptive amusia in a concert violinist who became severely aphasic, apparently as a result of left-hemisphere injury. In contrast to their other patient, this violinist lost his absolute pitch, had difficulty in appreciating tempo changes, was unable to analyze chord structure, and could not name familiar pieces. His performance was far from perfect, but he was able to pick out pieces on the violin with his nonparetic hand. Moreover, when accompanied on the piano, his performance improved. Thus, pursuing the analogy to the aphasias, here was a patient whose receptive problems were more striking than his expressive ones. Yet, while this dichotomy may aid in an effort to organize complex findings, the distinction between receptive and expressive factors remains problematic, particularly with reference to the violin player.

A second topic that can be probed only with case studies of musically talented individuals is the fate of music reading following damage to the brain. Intuitively, it might seem that linguistic and musical alexia should be closely allied. In fact, however, these two forms of reading have been dissociated from one another in a number of instances. Thus, Soukes and Baruk's (1930) patient, a severe Wernicke's aphasic, was wholly unable to read text while still able to read music at the piano. In contrast, Dorgueille (cited in Benton, 1977) reported a patient who, after a left hemisphere stroke, was no longer able to read music but could still read text.

A few other generalizations can be offered on the basis of the dozens of case studies carried out since the turn of the century. It is very rare to encounter individuals who have sustained significant aphasia without some loss in musical competence (Feuchtwanger, 1930; Ustvedt, 1937), even though the overlap between aphasia and amusia is very far from complete. There may be a rough association between receptive factors on the one hand and expressive on the other, but in general no set of factors is completely impaired without there being correlative difficulty with other factors. In nearly all cases, individuals prove better able to handle old, overlearned materials than new, unfamiliar materials. In fact, in some cases, patients perform almost perfectly with well-known materials, while showing little or no capacity to master new materials (Judd et al., 1983). This result may simply reflect the well-documented phenomenon that brain-damaged individuals have an inordinate amount of difficulty learning to master any new kinds of materials.

Of numerous case studies that have been conducted with competent musicians, several stand out in terms of the detail of reporting and the significance of the results. In the six reviewed here, relatively complete information existed about the premorbid level of skill; moreover, the examiners probed relevant issues about the organization of artistic capacities.

In three cases, a major composer suffered a stroke in the posterior region of the left hemisphere, thereby developing significant aphasic disturbance. The first, the renowned Russian composer Shebalin, became severely aphasic following a stroke; nonetheless, he continued his composing and teaching activities as before and was considered by critics to be as brilliant a composer as ever (Luria, Tsvetkova, & Futer, 1965).

A second individual was a major American composer of choral works. He initially suffered a fluent aphasia, which later cleared to the level of a moderate anomia. Like Shebalin, this musician's capacities to compose and to criticize performances of music returned rather quickly to a level approaching that of his premorbid skills (Judd et al., 1983). The condition of this composer is instructive in that he remained completely alexic for written language. As a result he had to institute various innovations to permit him to set text to music, for example, memorizing the text or having it read aloud as needed. His ability to read and write musical notation was much less severely impaired. Often, when unable to identify exact notes, he was still able to make shrewd guesses about what was wanted in a particular circumstance, and he could readily recognize scores, even when he could name neither the pitches nor the compositions. Here, then, is an instructive instance where the mechanics of musical performance and composition were impaired because of particular difficulty in the processing of visual symbols, while underlying musical intelligence was spared.

The well-known French composer Maurice Ravel had a tumor in the left hemisphere that left him with a permanent Wernicke's aphasia (Alajouanine, 1948). Ravel presented an interesting pattern of musical breakdown. He was able to recognize pieces he had known before his illness and could detect even minor faults in a performance. He still enjoyed listening to music after his illness and remained able to evaluate new pieces critically. However, he was never able to write or compose another piece, and he had great difficulty in playing the piano. Whether Ravel's inability to compose was due to mechanical difficulties of the sort that obtain in the Judd et al. case or to a more fundamental impairment of musical intelligence could not be determined with certainty, although it seems likely that his musical intelligence was at least to some extent compromised.

Another case provides further information on the relationship between left-hemisphere disease and amusia. A 64-year-old Swiss pianist suffered a form of Wernicke's aphasia in which word deafness was particularly pronounced. Despite this difficulty with language, his musical capacities remained essentially intact. He could instantly recognize pieces of music and make all necessary corrections in a performance. Moreover, he was able to play even new pieces with no noticeable mistakes. Only when tasks involved a linguistic capacity, such as identification of notes by names, did the patient exhibit difficulties (Assal, 1973).

Basso and Capitani (1985) treated an Italian musical conductor who had sustained severe left-hemisphere damage. Cortical and subcortical damage to the left posterior region of the brain left the patient with global aphasia and severe apraxia. He had difficulty with reading, writing, comprehension, and repetition beyond the single-word level; he exhibited ideomotor and buccofacial apraxia as well as "apraxia of use". Despite this constellation of deficits, however, the patient lost remarkably little of his musical competence. His ability to perceive and appraise music was intact. Remarkably, he continued to conduct orchestral pieces, communicating with members of the orchestra through gestures. Basso and Capitani argue that the patient's preserved abilities suggest that musical processing exists separately from linguistic processing and is capable of surviving even in the absence of linguistic support.

A final and highly instructive contrasting case is presented by a composer who suffered a stroke involving the right frontoparietal and temporal regions (T. Judd, A. Arslenian, L. Davidson, & S. Locke, unpublished research). Following his stroke, this composer's musical understanding remained intact. In fact, he wrote a musical textbook and also mastered two foreign languages after his stroke. Although musical testing uncovered some subtle perceptual defects, he was able to continue teaching at a school of music. In sharp contrast to the other musicians reviewed, however, he lost his interest in the creative process. He no longer felt motivated to compose; as he put it, he could no longer conjure up the appropriate atmosphere. He even reported that he could no longer "conceive of a whole piece." He indicated that he no longer listened to music for enjoyment as much as he had in the past and that he no longer experienced the rich set of associations while listening to music. His own postmorbid compositions he correctly judged as uninspired and uninspiring.

This case helps to clarify results obtained from individuals who have suffered an aphasia. With the possible exception of Ravel, musicians with language impairment caused by left-hemisphere disease have retained the capacity and the desire to engage in creative musical activity. In contrast, an individual with significant right-hemisphere disease, whose language remained on an extraordinarily high level and whose musical technique and technical skill had been largely spared, seemed to have undergone an alteration in his relationship to musical material and proved able to compose only in a very limited and uninspiring way.

On the basis of studies conducted with musicians who have suffered unilateral brain damage, and in light of studies conducted with both brain-damaged and healthy nonmusicians, complicated and sometimes conflicting patterns of findings have been reported. Nonetheless, a number of generalizations can be made. The most general statement that should be made is that both hemispheres are involved in music but that each hemisphere makes a different kind of contribution. Although the right hemisphere plays the most important role, it is rare to encounter an individual with severe aphasia who has not also suffered some loss in musical capacity.

The right hemisphere seems to be particularly important in four areas: the processing of the components of music (e.g., recognizing pitch, timbre); the internal representation of a melody that allows error detection; the production of music (e.g., combining notes into a recognizable melody, playing an instrument); and the individual's emotional relationship to music (e.g., motivation, inspiration, gratification sustained). The left hemisphere seems to be particularly important in those aspects of music most closely allied to language: reading musical notes and naming notes and entire pieces. It should be mentioned that the ability to read musical notation is dissociable from the ability to read linguistic text: Either one alone may be impaired as a result of left-hemisphere damage. It should also be stressed that, while the ability to read music and name pieces may be severely impaired, the individual's underlying musical intelligence may be spared. On the basis of this review, then, it seems possible to distinguish between a capacity to carry out tasks involving musical notation, and a capacity to engage in musical creation and to sustain certain kinds of emotional gratification from a relationship with works of music.

Drawing

The bulk of research on graphic competence conducted with both normal and gifted individuals documents a high degree of dissociation between graphic and linguistic capacity. Indeed, with the exception of Bay (1962, 1964), nearly all authorities agree that graphic competence can exist at a high level despite a significant aphasia and, correlatively, that graphic competence can be compromised even when language is spared.

A more promising way of conceptualizing graphic competence highlights the different contributions made to the graphic process by each cerebral hemisphere. As formulated by E. Kaplan (1982), the left hemisphere proves particularly important for providing the details in a copied or an original graphic production, while the right hemisphere contributes to the general configuration of a drawing. Caplan (in press) has broken the left hemisphere down in terms of the roles of the frontal lobe and the superior and inferior parietal lobules. Frontal lobe lesions in either hemisphere lead to carelessness and poor planning in executing drawings: Such patients often leave drawings unfinished. Patients with left inferior parietal lesions draw oversimplified figures with few details, but are able to copy drawings with little difficulty. These patients often have naming problems and/or alexia with agraphia. Left superior parietal lesions leave some patients with deficits in drawing people and body parts, concomitant with their difficulties in naming and describing these. Patients with right-hemisphere lesions, in contrast, tend to overemphasize detail but are impaired in drawing external form or structure. They often display constructional difficulties and a poor sense of proportion; patients with right parietal lesions often have severe left neglect and leave drawings incomplete or completely blank on the left side.

Other lateralized dissociations have also been reported. According to Kimura and Faust (1985), left-hemisphere–damaged patients often display greater deficits in spontaneous drawing than right-brain–damaged patients. The drawings of patients with left-hemisphere damage, particularly those of patients with anterior lesions, were smaller and less easily recognizable. This finding was particularly true of apraxic patients, who have difficulty in executing planned sequences of fine motor movements. Jones-Gotman and Milner (1977) found that the right hemisphere seems to play a role of particular importance in the fluency with which drawings are produced. When asked to draw an instance of a category (e.g., to draw a vegetable), a patient with an injury to the right hemisphere draws bizarre pictures that incorporate incorrect or extraneous information (e.g., a picture of a potato with a stem). In contrast, individuals with left anterior injury are able to draw prototypical members of a category, although various defects may also attend the performance of these language-impaired patients. Fluent aphasics, despite profound word-finding deficits, encounter little difficulty producing large numbers of pictures, although they often cannot name perfectly recognizable pictures that they have drawn (Grossman, 1980).

It is important to indicate that, although these differences in drawing performance can be documented in certain clearcut instances, in many other cases, overall level of drawing deteriorates to such an extent that the site of damage and the kind of drawing deficit become difficult to specify. Further difficulties in interpretation result from the natural variation in artistic ability among brain-damaged subjects. Nevertheless, attempts at localization of various art-related skills are worthwhile: They provide us with at least a rough map of the locations of some of the abilities that must be preserved for a person to create works of visual art.

On the receptive side, ample evidence suggests that the right hemisphere plays a principal role in the "reading of pictorial information," including paintings and drawings. Little information has been gathered on the abilities of brain-damaged patients to attend to those aspects of graphic symbols that contribute to their aesthetic significance, such as composition, balance, or expressiveness. However, one study (Gardner, 1975a) does document the role of the right hemisphere in "reading" the style of a work of art. Asked to put together those paintings that were made by the same artist, right-hemisphere–injured patients classify not by style but by subject matter. Patients with left–hemisphere damage, in contrast, show a normal or even a superior capacity to sort paintings by style, quite possibly because their orientation to the subject matter has been diminished by their pathology.

Examination of skilled artists who have suffered brain disease uncovers a number of suggestive phenomena. Studies of painters with left-hemisphere damage have revealed that the left hemisphere of the skilled individual may play a less crucial graphic role than it does in the unskilled. For instance, a major French painter studied by Alajouanine (1948) was rendered severely aphasic by a left-hemisphere stroke. After the stroke, his artistic activity did not decline and did not seem to change in its technique or tone. The painter poignantly described this split between his artistic self and his other selves:

> There are in me two men, the one who paints, who is normal while he is painting, and the other one who is lost in the mist, who does not stick to life. . . . I am saying very poorly what I mean. . . . There are inside me the one who grasps reality, life; there is the other one who is lost as regards abstract thinking. . . . These are two men, the one who is grasped by reality to paint, the other one, the fool who cannot manage words any more. (Alajouanine, 1948, p. 238)

The case of a Bulgarian painter, ZB, described by Zaimov, Kitov, and Kolev (1969), also supports the finding that the ability to paint is not necessarily affected by the loss of linguistic skills. ZB suffered a severe aphasia as well as paralysis of the right side of the body. Because of the paralysis, the painter began to teach himself to draw with his left hand. He gradually regained his fluency but, unlike the French painter described above, ZB had developed an entirely new style. In his prestroke work, he depicted events occurring over time—in the past, present, and future. His poststroke work was no longer in such a narrative style, but instead was characterized by strange and fantastic dreamlike images, clear colors, and symmetrical patterns. Although his style was clearly new, it was in no way worse than his prestroke style.

Studies of an aphasic patient seen in our lab at the Aphasia Research Center provide further evidence that severe left-hemisphere disease and resulting linguistic deficits do not necessarily compromise previously existing artistic skill. GM, a 62-year-old professional artist, suffered a large left-hemisphere stroke involving all of both Broca's and Wernicke's areas, as well as parts of the left frontal horn and left-hemisphere subcortical structures. Following the stroke he developed global aphasia, leaving him with poor auditory comprehension and virtually no speech save the words "yes" and "no" and a few stereotypes. A severe right hemiparesis left him unable to use his dominant right hand. With encouragement from friends and family, however, GM began to paint and draw again a few months after his stroke, using his left hand.

As is evident in Figures 11-1 through 11-4, GM's work showed some change in style subsequent to the stroke. An example of his painting prior to the stroke is shown in Figure 11.1. It shows complex use of form and line, and attention to depth and the interplay of shapes. His painting subsequent to the stroke (see Figure 11.2) continues to be concerned

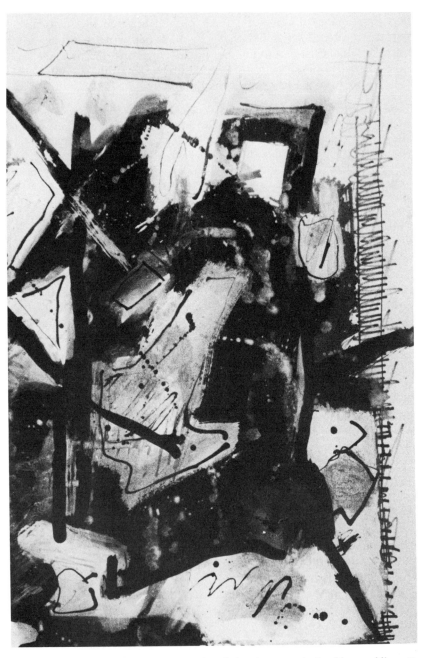

FIGURE 11.1. *This example of GM's prestroke painting shows complexity of form and line, attention to depth, and interplay of shapes.*

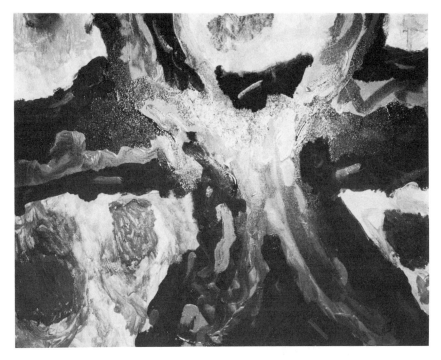

FIGURE 11.2. *This example of GM's poststroke painting has amorphous forms and little sense of depth.*

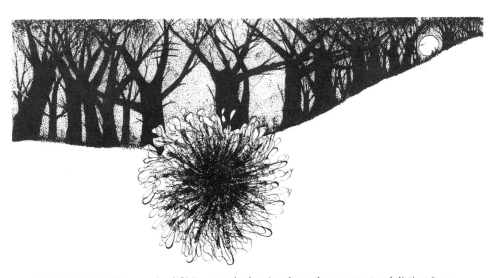

FIGURE 11.3. *This example of GM's prestroke drawing shows sharp contrast and distinct forms.*

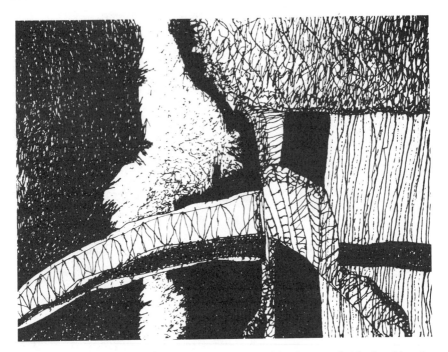

FIGURE 11.4. *This example of GM's poststroke drawing exhibits less control of depth and layering of shapes.*

with these graphic elements, but on a somewhat less sophisticated level: the forms seem amorphous and there is little sense of depth to the painting as a whole. His drawings show a similar but less dramatic change. GM's earlier drawing (Figure 11.3), executed just a few months before his stroke, relies on sharp contrast and clearly drawn forms to communicate its message to the viewer. Although his poststroke drawing (Figure 11.4) certainly contains these elements, they are less striking. The forms are not as masterfully drawn, and the artist does not exhibit the same control of depth and layering of shapes as in the earlier drawing. GM does, however, seem to have retained a good sense of overall composition.

The hypothesis that left-hemisphere damage leads to loss of detail in visual art does not appear to be strongly supported by GM's work. Although one might argue that his poststroke artwork is simpler overall, it is difficult to judge both because of the abstract nature of the work and because some simplification is attributable to the fact that he is working with his nondominant hand.

These differences between pre- and poststroke style do not mean that GM's art has diminished in expressiveness or power. In fact, many who have seen his poststroke work find it more interesting and emotionally evocative than his earlier work. GM continues to be highly critical of both his own work and that of others, communicating his opinions through gesture and facial expression. He is highly motivated to create, and has begun to pay particular attention to the improvement of his left-hand motor skills. His case clearly strengthens the hypothesis that artistic talent as well as artistic appreciation may persist and even flourish in the virtual absence of linguistic capacity. It is of note that GM does not use art to communicate in the same way that he would use language: Although his work may have grown more expressive emotionally, it does not communicate anything in a narrative sense. This supports the idea that, at least in trained artists, art and language skills do indeed exist as separate modes of expression.

One example of a skilled artist whose work WAS significantly affected by left-hemisphere damage was reported by Marsh and Philwin (1987). The patient, IK, was the victim of a fast-growing left posterior parietal tumor which left him transiently aphasic and manifested itself most strikingly in his painting, which showed right-sided neglect and constructional apraxia. The authors contrasted two paintings on the same theme; the painting done during IK's illness showed recognizable human figures only in the lower left hemifield, with progressive simplification from the left to the right side of the painting. These findings indicate that a tumor such as IK's may produce marked changes in visuospatial perception and in constructional ability. Such radical changes have not been reported in other cases of left-hemisphere disease, and may result as much from the nature of the tumor and its possible effects as from its focal location. IK's painting showed little change in terms of style or emotional quality; changes seem to have resulted solely from his perceptual difficulties.

The above case studies reveal that in skilled painters, graphic skills can function independently of language and most other left-hemisphere skills. As we saw earlier, this result appears to be less the case with unskilled individuals, in whom left-hemisphere damage results in an impoverishment of detail in their drawings. The hypothesis that left-hemisphere damage leads to loss of detail in visual art does not appear to be strongly supported by GM's work, or by the work of any artist in the case studies described above. Although one might argue that GM's poststroke artwork is simpler overall, it is difficult to judge both because of the abstract nature of the work and because some simplification is attributable to the fact that he is working with his nondominant hand. Whether the visual analysis of detail is preserved in the left-hemisphere–damaged artist because it is overlearned, or whether it is preserved because it is represented more widely in the brain, is not known. Since we do not have a comparable group of untrained left-hemisphere stroke victims who are matched to the artists in terms of lesion site, no strong conclusions can be drawn as to the difference between the role of the left hemisphere in normal and gifted draughtsmen.

Another case demonstrates that graphic ability may be impaired despite intact linguistic capacities and also that the ability to draw may be composed of two separable components. An investigation of a visually agnostic artist documented a striking dissociation of drawing skills (Wapner, Judd, & Gardner, 1978). This individual was unable to recognize objects that were presented to him, although he remained able to draw quite accurately from memory those objects as he had once known them. When asked to copy an object or picture placed in front of him, he was able to make exceedingly slavish copies of that object, ones of almost photographic accuracy; at the same time, he was unable to identify or name the object in question. In those rare cases where identification was possible or where the name was provided, he drew the objects in a very different, more schematic, and less slavish way.

The patient documents two separate forms of graphic competence in an artist: (a) a photographic copying mechanism in which every detail of an object is rendered just the way that it is perceived retinally, even at the cost of distortion (cf. Gombrich, 1960, who demonstrated that photographically accurate pictures may appear distorted), and (b) a more schematic way of rendering, in which the patient exploits some established pattern for representing an object. In the latter instance, the painter is prepared to sacrifice particular identifying features of the object in question in order to produce a more generally recognizable version of that object. Further confirmation of this dissociation can be found in the remarkable drawings by the autistic child Nadia (Selfe, 1977). This young girl could produce slavishly realistic representations, but she had no apparent knowledge of the objects involved and no generalized schemata that could be used to denote an entire class of objects.

The small amount of research carried out with major visual artists who have suffered strokes permits certain tentative generalizations. If a gifted artist suffers a left-hemisphere stroke, and is not completely paralyzed, he or she should be able to continue to draw in much the same style and also exhibit the same skills as in the premorbid state. In the case of regression, the style of depiction is likely to become more primitive but still be recognizable. Indeed, the clinical literature contains several descriptions of individuals who were allegedly able to draw better poststroke than prestroke; however, a certain romanticism may stimulate such claims (Gardner, 1975b).

It has proved possible to study the paintings of a few individuals who suffered significant right-hemisphere disease and yet still continued to paint (Jung, 1974). Two German expressionists, Lovis Corinth and Anton Räderscheidt, both resumed painting after partial recovery from significant right-hemisphere strokes. Initially, their paintings included neglect of the left side of space, irregular contours, misplaced detail, and general fuzziness in depiction. With recovery, the neglect of space was reduced; however, the drawings continued to exhibit fundamental differences in style. Specifically, the drawings became much more emotional, primitive, and bizarre, featuring rough lines and grotesque effects (Gardner, 1975b).

At the time that these drawings were first produced, art historians and critics spoke of a general change in style, one perhaps reflecting the patient's reaction to severe illness. However, it is possible to put forward an alternative explanation. Suppose, as several studies have suggested, that the right hemisphere is essential for emotional appropriateness; it may be that, as a result of their significant pathology, these patients were now affected by a different set of emotional concerns. Reflecting these concerns, they went on to produce paintings that were much more sensual and "raw" in appearance, or much less inhibited.

It is important to ascertain which account of the changed style of these painters is correct. If in fact painters, irrespective of their variety of brain damage, begin to paint in anomalous styles, then the "general reactive" interpretation gains in persuasiveness. If, however, as we believe, such painting changes occur only in individuals with significant right-hemisphere pathology, then the style alteration can be traced directly to a certain form of brain damage.

In sum, studies of both normal individuals who have suffered unilateral brain damage and gifted artists with brain damage reveal that, while both hemispheres play a role in the visual arts, the right hemisphere is dominant. In the case of average individuals, the left hemisphere is important for rendering the precise details of a represented object; the right hemisphere is important in enabling the artist to draw fluently, in capturing the overall form of an object, and in knowing what is and is not appropriate to include in a drawing. The graphic capabilities of the right hemisphere have been put to use in several aphasia therapy programs which encourage aphasics to communicate through drawing (for a review, see Lyon & Helm-Estabrooks, 1987).

In the case of gifted visual artists, the role of the left hemisphere is less clear. Painters with severe aphasia consequent to left-hemisphere damage have been able to continue painting, but the quality and style of their output may depend on the nature of the damage and on other factors that are difficult to pin down. A fast-growing parietal tumor causes deficits in visuospatial and constructional skills; although a massive left-hemisphere stroke may have little or no effect on the artist's skills, it may inspire a change in painting style or emotional quality. Despite the variety of sequelae of left-hemisphere damage in skilled artists, it is clear that graphic skills can function independently of linguistic and other left-hemisphere skills. When a painter suffers right-hemisphere damage, on the other hand, the paintings become altered in at least two ways: There is a noticeable neglect of the left side of the pictorial space, and, more importantly, the style of painting may become more emotional and direct.

Language and Literary Creativity

Research into the basic components of language—phonology, semantics, and syntax—has demonstrated that language is one of the most strongly lateralized functions. The central role of the left hemisphere in language is beyond dispute, and it is well known that damage to the left brain causes aphasias in the case of right-handed individuals. For a long time, it was commonly believed that ONLY the left hemisphere was involved in language processing. But there is by now a great deal of evidence that the right hemisphere also plays some role in language: The right brain is capable of uttering overlearned phrases (such as "How are you?") (Taylor, 1932); it can process vowels, intonation contours, and affectively tinged language (Blumstein & Cooper, 1974; Cicone, Wapner, & Gardner, 1980; Heilman, 1976; Kimura, 1973); and it may even possess some vocabulary and syntax (Gazzaniga, 1970; Sperry, 1974; Zaidel, 1973, 1977, 1978a, 1978b).

Despite all that is known about the organization of basic language skills, however, we cannot predict with confidence what will happen to literary skills after left-brain damage. Dealing with literature requires far more than syntax, semantics, or phonology. Indeed, the abilities most central to literary competence appear to lie in another area. For instance, to write or to appreciate a piece of literature, one must go beyond the literal and appreciate figurative forms of language involving metaphor, irony, or humor. And to perceive or produce a fictional work requires a sensitivity to the rules of narrative structure and an awareness of the boundary between fact and fiction. Thus, in evaluating the effects of left-hemisphere damage on literary skill, the important questions do not concern performance on standard linguistic tasks. Rather, one wants to know whether individuals understand metaphor and other types of nonliteral language, whether they know what a story is, and whether they grasp that a story is different from a journalistic account of an actual event. Put simply, might the spared abilities of the right hemisphere allow aphasics to interpret figurative language or to apprehend a story?

Two predictions are plausible. On the one hand, one might expect poor performance on literary tasks because such tasks tap higher order levels of language. However, clinical observations suggest that the right hemisphere may be particularly important in attending to the context and nuance. Given this, one might expect that just such artistic verbal abilities are spared after left-brain damage.

Presented with a description of a person having a "heavy heart," aphasics have difficulty explaining the meaning of this metaphor (Winner & Gardner, 1977). But this difficulty stems simply from an inability to put their understanding into words. Provided with a nonlinguistic response mode in which they may simply point to a picture that goes with such a metaphoric statement, patients with left-sided damage perform nearly as well as normal individuals (Winner & Gardner, 1977). The pictures that they were shown for "heavy heart" included a "literal" picture of a person staggering under the weight of a heavy, heart-shaped object; the correct choice was a picture of a person crying.

Left-hemisphere–damaged patients thus retain some literary sensitivity, suggesting that the right hemisphere contributes to the understanding of figurative language. Nevertheless, damage to the left hemisphere cripples the writer. The French poet Baudelaire, after suffering a left-hemisphere stroke, was never able to write again, and the only words that he could utter were an oath, *"cré-nom."* In situations where the aphasia recedes and some recovery is evidenced, the individual may go on to write again. The poet William Carlos Williams was able to write some poetry after his partial recovery from aphasia (Plimpton, 1977). Also, a number of physicians who have become aphasic and then recovered went on to write about their experiences (Gardner, 1975b). Not surprisingly, however, in no case has an aphasic writer demonstrated the ability to write in the face of a loss of ordinary language ability.

What happens to literary skill after right-hemisphere damage? On the surface, right-hemisphere–damaged patients appear to possess intact language. Yet closer inspection reveals subtle language difficulties. For instance, such individuals are often unable to relate a statement to its context and thus tend to misinterpret the speaker's meaning. Upon hearing someone reject an offer of help in hanging a picture by saying that "too many cooks spoil the broth," a right-hemisphere–damaged patient may fail to recognize that the import of this statement has to do with hanging pictures and not with cooking. Failure to relate this statement to its appropriate context leads to a literal interpretation.

The role of the right hemisphere in attending to context and intention suggests that this hemisphere may make an important contribution in the domain of the literary arts. When language is functioning aesthetically, it is often its nonliteral aspects that are the most crucial to apprehend. An inability to relate sentence to context ought to result in a tendency to interpret figurative language literally (taking "heavy hearted" to mean physically heavy) and to confuse the boundary between a fictive narrative and a straightforward description of actually occurring events (believing, for instance, that a story can only contain descriptions of events that may occur in reality). Indeed, investigation of the role of the right hemisphere in both metaphoric and narrative uses of language reveals just such difficulties.

Unlike left-hemisphere–damaged patients, those with right-hemisphere–damage often speak in a manner that sounds metaphoric (e.g., a patient might joke about a paralyzed arm, calling it his "old fin"). Yet, asked to paraphrase the metaphoric sentence "He had a very heavy heart," they are initially resistant, often insisting that such language is not proper English. After a bit of prodding, however, they reveal no difficulty in paraphrasing the sentence, explaining that it means that someone is sad. But, asked to point to the picture that goes with the description, right-hemisphere patients are as likely to choose the literal depiction as to choose the (correct) metaphoric one. Moreover, unlike lefthemisphere patients and non–brain-damaged individuals, they fail to find the literal pictures amusing. Nor do they notice the conflict between their verbal paraphrase and their literal picture choice (Winner & Gardner, 1977).

How can such results be explained? One way to understand these findings is to think of the left hemisphere as a "language machine," able to supply verbal paraphrases and definitions of any sentences or words it is given. Thus, the patient with a damaged right hemisphere and an intact left hemisphere has no problem paraphrasing metaphors. Where the right hemisphere appears to be particularly crucial is in alerting the listener to context—recognizing situations in which uttering a particular statement would or would not be appropriate. Thus, those with right-hemisphere damage are unable to select the picture depicting the situation in which one would ordinarily say "He had a very heavy heart."

Sensitivity to context is not only important in understanding the kind of language used in the verbal arts; it is also important in understanding fictional narrative. Understanding a narrative requires an ability to enter into the story, attending fully to the story line and its coherence, as well as picking up on events that are implied but not directly stated. Right-hemisphere–damaged patients have been shown to have difficulty with many of these higher order processing skills. In particular, these patients do not make appropriate use of contextual knowledge in making assumptions or predictions about what a speaker means. Furthermore, they are often reluctant to make the necessary revisions in their initial interpretations of sentences or situations when presented with new contextual information. These difficulties with prediction and revision, as well as other, related deficits, are a common result of right-hemisphere damage (Molloy, Brownell, & Gardner, 1990).

Several recent studies provide further evidence of the deficits shown by right-hemisphere–damaged patients in the processing of contextualized language. Investigations carried out at the Aphasia Research Center (Weylman, Brownell, Roman, & Gardner, 1989) and elsewhere (Foldi, 1987; Hirst, LeDoux, & Stein, 1984) suggest that right-hemisphere–damaged patients have difficulty interpreting indirect requests because they make inadequate use of the context provided. Hirst et al. showed left-hemisphere– and right-hemisphere–damaged patients videotaped episodes in which one actor asked another, "Can you X?"; the other actor responded by either doing what was requested or by saying, "Yes." Aphasics understood that it was appropriate to respond to such a question with an action if the context indicated that it was meant as an indirect request, but they proved unable to understand the literal meaning of the question. In contrast, right-hemisphere–damaged patients always interpreted the question literally, regardless of the context in which it was asked. Foldi (1987) also found that, relative to both aphasics and controls, right-hemisphere–damaged patients preferred literal interpretations of indirect requests over pragmatically appropriate ones. In Weylman et al.'s study (1989), subjects heard short stories with contextually appropriate indirect requests at the end; both right-hemisphere patients and aphasics had significantly more difficulty than controls in responding correctly to the requests; however, aphasics were at a clear disadvantage in this study because no visually presented information accompanied the text.

These findings suggest that, while aphasics are impaired in their literal understanding of language, they have retained the ability to use context in a meaningful way in interpreting language that they might otherwise be unable to understand. Right-hemisphere–damaged patients proved unable or unwilling to take contextual factors into account. Molloy et al. (1990) proposed that this may be reflective of a general deficit in linguistic prediction: right-hemisphere–damaged patients may not be able to use context predictively, and so cannot anticipate when sentence meaning and speaker meaning may diverge. Further support for this hypothesis comes from a study of sarcasm and irony by J. Kaplan, Brownell, Jacobs, and Gardner (1990). Right-hemisphere–damaged patients and normal controls heard short vignettes which ended with one of the characters making a remark to the other. When these remarks were literally false, they could best be interpreted as sarcastic (if one speaker were hostile to the other) or as being told on purpose to make the other person feel good (if the speaker was friendly with the listener). The right-hemisphere–damaged patients were less consistent than normal subjects in interpreting both of these types of remarks correctly. They proved to be somewhat insensitive to the relationship between the two characters, leaving them without strong guidelines in predicting what sort of an interaction these two people would likely have.

While the use of contextual information in the interpretation of stories is crucial, the apprehension of the various structural features that are particular to different types of narrative discourse also proves important. Bihrle, Brownell, Powelson, and Gardner (1986) found that right-hemisphere–damaged patients were deficient in their appreciation of the structure of jokes. Patients were presented with verbal short story jokes accompanied by cartoons, and were asked to select the best linguistic punchline. Right-hemisphere–damaged patients often chose non sequitur endings which preserved the element of surprise necessary for the punchline of a joke, but lacked coherence with the body of the joke. Aphasic patients sometimes confused straightforward endings with correct punchlines, but rarely chose non sequitur endings. This finding suggests that right-hemisphere damage creates a deficit in the ability to revise previously held interpretations, specifically the kind of revision that "getting" the punchline of a joke requires.

Further evidence for this type of revision-making deficit comes from studies of right-hemisphere–damaged patients' abilities to make inferences. Brownell, Potter, Bihrle, and Gardner (1986) presented patients with two-sentence stories, in which the second sentence provided information that would require the reader to revise his or her initial interpretation of the situation described. Right-hemisphere–damaged patients had difficulty reinterpreting the stories when given the second sentence.

Other studies of story comprehension reinforce the finding that right-hemisphere–damaged patients are insensitive to several key structural features of narratives (Delis, Wapner, Gardner, & Moses, 1983; Gardner, Brownell, Wapner, & Michelow, 1983; Joanette, Goulet, Ska, & Nespoulous, 1986; Moya, Benowitz, Levine, & Finklestein, 1986; Wapner, Hamby, & Gardner, 1981). These patients have no difficulty understanding and retaining the facts of a story, but they have trouble ordering events correctly, deriving the moral or main point from a narrative, and distinguishing between fact and fabrication. This last point is clearly illustrated in a study by Gardner et al. (1983) which assessed sensitivity to the insertion of noncanonical elements into stories. Normal controls generally judged these elements to be bizarre and did not incorporate them into their retellings of the stories. Aphasic patients altered the information so that it made sense within the context of the story. Right-hemisphere–damaged patients, however, accepted the bizarre elements as normal parts of the story and included them in their retellings, sometimes fabricating elaborate scenarios in an attempt to integrate all of the information. The results of this study and of the others mentioned above suggest that these patients have lost a sense of what elements make up the canonical form of a story.

With respect to the literary arts, we can conclude that literary creativity requires both an intact right and an intact left hemisphere. Severe aphasia, of course, cripples the literary artist. Nonetheless, despite the left hemisphere's undisputed dominance for language, the right hemisphere also plays a very important role in the literary arts. In particular, the right hemisphere is crucial in determining the intention behind an utterance and in relating an utterance to its linguistic, situational, and narrative context. Because patients with right hemisphere damage are often unable to recognize the context and the intention behind an utterance, they tend to misinterpret nonliteral language. Moreover, because of the right hemisphere's attention to context and narrative structure, this hemisphere plays a critical role in story understanding: without a sensitivity to these two elements, the right hemisphere–damaged patient is unable to accept a story as a fictional entity that must be taken on its own terms yet must also be clearly distinguished from "reality."

Conclusion

The symbol system of language has been shown to bear a different kind of relationship to each of the three art forms considered here. The relationship is never a simple one, and the pattern found often differs, depending on whether gifted or average individuals are under discussion. Still, despite the complexity of the findings, a few generalizations can be tentatively put forth.

Disorders of language appear in many cases to leave musical skill relatively unaffected. It is the right hemisphere that has a particularly important role to play, contributing not only to technical skill but also to the individual's affective relationship to music. Yet, it may well be that, in the case of the highly trained individual, left-hemisphere damage impairs the ability to perceive a piece of music in an analytic mode. Furthermore, the representation in the brain of musical abilities may differ greatly from one talented individual to another.

In the case of the visual arts, aphasias in the average individual appear to entail some loss of graphic ability. However, in the artist, in whom painting and drawing are overlearned skills, graphic ability continues to function largely independently of language and other left-hemisphere abilities. Once again, it is right-hemisphere damage that yields the most potent effects: Although it does not necessarily curtail artistic activity, it sometimes alters the style in which the artist paints.

It is, of course, in literary arts that one would expect the strongest relationship between aphasia and artistry. And, indeed, left-hemisphere damage affects the language of the writer no less than that of the average individual. Overlearning appears to be no protection against the ravages of aphasia, and the language abilities of the writer are indissoluably tied to linguistic competence per se.

The critical role of the left hemisphere in the case of the literary arts does not, however, mean that the right hemisphere is not involved. Indeed, the right hemisphere has been shown to be essential in governing attention to linguistic and extralinguistic context. Lacking such sensitivity, the right-hemisphere–injured individual often misinterprets nonliteral language and proves insensitive to the structural underpinnings of narrative materials such as jokes or stories.

The picture of symbolic functioning obtained from the study of organic patients yields certain implications for language therapy. Individuals with unilateral right-hemisphere lesions may well benefit from efforts to sensitize them to figurative or fictive uses of language, even as communication with these patients may initially proceed most effectively if their proclivity to take messages literally is borne in mind. Correlatively, even aphasic patients with severe compromise of ordinary language functions may retain basic understandings of verbal humor and narrative constructions (Bihrle et al., 1986; Gardner et al., 1983; cf. Stachowiak, Huber, Poeck, & Kerschensteiner, 1977). Upon these spared capacities, it may be possible to build, or to resurrect, enhanced understanding of the messages of daily life, as well as provide an entry to simple works of literature.

Acknowledgments

Preparation of this chapter was supported by the Veterans Administration; the National Institutes of Neurological Diseases, Communication Disorders, and Stroke (MS 11408); and Harvard Project Zero. We thank Hiram Brownell, Andrew Ellis, and Dee Michel for their thoughtful comments on an earlier version.

References

Alajouanine, T. (1948). Aphasia and artistic realization. *Brain, 71*, 229–241.

Assal, G. (1973). Aphasie de Wernicke chez un pianiste. *Revue Neurologique, 29*, 251–255.

Basso, A., & Capitani, E. (1985). Spared musical abilities in a conductor with global aphasia and ideomotor apraxia. *Journal of Neurology, Neurosurgery and Psychiatry, 48*, 407–412.

Bay, E. (1962). Aphasia and non-verbal disorders of language. *Brain, 85*, 411–426.

Bay, E. (1964). Present concepts of aphasia. *Geriatrics, 19*, 319–331.

Benton, A. L. (1977). The amusias. In M. Critchley & R. A. Henson (Eds.), *Music and the brain*. London: Heinemann.

Bever, T., & Chiarello, R. (1974). Cerebral dominance in musicians and non-musicians. *Science, 185*, 357–359.

Bihrle, A. M., Brownell, H. H., Powelson, J. A., & Gardner, H. (1986). Comprehension of humorous and non-humorous materials by left and right brain-damaged patients. *Brain and Cognition, 5*, 399–411.

Blumstein, S., & Cooper, W. E. (1974). Hemispheric processing of intonation contours. *Cortex, 10*, 146–158.

Bogen, J., & Gordon, H. (1971). Musical tests for functional lateralization with intra-carotid amabarbital. *Nature (London), 230*, 524–525.

Botez, M. I., & Wertheim, N. (1959). Expressive aphasia and amusia following right frontal lesion in a right handed man. *Brain, 82*, 186–201.

Brownell, H. H., Ostrove, J. M., Postlethwaite, W. A., Seibold, M. S., Roman, M., MacDougall, D. L., & Gardner, H. (submitted). Sensitivity to tonal goodness and pitch height in unilaterally left- and right-hemisphere brain-damaged patients.

Brownell, H. H., Potter, H. H., Bihrle, A. M., & Gardner, H. (1986). Inference deficits in right brain-damaged patients. *Brain and Language, 27*, 310–321.

Caplan, L. R. (in press). Drawing, copying and brain lesions. In A. Shindler (Ed.), *Art and the brain*.

Cicone, M., Wapner, W., & Gardner, H. (1980). Sensitivity to emotional expressions and situations in organic patients. *Cortex, 16*, 145–158.

Delis, D. C., Wapner, W., Gardner, H., & Moses, J. A. (1983). The contributions of the right hemisphere to the organization of paragraphs. *Cortex, 19*, 43–50.

Deutsch, D. (Ed.). (1982). *The psychology of music*. New York: Academic Press.

Dowling, W. J. (1978). Scale and contour. Two components of a theory of memory for melodies. *Psychological Review, 85*, 341–354.

Dowling, W. J. (1979). *Mental structures through which music is perceived*. Paper presented at the National Symposium on the Applications of Psychology to the Teaching and Learning of Music, Ann Arbor, MI.

Feuchtwanger, E. (1930). *Amusie*. Berlin: Springer-Verlag.

Foldi, N. S. (1987). Appreciation of pragmatic interpretations of indirect commands: Comparison of right and left hemisphere brain-damaged patients. *Brain and Language, 31,* 88–108.

Galin, D. (1974). Implications for psychiatry of left and right cerebral specialization. *Archives of General Psychiatry, 35,* 572–583.

Gardner, H. (1975a, October). *Artistry following aphasia.* Paper presented at the Academy of Aphasia, Victoria, B.C.

Gardner, H. (1975b). *The shattered mind.* New York: Alfred Knopf.

Gardner, H. (1982). *Art, mind, and brain.* New York: Basic Books.

Gardner, H. (1985). *The mind's new science: A history of the cognitive revolution.* New York: Basic Books.

Gardner, H., Brownell, H. H., Wapner, W., & Michelow, D. (1983). Missing the point: The role of the right hemisphere in the processing of complex linguistic materials. In E. Perecman (Ed.), *Cognitive processing in the right hemisphere.* New York: Academic Press.

Gardner, H., & Denes, G. (1973). Connotative judgments by aphasic patients on a pictorial adaptation of the semantic differential. *Cortex, 9,* 183–196.

Gardner, H., & Perkins, D. (Eds.). (1989). *Art, mind, and education.* Chicago: University of Illinois Press.

Gardner, H., Silverman, J., Denes, G., Semenza, C., & Rosenstiel, A. (1977). Sensitivity to musical denotation and connotation in organic patients. *Cortex, 13,* 243–256.

Gazzaniga, M. (1970). *The bisected brain.* New York: Appleton.

Gombrich, E. H. (1960). *Art and illusion.* Princeton, NJ: Bolligen.

Goodglass, H., & Kaplan, E. (1972). *The assessment of aphasia and related disorders.* Philadelphia, PA: Lea & Febiger.

Goodman, N. (1968). *Languages of art.* Indianapolis, IN: Bobbs-Merrill.

Goodman, N. (1972). *Problems and projects.* Indianapolis, IN: Bobbs-Merrill.

Goodman, N. (1979). *Ways of worldmaking.* Indianapolis, IN: Hackett Publishing.

Gordon, H. W. (1970). Hemispheric asymmetries in the perception of musical chords. *Cortex, 6,* 387–398.

Gordon, H. W. (1980). Degree of ear asymmetries for perception of dichotic chords and for illusory levels of competence. *Journal of Experimental Psychology: Human Perception and Performance, 6,* 516–527.

Grossman, M. (1980, February). *Figurative referential skills after brain damage.* Paper presented at the International Neuropsychological Society, San Diego, CA.

Heilman, K. (1976, October). *Affective disorders associated with right hemisphere disease.* Invited address to Aphasia Academy, Miami, FL.

Helm-Estabrooks, N. (1983). Exploiting the right hemisphere for language rehabilitation: Melodic intonation therapy. In E. Perecman (Ed.), *Cognitive processing in the right hemisphere.* New York: Academic Press.

Hirst, W., LeDoux, J., & Stein, S. (1984). Constraints on the processing of indirect speech acts: Evidence from aphasiology. *Brain and Language, 23,* 26–33.

Joanette, Y., Goulet, P., Ska, B., & Nespoulous, J.-L. (1986). Informative content of narrative discourse in right-brain-damaged right-handers. *Brain and Language, 29,* 81–105.

Jones-Gotman, M., & Milner, B. (1977). Design fluency: The invention of nonsense drawings after local cortical lesions. *Neuropsychologia, 15,* 653–674.

Judd, T., Gardner, H., & Geschwind, N. (1983). Alexia without agraphia in a composer. *Brain, 106,* 435–457.

Jung, R. (1974). Neuropsychologie und Neurophysiologie des Kontur—Formensehens in Zeichung und Malerei. In H. H. Wieck (Ed.), *Psychopathologie Musischer Gestaltungen.* Stuttgart: Schattauer-Verlag.

Kaplan, E. (1982). Process and achievement revisited. In S. Wapner & B. Kaplan (Eds.), *Towards holistic developmental psychology.* Hillsdale, NJ: Erlbaum.

Kaplan, J., Brownell, H. H., Jacobs, J. R., & Gardner, H. (1990). The effects of right hemisphere damage on the pragmatic interpretation of conversational remarks. *Brain and Language* **38,** 315–333.

Kaplan, J., & Gardner, H. (1989). Artistry after unilateral brain disease. In F. Boller & J. Grafman (Eds.), *Handbook of neuropsychology* (Vol. 2). Amsterdam: Elsevier.

Kimura, D. (1973). The asymmetry of the human brain. *Scientific American, 228,* 70–78.

Kimura, D. & Faust, R. (1985). Spontaneous drawing in an unselected sample of patients with unilateral cerebral damage. Research Bulletin # 624, Dept. of Psychology, University of Western Ontario. London, Ontario.

Kleist, K. (1962). *Sensory aphasia and amusia.* Oxford: Pergamon.

Krumhansl, C. (1979). The psychological representation of musical pitch in a tonal context. *Cognitive Psychology, 11,* 346–374.

Lerdahl, F., & Jackendoff, R. (1983). *A generative theory of tonal music.* Cambridge, MA: MIT Press.

Luria, A. R., Tsvetkova, L. S., & Futer, D. S. (1965). Aphasia in a composer. *Journal of Neurological Science, 2,* 288–292.

Lyon, J. G., & Helm-Estabrooks, N. (1987). Drawing: Its communicative significance for expressively restricted aphasic adults. *Topics in Language Disorders, 8,* 61–71.

Marin, O. S. M. (1982). Neurological aspects of music perception and performance. In D. Deutsch (Ed.), *The psychology of music.* New York: Academic Press.

Marsh, G. G., & Philwin, B. (1987). Unilateral neglect and constructional apraxia in a right-handed artist with a left posterior lesion. *Cortex, 23,* 149–155.

Meyer, L. (1956). *Emotion and meaning in music.* Chicago, IL: University of Chicago Press.

Milner, B. (1962). Laterality effects in audition. In V. B. Mountcastle (Ed.), *Interhemispheric relations and cerebral dominance.* Baltimore, MD: Johns Hopkins Press.

Molloy, R., Brownell, H. H., & Gardner, H. (1990). Discourse comprehension by right hemisphere stroke patients: Deficits of prediction and revision. In Y. Joanette & H. H. Brownell (Eds.), *Discourse ability and brain damage: Theoretical and empirical perspectives.* New York: Springer-Verlag.

Moya, K. L., Benowitz, L. I., Levine, D. N., & Finklestein, S. (1986). Covariant deficits in visuospatial abilities and recall of verbal narrative after right hemisphere stroke. *Cortex, 22,* 381–397.

Nebes, R. (1974). Hemispheric specialization in commissurotomized man. *Psychological Bulletin, 81,* 1–14.

Plimpton, G. (Ed.). (1977). *Writers at work* (Vol. 3). New York: Penguin Books.

Ross, E., & Mesulam, M. (1979). Dominant language functions of the right hemisphere: Prosody and emotional gesturing. *Archives of Neurology (Chicago), 36,* 144–148.

Selfe, L. (1977). *Nadia.* New York: Academic Press.

Shankweiler, D. (1966). Effects of temporal lobe damage on perception of dichotically presented melodies. *Journal of Comparative and Physiological Psychology, 62,* 115.

Shanon, B. (1980). Lateralization effects in musical decision tasks. *Neuropsychologia, 18,* 21–31.

Shapiro, B., Grossman, M., & Gardner, H. (1981). Selective musical processing deficits in brain damaged populations. *Neuropsychologia, 19,* 161–169.

Sidtis, J. J., & Volpe, B. T. (1981, February). *Right hemisphere lateralization of complex pitch perception: A possible basis for amusia.* Paper presented at the International Neurological Society.

Sloboda, J. A. (1985). *The musical land.* Oxford: Clarendon Press.

Sloboda, J. A. (Ed.). (1988). *Generative processes in music.* Oxford: Oxford University Press (Clarendon).

Soukes, A., & Baruk, H. (1930). Autopsie d'un cas d'amusie (avec aphasie) chez un professeur de piano. *Revue Neurologique, 1,* 545–556.

Sperry, R. (1974). Lateral specialization in the surgically separated hemispheres. In F. O. Schmitt & F. Worden (Eds.), *The neurosciences: Third study program.* Cambridge, MA: MIT Press.

Stachowiak, F. J., Huber, W., Poeck, K., & Kerchensteiner, M. (1977). Text comprehension in aphasia. *Brain and Language, 4,* 177–195.

Taylor, J. (Ed.). (1932). *Selected writings of John Hughlings Jackson* (Vols. 1 and 2). London: Hodder & Stoughton.

Ustvedt, H. (1937). Über die untersuchung der musikalischen funktionen bei patienten mit gerhirnleiden, besonders bei patienten mit aphasie. *Acta Medica Scandinavica, Supplementum, 86.*

Wapner, W., Hamby, S., & Gardner, H. (1981). The role of the right hemisphere in the organization of complex linguistic materials. *Brain and Language, 14,* 15–33.

Wapner, W., Judd, T., & Gardner, H. (1978). Visual agnosia in an artist. *Cortex, 14,* 343–364.

Wertheim, N., & Botez, M. (1961). Receptive amusia. *Brain, 84,* 19–30.

Weylman, S. T., Brownell, H. H., Roman, M., & Gardner, H. (1989). Appreciation of indirect requests by left- and right-brain-damaged patients: The effects of verbal context and conventionality of wording. *Brain and Language, 36,* 580–591.

Winner, E. (1982). *Invented worlds: The psychology of the arts.* Cambridge, MA: Harvard University Press.

Winner, E., & Gardner, H. (1977). The comprehension of metaphor in brain damaged patients. *Brain, 100,* 719–727.

Zaidel, E. (1973). *Linguistic competence and related functions in the right hemisphere of man following cerebral commissurotomy and hemispherectomy.* Unpublished doctoral dissertation, California Institute of Technology, Pasadena.

Zaidel, E. (1977). Unilateral auditory language comprehension on the Token Test following cerebral commissurotomy and hemispherectomy. *Neuropsychologia, 15,* 1–8.

Zaidel, E. (1978a). Auditory language comprehension in the right hemisphere following cerebral commissurotomy and hemispherectomy: A comparison with child language and aphasia. In A. Caramazza & E. B. Zurif (Eds.), *Language acquisition and language breakdown: Parallels and divergences.* Baltimore, MD: Johns Hopkins Press.

Zaidel, E. (1978b). The elusive right hemisphere of the brain. *Engineering and Science, 42.*

Zaimov, K., Kitov, D., & Kolev, N. (1969). Aphasie chez un peintre. *Encephale, 68,* 377–417.

Zattore, R. J. (1979). Recognition of dichotic melodies by musicians and nonmusicians. *Neuropsychologia, 17,* 607–617.

Zatorre, R. J. (1984). Musical perception and cerebral function: A critical review. *Music Perception, 2,* 196–221.

12

Language in Aging and Dementia

RHODA AU, LORAINE K. OBLER, and MARTIN L. ALBERT

Research on language in the aged has proliferated in the past decade. In 1980 when Obler and Albert provided a comprehensive overview of language in aphasia and dementia, few experimental studies had been published. Over these last 10 years, numerous projects from various disciplines have reported on language in the elderly. As a result, it becomes a challenge to present a comprehensive review of the entire literature. Consequently, in this chapter we focus on selected issues related to language in the elderly.

First, we discuss the language abilities of normal elderly adults. It is important to understand the patterns of language change that occur during normal aging, both to further our knowledge of the brain bases of language and to appreciate the language profiles of elderly populations with cerebral dysfunction. Second, we present evidence suggesting that different age groups may be more or less susceptible to specific types of aphasia. Moreover, patterns of recovery from aphasia may be influenced by age-related factors. In the third section we describe the general pattern of language change that accompanies the progressive decline of dementia of the Alzheimer's type (DAT). In the final section we address the issue of whether the language of DAT can, or should be, characterized as aphasia.

Language in Normal Aging

Early research on language in normal adults reported no age-related differences. Botwinick and Storandt (1974) administered the Wechsler Adult Intelligence Scale (WAIS) Vocabulary subtest to both young (17- to

20-year-old) and elderly (62- to 83-year-old) subjects, and reported no differences between the two groups. They concluded that language did not change in normal aging. This conclusion, however, was premature.

In a later study, Botwinick, West, and Storandt (1975) found qualitative age-related differences for performance on the WAIS Vocabulary subtest. Using a scoring system that quantified the qualitative responses, they reported that younger subjects (20- to 59-year-olds) produced significantly more superior antonyms than did elderly subjects (60- to 79-year-olds). Furthermore, elderly subjects' responses contained more words than those of young subjects. These qualitative differences existed, despite the fact that on the quantitative measures of vocabulary, no age-related differences were evidenced.

Botwinick, West, and Storandt's (1975) findings challenged their original hypothesis that language did not change as people aged. Subsequently, numerous studies have supported the alternative theory that the language of normal elderly adults differs subtly from the language of young adults (Emery, 1985, 1986; Kynette & Kemper, 1986; Light & Burke, 1988; Obler & Albert, 1980; Sandson, Obler, & Albert, 1987). In the remainder of this section, we focus on age-related differences that have been found in different areas of language.

Naming Abilities in Normal Aging

Naming involves retrieving the word label for a concept whose semantic representation has been activated. One test of naming is the Boston Naming Test (BNT; Kaplan, Goodglass, & Weintraub, 1976). In this test, subjects are shown line drawings of objects and are asked to identify them. Borod, Goodglass, and Kaplan (1980) administered the BNT to normal adults ranging in age from under 40 to 85 years and found that naming performance declined significantly after age 69. Nicholas, Obler, Albert, and Goodglass (1985) demonstrated that this age-related naming deficit was not limited to the naming of objects; they found a similar pattern of decline for naming of action pictures among subjects whose ages ranged from 30 to 79 years. On both tests, elderly subjects produced significantly fewer names than did young subjects. More recently, Au, Obler, Joung, and Albert (1990) analyzed longitudinally collected naming data that confirmed that the age-related DIFFERENCES in naming reported in cross-sectional studies were, in fact, age-related CHANGES. Over a 7-year period, 66 subjects, initially aged 30 to 75, demonstrated a slow, progressive decline in naming, despite the fact that these subjects had been given the same set of pictured stimuli at each of three test sessions.

Additional naming studies using different paradigms have also found an age-related decline in naming. Cohen and Faulkner (1986) asked young (20- to 39-year-old), middle-aged (40- to 59-year-old), and old (60- to 80-year-old) subjects to record the next instance when they were unable to recall a word name. When a name block occurred, subjects filled out a questionnaire which probed for information about the target word. In responding to the questions, the subjects described target word characteristics, such as phonological, orthographic, or semantic information. Cohen and Faulkner found that old subjects produced significantly more responses that contained conceptual information about the target word than did young or middle-aged subjects. On the other hand, old subjects' responses were significantly less likely to contain phonological information that corresponded to the target word than those of young or middle-aged subjects. Cohen and Faulkner concluded that the decline found in naming in normal aging could be attributed to retrieval failure rather than to a loss in representational memory.

The tip-of-the-tongue (TOT) phenomenon (i.e., knowing a word without being able to name it) provides another means of looking at naming deficits in elderly adults. Burke, Worthley, and Martin (1988) conducted a diary study examining TOTs in two sets of subjects, the first having a mean age of 19.7 and the second having a mean age of 70.5. They reported retrieval patterns similar to those reported by Cohen and Faulkner. They asked subjects to record TOT occurrences over a 4-week interval. Elderly subjects experienced significantly more TOTs than younger subjects. Both young and old subjects, however, were able to resolve most TOTs, suggesting again that the naming problem is a retrieval problem rather than a representational one.

The nature of the retrieval failure in naming among elderly adults was investigated by Bowles and Poon (1985) who used a naming-to-definition paradigm. Subjects were presented a definition, thereby activating a concept in semantic memory, and were asked to name the defined word. Preceding each definition was one of several primes. These primes varied in the amount of phonological–orthographic information they provided about the target word. Bowles and Poon found that the naming deficit evidenced in elderly subjects (aged 66 to 80 years) was maximized in the absence of orthographic–phonological information. When orthographic–phonological information was provided, the naming deficit was minimal. Bowles and Poon concluded that elderly subjects were able to activate the correct semantic representation elicited from the definition, but had difficulty retrieving the correct name from the lexicon. Nicholas, Obler, Albert, and Goodglass (1985) reported evidence that supports Bowles and Poon's conclusion. As discussed above, elderly subjects in their study performed worse on a picture naming test than did young adult subjects. When subjects were unable to retrieve a target word spontaneously, a phonological cue was provided (i.e., the initial phoneme of the target word). As shown before, elderly subjects required more phonological cues than did younger subjects. When a cue was provided, however, young and old subjects were equally likely to benefit from the cue. In other words, the target word information was equally available in both young and old adults, but old subjects had more difficulty accessing that information via semantic routes.

Converging evidence thus suggests that the language changes in normal aging include naming deficits related to accessing the lexicon via the semantic network. The language changes of normal aging are not confined to changes in naming, however. In the following section we discuss how discourse patterns of normal elderly adults differ from those of young adults.

Discourse in Normal Aging

In certain cultures, normal elderly adults are recognized and admired for their story-telling skills (Obler, 1980). Their stories are often rich in context, stemming from increased elaborateness that includes using more repetition, more modifiers, and artful chunking of sentences. It is important to realize that age-related changes in language do not necessarily imply impairment.

Indeed, Sandson et al. (1987) were able to demonstrate ways in which elderly (60- to 79-year-old) adults produced more elaborate speech than younger (30- to 39-year-old and 50- to 59-year-old) adults. They asked their younger and older subjects to describe a pictured story (Cookie Theft picture from the Boston Diagnostic Aphasia Examination; Goodglass & Kaplan, 1972, 1983). Analysis of the oral descriptions revealed that older subjects used more words per content unit than did younger subjects. This "elaborate" speech could be qualitatively characterized by filler phrases (e.g., "you know"), deictic references ("this," "that"), comments (e.g., "Isn't that funny?"), modifiers (adjectives and adverbs), and circumlocutions.

Not all discourse changes associated with age are considered positive, however. Kynette and Kemper (1986) recorded 20-min speech samples from both middle-aged (50- to 69-year-old) and older (70- to 89-year-old) subjects. They analyzed the sentences for simple versus complex grammatical form and syntactic structures. Elderly subjects produced a significantly reduced range of complex sentences compared with younger subjects. In addition, older subjects generated significantly more right-branching sentences than did younger subjects. These appear to place less demand on working memory than center-embedded or left-branching sentences. Finally, older adults made more errors than younger subjects. For example, they sometimes omitted the obligatory grammatical morphemes within syntactically simple sentences, whereas the younger subjects did not. By this analysis, the discourse of older adults is impaired. Indeed, in another type of task, a prose recall task, older adults gave significantly shorter responses than younger subjects. This shortening was related to their poorer recall of specific items (e.g., Cohen, 1979; Obler, 1980).

These results, and those of Kynette and Kemper (1986), do not address the increased elaborateness that is associated with story-telling by elderly adults. We may conclude, however, that elderly adults' discourse differs qualitatively from that of younger adults. Depending on the task and modes of analyses, the differences may be considered "deficits" or "improvements." Although discourse content changes with age, the ability to communicate does not. This distinction is important. Elderly populations demonstrate language changes, but not necessarily a decline in functional communication.

Thus far, our discussion of language in normal aging has focused on language production. Next, we discuss language comprehension. Language competence is measured by tests of comprehension, as well as by tests of language production. The following section reviews studies that investigate comprehension in normal aging.

Comprehension in Normal Aging

Numerous studies on comprehension in normal aging have reached the conclusion that comprehension abilities decline with increasing age (Cohen, 1979; Davis & Ball, 1989; Feier & Gerstman, 1980; Hasher & Zacks, 1988; Obler, Fein, Nicholas, & Albert, submitted; Obler, Nicholas, Albert & Woodward, 1985). On the other hand, some studies have reported no age-related differences in comprehension (LeDoux, Blum, & Hirst, 1983; Light & Burke, 1988; Meyer & Rice, 1981; Sasanuma et al., 1985). Light and Burke (1988) and Hasher and Zacks (1988) suggested a working memory hypothesis which can, in part, account for these conflicting results. They suggested that comprehension deficits in normal aging may be evidenced when working memory demands are high. If a comprehension task involves multiple processes that use working memory, then these processes may interfere with comprehension processes. They claimed that when memory demands are minimized, no age-related differences in comprehension will occur.

Comprehension is typically tested in one of two ways: orally or in written form. Oral comprehension is tested either by asking subjects to respond to sentences that vary in syntax, or by presenting subjects with paragraph-length material and then asking them questions about it. Written comprehension, on the other hand, is tested by having subjects read sentences or paragraphs and then asking questions that require them to make inferences.

Studies that use syntactic manipulation to test comprehension vary in their definition of syntactic complexity. Sentence structures that result in more response errors or slower reaction times are generally considered more complex than sentences that result in few errors or fast response times. Obler et al. (submitted) presented taped sentences of varied syntax to young (30- to 39-year-old and 50- to 59-year-old) and elderly (60- to 79-year-old) subjects. After each sentence presentation, a yes–no question followed. Elderly subjects gave fewer correct responses for syntactically complex sentences than for sentences that were less complex. Although this same pattern held for younger subjects, elderly subjects performed significantly worse across all syntactic conditions than younger subjects.

Manipulation of sentence syntax is a common method of testing comprehension among the elderly. Other researchers who have manipulated sentence syntax also report age-related differences (Davis & Ball, 1989; Emery, 1985, 1986; Feier & Gerstman, 1980; Obler et al., 1985). Consistently, elderly subjects perform worse across all syntactic conditions, and substantially worse on sentences of high syntactic complexity.

Reaction time measures have been used in other research to estimate working memory demands. Increases in reaction times are often assumed to reflect greater involvement of working memory processes. In a submitted study, Obler et al. reported that mean response times differed across syntactic conditions, which may, in turn, reflect variable demands on working memory. Those sentences that led to longer response times, such as those containing double negatives, may place greater demands on working memory than sentences that permitted shorter response times.

Another common method of measuring comprehension is to use tests of inferential reasoning. Results using such tests, however, have been less consistent than results using tests manipulating syntax. Age-related differences and the absence of age-related differences have both been found on tests of inferential reasoning.

Age-related differences in recall of implicit information have been reported in several studies. Cohen (1979), for example, presented sentences and paragraphs to both young (20- to 29-year-old) and old (65- to 79-year-old) subjects. After reading the test stimuli aloud, Cohen asked subjects questions that involved implicit versus explicit information. She found that age-related differences emerged for implicit information that must be extracted from the questions, but not for explicit information that was immediately available. The difference between the implicit and explicit conditions may include working memory factors. Questions that draw on implicit information require constructive processing, which must co-occur in working memory with comprehension processes. On the other hand, questions that rely on explicit information do not involve additional constructive processes that can interfere with comprehension (see Light & Burke, 1988, for review).

This working memory hypothesis can be applied to results from other studies of inferential reasoning. Hasher, Zacks, and colleagues conducted a series of studies, which included the presentation of oral and written materials (Hasher & Zacks, 1988; Zacks & Hasher, 1988; Zacks, Hasher, Doren, Hamm, & Attig, 1987). Both young (university students) and elderly (63- to 90-year-old) subjects were asked to listen to or read a paragraph and recall information that was explicitly stated, implied by the context, or not expected from the context. In the last condition, the researchers assumed that subjects would have to reevaluate the information that was presented, since the outcome was unexpected. This reevaluation was expected to place great demands on working memory in the oral presentation condition, because subjects had to retrieve stored information. For written presentation, this reevaluation was expected to place limited demands on working memory, since the information was still available in written form. Hasher, Zacks, and colleagues reported that young and elderly subjects were equally likely to recall explicit information in either presentation modality. When the material was presented orally, age-related differences emerged when recall required making the expected or unexpected inference. In the written condition, however, elderly subjects were able to make both expected and unexpected inferences. Hence, the researchers concluded that comprehension performance in normal elderly adults is dependent on working memory demands. If the comprehension task places high demands on working memory, elderly adults will perform significantly worse than young adults. Conversely, if the working demands are minimal, no age differences will emerge.

Other studies that minimized constructive processes in inferential reasoning tasks reported no differences in comprehension performance between young and old subjects (LeDoux et al., 1983; Sasanuma et al., 1985). Thus, research on comprehension highlights the importance of other influences on language in normal aging. It is invariably necessary to consider ways in which cognitive factors may affect linguistic performance.

Aphasia and Aging

Because aging affects language performance in normal elderly adults, perhaps it is not surprising that age is also related to the type of aphasia a stroke victim is likely to develop. Research has demonstrated that certain types of aphasia predominate within specific age groups (Obler, Albert, Goodglass, & Benson, 1978; Basso, Capitani, Laiacona, & Luzzatti, 1980; De Renzi, Faglioni, & Ferrari, 1980; Eslinger & Damasio, 1981; Pashek & Holland, 1988). Moreover, age may also be an important factor in determining recovery patterns. In this section, we describe the relationship between age and aphasia type, and present evidence that suggests that the prognosis for recovery of function may also be related to age.

Aging and Aphasia Type

Younger stroke patients are more likely to develop nonfluent aphasia than fluent aphasia. As people get older, the likelihood of developing fluent aphasia increases. Obler et al. (1978) studied a patient pool of 167 subjects that included adults with Broca's, Wernicke's, anomic, conduction, and global aphasia. They found that, on the average, individuals with Broca's aphasia were significantly younger (mean age 51) than those with Wernicke's aphasia (mean age 63). Furthermore, they reported that the relative proportion of patients with Wernicke's aphasia increased as age increased.

Several other teams of researchers have since confirmed Obler et al.'s findings (Basso et al., 1980; Harasymiw, Halper, & Sutherland, 1981; Pashek & Holland, 1988). Brown and Jaffe (1975) posited a theory of continuous lateralization which might account for the relationship between age and aphasia type. They proposed that the lateralization of neuropsychological functions evolved across the lifespan such that a 50-year-old and a 70-year-old with identical lesions would present with different patterns of deficits. Eslinger and Damasio (1981) adopted Brown and Jaffe's arguments and suggested that in the later decades, changes occur within the middle cerebral artery itself, such that strokes are likely to occur more posteriorly or envelop a larger area of the territory of the middle cerebral artery.

To test Brown and Jaffe's hypothesis, Basso, Bracchi, Capitani, Laiacona, and Zanobio (1987) recorded the age and aphasia type of 198 patients. They confirmed previous reports that subjects with nonfluent aphasia are, on average, younger than those with fluent aphasia. Moreover, patient computerized tomographic (CT) scans revealed no age differences in lesion sites. In fact, half the older patients who presented with a fluent aphasia had anterior lesions, whereas younger patients with similar anterior lesions had nonfluent aphasia. In an earlier study Basso et al. (1980) cautioned that, although a correlation between age and aphasia type exists, other differences between young and old age groups must also be considered. Although they also reported that subjects with fluent aphasia were older than subjects with nonfluent aphasia, they suggested that these results may reflect the fact that there is an age bias for survivability. Because nonfluent aphasia correlates with larger lesions than fluent aphasia, older persons who have larger lesions may not survive, whereas young patients may prove more resilient. Basso et al. (1987), however, did not report any significant data that support their argument.

It seems clear that processes of aging modify the neurologic substrate of language such that different aphasia syndromes occur with greater frequency in younger and older persons. The nature of these neurobiologic changes remains to be determined.

Aging and Recovery of Function

Although it is often assumed that elderly patients do not recover from aphasia as well as younger persons, in fact, the effect of aging on recovery of function has not been widely addressed. Sarno (1980) noted that contradictory findings have been reported, even within her own research. In one study, Sands, Sarno, and Shankweiler (1969) reported that age was the single most important factor that determined the extent of recovery of function. Younger patients with aphasia, on average, recover to a greater extent than older subjects. Their results from this study concur with those from Vignolo's (1964) earlier study, where he reported a correlation between age and recovery. Younger patients were significantly more likely to demonstrate some recovery than patients over 65 years of age. More recently, Sasanuma (1989) and Holland, Greenhouse, Fromm, and Swindell (1989) documented that geriatric patients with aphasia showed significantly less functional improvement with speech therapy than did younger adults with aphasia.

In contrast, numerous studies have indicated that no direct relationship exists between age of onset and extent of recovery (Culton, 1971; Kenin & Swisher, 1972; Kertesz & McCabe, 1977; Sarno, 1980; Sarno & Levita, 1971; Sarno, Silverman, & Levita, 1970). Kertesz and McCabe (1977), for example, reported that although age correlated positively with recovery of function, the correlation was not significant. Severity of aphasia, however, did correlate significantly with recovery.

The more severe the aphasia, the less promising the prognosis for recovery. Although, Kertesz and McCabe concluded that age was not an important factor in determining prognosis, they could not rule out that it did not contribute to recovery. Age, severity, and recovery may be interrelated. The prognosis for spontaneous recovery of a young patient with mild aphasic symptoms is generally good. In contrast, an elderly patient with severe aphasia most likely has a low probability for significant spontaneous recovery.

In light of the contradictory findings, it may be premature to rule out all age effects on recovery of function in aphasia. Research on recovery has also indicated that individuals with different aphasia types recover at different rates. Moreover, the pattern and extent of recovery varies with different types of aphasia. We have already presented evidence indicating that age relates to aphasia type; therefore, if age affects aphasia type, and different aphasia types have different patterns of recovery, it holds that age would have at least an indirect influence on recovery of function.

Consider the findings of Kertesz and McCabe (1977), for example, who documented both rate and extent of recovery for different types of aphasia. They noted that patients with Broca's aphasia recovered at the fastest rate, and those with conduction aphasia recovered more slowly than those with Broca's aphasia, but on average faster than patients with other types of aphasia. Those with untreated global aphasia and anomic aphasia recovered most slowly. Although recovery from anomic aphasia was slow, the extent of recovery of function in these patients was the greatest. In general, patients with conduction and Broca's aphasia also demonstrated significant recovery. Among patients with Broca's aphasia, age was a factor in recovery: Younger patients experienced greater recovery than older patients. Patients who had Wernicke's aphasia showed a bimodal distribution of recovery. Those patients who produced jargon speech showed little improvement over time, whereas those who used little jargon (and had low aphasia severity scores) showed substantial recovery of function. Subjects with global aphasia showed the least amount of recovery. These data support our contention that age at least indirectly influences recovery. Since a higher incidence of Broca's aphasia occurs among younger patients, and those with Broca's aphasia demonstrate significant recovery, it follows that younger patients have a better prognosis for recovery than older patients.

Age may also influence recovery of function in multilinguals. Two hypotheses that predict which language is most likely to recover poststroke have been proposed. Ribot's (1881) rule suggests that the first language returns first, whereas Pitres's (1895) rule predicts that the language used most recently will recover first. Obler and Albert (1977) reviewed the data on 106 case studies of multilinguals to determine which rule was viable, and whether age was a factor in predicting which language would recover. For the group as a whole, only Pitres's rule was followed with significantly greater than chance likelihood. Pitres's rule was applicable for young adult and middle-aged subjects (under age 65). When the oldest subjects were considered separately, however, those over age 65 were no more or less likely to recover the language they were speaking at the time of the aphasia-provoking incident than any other language they had used previously.

These observations suggest that until the 60s, "practice" influences accessibility of a language, but among older subjects with aphasia, additional and complex factors are operating. One of these factors, not yet subjected to experimental study, is the extent to which dementia may play a role in recovery patterns.

Language in Dementia of the Alzheimer's Type

The language of dementia of the Alzheimer's type (DAT) can be distinguished from language patterns in normal aging and in aphasia. One primary symptom of DAT is a progressive decline in language and other cognitive functions, especially memory. This decline may occur rapidly or at variable rates (Cummings & Benson, 1983; Martin et al., 1986), but its progressive nature distinguishes it from classical, stroke-induced aphasia syndromes. Numerous studies have documented the language patterns that accompany dementing disorders, in particular DAT (Appel, Kertesz, & Fisman, 1982; Bayles & Kaszniak, 1987; Cummings, Benson, Hill, & Read, 1985; Kaszniak & Wilson, 1985; Kertesz, Appell, & Fisman, 1986; Obler & Albert, 1981, 1984; Sasanuma et al., 1985; Selnes, Carson, Rovner, & Gordon, 1988). Obler and Albert (1984) proposed a three-stage model to describe the general pattern of language change in dementia. Although this pattern has been confirmed in other studies, Martin et al. (1986) cautioned that the overall presenting symptoms in dementia, particularly in DAT, vary from case to case. They identified neuropsychological subtypes of Alzheimer's disease that could be characterized by different patterns of progressive decline. For example, one group might demonstrate more rapid motor decline relative to other functions, whereas another group might show significant impairment in memory and relative preservation of language. Despite variability in the extent of the deficits and the rate of decline, a general pattern of language change in DAT has been documented. See Bayles and Kasniak (1987) and Kertesz and Kertesz (1988) for additional reviews.

Language in early to early-mid stages of Alzheimer's disease is marked by deficits in naming. Speech is often circumlocutory and contains verbal paraphasias, that is, errors associated with word-finding difficulties (Nicholas, Obler, Albert, & Helm-Estabrooks, 1985). However, speech is also well articulated, fluent, prosodic, and syntactically preserved. Other language areas, such as comprehension and repetition, appear to be relatively intact.

Mid to mid-late stages in Alzheimer's disease are marked by significant changes in language. Naming is severely impaired and marked by speech errors, including verbal and literal paraphasias, neologisms, perseverations, and unrelated responses. Speech, although well articulated, becomes hyperfluent, paragrammatic, fragmented, and tangential. Writing mirrors spoken output, and comprehension is mildly to moderately impaired.

In the late stage of Alzheimer's disease, language is severely impaired in all aspects, and at the end stages may become markedly reduced. Sandson et al. (1987) characterized language in the late stage as nonfluent, palilalic, echolalic, and perseverative. Comprehension, reading, and writing were severely impaired. Causino, Obler, Knoefel, and Albert (submitted), however, noted that some pragmatic communication skills were preserved in the late stages. This permitted limited interaction between the patient and the caretaker. Hier, Hagenlocker, and Shindler (1985) documented that patients with late-stage Alzheimer's disease retain minimal repetition skills. Few data have been available on the language deficits in the late to end stages of Alzheimer's disease because testing becomes virtually impossible.

It is interesting to note that each stage of the three-stage pattern of language in dementia corresponds to different aphasic syndromes. The relatively isolated word-finding problems that characterize the early to early-mid stages of Alzheimer's disease are similar to those of anomic aphasia. Nicholas, Obler, Albert, and Helm-Estabrooks (1985) compared the naming deficits of anomic aphasia and those of the early to early-mid stages of Alzheimer's disease and found no significant differences between the two groups. Other researchers have also noted the similarity in naming performances between anomic aphasia and early to early-mid stages of Alzheimer's disease (Albert, 1980; Gewirth, Shindler, & Hier, 1984; Hier et al., 1985; Kertesz & Kertesz, 1988; Schwartz, Marin, & Saffran, 1979).

The language deficits documented in the mid to mid-late stages of

Alzheimer's disease have been compared with those of Wernicke's aphasia and transcortical sensory aphasia. The fluent speech that contains paraphasic errors and the impaired comprehension characteristics of mid to mid-late stages of Alzheimer's disease resemble the impairments found in the fluent aphasias. Wernicke's aphasia and transcortical sensory aphasia are distinguished by the impairment of repetition in the former and its sparing in the latter. The preservation of repetition abilities in Alzheimer's disease has not been consistently reported, however. Cummings et al. (1985) reported that patients with mid to mid-stage Alzheimer's disease demonstrate impaired repetition skills. The results of other studies are consistent with these findings (Albert, 1980; Appell et al., 1982; Kertesz & Kertesz, 1988). Relative to other language abilities, repetition may appear to be spared, however, especially in echolalic patients.

The late stages of Alzheimer's disease are marked by severe deficits in all language areas, not unlike global aphasia (Kertesz et al., 1986). We have been intrigued by the clinical observation that severe nonfluent aphasia virtually never occurs in DAT until the late stages. This clinical observation may serve as a diagnostic clue in distinguishing among dementia syndromes. If the dementia syndrome is mild or moderate, and if the patient has a nonfluent aphasia, the diagnosis is not likely to be Alzheimer's disease.

Aphasia in Dementia

The similarity between language changes in Alzheimer's disease and in certain aphasic syndromes has generated a debate as to whether the language changes found in DAT should be called aphasia. Those researchers who argue in favor of labeling the language of DAT as aphasia point to the similar patterns of impairment in patients with Alzheimer's disease and those with aphasia (Cummings & Benson, 1983; Cummings et al., 1985; Faber-Langendoen et al., 1988; Hier et al., 1985; Kertesz & Kertesz, 1988; Murdoch, Chenery, Wilks, & Boyle, 1987; Wechsler, 1977). In contrast, those who argue against labeling the language of DAT as aphasia focus on the qualitative differences in the responses that are produced by subjects with DAT versus those with aphasia (Bayles, 1984; Bayles & Kaszniak, 1987; Bayles & Tomoeda, 1989).

Gonzalez-Rothi (1988) identified two central problems that contribute to the controversy of whether the language of DAT should be called aphasia. One problem revolves around the definition of aphasia, and the second involves qualitative differences between neurologic syndromes caused by focal lesions and those associated with multifocal brain damage. She observed that the professional discipline of the person doing the labeling was a major factor in determining the response. Neurologists generally view aphasia as a behavioral syndrome, characterized by certain signs, and independent of etiology or neuropathology. Nonneurologists, and particularly speech–language pathologists, maintain that aphasia is a syndrome of language deficits that necessarily includes etiology and neuropathology. Moreover, these language deficits occur in the relative absence of other cognitive impairments. Gonzalez-Rothi concluded that a diagnosis of aphasia should not depend on the absence of cognitive deficits. Au (1989) pointed out that language and cognition are not mutually exclusive. In fact, current measures of language performance do not exclude cognitive variables, and vice versa.

Another important consideration in this debate is that the classification of aphasia is still evolving. Clustering aphasic signs into different syndromes developed from the experience of clinicopathological observations, and was used to help increase our understanding of brain–language relationships. Those relationships are still not fully determined. Contemporary techniques of neuroimaging and emerging theories of cognitive neuroscience are leading to revisions in classic dogmas of aphasia classification.

Moreover, studies of communication breakdown in DAT can provide complementary information to that from patients with gross focal lesions (Sasanuma, 1988). It would be naive to think that a connectionist model, derived from studies of focal lesion patients, accurately reflects cell-level structural and functional neurologic organization. Studies of language in DAT can highlight areas of language deficit that occur with no clear correlation with lesion location, and that are possibly related to pharmacosystems dysfunction.

Au, Albert, and Obler (1988) proposed that advances made in the study of DAT may prove useful in the treatment of aphasia. A pilot test conducted by Albert, Bachman, Morgan, and Helm-Estabrooks (1988) has already made advances in this direction. Albert and colleagues administered bromocriptine to a subject with aphasia. The impetus for this pharmacotherapy treatment stemmed from research on pharmacosystems in DAT. Albert et al. (1988) found that when a patient with nonfluent aphasia was given bromocriptine, he performed better on language tests than when he was not medicated. The limited success of this pilot study highlights the advantages that an integration of research from DAT and aphasia will provide. We maintain that this synthesis will serve only to enhance our understanding of brain–behavior relationships.

Summary

We have addressed several key areas related to language changes in aging. Within the normal aging population, we find age-related differences on naming, discourse, and comprehension tasks. Age also plays a role in language patterns that are characteristic of patients with neurologic dysfunction. Among patients with focal lesions, the type of aphasic syndrome that is likely to develop is related to factors associated with the process of aging. Nonfluent aphasias are more likely to occur among younger patients, whereas fluent aphasias increase in frequency as people get older. The role of age with respect to recovery of function is still unclear. A number of studies indicate that younger patients, on average, show greater recovery than older patients; however, whether this correlation is directly related to age per se, or is a consequence of other variables such as aphasia type, has yet to be determined.

The progressive decline of DAT is accompanied by characteristic changes in language. Current debates among researchers and clinicians include discussions concerning whether the language of DAT should be called aphasia. The benefits in doing so will be to bring together ideas about brain–behavior relationships that were developed in parallel, within different scientific disciplines, and to use them to explore new directions for research and treatment.

As the elderly population continues to grow, the need to achieve a better understanding of language behavior in an aging population will increase. Pragmatic implications of this line of investigation include improving communication with and among a normal aging population, and developing new and effective treatment techniques for those elderly persons who are neurologically impaired.

Acknowledgments

Preparation of this paper was supported in part by the Veterans Administration Medical Research Service, NIH Program Project DC00081-25, and the Seidel Fund for Research in Dementia.

References

Albert, M. L. (1980). Language in normal and dementing elderly. In L. K. Obler & M. L. Albert (Eds.), *Language and communication in the elderly.* Boston, MA: D. C. Heath.

Albert, M. L., Bachman, D., Morgan, A., & Helm-Estabrooks, N. (1988). Pharmacotherapy for aphasia. *Neurology, 38,* 877–879.

Appell, J., Kertesz, A., & Fisman, M. (1982). A study of language functioning in Alzheimer patients. *Brain and Language, 17,* 73–91.

Au, R. (1989). Cognitive cloud: Thunderheads on the horizon? *Aphasiology, 3,* 751–753.

Au, R., Albert, M. L., & Obler, L. K. (1988). The relation of aphasia to dementia. *Aphasiology, 2,* 161–173.

Au, R., Obler, L. K., Joung, P., & Albert, M. L. (1990). Naming in normal aging: Age-related differences or age-related changes? *Journal of Clinical and Experimental Neuropsychology, 12,* 30.

Basso, A., Bracchi, M., Capitani, E., Laiacona, M., & Zanobio, M. E. (1987). Age and evolution of language area functions: A study of adult stroke patients. *Cortex, 23,* 475–483.

Basso, A., Capitani, E., Laiacona, M., & Luzzatti, C. (1980). Factors influencing type and severity of aphasia. *Cortex, 16,* 631–636.

Bayles, K. A. (1984). Language and dementia. In A. Holland (Ed.), *Language disorders in adults.* San Diego, CA: College-Hill Press.

Bayles, K. A., & Kaszniak, A. W. (1987). *Communication and cognition in normal aging and dementia.* Boston, MA: College Hill Press.

Bayles, K. A., & Tomoeda, C. (1989). *Are the communications disorders of dementia appropriately characterized as aphasia?* Presented at the American Speech-Language-Hearing Association Meeting, Boston, MA.

Borod, J., Goodglass, H., & Kaplan, E. (1980). Normative data on the Boston Diagnostic Aphasia Examination, Parietal Lobe Battery, and the Boston Naming Test. *Journal of Clinical Neuropsychology, 2,* 209–215.

Botwinick, J., & Storandt, M. (1974). Vocabulary ability in later life. *Journal of Genetic Psychology, 125,* 303–308.

Botwinick, J., West, R., & Storandt, M. (1975). Qualitative vocabulary test responses and age. *Journal of Gerontology, 30,* 574–577.

Bowles, N. L., & Poon, L. W. (1985). Aging and retrieval of words in semantic memory. *Journal of Gerontology, 40,* 71–77.

Brown, J., & Jaffe, J. (1975). Hypothesis on cerebral dominance. *Neuropsychologia, 13,* 107–110.

Burke, D., Worthley, J., & Martin, J. (1988). I'll never forget what's-her-name: Aging and tip of the tongue experiences in everyday life. In M. M. Gruenberg, P. E., Morris, and R. N. Sykes (Eds.), *Practical aspects of memory* (Vol. 2, pp. 113–118). Chichester: Wiley.

Causino, Obler, L. K., Knoefel, J., & Albert, M. L. (submitted). Pragmatic ability in late-stage dementia.

Cohen, G. (1979). Language comprehension in old age. *Cognitive Psychology, 11,* 412–429.

Cohen, G., & Faulkner, D. (1986). Memory for proper names: Age differences in retrieval. *British Journal of Developmental Psychology, 4,* 187–197.

Culton, G. L. (1971). Reaction to age as a factor in chronic aphasia in stroke patients (letter). *Journal of Speech and Hearing Disorders, 36,* 563–564.

Cummings, J. L., & Benson, D. F. (1983). *Dementia, a clinical approach.* Boston, MA: Butterworth.

Cummings, J. L., Benson, D. F., Hill, M. A., & Read, S. (1985). Aphasia in dementia of the Alzheimer type. *Neurology, 35,* 394–397.

Davis, G. A., & Ball, H. (1989). Effects of age on comprehension of complex sentences in adulthood. *Journal of Speech and Hearing Research, 32,* 143–150.

De Renzi, E., Faglioni, P., & Ferrari, P. (1980). The influence of sex and age on the incidence and type of aphasia. *Cortex, 16,* 627–630.

Emery, O. (1985). Language and aging. *Experimental aging research* (Monograph). Mount Desert, ME: Beech Hill Publishing.

Emery, O. (1986). Linguistic decrement in normal aging. *Language and Communication, 6,* 47–64.

Eslinger, P. J., & Damasio, A. R. (1981). Age and type of aphasia in patients with stroke. *Journal of Neurology, Neurosurgery and Psychiatry, 44,* 377–381.

Faber-Langendoen, K., Morris, J. C., Knesevich, J. W., LaBarge, E., Miller, J. P., & Berg, L. (1988). Aphasia in senile dementia of the Alzheimer type. *Annals of Neurology, 23,* 365–370.

Feier, C. D., & Gerstman, L. J. (1980). Sentence comprehension abilities throughout the adult life span. *Journal of Gerontology, 35,* 722–728.

Gewirth, L. R., Shindler, A. G., & Hier, D. B. (1984). Altered patterns of word association in dementia and aphasia. *Brain and Language, 21,* 307–317.

Gonzalez-Rothi, L. (1988). *Argument for and against characterizing the communication disorders of dementia as aphasia: From the perspective of behavioral neurology and neuropsychology.* Presented at the American Speech-Language and Hearing Association meeting, Boston, MA.

Goodglass, H., & Kaplan, E. (1972). *Boston diagnostic aphasia examination* (1st ed.). Philadelphia, PA: Lea & Febiger.

Goodglass, H., & Kaplan, E. (1983). *Boston Diagnostic Aphasia Examination* (2nd ed.). Philadelphia, PA: Lea & Febiger.

Harasymiw, S., Halper, A., & Sutherland, B. (1981). Sex, age, and aphasia types. *Brain and Language, 12,* 190–198.

Hasher, L., & Zacks, R. T. (1988). Working memory, comprehension, and aging: A review and a new view. In G. Bauer (Ed.), *The Psychology of Learning and Motivation: Advances in Research and Theory* (Vol. 22, pp. 193–225). San Diego, CA: Academic Press.

Hier, D. B., Hangelocker, K., & Shindler, A. G. (1985). Language disintegration in dementia: Effects of etiology and severity. *Brain and Language, 25,* 117–133.

Holland, A. L., Greenhouse, J. B., Fromm, D., & Swindell, C. S. (1989). Predictors of language restitution following stroke: A multivariate analysis. *Journal of Speech and Hearing Research, 32,* 232–238.

Kaplan, E., Goodglass, H., & Weintraub, S. (1976). *The Boston Naming Test* (Exp. ed.). Aphasia Research Center, Boston University, Boston, MA.

Kaszniak, A. W., & Wilson, R. S. (1985). *Longitudinal deterioration of language and cognition in dementia of the Alzheimer's type.* Symposium: Communication and Cognition in Dementia: Longitudinal Perspectives. International Neuropsychological Society Meeting, San Diego, CA.

Kenin, M., & Swisher, L. P. (1972). A study of pattern of recovery in aphasia. *Cortex, 8,* 56–58.

Kertesz, A., Appell, J., & Fisman, M. (1986). The dissolution of language in Alzheimer's disease. *Canadian Journal of Neurological Science, 13,* 415–418.

Kertesz, A., & Kertesz, M. (1988). Memory deficit and language dissolution in Alzheimer's disease. *Journal of Neurolinguistics, 3,* 103–114.

Kertesz, A., & McCabe, P. (1977). Recovery patterns and prognosis in aphasia. *Brain, 100,* 1–18.

Kynette, D., & Kemper, S. (1986). Aging and the loss of grammatical forms: A cross-sectional study of language performance. *Language and Communication, 6,* 65–72.

LeDoux, J. F., Blum, C., & Hirst, W. (1983). Inferential processing of context: Studies of cognitively impaired subjects. *Brain and Language, 19,* 216–224.

Light, L. L., & Burke, D. M. (1988). Patterns of language and memory in old age. In L. L. Light & D. M. Burke (Eds.), *Language, memory, and aging.* New York: Cambridge University Press.

Martin, A., Brouwers, P., LaLorde, F., Cox, C., Teleska, P., & Fedio, P. (1986). Towards a behavioral typology of Alzheimer's patients. *Journal of Clinical and Experimental Neuropsychology, 8,* 594–610.

Meyer, B. J. F., & Rice, G. E. (1981). Information recalled from prose by young, middle and old adult readers. *Experimental Aging Research, 7,* 253–268.

Murdoch, B. E., Chenery, H. J., Wilks, V., & Boyle, R. S. (1987). Language disorders in dementia of Alzheimer type. *Brain and Language, 31,* 122–137.

Nicholas, M., Obler, L. K., Albert, M. L., & Goodglass, H. (1985). Lexical retrieval in healthy aging. *Cortex, 21,* 595–606.

Nicholas, M., Obler, L. K., Albert, M. L., & Helm-Estabrooks, N. (1985). Empty speech in Alzheimer's disease, healthy aging, and aphasia. *Journal of Speech and Hearing Research, 28,* 405–410.

Obler, L. K. (1980). Narrative discourse style in the elderly. In L. K. Obler & M. L. Albert (Eds.), *Language and communication in the elderly: Clinical, therapeutic, and experimental issues.* Lexington, MA: D. C. Heath.

Obler, L. K., & Albert, M. L. (1977). Influence of aging on recovery from aphasia in polyglots (note). *Brain and Language, 4,* 460–463.

Obler, L. K., & Albert, M. L. (Eds.). (1980). *Language and communication in the elderly: Clinical, therapeutic, and experimental issues.* Lexington, MA: D. C. Heath.

Obler, L. K., & Albert, M. L. (1981). Language in the elderly aphasic and in the dementing patient. In M. T. Sarno (Ed.), *Acquired aphasia.* New York: Academic Press.

Obler, L. K., & Albert, M. L. (1984). Language in aging. In M. L. Albert (Ed.), *Clinical neurology of aging.* New York: Oxford University Press.

Obler, L. K., Albert, M. L., Goodglass, H., & Benson, D. F. (1978). Aphasia type and aging. *Brain and Language, 6,* 318–322.

Obler, L. K., Fein, D., Nicholas, M., & Albert, M. L. (submitted). Auditory comprehension and aging: Decline in syntactic processing.

Obler, L. K., Nicholas, M., Albert, M. L., & Woodward, S. (1985). On comprehension across the adult lifespan. *Cortex, 21,* 273–280.

Pashek, G. V., & Holland, A. L. (1988). Evolution of aphasia in the first year post-onset. *Cortex, 24,* 411–423.

Pîtres, A. (1895). Etude sur l'aphasie. *Revue de Médécine (Paris), 15,* 873–899.

Ribot, T. (1881). *Les maladies de la mémoire* (pp. 146–147). Paris: Librairie Germer Baillière et Cie.

Sands, E., Sarno, M. T., & Shankweiler, K. (1969). Long term assessment of language function in aphasia due to stroke. *Archives of Physical Medicine and Rehabilitation, 50,* 202–207.

Sandson, J., Obler, L. K., & Albert, M. L. (1987). Language changes in healthy aging and dementia. In S. Rosenberg (Ed.), *Advances in applied psycholinguistics* (Vol. 1). New York: Cambridge University Press.

Sarno, M. T. (1980). Language rehabilitation outcome in the elderly aphasia patient. In L. K. Obler & M. L. Albert (Eds.), *Language and communication in the elderly: Clinical, therapeutic, and experimental issues.* Lexington, MA: D. C. Heath.

Sarno, M. T., & Levita, E. (1971). Natural course of recovery in severe aphasia. *Archives of Physical Medicine and Rehabilitation, 52,* 175–179.

Sarno, M. T., Silverman, M., & Levita, E. (1970). Psychosocial factors and recovery in geriatric patients with severe aphasia. *Journal of the American Geriatrics Society, 18,* 405–409.

Sasanuma, S. (1989). Studies of dementia: In search of the linguistic/cognitive interaction underlying communication. *Aphasiology, 2,* 191–193.

Sasanuma, S. (1989). Aphasia rehabilitation in Japan: State of the art. In M. T. Sarno & D. E. Woods (Eds.), *Aphasia rehabilitation in Asia and the Pacific Region: Japan, China, India, Australia, and New Zealand.* New York: World Rehabilitation Fund.

Sasanuma, S., Itoh, M., Watamori, T. S., Fukuzawa, K., Sakuma, N., Fukusako, Y., & Monoi, H. (1985). Linguistic and nonlinguistic abilities of the Japanese elderly and patients with dementia. In H. K. Ulatowska (Ed.), *The aging brain: Communication in the elderly.* San Diego, CA: College-Hill Press.

Schwartz, M. F., Marin, O. S. M., & Saffran, E. M. (1979). Dissociations of language function in dementia: A case study. *Brain and Language, 7,* 277–306.

Selnes, O. A., Carson, K., Rovner, B., & Gordon, B. (1988). Language dysfunction in early- and late-onset possible Alzheimer's disease. *Neurology, 38,* 1053–1056.

Vignolo, L. A. (1964). Evolution of aphasia and language rehabilitation: A retrospective exploratory study. *Cortex, 1,* 344–367.

Wechsler, A. F. (1977). Presenile dementia presenting as aphasia. *Journal of Neurology, Neurosurgery and Psychiatry, 40,* 303–305.

Zacks, R. T., & Hasher, L. (1988). Capacity theory and the processing of inferences. In L. L. Light & D. M. Burke (Eds.), *Language, memory, and aging.* New York: Cambridge University Press.

Zacks, R. T., Hasher, L., Doren, B., Hamm, V., & Attig, M. S. (1987). Encoding and memory of explicit and implicit information. *Journal of Gerontology, 42,* 418–422.

13

Acquired Aphasia in Children

DOROTHY M. ARAM

Introduction

Children Versus Adults

Language disruptions secondary to acquired central nervous system (CNS) lesions differ between children and adults in multiple respects. Chief among these differences are the developmental stage of language acquisition at the time of insult and the developmental stage of the CNS.

In adult aphasia premorbid mastery of language is assumed, at least to the level of the aphasic's intellectual ability and educational opportunities. Acquired aphasia sustained in childhood, however, interferes with the developmental process of language learning and disrupts those aspects of language already mastered. The investigator and clinician thus are faced with sorting which aspects of language have been lost or impaired from those yet to emerge, potentially in an altered manner. Complicating research and clinical practice in this area has been the need to continually account for the developmental stage of that aspect of language under consideration for each child. In research, stage-appropriate language tasks must be selected, and comparison must be made to peers of comparable age and language stage. Also, appropriate controls common in adult studies, such as social class and gender, are critical. These requirements present no small challenge, as most studies involve a wide age range of children and adolescents. In clinical practice, the question is whether assessment tools used for developmental language disorders should be employed or whether adult aphasia batteries should be adapted for children. The answer typically depends upon the age of the child and the availability of age- and stage-appropriate measures. With childhood acquired aphasias, the question of how language is altered following a CNS insult is inextricably related to how language learning proceeds.

The second major difference between adults and children sustaining language-disrupting neurological insults is the stage of maturity of the CNS at the time of insult. The controversy relating to the degree of early hemispheric specialization versus equipotentiality for language (e.g., Kinsbourne & Hiscock, 1977; Lenneberg, 1967) has sparked much of the research in this area during the past 20 years. Although most of the data appear to evidence considerable early brain specialization for language and other higher cognitive functions (Best, 1988; Molfese & Segalowitz, 1988), the remarkable capacity of young children to recover from major cortical insults has been reported repeatedly. That children recover much more rapidly and completely from focal brain lesions than do adults with comparable insults has become a truism that is generally, although not universally, supported. The rapidity and level of language recovery in young brain-injured children evidence a degree of functional and presumed neural plasticity far exceeding that in adults (Aram & Eisele, in press). An immature CNS at the time of insult does not necessarily lead, however, to a more favorable outcome. In some instances— for example, conditions resulting in diffuse brain involvement—a brain insult incurred at a young age may be more, rather than less, deleterious, a topic returned to later in this chapter. The essential concern here is that just as the child's language system is in the process of development, so too is the central nervous system, processes that are complete or declining in the adult. While in many instances the immaturity of the child's CNS supports alternatives for greater functional recovery, at other times early insults appear to interfere with primary skills, thus precluding later achievements.

Terminology

ACQUIRED VERSUS DEVELOPMENTAL APHASIA

The term ACQUIRED is used to modify the term APHASIA in children to distinguish language disorders accompanied by known CNS insults from the much more common form of DEVELOPMENTAL APHASIA. Developmental aphasia, also referred to as developmental language disorders or specific language disorders, is manifest when a child fails to learn to talk normally, but a frank neurological basis is not apparent. Indeed, the presence of a frank neurological abnormality typically is established as an exclusionary criterion for the diagnosis of developmental aphasia or developmental language disorder (Benton, 1964; Tallal, 1988). Although many researchers assume abnormal neurological functions give rise to the developmental aphasias (Rapin & Allen, 1988), the search for identifiable brain lesions to account for these developmental disorders has been largely unproductive. This chapter addresses the language abilities only in children with known brain insults, that is, those with acquired aphasia.

ACQUIRED LANGUAGE LOSS VERSUS
ACQUIRED BRAIN LESION

According to the literature bearing on the topic of acquired aphasia in children, although the lesion is generally acquired—through stroke, tumor, trauma, or some other form of CNS insult—the language loss is not necessarily "acquired," as frequently the insult occurs before much language has been acquired and therefore not much can be "lost." Very few studies have been confined to older children with relatively well-developed language at the time of insult; rather most have involved a wide age range at lesion onset, typically extending from pre- or perinatal insults to those incurred during adolescence. Indeed, many studies compare outcome as a function of whether the lesion was sustained prior to 1 year of age (the somewhat arbitrary demarcation for the onset of language) or after 1 year of age, with a broad range of onset ages included in the latter group. Therefore, acquired aphasia, as used here, refers to language discrepancies or abnormalities accompanied by a known brain lesion, irrespective of when during the course of language development that lesion occurred.

Nature of the Studies Available

Although a more homogeneous age of lesion onset would be desirable in reports of acquired aphasia in children, age is only one of several, markedly heterogeneous variables complicating interpretation of the majority of studies addressing this topic. The major methodological problems confounding review of work in this area have been reviewed elsewhere (Aram & Whitaker, 1988). Five variables, typically noncomparable both within and across studies, are of particular note:

1. AGE OF LESION ONSET has been discussed above and generally involves a broad spectrum of age.

2. The NATURE OF THE NEUROLOGICAL INSULTS included within studies are typically diverse, and often include such disparate conditions as tumors, head trauma, herpes encephalitis, and cerebral vascular accidents in a single study. This chapter draws not only from studies specifically addressing acquired CNS insults and aphasias in children, but also from studies of infantile or childhood hemiplegias, as the overlap between children included in these studies is considerable. In an effort to reduce the wide diversity of conditions considered, this chapter does not treat the hemispherectomy or epileptic aphasia literature except when an occasional hemispherectomized or epileptic aphasic child has been included in a group study.

3. EXTENSIVENESS OF BRAIN INVOLVEMENT also varies widely from circumscribed focal lesions to diffuse white and gray matter involvement. Often specification of the degree of actual brain involvement is lacking and can only be inferred from the etiology or clinical pattern. This topic is discussed more fully later in this chapter.

4. AGE AT FOLLOW-UP varies both with respect to chronological age and with respect to time elapsed since lesion onset. A few studies have described language during the acute period of recovery, although most have assessed language status years after lesion onset.

5. The METHOD OF EVALUATION used in various studies has differed. Until the past 10 years, most statements pertaining to language ability were based on nonsystematic clinical observations or verbal intelligence scores. During the past 10 years studies have begun to report standardized language tests, yet few have initiated a more experimental or hypothesis testing approach to the study of acquired aphasia in children.

Because very few experimentally rich or methodologically sound studies of relatively homogeneous groups of lesioned children exist, the present review is not restricted to those few studies. Rather, an attempt has been made to cull from the diverse studies available and to interpret contradictory findings in light of the differences among studies.

In this chapter, I first review language characteristics of children with acquired aphasia, including language comprehension, language production, reading, writing, and spelling. I then discuss factors related to recovery, centering on differences in the degree of brain involvement, etiology, lesion laterality, site of lesion within a hemisphere, lesion size, and presence or absence of seizures. Finally, I derive speculations concerning the process of recovery from the limited evidence available from dichotic listening tests, sodium amytal studies, and electrophysiological findings.

The Clinical Picture: Language Characteristics

Comprehension

Comprehension is probably the least studied aspect of language in children with acquired aphasia. Despite pronouncements that receptive disorders are rare or that beyond the acute period comprehension disorders disappear rapidly and virtually completely (Hécaen, 1976, 1983), until recently few studies provided objective data substantiating these claims. Guttmann (1942) appears to be one of the few early observers noting long-standing receptive as well as expressive deficits following temporal lobe lesions in children. Alajouanine and Lhermitte (1965), although commenting that receptive disorders were rare, reported that 4 of 32 children with acquired aphasia presented marked comprehension disorders. Recently, several case studies have detailed the recovery of comprehension abilities during the acute period, usually (Aram, Rose, Rekate, & Whitaker, 1983; Ferro, Martins, Pinto, & Castro-Caldas, 1982; Martins, Ferro, & Trindade, 1987; Pohl, 1979), but not always (Dennis, 1980; Oelschlaeger & Scarborough, 1976), demonstrating complete or relatively good recovery of comprehension skills. Except for the exemplary work of Dennis and her colleagues with young hemispherectomy patients, prior to the past 10 years there appear to be no studies other than IQ results in which findings are detailed relative to comprehension abilities among children with acquired aphasia. These relatively recent studies have focused predominantly on syntactic and lexical comprehension.

SYNTACTIC COMPREHENSION

Dennis (1980) provided a comprehensive study of the acute language status of a 9-year-old girl with a left temporoparietal infarct at 2 weeks and at 3 months after lesion onset. Drawing from an array of standardized and experimental tasks, Dennis (1980) concluded that, although improvement had been observed, at 3 months after lesion onset, the child's comprehension of longer, nonredundant oral commands continued to be impaired, and lower level syntactic structures were better preserved than were more complex structures involving supraordinate schemata such as embeddings. On a metalinguistic judgment task in which the interrelatedness of words was assessed, the child seemed to adopt a simplified surface and linear processing strategy for complex utterances. Although still relatively early in recovery, this case study demonstrated significant disruption in all aspects of language, including comprehension, expression, and communicative intent; unfortunately, language status after 3 months was not reported. Other case studies have reported notable syntactic comprehension deficits acutely but with relatively good recovery within the first several months following lesion onset (Aram et al., 1983; Ferro et al., 1982; Pohl, 1979).

Several group studies of children with brain lesions studied well beyond the acute period have assessed syntactic comprehension and generally found subtle yet persistent comprehension deficits. Findings between studies vary somewhat, presumably reflecting differences in subject variables, notably the nature and diffuseness of the lesion, concomitant seizure disorders, and overall intellectual level. Levine, Huttenlocher, Banich, and Duda (1987) found that well after lesion onset, all four groups of children with left, right, congenital, and acquired hemiplegias performed below average on the Northwestern Syntax Screening Test (Lee, 1969); it should be noted, however, that these children's intelligence also was below average and half had ongoing seizure disorders. In contrast, Kiessling, Denckla, and Carlton (1983), studying groups of left- or right-hemiplegic children selected because they were functioning well in school, found a significant correlation between right-hand function on the Annett pegboard (used as a measure of left-hemisphere function) and performance on a syntactic awareness task.

Token Test (De Renzi & Vignolo, 1962) results have been reported by several groups of investigators, with findings apparently reflecting the variable subject groups under test. Woods and Carey (1979) reported that left-lesioned subjects differed from controls on the Token Test if lesion onset occurred after but not before 1 year of age. Vargha-Khadem, O'Gorman, and Watters (1985) reported that irrespective of age of onset their three left-lesioned subject groups (prenatal, early postnatal, and late postnatal) but not the three respective right-lesioned groups performed worse than control subjects. Similarly, Aram and Ekelman (1987) found performance of left- but not right-lesioned subjects to be significantly lower than that of controls and identified no relationship between age of lesion onset and revised Token Test (McNeil & Prescott, 1978) performance among lesioned subjects. Variable performance depending upon the Token Test subtest has been noted. Left-hemisphere–lesioned children have been reported to have particular difficulty with subtests that assess syntactic components (Aram & Ekelman, 1987; Cooper & Flowers, 1987; Riva, Cazzaniga, Pantaleoni, Milani, & Fedrizzi, 1986) or that tax verbal memory (Aram & Ekelman, 1987; Rankin, Aram, & Horwitz, 1981), whereas right-hemisphere–lesioned subjects have been reported to do more poorly on items requiring spatial skills (Aram & Ekelman, 1987; Riva et al., 1986). Van Dongen and Loonen (1977), studying a group of acquired aphasic children with mixed etiologies, reported that comprehension deficits on the Token Test during the acute stage were associated with a poor prognosis for recovery.

In summary, the data suggest that syntactic comprehension often is impaired following left-brain involvement. Poor subject performance by right-hemisphere–lesioned subjects appears to be related to spatial demands of the task and/or more generalized brain involvement. Beyond the acute period, most but not all syntactic comprehension deficits are mild. Poor syntactic comprehension in the acute period appears to be related to a poor prognosis for recovery. Age of lesion onset has not been found to have a consistent relationship to syntactic comprehension.

LEXICAL COMPREHENSION

Except for a few detailed case studies, lexical comprehension skills among children with acquired aphasia have been studied very little beyond the administration of the Peabody Picture Vocabulary Test (PPVT; Dunn, 1965). In a 10-year-old girl sustaining diffuse traumatic brain involvement following a fall from a horse, Oelschlaeger and Scarborough (1976) documented significant limitations in lexical comprehension 1 year after the trauma was sustained. Most group reports do not indicate deficits as pronounced as that observed by Oelschlaeger and Scarborough (1976), but do evidence mild long-standing deficits in lexical comprehension. Using the PPVT, Aram, Ekelman, Rose, and Whitaker (1985), Cooper and Flowers (1987), Levine et al. (1987), and Riva et al. (1986) all have reported lower performance by the lesioned than the control subjects. Although Kiessling et al. (1983) reported a correlation between right-hand function and PPVT performance, most studies (Aram et al., 1985; Levine et al., 1987; Riva et al., 1986) have failed to find a lateralized hemisphere effect on PPVT performance.

Using a parent informant inventory, the Language and Gesture Inventory (Bates et al., 1985), Bates and her colleagues are collecting longitudinal data detailing the emergence of language, including comprehension in very young hemiplegic children. Although the study is currently in progress and the number of children yet studied is small, thus far some interesting trends have been reported. Four of the 5 infants studied (up to 16 months of age) were delayed in lexical comprehension, irrespective of lesion laterality (Marchman, Miller, & Bates, 1989). Of the 15 children studied as toddlers (1 to $2\frac{1}{2}$ years of age), several had achieved normal or near-normal profiles of receptive lexical ability. Whereas among right-lesioned children lexical comprehension and production tended to be comparable or production exceeded comprehension, left-lesioned children tended to present marked disparity between relatively well-developed lexical comprehension and marked delays in lexical production (Thal, Marchman, & Bates, 1989).

Finally, one of the few studies (Cooper & Flowers, 1987) to examine lexical comprehension beyond single-word representation assessed meaning in context using the Processing Spoken Paragraphs subtest of the Clinical Evaluation of Language Functions (Semel-Mintz & Wiig, 1982). On this test, significant deficits among the group of chronic–brain-injured children were reported, although, due to the diffuse nature of brain involvement for most of the subjects, no attempt was made to relate findings to laterality of brain involvement.

In summary, based upon studies predominantly assessing single-word comprehension, at least mild lexical deficits have been noted in most groups of children with acquired aphasia. Lexical comprehension deficits generally have not been found to be lateralized to either left or right lesions. It has been suggested, however, that discrepancy between lexical comprehension and production may be more pronounced following left than right lesions.

Language Production

In contrast to comprehension, language production is the most extensively studied aspect of acquired childhood aphasia. Although descriptions tend to center upon reduced verbal output, descriptions of more fluent-type aphasia and paraphasic behaviors have been reported. Limited work has also addressed lexical retrieval and phonological production.

REDUCED VERBAL PRODUCTION

· Most early reports of acquired aphasia focused upon diminished speech output and telegraphic speech thought to characterize acquired aphasia in children (Alajouanine & Lhermitte, 1965; Guttmann, 1942; Hécaen, 1976, 1983). Early descriptions emphasized the striking feature of reduced verbal output, ranging from mutism to a reluctance to speak, and stated that syntax was simplified rather than erroneous (Alajouanine & Lhermitte, 1965; Guttmann, 1942; Hécaen, 1976, 1983). Equally impressive to many early observers was the rapid recovery of expressive abilities, the absence of fluent Wernicke-type aphasias, and the infrequency of paraphasias (Alajouanine & Lhermitte, 1965; Guttmann, 1942; Hécaen, 1976, 1983). Although fluent aphasias with neologistic, semantic, and phonemic paraphasias have since been described (see the next section), reduced output continues to be regarded as the dominant feature of acquired aphasia in children (Cranberg, Filley, Hart, & Alexander, 1987; Martins & Ferro, 1987).

Woods and Carey (1979) provided what appears to be the first experimental study of productive syntax in left-hemisphere–lesioned patients. Using a series of syntactic production tasks, including identifying and correcting anomalous sentences employing "that" clauses, using ask– tell distinctions, and utilizing the sentence completion task from the Boston Diagnostic Aphasia Examination (Goodglass & Kaplan, 1983), left-lesioned childhood aphasics, sustaining lesions after but not before 1 year of age, were found to differ significantly from control subjects.

Most subsequent studies of children with acquired lesions have found syntactic limitations to be associated with predominantly left but not right lesions. For example, both Kiessling et al. (1983) in a study of hemiplegic children and Riva et al. (1986) in a study of acquired lesions due to diverse etiologies, found left-hemisphere–lesioned children to perform more poorly than right-lesioned or control subjects on sentence repetition tasks. In an analysis of the spontaneous conversational language of left- and right-lesioned children studied well beyond the acute period, Aram, Ekelman, and Whitaker (1986) found left- but not right-lesioned children to perform less well on a range of measures of simple and complex sentence structure. Deficits in syntactic production rarely are reported following right lesions except in cases thought to represent crossed aphasia (Martins et al., 1987). An exception has been a recent study using a speech shadowing task (Woods, 1987) in which sentences were to be repeated in correct and reversed word order. On this task both left- and right-lesioned subjects performed more poorly than controls, despite the right-lesioned subjects' normal performance on other language measures. Woods (1987) suggested that the shadowing task tapped skills dependent upon global cerebral function, rather than more narrowly defined language functions.

Thus, it appears that reduced output and simplified syntax are the typical presentation following left-hemisphere lesions and that syntactic deficits may persist for years.

FLUENT VERBAL PRODUCTION

Many of the early descriptions of acquired aphasia in children stated that fluent aphasias did not occur or were extremely rare in children younger than 10 years of age (Alajouanine & Lhermitte, 1965; Guttmann, 1942; Hécaen, 1976). The absence of fluent aphasia in young children was ascribed to an underdeveloped or underautomatized Broca's area controlling expressive language which was incapable of "running on" in the absence of appropriate input from posterior language areas. More recently, however, several examples of fluent aphasias with jargon or logorrhea have been described in young children. Woods and Teuber (1978) appear to be one of the first to have described jargon aphasia, defined as jabbering away with unintelligible sounds as though understood, in a single 5-year-old among the 65 children studied. Additional case studies of fluent aphasias have been reported by Van Hout and Lyon (1986) and van Dongen, Loonen, and van Dongen (1985). These studies detailed young children with logorrheic speech, a high proportion of neologisms, and significant comprehension disorders. Van Dongen et al.'s (1985) 3 cases also presented a phrase length of at least seven words; a speaking rate of more than 90 words per minute; and normal prosody, articulation, pauses, and effort. These patients also exhibited frequent paraphasias.

PARAPHASIAS

Just as fluent aphasia was thought to be rare or absent among childhood acquired aphasics, paraphasias were considered to be exceptional (Alajouanine & Lhermitte, 1965; Hécaen, 1976). Their occurrence, however, has been described in recent years among children with reduced verbal productions, and particularly among the few with more fluent verbal production. Paraphasias appear to be more common during the acute period following acquired brain lesions, and have been described as especially notable and persistent among children with diffuse brain involvement, as opposed to more focal or lateralized brain lesions. Visch-Brink and Sandt-Koenderman (1984) and van Dongen and Visch-Brink (1988) have provided detailed descriptions of neologisms, literal paraphasias, and verbal paraphasias in spontaneous speech and naming tasks in first 2 and then 6 children who were 5 years and older at the age of insult. In addition, they presented a single case of phonemic jargon aphasia. These case studies exemplify the early appearance of neologisms and paraphasias after lesion onset and their rapid disappearance, usually within 2 or 3 weeks of lesion onset, at least among head-injured patients.

Van Hout, Evrard, and Lyon (1985) also summarized the verbal and paraphasic errors among 11 children with acquired aphasia. They divided their patients into three groups according to the evolution of their paraphasias, which also coincided with the severity of associated problems. For Groups I and II, the paraphasias resolved in a matter of days and over a few months, respectively, and for Group III the paraphasias persisted for more than a year. Particularly notable among Van Hout's patients was the severity of associated problems in all but Group I and the diffuse nature of brain involvement in all patients. Three of the 4 patients in Group III, the most severely impaired group, had herpes encephalitis, and the fourth incurred cerebral trauma followed by a Stage III coma for 1 month with decerebrate posturing. All had significant associated problems and appeared to be grossly demented. Although paraphasic errors may occur in the acute period following acquired focal lesions in young children with either reduced or fluent verbal outputs, in general their persistence appears to be associated with more pervasive cognitive disorders as a consequence of diffuse brain involvement.

NAMING AND LEXICAL RETRIEVAL

Although a few studies (van Dongen & Visch-Brink, 1988) have described paraphasic errors on naming tasks, the majority of studies addressing naming and lexical retrieval have simply recorded the correctness of response. Most have reported reduced naming abilities among children with left- but not right-brain lesions. For example, Hécaen (1976, 1983) reported that 44% of left-lesioned but none of the right-lesioned children had naming disorders that were described as being impoverished. Similarly, van Dongen and Visch-Brink (1988) reported no naming problems in the spontaneous speech or on naming tasks among right-lesioned children. Among those with left lesions, they differentiated between children with head injury who demonstrated a successive decrease in neologisms and recovery of all naming errors by 6 months of age, and non–head-injured children (CVA, subdural empyema, encephalitis) who presented more severe and persistent aphasic symptoms with irregular distribution of types of naming errors during recovery. Riva et al. (1986) appear to have provided one of the few studies documenting expressive vocabulary deficits among right- as well as left-lesioned subjects.

Aram, Ekelman, and Whitaker (1987) administered the Word Finding Test (Wiegel-Crump & Dennis, 1984) and the Rapid Automatized Naming Test (RAN; Denckla & Rudel, 1976) to left-lesioned, right-lesioned, and control subjects. On the Word Finding Test, left-lesioned subjects were slower than other subjects in latency of response when given semantic or visual cues and they made more errors when given rhyming cues. On the RAN, left-lesioned subjects were significantly slower than controls in naming all semantic categories (colors, numbers, objects, and letters). In contrast, right-lesioned subjects responded as quickly as or more quickly than control subjects in all access and semantic category conditions, yet produced more errors than controls, suggesting a speech–accuracy trade-off. Although types of errors were analyzed, the overwhelming error type was "no response" and few error types among the lesioned subjects differed appreciably from those of controls. Lesioned subjects, however, were all assessed at least 1 year and often several years following lesion onset.

Age of lesion onset has been equivocally related to naming deficits among left-lesioned subjects. Woods and Carey (1979) found left-lesioned subjects with lesions sustained after but not prior to 1 year of age to be impaired on naming tasks. However, Vargha-Khadem et al. (1985) found left-lesioned subjects, irrespective of the age when the lesion was sustained (congenital, early, or late acquired), to perform more poorly than right-lesioned subjects on the Oldfield–Wingfield Object Naming Task (Oldfield & Wingfield, 1964). Similarly, Aram et al. (1987) found no relationship between age of lesion onset and lexical retrieval abilities among either left- or right-lesioned children.

In summary, it appears that naming and lexical retrieval deficits are common after left- but not right-hemisphere lesions and for the most part do not appear to be related to age of lesion onset. Paraphasic errors have been described especially in the acute period after lesion onset. Although paraphasic errors may persist for some aphasic children, they do not appear to be a common feature later in recovery.

PHONOLOGICAL AND ARTICULATORY PRODUCTION

Aside from the few case reports of phonemic paraphasias (Van Hout et al., 1985; Visch-Brink & Sandt-Koenderman, 1984), very little detail has been offered relative to phonological production or articulatory abilities among children with acquired aphasia. No consensus appears regarding the occurrence of phonological and/or articulatory problems. Early studies suggested that articulatory disturbances were common. Alajouanine and Lhermitte (1965) stated that if the lesion occurred before 10 years of age, disorders of articulation were always present; these disorders were described as a phonetic disintegration no different from those observed in adults, if the stage of development was taken into account. Hécaen (1976) suggested that articulatory disturbances occurred following either left- or right-hemisphere lesions and were frequent in children younger than 10 years of age at lesion onset. Hécaen (1983) also reported that articulatory problems occurred 81% of the time following left anterior lesions versus 20% following left posterior lesions. The common occurrence of articulatory disorders has not been substantiated in most recent reports, or after the acute period. For example, Cranberg et al. (1987) reported that only one in eight children with acquired aphasia exhibited dysarthria at follow-up; Dennis (1980) noted dramatic improvement in articulation by 3 months following lesion onset in her 9-year-old child with a left posterior infarct; and Kershner and King (1974) found articulation errors to be no more common among left- or right-hemiplegic children than among controls.

The limited work on productive phonology is inconclusive. Aram et al. (1987) reported that in response to rhyming (phonemic) cues, left- but not right-lesioned children made more errors in word retrieval than did control children; however, Woods and Carey (1979) reported that left-lesioned children did not differ from controls on a task requiring rhyming and completing nursery rhymes. Clearly, very little systematic investigation of phonology or articulation has been pursued among children with acquired aphasia; the data are not available to generalize as to conditions that may relate to the presence or absence of phonological and/or articulatory problems.

Reading

Despite relatively good recovery for spoken language, long-term reading and writing problems are often, although not always, reported to persist. Alajouanine and Lhermitte (1965) reported that none of their 32 children with acquired aphasia were able to follow normal progress at school; although they were able to regain what they had previously learned, they had difficulty learning new information. Eighteen of the 32 experienced persistent reading problems: 9 were totally unable to read; 5 had a severe alexia for letters, syllables, and words; and 4 had alexia for letters and somewhat better reading of words. Similarly, both Cranberg et al. (1987) and Cooper and Flowers (1987) found sizable numbers of their acquired aphasic children to have long-term word recognition or reading comprehension deficits.

Although reading usually is reported as more impaired than spoken language among children with acquired aphasia, this is not always the case at least acutely. For example, Dennis (1980) reported that at 2 weeks following lesion onset for a 9-year-old child, reading was higher than oral language; at 3 months, reading but not oral language was age appropriate. This case demonstrated that, even among children with acquired aphasia, a dissociation between auditory and reading comprehension may exist. Hécaen (1976, 1983) is one of the few to suggest that, although reading problems may occur in the acute period, especially following left-hemisphere insults, reading problems usually disappear rapidly and completely.

Findings relating reading deficits to lesion laterality and age of onset are somewhat equivocal. Several investigators have compared reading in children with predominantly left- or right-hemisphere lesions. Although some researchers reported no difference between left or right congenitally hemiplegic children on the Wide Range Achievement Test (WRAT; Jastak & Jastak, 1978), a test of single-word recognition (Kershner & King, 1974; Reed & Reitan, 1969), others found WRAT word recognition to be related to adequacy of right-hand performance, that is, reflecting left-hemisphere functioning (Kiessling et al., 1983). Vargha-Khadem, Frith, O'Gorman, and Watters (1983) reported that children with either left or right lesions tended to have more difficulty than control subjects on measures of reading speed and reading comprehension, whereas those with left-hemisphere lesions acquired postnatally were most impaired in their reading skills. Aram, Gillespie, and Yamashita (in press) reported few significant mean group differences between left-lesioned children and their controls or between right-lesioned children and their controls on a battery of phonetic analysis, word recognition, and reading comprehension tests, although mean performance of the lesioned subjects was consistently below that of controls. Notable individual differences were present, however, within the lesioned subject groups, with 5 of 20 left- and 2 of 10 right-lesioned children presenting marked reading deficits, in contrast to only 1 of 30 control subjects. Age of lesion onset was not found to differentiate between those with and without reading problems, although a family history for reading disorders or involvement of specific subcortical structures was present for all subjects with reading problems.

Overall, it appears that long-standing reading problems involving phonetic analysis, decoding, and comprehension may occur for a sizable proportion of children with acquired aphasia. Although reading problems have been reported following a variety of acquired lesions, they appear to be most common among the children with postnatally acquired left lesions.

Writing and Spelling

Although it has been suggested that written language skills are particularly impaired among children with acquired aphasia, there appear to be no detailed reports of these children's writing ability. Alajouanine and Lhermitte (1965) reported that written language was always more severely disturbed than oral language. Among their 32 children with acquired aphasia, severe alterations in writing were noted in 19, of whom 8 could only copy words and 5 were said to be "dysorthographic" in their spontaneous writing. Even Hécaen (1976, 1983), who considered oral language and reading problems to disappear "rapidly and completely," noted that writing problems among children with acquired aphasia tended to persist, even permanently. Beyond a few case study examples in which writing skills were only one aspect described (e.g., Dennis, 1980; Ferro et al., 1982), however, apparently no studies explore the nature of these written language impairments.

Spelling deficits, reported to be relatively common among children with acquired aphasia, also have not been described extensively. Cranberg et al. (1987) and Cooper and Flowers (1987) reported spelling problems in 3 of 8 and 8 of 15, respectively, of their children with acquired aphasia. Woods and Carey (1979) reported that children with left-hemisphere lesions prior to as well as after 1 year of age were significantly poorer than controls in spelling a series of eight words. Vargha-Khadem et al. (1983) also found that children with left-hemisphere lesions performed more poorly on spelling tasks than those with right lesions or control subjects, especially children with postnatally acquired left lesions. This group had notable difficulty with infrequently occurring words, while findings for frequently occurring words were less clear-cut. Vargha-Khadem et al. (1983) appear to be one of the few who have provided qualitative data describing the spelling errors made by aphasic children, which were categorized as morphophonemic, orthographic, or preservation of the sound frame.

Thus, although writing and spelling problems appear to be relatively frequent and persistent among children with acquired aphasia, especially those with postnatally sustained left-hemisphere lesions, the problems presented have not been detailed.

Summary of Language Characteristics

Although typically less severe than the deficits observed among adults with acquired aphasia, a range of language deficits have been described in both the acute period and the long term among children with a variety of acquired brain lesions. Syntactic comprehension disorders, while more pronounced in the acute phase, have been shown to persist long term following predominantly left-hemisphere lesions. Lexical comprehension deficits also tend to persist, but have been associated with either left- or right-hemisphere lesions. Reduced, syntactically simplified language output is the most commonly described expressive language characteristic observed among children with acquired aphasia, particularly subsequent to predominantly left-hemisphere involvement. Paraphasias and more fluent-type aphasias, however, have been described usually during the acute phase of recovery or following diffuse brain involvement. Impaired naming and lexical retrieval exemplified by paraphasias, impoverished vocabularies, and slow rate of retrieval have been detailed both in the acute and long-term periods, especially following left-hemisphere lesions. Data addressing phonological production and articulation are equivocal, with insufficient detail available to resolve the contradictory reports. Reading, writing, and spelling deficits are seen as the most frequent, persistent, and significant sequelae among children with acquired aphasia. Reading deficits involving phonetic analysis, word recognition, and reading comprehension have been described, typically in association with left-hemisphere lesions. Writing and spelling limitations also often appear to be long-standing problems, predominantly associated with left-hemisphere lesions, yet data detailing either limitation are sparse.

Factors Related to Recovery of Language Abilities

Clearly, recovery of language skills among children with acquired lesions is variable, both within and across studies. The primary factors thought to be associated with how well a child recovers involve the nature of the neurological insult and the age of the child at lesion onset.

Nature of the Neurological Insult

The nature of the neurological insult appears to account for much of the variability in outcome reported for children with acquired aphasias. Several aspects relating to the neurological insult will be examined here: the degree of brain involvement, the etiology of the lesion, lesion laterality (i.e., involvement of the left or right hemisphere), the specific site of lesion (i.e., the actual structures involved within a hemisphere), the size or extensiveness of the lesion within a hemisphere, and the presence and severity of an accompanying seizure disorder.

DEGREE OF BRAIN INVOLVEMENT

Unlike most of the adult aphasia literature, the majority of studies addressing acquired aphasia in children are not confined to focal, more circumscribed lesions. Rather, most have included at least some children with known or presumed diffuse brain involvement, for example, secondary to asphyxia, head trauma, infectious processes, or cranial radiation and/or chemotherapy for the treatment of tumors. Often, however, the degree of more generalized involvement is not addressed; instead, lesions are treated as if the effect were confined solely to a focal area, for example, the location of a subdural hematoma following head trauma, or of a tumor with no mention of cranial radiation or chemotherapy. When results in these studies vary from findings following more circumscribed lesions, the findings need to be interpreted in light of some degree of probable diffuse brain involvement.

The few studies that have explicitly contrasted the effects of diffuse versus focal brain involvement on children's cognitive abilities, have consistently identified bilateral and/or diffuse hemispheric involvement as a poor prognostic sign (Hécaen, 1976; Janowsky & Nass, 1987; Loonen & van Dongen, in press; Van Hout et al., 1985). For example, as noted above, most of the children with severe comprehension disorders and persistent paraphasias (Van Hout et al., 1985) typically incurred diffuse brain involvement. Annett (1973) apparently was one of the first to study the relationship between the degree of more diffuse brain involvement and higher cognitive functions, including language. She reported an association between a decline in intelligence scores and increased impairment of the nonhemiplegic hand, thus demonstrating involvement of both hemispheres, not merely the more apparent side of hemiplegia. More recently, Loonen and van Dongen (in press) reported an inverse relationship between recovery of spontaneous language and auditory comprehension skills and the degree of bilateral brain involvement. In general, then, it appears that lesions involving focal areas of the brain are associated with better recovery than are lesions involving diffuse areas of the brain.

ETIOLOGY

Closely related to the degree of brain involvement is the etiology of the brain lesion. In a review of 47 cases of acquired aphasia, Martins and Ferro (1987) reported that the prognosis for vascular and traumatic lesions was better than for encephalitis and tumor. Similarly, Van Hout et al. (1985) found a high incidence of infections, in particular herpes encephalitis, among her patients with the most severe and persistent language deficits. Many investigators have documented the deleterious effects on higher cognitive function of cranial radiation and chemotherapy for CNS tumors in children due to the diffuse effects of these treatments (Fletcher & Copeland, 1988). Guttmann (1942), van Dongen and Loonen (1977), and van Dongen and Visch-Brink (1988) have suggested that children with aphasic symptoms recover more rapidly from head trauma than from vascular lesions; however, one might question the severity of their patients' head trauma, as the severity of head trauma is thought to be the single most important variable in determining recovery (Fletcher & Levin, 1988). When considering prognosis as it relates to etiology, severity of the injury or disease process must be considered, as well as concomitant treatment. Thus, in general, etiologies implicating more diffuse brain involvement, including infectious processes, tumors treated with cranial radiation therapy and chemotherapy, and severe head injury, are related to poorer outcome than more focal lesions as a result of vascular problems. Even within groups of children with focal lesions, however, outcome is variable. In these cases, the additional variables of lesion laterality, size, site, and presence of seizures need to be considered.

LESION LATERALITY

Woods and Teuber (1978) reported what is probably the landmark paper addressing lesion laterality and acquired aphasia in children. These investigators noted that since the introduction of antibiotics and mass immunization programs in the 1930s and 1940s, stemming previously common forms of diffuse brain involvement in children, the incidence of aphasia arising from right-hemisphere lesions is no higher than that reported in adults. Excluding earlier studies in which reports of diffuse brain involvement were frequent, these investigators reported that the incidence of aphasia associated with right-hemisphere lesions was less than 10%. If left handers were excluded, the incidence dropped to 5%. Others have since substantiated that the incidence of aphasia following left lesions is comparable for right-handed children and adults, and the risk is substantially greater following left than right lesions at any age (Carter, Hohenegger, & Satz, 1982; Satz & Bullard-Bates, 1981). Such data prompted Hécaen to change his view regarding the lack of language lateralization in children and state, "One could reasonably conclude, therefore, that studies of acquired aphasia in children support the notion of early cerebral lateralization and even innate cerebral organization for the presentation of language" (1983, p. 586). In this chapter, deficits in language comprehension, syntactic production, and naming and lexical retrieval were all associated with left- and not right-hemisphere lesions. Thus, it appears that when lesions in children are confined to one hemisphere, just as in adults, aphasia is associated predominantly with left-hemisphere involvement.

SITE OF LESION WITHIN A HEMISPHERE

Unlike most studies of adult aphasics, until very recently few studies with children provided sufficient evidence of lesion localization. In the past 10 years, studies have begun reporting computerized tomographic (CT) scan data for the majority of subjects, yet even these reports fail to define adequately the involvement of subcortical areas or to address actual brain function. Nonetheless, some preliminary attempts toward localization have been offered.

Prior to the availability of CT scans and other noninvasive radiological evidence, findings were based on an array of laboratory findings (e.g., pneumocephalograms, arteriograms, surgery) and clinical findings (e.g., sensory and motor abnormalities), with little consensus among reports. For example, Guttmann (1942) suggested that posterior left lesions resulted in more pronounced language deficits, whereas Hécaen (1983) concluded the converse, that anterior lesions produced more severe language deficits than did posterior lesions. The availability of CT scan data has not appreciably clarified the relationship between lesion location and language symptomatology. For example, Cranberg et al. (1987) found nonfluent aphasias to occur following either anterior or posterior lesions, and Visch-Brink and Sandt-Koenderman (1984) were unable to identify a relationship between lesion location as determined by CT scans and the occurrence of paraphasias. Similarly, in our series of studies assessing aspects of language among children with unilateral brain lesions (reviewed in Aram, 1988), we have been unable to identify involvement of localized cortical areas associated with specific language symptomatology beyond a slight trend for somewhat greater deficits following posterior left lesions, although this finding may interact with lesion size. In a series of recent studies (Aram, Ekelman, & Gillespie, 1989; Aram et al., under review), however, we have presented evidence of particularly pronounced language deficits for a small group of children with involvement of specific subcortical nuclei (the head of the caudate and the putamen) and the adjacent white matter tracts, suggesting that children with involvement of these structures may not recover as well as those with involvement of other portions of the left hemisphere. Whether these findings will be substantiated in further work with larger groups of children remains to be seen.

LESION SIZE WITHIN A HEMISPHERE

Several recent studies have quantified lesion size based on CT scans and have attempted to draw relationships between lesion size and language sequelae, but with contradictory results. Several have suggested that the larger the lesion, the poorer the cognitive performance (Cohen & Duffner, 1981; Levine et al., 1987; Riva et al., 1986), whereas others have found little relationship between lesion size and recovery (Loonen & van Dongen, in press; Thal et al., 1989; Vargha-Khadem et al., 1985). Some investigators have suggested that lesion size may be important in older but not younger age groups (Kornhuber, Bechinger, Jung, & Sauer, 1985). At this point the role lesion size plays in determining recovery is not clear, although it may be that size interacts with site and possibly age of onset.

PRESENCE OF SEIZURES

Most studies demonstrate poorer outcomes when seizures accompany acquired brain injury than when seizures are not present (e.g., Aicardi, Amsili, & Chevrie, 1969; Annett, 1973; Solomon, Hilal, Gold, & Carter, 1970; van Dongen & Loonen, 1977). Levine et al. (1987), on the other hand, reported that IQ deficits correlated with the presence of electroencephalographic (EEG) abnormalities. When lesion size was entered as a covariate, the relationship between IQ and EEG abnormalities no longer maintained, suggesting that lesion size rather than EEG abnormalities was a more powerful predictor of cognitive recovery. However, most clinicians and investigators apparently view the presence of seizures as having a negative effect on outcome. This adverse effect most probably can be related to the spread of abnormal electrical activity, thus implicating more diffuse brain involvement than the more circumscribed effects of the original lesion. In addition, prognosis for language recovery in children with seizures accompanying their acquired aphasia needs to take into account the frequency, severity, and type of seizures, as well as the effectiveness, dosage, and number of anticonvulsants.

Age of Insult

Because children with acquired aphasia usually recover more rapidly and completely than adults, age is assumed to be an important factor in determining outcome. The presumed plasticity possible in the immature brain has typically been seen as the mechanism responsible for age-dependent recovery (e.g., Lenneberg, 1967). Also, much of the earlier work with animals suggested better recovery of functions following early rather than later lesions (Kennard, 1936), a position often referred to as the "Kennard principle."

Evidence from children with acquired aphasia, however, is highly contradictory, and no single relationship between age at lesion onset and outcome is supported. Some researchers have suggested that lesions sustained prior to the onset of language do not have as significant an effect on language as those sustained after 1 year of age (e.g., Woods & Carey, 1979). Others have suggested that earlier lesions have more pervasive effects on development of higher cognitive functions than do later lesions (Basser, 1962). Most have failed to identify a clear relationship between age of lesion onset and recovery (Aram, 1988; Hécaen, 1976; Loonen & van Dongen, in press; Woods & Teuber, 1978). Some have suggested that the variable effect of age on outcome may be explained by other factors, for example, different etiologies among the age groups (Martins & Ferro, 1987). Finally, some have suggested that the importance of age at lesion onset is not for predicting the rapidity or completeness of recovery, but for understanding the specificity of the lesion's effect dependent upon the stage of language development at the time. For example, Alajouanine and Lhermitte (1965) have contrasted language characteristics of children with lesions before versus after 10 years of age, stating that reduced verbal expression, disordered articulation, and comprehension deficits are characteristic of the effects of lesions prior to 10 years of age, whereas paraphasias and written language disturbances are common when lesions are sustained after 10 years of age.

Thus, it does not appear that a single relationship between age of lesion onset and prognosis for language recovery holds; rather, age may interact with other variables, such as etiology, and may exert a variable effect on language depending on the stage at which language is disrupted.

How Language Recovers

Although considerable theorizing has been offered to explain language recovery among children with acquired aphasia, how and where language recovers are still largely speculative issues. Several mechanisms have been suggested, such as FUNCTIONAL SUBSTITUTION of "uncommitted" portions of the same or the opposite hemisphere, or REDUNDANT NEURAL REPRESENTATIONS that make possible the release of existing, but previously suppressed pathways (see Aram & Eisele, in press, for a review of mechanisms proposed for recovery). Much of the evidence for functional reorganization following brain lesions has been derived from work with animals. The limited data available pertaining to reorganization of language functions among children with acquired aphasia have addressed only which hemisphere continues to be active during language tasks, as opposed to where within a hemisphere language functions occur. The few studies available with individuals with early lateralized lesions have employed dichotic listening, sodium amytal, or electrophysiological procedures.

Evidence from Dichotic Listening Tests

Several investigators have used dichotic listening tasks to infer hemispheric laterality following early lateralized lesions. The dichotic paradigm presents different stimuli independently but simultaneously to each ear; the hemisphere contralateral to the ear through which the higher score of accurate recognition is obtained, is considered to be dominant for that aspect of language (Berlin & McNeil, 1976). By presenting two-digit dichotic pairs to children and adolescents with lateralized seizures and hemiplegia, Goodglass (1967) found a dramatic inferiority of report from the ear opposite the injured hemisphere in most cases, with several instances of total suppression. Distinguishing between a "cerebral dominance effect," which usually favored one ear by only a small difference, and "a lesion effect," where differences ranged up to 100%, Goodglass suggested a parallel between lateralized suppression of auditory input and visual or tactile neglect, extinction, and displacement.

Subsequently, several other investigators have reported similar findings of inferiority of verbal recognition contralateral to the lesioned hemisphere and instances of total auditory suppression (Ferro et al., 1982; Martins et al., 1987; Pohl, 1979; Yeni-Komshian, 1977). Both Pohl (1979) and Yeni-Komshian (1977) administered dichotic tests during the course of recovery and related dichotic findings to language improvement. Pohl (1979) studied a 6-year-old boy with a left middle cerebral artery occlusion at 8 months and again at 13 months following lesion onset. Under dichotic testing conditions, total right-ear extinction was found at both times, and was not modified through verbal training. At 13 months, however, the right-ear extinction disappeared if words were presented monaurally to the right ear with white noise on the left. Pohl interpreted the right-ear extinction as signaling a switch in hemisphere dominance for speech from the left to the right hemisphere. Similarly, Yeni-Komshian (1977) described dichotic findings and language skills over time for four children with acquired brain damage. The three with bilateral brain involvement all showed marked right-ear advantage initially and were unable to process competing stimuli, although they regained some capacity to do so over time. A relationship between the degree of language loss and the ability to process two competing stimuli was noted. Yeni-Komshian interpreted the pronounced right-ear advantage, which coincided with significant recovery of language, as an indication that language was originally represented in the left hemisphere and that recovery also took place in the damaged left hemisphere. In contrast, her fourth child, an 11-year-old boy with a total destruction of the left hemisphere, persisted in demonstrating a marked left-ear advantage, and, despite intensive therapy, a severe aphasia remained at 14 months following lesion onset. Yeni-Komshian proposed that the strong left-ear advantage was suggestive that language recovery, although impaired, was taking place in the right hemisphere.

These studies demonstrate the utility of dichotic listening tasks in providing one approach for identifying which hemisphere assumes language functions following acquired lesions.

Evidence from Sodium Amytal Studies

Probably the strongest evidence of hemispheric dominance for language comes from sodium amytal studies, also referred to as the "Wada procedure" after the neurologist who developed the technique. This technique uses a short-acting barbiturate injected into either the left or the right internal carotid artery, and on a separate occasion repeated in the alternate carotid artery. During the short period in which the drug circulates through the hemisphere, functions normally sustained by that hemisphere are significantly impaired, thus permitting determination of that hemisphere's role in a specific function. Because of the invasive nature of the technique, sodium amytal studies are usually restricted to preliminary assessment prior to surgical resection of the brain to relieve intractable seizure disorders, in order to determine the effect of the surgery on language and memory functions. Thus, the patients for whom these data are available consist predominantly of persons with severe and often long-standing seizure disorders; nonetheless, for these patients a direct indication of hemisphere dominance for language can be obtained.

Rasmussen and Milner (1977) have provided one of the most comprehensive summaries of sodium amytal findings as they pertain to lateralization of language functions following left-hemisphere lesions sustained early in life. In a review of 134 patients in whom the epileptogenic lesions all occurred prior to 6 years of age, and in most instances from the prenatal period, the following was reported. First, 81% of their left-lesioned patients who remained right handed were also left-hemisphere dominant for speech, thus suggesting that an early left-hemisphere lesion that does not modify hand preference is unlikely to change hemispheric dominance for language. In contrast among the non–right-handed subjects with left-hemisphere lesions, 53% had right-hemisphere language representation and 19% had evidence of bilateral representation. Second, Rasmussen and Milner reported that speech could be mediated asymmetrically in the two hemispheres with the anterior speech areas in one hemisphere and the posterior areas in the other hemisphere. Third, even gross lesions that did not involve the primary speech zone (the inferior frontal and posterior temporoparietal regions of the left hemisphere) rarely altered speech lateralization, whereas damage to either of these critical areas usually resulted in right or bilateral speech representation. Finally, they speculated that after 5 years of age recovery is achieved by intrahemispheric reorganization rather than by shift of hemispheric dominance, and suggested that upward displacement of the posterior speech zone to include more of the parietal cortex may provide such a compensatory mechanism.

A more recent sodium amytal study (Mateer & Dodrill, 1983) likewise found that left-hemisphere lesions involving the inferior frontal and posterior temporoparietal regions usually resulted in right-hemisphere or, more rarely, bilateral-hemispheric representation for language. In addition, Mateer and Dodrill reported that for their group of patients with bilateral speech representation, the early brain injuries appeared to be diffuse and not lateralized to a single hemisphere. However, they pointed out that all instances of bilateral damage did not necessarily result in bilateral language representation. These investigators suggested that early diffuse injury may either actively inhibit language lateralization or possibly require contributions from both hemispheres for the support of language development.

In general, the data from sodium amytal studies do provide evidence for right or bilateral representation of language functions for some left-lesioned subjects, particularly when the patient is left handed, when the primary speech zones are involved, and when injury occurs at a young age. Yet this data is derived for a small subgroup of individuals with intractible seizure disorders and requires an invasive procedure for determining lateralization.

Evidence from Electrophysiological Findings

Electrophysiological procedures such as those involving auditory evoked potentials provide a noninvasive means of determining brain activity in response to language stimuli. As of yet, however, it appears that few investigators have applied these techniques to the study of brain organization for language of children with acquired aphasia. Recently, Papanicolaou, DiScenna, Gillespie, and Aram (1990) reported the use of the probe evoked potential paradigm (Papanicolaou & Johnstone, 1984) with a group of children with unilateral left lesions in the absence of seizure disorders. The left-lesioned children in this study displayed the normal pattern of predominantly left-hemisphere engagement in a language task and right-hemisphere engagement in a visuospatial task; thus, among this group of left-lesioned subjects it appeared that language restitution and development involved intra- rather than interhemispheric functional reorganization. That 9 of the 14 children in this study were left handed at the time of study is not consistent with Rasmussen and Milner's (1977) findings reported with the sodium amytal procedure; however, differences may relate to the fact that in Papanicolaou et al.'s patients, lesions were focal and not accompanied by seizures, as opposed to Rasmussen and Milner's patients with intractible seizure disorders. Also, in the evoked potential study, the language tasks involved only a phonological target detection task, signaled by raising the index fingers, whereas the tasks used in Rasmussen and Milner's sodium amytal study involved naming and sequential speech. Thus the task used in the evoked potential study did not require any language production and thus may not have tapped more anterior speech areas. Therefore, the Papanicolaou et al. findings cannot preclude the possibility, suggested by Rasmussen and Milner (1977), that speech functions among early lesioned subjects may be mediated asymmetrically by the hemispheres. Had a language production task been included, it is possible that results for that task may have been different than for the phonological detection task.

Clearly, much remains to be learned about how language recovers among children with acquired aphasia. The few studies available suggest that both intra- and interhemispheric reorganizations occur. With the application of noninvasive techniques, such as evoked potentials, and more dynamic imaging techniques, such as positron emission topography, greater understanding of factors related to the process of recovery from acquired aphasia in childhood hopefully will be forthcoming.

Acknowledgment

Preparation of this chapter was supported by NIH grant NS17366 to the author. The author wishes to thank Meg Guncik for her help in the preparation of this manuscript.

References

Aicardi, J., Amsili, J., & Chevrie, J. J. (1969). Acute hemiplegia in infancy and childhood. *Developmental Medicine and Child Neurology, 11,* 162–173.

Alajouanine, T. H., & Lhermitte, F. (1965). Acquired aphasia in children. *Brain, 88*(4), 653–662.

Annett, M. (1973). Laterality of childhood hemiplegia and the growth of speech and intelligence. *Cortex, 9,* 4–33.

Aram, D. M. (1988). Language sequelae of unilateral brain lesions in children. In F. Plum (Ed.), *Language, communication and the brain* (pp. 171–197). New York: Raven Press.

Aram, D. M., & Eisele, J. A. (In press). Plasticity and recovery of higher cortical functions following early brain injury. In I. Rapin & S. J. Segalowitz (Eds.), *Handbook of neuropsychology: Child neuropsychology.* New York: American Elsevier.

Aram, D. M., & Ekelman, B. L. (1987). Unilateral brain lesions in childhood: Performance on the Revised Token Test. *Brain and Language, 32,* 137–158.

Aram, D. M., Ekelman, B. L., & Gillespie, L. L. (1989). Reading and lateralized lesions in children. In K. von Euler, I. Lundberg, & G. Lennerstrand (Eds.), *Brain and reading* (pp. 61–75). Hampshire, England: Macmillan Press Ltd.

Aram, D. M., & Ekelman, B. L., Rose, D. F., & Whitaker, H. A. (1985). Verbal and cognitive sequelae following unilateral lesions acquired in early childhood. *Journal of Clinical and Experimental Neuropsychology, 7,* 55–78.

Aram, D. M., Ekelman, B. L., & Whitaker, H. A. (1986). Spoken syntax in children with acquired unilateral hemisphere lesions. *Brain and Language, 27,* 75–100.

Aram, D. M., Ekelman, B. L., & Whitaker, H. A. (1987). Lexical retrieval in left and right brain lesioned children. *Brain and Language, 31,* 61–87.

Aram, D. M., Gillespie, L. L., & Yamashita, T. S. (In press). Reading among children with left and right brain lesions. *Developmental Neuropsychology, 6*(4).

Aram, D. M., Rose, D. F., Rekate, H. L., & Whitaker, H. A. (1983). Acquired capsular/striatal aphasia in childhood. *Archives of Neurology (Chicago), 40,* 614–617.

Aram, D. M., & Whitaker, H. A. (1988). Cognitive sequelae of unilateral lesions acquired in early childhood. In D. L. Molfese & S. J. Segalowitz (Eds.), *The developmental implications of brain lateralization* (pp. 417–436). New York: Guilford Press.

Basser, L. S. (1962). Hemiplegia of early onset and the faculty of speech with special reference to the effects of hemispherectomy. *Brain, 85,* 427–460.

Bates, E., Beeghley, M., Bretherton, I., McNew, S., Oakes, L., O'Connell, B., Reznick, S., Shore, C., Snyder, L., Volterra, V., & Whitesell, L. (1985). *Language and gesture inventory.* Unpublished test materials, University of California, San Diego.

Benton, A. L. (1964). Developmental aphasia and brain damage. *Cortex, 1,* 40–52.

Berlin, C., & McNeil, M. (1976). Dichotic listening. In N. J. Lass (Ed.), *Contemporary issues in experimental phonetics* (pp. 327–387). New York: Academic Press.

Best, C. T. (1988). The emergence of cerebral asymmetries in early human development: A literature review and a neuroembryological model. In D. L. Molfese & S. J. Segalowitz (Eds.), *The Developmental Implications of Brain Lateralization* (pp. 5–34). New York: Guilford Press.

Carter, R. L., Hohenegger, M. K., & Satz, P. (1982). Aphasia and speech organization in children. *Science, 219,* 797–799.

Cohen, M. E., & Duffner, P. K. (1981). Prognostic indicators of hemiparetic cerebral palsy. *Annals of Neurology, 9,* 353–357.

Cooper, J. A., & Flowers, C. R. (1987). Children with a history of acquired aphasia: Residual language and academic impairments. *Journal of Speech and Hearing Disorders, 52,* 251–262.

Cranberg, L. D., Filley, C. M., Hart, E. J., & Alexander, M. P. (1987). Acquired aphasia in childhood: Clinical and CT investigations. *Neurology, 37*(7), 1165–1172.

Denckla, M. B., & Rudel, R. G. (1976). Rapid "automatized" naming (R.A.N.): Dyslexia differentiated from other learning disabilities. *Neuropsychologia, 14,* 471–479.

Dennis, M. (1980). Strokes in childhood. I: Communicative intent, expression, and comprehension after left hemisphere arteriopathy in a right-handed nine-year old. In R. W. Rieber (Ed.), *Language development and aphasia in children* (pp. 45–67). New York: Academic Press.

De Renzi, E., & Vignolo, L. A. (1962). The Token Test: A sensitive test to detect receptive disturbances in aphasics. *Brain, 85,* 665–678.

Dunn, L. M. (1965). *Peabody picture vocabulary test.* Circle Pines, MN: American Guidance Service.

Ferro, J. M., Martins, I. P., Pinto, F., & Castro-Caldas, A. (1982). Aphasia following right striato-insular infarction in a left-handed child: A clinico-radiological study. *Developmental Medicine and Child Neurology, 24,* 173–182.

Fletcher, J. M., & Copeland, D. R. (1988). Neurobehavioral effects of central nervous system prophylactic treatment of cancer in children. *Journal of Clinical and Experimental Neuropsychology, 10*(4), 495–538.

Fletcher, J. M., & Levin, H. S. (1988). Neurobehavioral effects of brain injury in children. In D. K. Routh (Ed.), *Handbook of pediatric psychology* (pp. 258–295). New York: Guilford Press.

Goodglass, H. (1967). Binaural digit presentation and early lateral brain damage. *Cortex, 3,* 195–306.

Goodglass, H., & Kaplan, E. (1983). *The assessment of aphasia and related disorders* (2nd ed.). Philadelphia, PA: Lea & Febiger.

Guttmann, E. (1942). Aphasia in children. *Brain, 65,* 205–219.

Hécaen, H. (1976). Acquired aphasia in children and the ontogenesis of hemispheric functional specialization. *Brain and Language, 3,* 114–134.

Hécaen, H. (1983). Acquired aphasia in children: Revisited. *Neuropsychologia, 21*(6), 581–587.

Janowsky, J. S., & Nass, R. (1987). Early language development in infants with cortical and subcortical perinatal brain injury. *Developmental and Behavioral Pediatrics, 8*(1), 3–7.

Jastak, J. F., & Jastak, S. (1978). *The wide range achievement test.* Wilmington, DE: Jastak Associates.

Kennard, M. A. (1936). Age and other factors in motor recovery from precentral lesions in monkeys. *American Journal of Physiology, 115,* 138–146.

Kershner, J. R., & King, A. J. (1974). Laterality of cognitive functions in achieving hemiplegic children. *Perceptual and Motor Skills, 39,* 1283–1289.

Kiessling, L., Denckla, M., & Carlton, M. (1983). Evidence for differential hemispheric function in children with hemiplegic cerebral palsy. *Developmental Medicine and Child Neurology, 25,* 724–734.

Kinsbourne, M., & Hiscock, M. (1977). Does cerebral dominance develop? In S. J. Segalowitz & F. A. Gruber (Eds.), *Language development and neurological theory* (pp. 171–191). New York: Academic Press.

Kornhuber, H. H., Bechinger, D., Jung, H., & Sauer, E. (1985). A quantitative relationship between the extent of localized cerebral lesions and the intellectual and behavioural deficiency in children. *European Archives of Psychiatry and Neurological Sciences, 235,* 129–133.

Lee, L. (1969). *Northwestern syntax screening test.* Evanston, IL: Northwestern University Press.

Lenneberg, E. (1967). *Biological foundations of language.* New York: Wiley.

Levine, S. C., Huttenlocher, P., Banich, M. T., & Duda, E. (1987). Factors affecting cognitive functioning of hemiplegic children. *Developmental Medicine and Child Neurology, 29,* 27–35.

Loonen, M. C. B., & van Dongen, H. R. (in press). Acquired childhood aphasia: Course and outcome.

Marchman, V., Miller, R., & Bates, E. (1989). *Prespeech and babble in children with focal brain injury.* Paper presented at the Society for Research in Child Development Bicentennial Conference, Kansas City, MO.

Martins, I. P., & Ferro, J. M. (1987). *Acquired hemispheric lesions in children.* Paper presented at the International Neuropsychological Society meetings, Barcelona, Spain.

Martins, I. P., Ferro, J. M., & Trindade, A. (1987). Acquired crossed aphasia in a child. *Developmental Medicine and Child Neurology, 29,* 96–109.

Mateer, C. A., & Dodrill, C. B. (1983). Neuropsychological and linguistic correlates of atypical language lateralization: Evidence from sodium amytal studies. *Human Neurobiology, 2,* 135–142.

McNeil, M. R., & Prescott, T. E. (1978). *Revised token test.* Austin, TX: Pro-Ed.

Molfese, D. L., & Segalowitz, S. J. (Eds.). (1988). *Brain lateralization in children.* New York: Guilford Press.

Oelschlaeger, M. L., & Scarborough, J. (1976). Traumatic aphasia in children: A case study. *Journal of Communication Disorders, 9,* 281–288.

Oldfield, R. C., & Wingfield, A. (1964). The time it takes to name an object. *Nature (London), 202,* 1031–1032.

Papanicolaou, A. C., DiScenna, A., Gillespie, L. L., & Aram, D. M. (1990). Probe evoked potential findings following unilateral left hemisphere lesions in children. *Archives of Neurology, 49,* 562–566. (Chicago).

Papanicolaou, A. C., & Johnstone, J. (1984). probe evoked potentials: Theory, method and applications. *International Journal of Neuroscience, 24,* 107–131.

Pohl, P. (1979). Dichotic listening in a child recovering from acquired aphasia. *Brain and Language, 8,* 372–379.

Rankin, J. M., Aram, D. M., & Horwitz, S. J. (1981). Language ability in right and left hemiplegic children. *Brain and Language, 14,* 292–306.

Rapin, I., & Allen, D. A. (1988). Syndromes in developmental dysphasia and adult aphasia. In F. Plum (Ed.), *Language, communication and the brain* (pp. 57–76). New York: Raven Press.

Rasmussen, T., & Milner, B. (1977). The role of early left-brain injury in determining lateralization of cerebral speech functions. *Annals of the New York Academy of Sciences, 299,* 335–369.

Reed, J. C., & Reitan, R. M. (1969). Verbal and performance differences among brain-injured children with lateralized motor deficits. *Perceptual and Motor skills, 29,* 747–752.

Riva, D., Cazzaniga, L., Pantaleoni, C., Milani, N., & Fedrizzi, E. (1986). Acute hemiplegia in childhood: The neuropsychological prognosis. *Journal of Pediatric Neurosciences, 4,* 239–240.

Satz, P., & Bullard-Bates, C. (1981). Acquired aphasia in children. In M. T. Sarno (Ed.), *Acquired aphasia* (pp. 399–426). New York: Academic Press.

Semel-Mintz, E., & Wiig, E. H. (1982). *Clinical evaluation of language functions.* San Antonio, TX: The Psychological Corp.

Solomon, G. E., Hilal, S. K., Gold, A. P., & Carter, S. (1970). Natural history of acute hemiplegia of childhood. *Brain, 93,* 107–120.

Tallal, P. (1988). Developmental language disorders. In J. F. Kavanaugh & T. J. Truss (Eds.), *Learning disabilities: Proceedings of the national conference* (pp. 181–272). Parkton, MD: York Press.

Thal, D., Marchman, V., & Bates, E. (1989). *Early communication and language.* Paper presented at the Society for Research in Child Development Bicentennial Conference, Kansas City, MO.

van Dongen, H. R., & Loonen, M. C. B. (1977). Factors related to prognosis of acquired aphasia in children. *Cortex, 13,* 131–136.

van Dongen, H. R., Loonen, M. C. B., and van Dongen, K. J. (1985). Anatomical basis for acquired fluent aphasia in children. *Annals of Neurology, 17,* 306–309.

van Dongen, H. R., & Visch-Brink, E. G. (1988). Naming in aphasic children: Analysis of paraphasic errors. *Neuropsychologia, 26,* 629–632.

Van Hout, A., Evrard, P., & Lyon, G. (1985). On the positive semiology of acquired aphasia in children. *Developmental Medicine and Child Neurology, 27,* 231–241.

Van Hout, A., & Lyon, G. (1986). Wernicke's aphasia in a 10-year old boy. *Brain and Language, 29*, 268–285.

Vargha-Khadem, F., Frith, U., O'Gorman, A. M., & Watters, G. V. (1983). *Learning disabilities in children with unilateral brain damage.* Paper presented at the International Neuropsychological Society meetings, Lisbon, Portugal.

Vargha-Khadem, F., O'Gorman, A. M., & Watters, G. V. (1985). Aphasia and handedness in relation to hemispheric side, age at injury and severity of cerebral lesion during childhood. *Brain, 108*, 677–696.

Visch-Brink, E. G., & Sandt-Koenderman, M. (1984). The occurrence of paraphasias in the spontaneous speech of children with an acquired aphasia. *Brain and Language, 23*, 258–271.

Wiegel-Crump, C. A., & Dennis, M. (1984). *The word-finding test* (Exp. ed.: unpublished test). Toronto: The Hospital for Sick Children.

Woods, B. T. (1987). Impaired speech shadowing after early lesions of either hemisphere. *Neuropsychologia, 26*, 519–525.

Woods, B. T., & Carey, S. (1979). Language deficits after apparent clinical recovery from childhood aphasias. *Annals of Neurology, 6*(5), 405–409.

Woods, B. T., & Teuber, H. L. (1978). Changing patterns of childhood aphasia. *Annals of Neurology, 3*, 273–280.

Yeni-Komshian, G. H. (1977). *Speech perception in brain injured children.* Paper presented at the Conference on the Biological Bases of Delayed Language Development, New York.

14

Aphasia After Head Injury

HARVEY S. LEVIN

Closed Head Injury and Missile Wounds of the Brain

Epidemiology and Mechanisms of Injury

In contrast to the frequent occurrence of open head injuries from penetrating missile wounds (e.g., bullets, shell fragments) in casualties of war, closed head injury (CHI) predominates in civilian head trauma. The term CHI is used here to refer to head trauma in which the primary mechanism of injury is a sudden acceleration–deceleration imparted to the freely moving head. Impact of a blunt object is another common mechanism of CHI. The primary cause of CHI in many areas of the United States is vehicular accident (Kraus et al., 1984), whereas assault is a more frequent mechanism in some urban areas. Falls also are a common cause of head injury in young children. Kraus and coworkers (1984) reported incidence data based on all hospital admissions for traumatic brain injury in San Diego County. Using case ascertainment criteria, such as acute impairment of consciousness, Kraus et al. found an overall incidence of 180/100,000 population, which closely approximates previous findings reported for Olmsted County, Minnesota, over the period from 1935 to 1974 (Annegers, Grabow, Kurland, & Laws, 1980). As shown in the age- and sex-specific incidence curve (Figure 14.1), the incidence of head injury rises sharply in late childhood and reaches a peak exceeding 400/100,000 population in adolescent and young adult males. A second peak in incidence is seen in older adults, which could have an impact on rehabilitation services because of the shift in the age

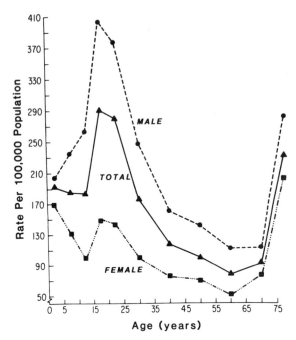

FIGURE 14.1. *Age- and sex-specific incidence rates of brain injury per 100,000 population, San Diego County, California, 1981. From Kraus et al. (1984). Reproduced with permission of the author and publisher.*

distribution of the general population. Although males predominate during most of the age span in hospital admissions of adults with CHI, the male–female disparity in head injury is low in young children and in adults over 70 years of age (Kraus et al., 1984).

An important epidemiologic finding in the San Diego study is that mild to moderate head injury accounts for about three-fourths of all admissions of acute head trauma. Consequently, the impressions gained from rehabilitation studies about the frequency of aphasia probably reflect selection of more severely injured patients. At the other end of the continuum, available data underestimate the incidence of mildly injured patients who are treated and released from emergency rooms.

Neuropathologic investigation of the traumatized human brain (see Adams, Mitchell, Graham, & Doyle, 1977) and studies employing experimental models of head injury in animals (see Ommaya & Gennarelli, 1974) have suggested that a primary mechanism of CHI is rotational acceleration of the skull, which produces shear strains within the intracranial contents. Histological study of the brains of patients dying soon after CHI has disclosed diffuse injury to the cerebral white matter, which apparently results from shearing and stretching of nerve fibers at the moment of impact (Adams et al., 1977). Pertinent to the development of hemispheric disconnection, the corpus callosum is especially vulnerable to diffuse mechanically induced shear strains. Ommaya and Gennarelli (1974) postulated that the severity of diffuse CHI follows a centripetal gradient; that is, the injury extends to the rostral brain stem only in cases with severe diffuse hemispheric injury. The bulk of cerebral white matter may be reduced further by delayed degeneration, which results in ventricular enlargement. Complications contributing to the severity of generalized CHI include brain swelling, increased intracranial pressure, hypoxia, and infection.

Focal lesions after CHI result from contusion of the brain surface by transient in-bending of the skull or by penetration of bone fragment in cases of depressed skull fracture, which may also produce brain laceration (Gurdjian & Gurdjian, 1976). Focal areas of ischemia are frequently present in the neocortex and basal ganglia (Graham & Adams, 1971). Stresses of the impact may cause arterial and venous tears resulting in intracerebral (see Figure 14.2) or extracerebral hematomas. The orbital surfaces of the frontal and temporal lobes are particularly vulnerable to contusion by impaction against the bony sphenoid wing. Formation of hematomas is also common in this area. Large mass lesions may produce contralateral shift of midline structures and tentorial herniation of the temporal lobe, possibly involving the uncus and hippocampus.

Blunt head injury often produces a period of amnesia, if not loss of consciousness, immediately after impact. The acute severity of diffuse CHI is measured by the degree and duration of altered consciousness. Teasdale and Jennett (1974) developed the Glasgow Coma Scale (GCS) (see Table 14.1) for the assessment of coma. This scale consists of three components: the minimal stimulus necessary to elicit eye opening, the best motor response to command or to painful stimulation, and the best verbal response. Summation of the component scores of the GCS yields a total score, which can range from 3 to 15. Jennett et al. (1977) defined a severe acute CHI as one that results in no eye opening, inability to obey commands, and no comprehensible speech, that is, a GCS score of 8 or less for a period of at least 6 hr. Recent outcome research has typically defined a moderate CHI primarily by impaired consciousness (i.e., a GCS score from 9 to 12) which does not produce coma, whereas a mild CHI is reflected by confusion and disorientation (a GCS score from 13 to 15).

Recent evidence raises a question concerning the contribution of acute linguistic disturbance to duration of impaired consciousness. To investigate the relationship between lateralization of focal parenchymal lesion

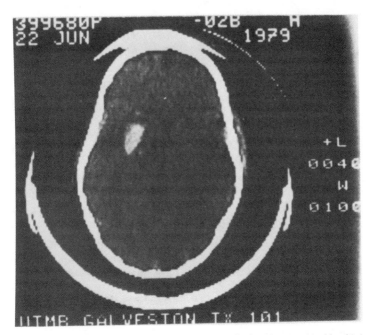

FIGURE 14.2. *Computerized tomographic scan obtained on the day of severe closed head injury in a 12-year-old girl struck by a car. The scan shows a left-hemisphere intracerebral hematoma in the putamen and anterior limb of the internal capsule. This left-handed patient had a right hemiplegia and was mute for 6 weeks after regaining consciousness.*

and impaired consciousness, Levin, Gary, and Eisenberg (1989) serially assessed selected patients from the Traumatic Coma Data Bank who had unilateral intracerebral lesions of at least 15 cc until they recovered from coma. When the criterion for resolution of coma was the return of the ability to obey simple commands, patients with left-hemisphere lesions were found to have a more prolonged period (mean = 32.8 days) of

TABLE 14.1
The Glasgow Coma Scale

Best Eye Opening		*Best Motor Response*		*Best Verbal Response*	
4	Spontaneous	6	Obeys Commands	5	Oriented
3	To Speech	5	Localizes to Pain	4	Confused
2	To Pain	4	Flexion–Withdrawal to Pain	3	Inappropriate Words
1	None	3	Abnormal Flexion to Pain	2	Incomprehensible
		2	Extension to Pain	1	None
		1	None		

impaired consciousness than were patients who sustained focal right-hemisphere insults (mean = 8.8 days). In contrast, lateralization of lesion had no effect when localization of a painful stimulus (e.g., moving an arm toward the site of supraorbital pressure) was the criterion for improved consciousness in patients who were initially comatose. The investigators interpreted these findings as evidence for the contribution of acute disturbance of receptive language to the impression of more prolonged impaired consciousness in CHI patients with left-hemisphere lesions. An implication is that nonverbal modes of response and processing are necessary to evaluate recovery of consciousness in head-injured patients with left-hemisphere lesions.

Confusion and anterograde amnesia (i.e., the inability to consolidate information about ongoing events) usually persist for a varying duration after the patient emerges from coma (Russell & Smith, 1961). The duration of posttraumatic amnesia (PTA) may range from a few minutes after mild CHI that produces no coma to several months following severe CHI. The duration of PTA is assessed directly by questioning the patient concerning orientation and recent events (Levin, O'Donnell, & Grossman, 1979) and is estimated retrospectively by inquiring of the period for which the patient has no remembrance (Russell & Smith, 1961). Focal brain lesions (e.g., hematomas) may occur in the presence of relatively mild or moderate diffuse CHI, as reflected by the period of coma and PTA.

Missile injury causes tearing of the scalp, depression or fracture of the skull, and possibly wounding of brain tissue in the track of the foreign body (see Figure 14.3). A small shower of bone fragments is often projected into the brain from the point of impact; the extent of dural penetration and loss of brain tissue are indexes of injury severity (Newcombe, 1969). As a consequence of dural penetration, posttraumatic seizure disorder is more strongly associated with aphasia secondary to missile wounds than in cases of CHI (Russell & Espir, 1961).

To determine the locus of lesion, Russell and Espir (1961) used surgical findings and lateral and anteroposterior skull X-rays to chart the entry wound and missile track on a lateral sagittal diagram of the hemisphere (see Figure 14.4). Verification of lesion localization by postmortem data suggested that this was a fairly accurate method. Although missile wounds tend to be more circumscribed than diffuse CHI and produce little or no coma, metal fragments can spread far from the primary locus of injury. Furthermore, Mohr et al. (1980) found that missile injury that produced language disorder was frequently associated with a period of unconsciousness, suggesting that diffuse effects were contributory. Missile injury that results in aphasia also commonly

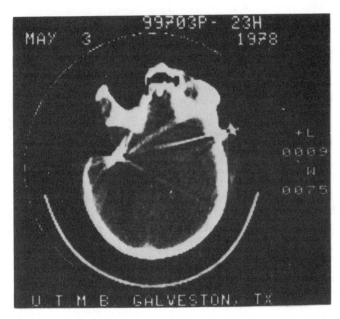

FIGURE 14.3. *Gunshot wound of the right frontotemporal region visualized by computerized tomography. Note the path of the bullet and bone fragments which traversed to the left temporal area. Wernicke's aphasia with jargon persisted for 18 months postinjury in this woman.*

produces motor and/or sensory deficit contralateral to the dominant hemisphere; this association is stronger than in the case of CHI (Levin, Grossman, & Kelly, 1976).

From this summary of the pathophysiology of head injury, we may infer that clinical data concerning the extent of focal brain injury and the severity of diffuse cerebral disturbance are pertinent to the assessment of posttraumatic aphasia.

Distinctive Features of Traumatic Aphasia

One distinctive feature of acute aphasia after CHI is the predominance of anomia (Heilman, Safran, & Geschwind, 1971). Fluent speech is often associated with verbal paraphasia and circumlocution; comprehension and repetition are relatively spared, whereas naming is markedly defective, especially to confrontation. Anomic errors include semantic approximation (e.g., "snout" for the tusks of an elephant), circumlocution (e.g., "to make music" for pedals of a piano), and concrete representation (e.g., "orange" for a circle). Anomic aphasia after

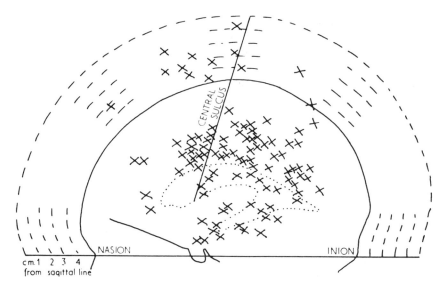

FIGURE 14.4. *Chart indicating the center of injury for missile wounds to the left hemisphere that caused aphasia. Cases with foreign bodies in remote regions of the brain were excluded from this map. Localization of missile wounds on the outline of a normal lateral skull was based on skull X-rays and surgical findings. From Russell and Espir (1961).*

CHI is distinguished from nonaphasic misnaming (Weinstein & Kahn, 1955) insofar as the former is not restricted to names of objects related to the patient's illness (e.g., wheelchair) and may be apparent during spontaneous speech (Heilman et al., 1971).

Wernicke's aphasia is the second most common language disorder following CHI. Although an acute picture of fluent paraphasic speech, poor comprehension for oral and written language, and impaired repetition has been described in CHI cases with left temporal lesions (Heilman et al., 1971; Stone, Lopes, & Moody, 1978; Thomsen, 1976), restoration of comprehension may be rapid after a hematoma resolves or is surgically removed (cf. Stone et al., 1978). A case of transient Wernicke's aphasia was observed after a relatively mild diffuse injury (as reflected by the GCS) concomitant with a suspected left-hemisphere mass lesion that was not directly visualized by computerized tomography (CT).

A 17-year-old right-handed student sustained blunt head trauma in a motorcycle accident on 23 December 1979. When admitted to the neurosurgery service in Galveston on the day of injury, he had a GCS score of 11 and no focal motor or sensory deficit. CT showed compression of the left lateral ventricle, which resolved during the course of hospitalization. The patient's speech was fluent at a rate faster than normal and was contaminated by jargon (e.g., "ruby baby"). Comprehension was grossly impaired, and the patient's mood was characterized by excitement and agitation. Throughout the first 2 weeks of his hospitalization, he was grossly disoriented and continued to exhibit Wernicke's aphasia. Stereotyped phrases and expletives were relatively spared. The patient's orientation began to improve 3 weeks postinjury and reached a normal level by 14 January. Although a clinical interview showed substantial improvement in his comprehension, the Multilingual Aphasia Examination on 17 January disclosed defective visual naming (e.g., he described a rectangle as a "long square"), inability to repeat sentences presented orally, and decreased word finding. Follow-up assessment 6 months postinjury revealed total recovery of language (see Figure 14.5).

Most published studies of aphasia after missile wounds to the brain are based on detailed observations of servicemen who were treated at the Military Hospital for Head Injuries in Oxford during and after World War II (Newcombe, 1969; Russell & Espir, 1961; Schiller, 1947). Mohr et al. (1980) and Ludlow and coworkers (1986) extended this research to include servicemen who sustained penetrating head injuries in Viet Nam. These authors have frequently described linguistic disturbance characteristic of Broca's aphasia which is typically seen after occlusion of the left middle cerebral artery.

Russell and Espir (1961) obtained information on localization of injury by separately studying aphasics who had circumscribed left-hemisphere wounds without foreign bodies in remote areas of the brain (see Figure 14.4). In contrast to the rare occurrence of nonfluent agrammatic language disturbance after CHI, Russell and Espir (1961) reported that 12% of aphasics with missile wounds had Broca's aphasia, which was typically associated with right-sided weakness and a focal injury to the frontal or Rolandic area. In a related study Schiller (1947) linked a disturbance of articulation, inflection, and rate of speech with a wound at the foot of the precentral convolution. He observed that agrammatism, disturbed prosody, and perseveration were present in patients with left frontotemporal missile wounds. Russell and Espir found focal missile wounds in the dominant parietal lobe to result frequently in a global aphasia, although small posterior parietal lesions resulted in specific anomia, alexia, and agraphia. Similarly, Mohr et al. (1980) noted that parietal injury was more likely to produce aphasia than was a focal wound of any other lobe. Global aphasia with jargon, prolonged posttraumatic amnesia, and residual memory deficit has been observed during the early stage of recovery from penetrating injury of the left tem-

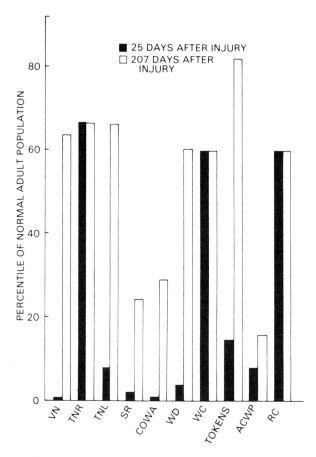

FIGURE 14.5. *Profile of language test scores obtained 1 and 6 months postinjury in a 17-year-old student who had a Wernicke's aphasia that completely resolved. VN, Visual Naming; TNR, Tactile Naming, Right Hand; TNL, Tactile Naming, Left Hand; SR, Sentence Repetition; COWA, Controlled Word Association; WD, Writing to Dictation; WC, Writing–Copying; TOKENS, Token Test; ACWP, Auditory Comprehension of Words and Phrases; and RC, Reading Comprehension.*

poral lobe (Russell & Espir, 1961). Focal temporal wounds damaging the optic radiations resulted in a visual field defect in addition to global aphasia. Impairment of reading was common in these patients.

Russell and Espir (1961) analyzed the occurrence of aphasia after unilateral brain wounds separately for right and left handers. The authors defined handedness in terms of preference for a majority of motor skills. As anticipated from other sources of data concerning cerebral dominance, only 1% of right handers became aphasic after right-hemisphere wounds, whereas 17% of left handers became aphasic after right-hemisphere wounds. Also consistent with other lines of evidence for cerebral dominance, unilateral left-hemisphere wounds more frequently produced aphasia in right handers (65%) than in sinistrals (38%). The overall figures for aphasia after unilateral injury of either hemisphere were 37% for right and 27% for left handers. Although these figures are incompatible with the concept that sinistrals are more likely to become aphasic, the comparative data presented by Russell and Espir included right-handed patients with lesions outside the speech territory. Of the right-hemisphere wounds that resulted in aphasia in sinistrals, the frontal or parietal lobes were involved in all cases.

In summary, the pattern of aphasia observed after missile wounds to the brain conforms fairly well to the localization of language in patients with cerebrovascular disease (see chapter 3 for background). The localizing significance of missile wounds is greatly enhanced by identifying patients in whom there is no evidence of additional brain penetration by fragments in remote areas (see Figure 14.4).

Prognosis for Recovery

Reports based on large numbers of servicemen with penetrating missile wounds suggest a favorable prognosis for recovery from aphasia (Mohr et al., 1980; Russell & Espir, 1961). Although the results of these studies suggest more rapid restitution of language than in aphasia secondary to cerebral vascular disease, the young age of brain-injured servicemen may also be a contributing factor. Recovery of language after missile wounds has been especially rapid and complete in cases of nonfluent, expressive aphasia ("motor aphasia") produced by focal left frontal injury or lesions situated in the lower part of the rolandic area (Mohr et al., 1980; Russell & Espir, 1961). Although resolution of right-sided weakness generally parallels the recovery of language in dysfluent aphasics, more deficit may persist after restitution of language. Russell and Espir noted that rolandic lesions also frequently resulted in residual sensory defect.

Mohr et al. (1980) observed that over the course of at least a year the aphasia produced by left parietal injury evolved into a residual expressive disorder characterized by reduced fluency. In patients with left posterior parietal lesions, Russell and Espir (1961) observed that anomia, alexia, and impaired spelling were the characteristic sequelae. Mohr et al.'s follow-up findings in patients with acute Wernicke's aphasia secondary to left temporal missile injury showed, however, that impaired comprehension persisted in more than three-fourths of these patients.

Studies reporting on the rate of recovery from aphasia after left-hemisphere missile wounds have not been in close agreement. This disparity may reflect differences in the site of injury, selection criteria, assessment techniques, and follow-up interval across the various series. Whereas Mohr et al. contended that most recovery of language occurs within 1 year after injury, Walker and Jablon (1961) observed recovery of language within 9 months after injury in nearly one-third of their cases. By 7 to 8 years postinjury, however, more than one-half of the servicemen who had been aphasic continued to exhibit language disturbance.

The 15-year outcome of nonfluent aphasia resulting from penetrating missile wounds of the left hemisphere was elucidated in a detailed study by Ludlow et al. (1986). The selection criteria included persistence of nonfluent aphasia 6 months after injury and absence of confounding complications such as bilateral hearing loss. Of the 39 servicemen who returned for follow-up, two-thirds had fully recovered, whereas one-third had residual nonfluent aphasia according to the results of standardized tests, including the Boston Diagnostic Aphasia Examination (Goodglass & Kaplan, 1983). The conversation of the nonrecovered men was characterized by simple sentences, a high proportion of automatic phrases, and relatively well-preserved retrieval of vocabulary. Comparison of the follow-up CT scans in these groups disclosed that left-hemisphere lesions encroaching on posterior cortex (Wernicke's area and supramarginal gyrus) most clearly separated the nonrecovered (92%) from the recovered (42%) patients. Other lesion sites that distinguished the residual aphasics included the posterior white matter and basal ganglia. In contrast, 77% of both groups had anterior cortical lesions involving Broca's area. Consistent with this lesion localization, right hemiparesis was present in 75% of the nonrecovered patients compared with 36% of the recovered group. Interestingly, 19% of the recovered patients were left handed prior to injury, whereas none of the patients with residual aphasia were sinistrals. Ludlow and coworkers (1986) postulated that bilateral speech representation in the left handers enhanced their recovery from nonfluent aphasia. In summary, the findings of these investigators suggest that lesions restricted to the left anterior region portend recovery from nonfluent aphasia (especially in left handers) following left-hemisphere missile injury.

In a broader study of long-term outcome after missile injury, Newcombe (1969) found that nearly one-third of the Oxford patients with left-hemisphere wounds continued to evidence aphasic symptoms when examined at the time of follow-up. Word fluency, measured by retrieval of items from a given category (e.g., colors), was reduced in the total series of left-hemisphere–injured patients, although the deficit was more severe in patients with residual aphasic symptoms. Defects in vocabulary, reading, spelling, and writing were confined to patients considered to be aphasic. In contrast, more than half of the total series (including nonaphasic patients with left-hemisphere wounds) continued to complain of "being at a loss for a word." Residual impairment of verbal memory was found in patients with left-hemisphere injury, including those who were nonaphasic at the time of follow-up. In summary, most patients rendered aphasic by missile injury exhibit relatively permanent aphasic symptoms or more subtle defects in verbal skills and memory.

Investigators only recently have studied the early recovery of communicative skills after prolonged coma in patients with severe CHI. Najenson, Sazbon, Fiselzon, Becker, and Schechter (1978) plotted recovery curves for communicative skills during the first 18 months after severe CHI in 15 patients with prolonged coma (undefined) who were referred to a rehabilitation unit. The authors developed a scale, shown in Table 14.2, to rate expressive and receptive functions because the patients were unable to cooperate with standardized tests usually employed during later stages of recovery. As shown in Table 14.2, this scale consists of six major functions, and each is divided into specific communicative skills. At evaluation, each specific test is assigned a score ranging from 0 to 4. The total score for each major function is summed and expressed as a percentage of the maximum possible score. Najenson et al. plotted the percentage scores monthly to depict the course of recovery. Six patients in this study remained in a vegetative state, whereas 9 cases had partial or full restitution of language. The authors observed a consistent sequence of recovery. Comprehension of gestures and oral language appeared first, usually between 3 weeks and 5 months after trauma. Oral expression, reading, and writing were slower to recover, and motor defects in speech (e.g., articulation, respiratory control, and phonation) were often persistently impaired. Of the 9 patients who recovered communication, 8 had dysarthric speech. The authors observed that the recovery of communicative ability corresponded to progressive improvement in locomotion.

In a study of outcome after severe diffuse CHI (coma > 24 hrs), Thomsen (1975) administered a follow-up (mean interval = 31 to 33 months after injury) language examination of her own design to 12 patients who had been acutely aphasic. Four patients, including 2 sinistrals, had no signs of aphasia. In the others, amnestic aphasia (slow rate of speech, slow repetition of words or phrases, verbal paraphasia, and perseveration) was frequently present. Thomsen noted a residual decline in complex verbal skills, such as detailed verbal description and

TABLE 14.2

Assessment of Communication Functions After Prolonged Coma[a]

Auditory comprehension	*Oral expression*
Awareness of gross environmental sounds	Voicing
Awareness of speech	Saying vowels
Ability to indicate yes and no	Saying consonants
Understanding own name	Saying own name
Recognition of family names	Saying nouns
Understanding simple verbal orders	Saying verbs
Recognition of names of familiar objects	Saying noun–verb combinations
Recognition of colors	Saying short sentences (automatic)
Recognition of forms	Saying short sentences (nonautomatic)
Understanding use of familiar objects	Conversational speech
Visual comprehension	*Reading*
Awareness of visual stimulation	Reading own name
Understanding gesture direction	Reading family names
Association of identical objects	Reading single words
Association of identical forms	Reading simple sentences
Association of similar objects	Reading newspaper headlines
Categorization	Reading newspaper articles
Speech	*Writing*
Articulation	Writing own name
Respiration	Writing family names
Voice	Writing words
	Writing simple sentences
	Writing a letter

[a]From Najenson, Sazbon, Fiselzon, Becker, and Schecter (1978). Reproduced with permission of the authors and publisher.

the use of antonyms, synonyms, and metaphors. Impaired reading was found in 4 cases, but no patient was totally alexic. Although these findings agree with the view that aphasia secondary to CHI has a good prognosis, Thomsen emphasized that residual linguistic defects and dysarthria were present. Moreover, she pointed out that the manifestations of "subclinical" language problems depend on the recovery of memory and general cognitive function.

In a second investigation, Thomsen (1976) reexamined the language of 15 patients who had focal mass lesions (in which temporal lobe damage predominated) or extensive destruction of the left hemisphere and who had been aphasic during the initial hospitalization. When tested at least 1 year after injury (mean interval = 29 months), an overall trend of improvement was evident, although all patients exhibited residual language deficits. The course of recovery was characterized by improved comprehension of oral and written language and less severe agraphia. As in Thomsen's (1975) study of diffuse CHI patients, amnestic aphasia and perseveration persisted in nearly all patients. Global aphasia with gross impairment of all language functions typically evolved into receptive aphasia, whereas patients who initially had a receptive aphasia frequently evidenced improvement in comprehension despite residual anomia. Although Thomsen concluded that nearly all patients with focal left-hemisphere lesions made some improvement, she noted that "half the patients had severe or moderate aphasia two and a half years after the trauma and a few had not been able to pass the level of automatic language (e.g., expletives, stereotyped phrases)" (p. 376).

Groher (1977) administered the Porch Index of Communicative Ability to 14 consecutively admitted, comatose CHI patients at 1-month intervals beginning shortly after termination of coma (mean duration = 17 days). He reported progressive improvement in expressive and receptive skills over a 4-month period. Naming to confrontation recovered in all patients, whereas spelling errors, incomplete sentence construction, and syntax errors persisted. The degree of recovery suggested by this study appears to be greater than the impression conveyed by other investigators of aphasia after severe CHI. This finding may be attributed to Groher's inclusion of a consecutive series of comatose patients instead of confining the study to acutely aphasic cases.

When consecutive referrals of CHI patients to a rehabilitation program are considered, a different view of outcome emerges which may reflect the severity of injuries requiring intensive retraining. Sarno, Buonaguro, and Levita (1986) described the results of administering the Neurosensory Center Comprehensive Examination for Aphasia (NCCEA) to 125 patients after an average postinjury interval of 45 weeks. The series, which included a wide range of coma duration (15 min to 6 months), consisted of CHI produced by motor vehicle accidents in about half of the cases. Consistent with earlier findings (Sarno, 1980, 1984) Sarno et al. reported that language disorder and/or dysarthria were present in all patients. Of interest were the distinctions among classic aphasia ($n = 37$), dysarthria with subclinical aphasia ($n = 43$), and subclinical aphasia ($n = 45$). Sarno et al. diagnosed dysarthria and classic aphasia on the basis of spontaneous speech and comprehension during an interview. The investigators used the term SUBCLINICAL APHASIA DISORDER to refer to evidence of linguistic processing deficits on testing in the absence of clinical manifestations of linguistic impairment. Applying this broad classification, Sarno et al. found that all patients in the series had residual speech or language defects. The aphasic group was older (mean age = 38 years) than the dysarthric (mean = 24 years) and subclinical (mean = 28 years) patients. Right hemiplegia was more common among aphasics, whereas quadriplegia was more frequent in dysarthrics. The quantitative test results obtained by Sarno et al. are illustrated in Figure 14.6, which shows percentile scores based on an aphasic population. The subclinical linguistic deficits involved visual naming, word fluency, and comprehension of multistage commands (Token Test;

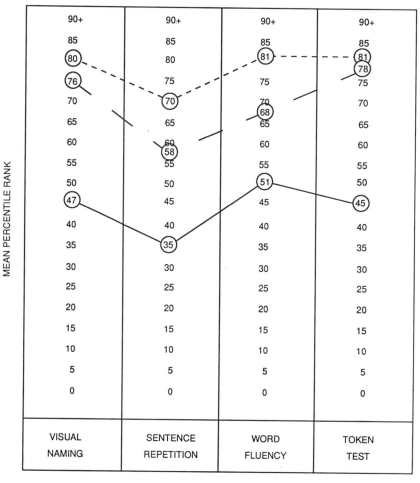

FIGURE 14.6. *Mean percentile rank of aphasic and subclinical language disorder groups on subtests of the Neurosensory Center Examination for Aphasia.* ———, *Aphasic;* — —, *dysarthric and subclinical;* – – –, *subclinical. Note that the percentile scores are based on results obtained in an aphasic population. From Sarno, Buonaguro, and Levita (1986). Reproduced with permission by the author and publisher.*

see Figure 14.6). The findings obtained by Sarno et al. confirmed Thomsen's (1975) findings in showing that subtle language disturbance is common after CHI even in the absence of unequivocal aphasia.

In the course of a long-term study of patients with severe CHI who had been acutely aphasic, Levin, Grossman, Sarwar, and Meyers (1981) assessed recovery from aphasia in 21 patients. The results of initial CT and findings from surgery disclosed evidence of primary left-hemisphere injury in 8 cases, focal lesions of the right hemisphere in 4 cases, bilateral injury in 2 patients, and diffuse CHI in the remaining patients. The Multilingual Aphasia Examination (MAE) (Benton, 1967) and portions of the aphasia battery of Spreen and Benton (1969) were administered at the time of follow-up. Nine patients fully recovered from acute aphasia as reflected by uniformly normal scores and intact conversational speech. The 12 patients with residual language deficit (indicated by at least one grossly defective score) were equally divided between cases with a persistent impairment of both expressive and receptive abilities and cases of specific language deficit. Anomia and decreased word finding were the most common isolated defects. Patients who fully recovered from acute aphasia or exhibited a specific language disturbance at the time of follow-up were generally functioning within the average range of intelligence, whereas patients with generalized language impairment evidenced intellectual deficit on both the Verbal and the Performance scales of the Wechsler Adult Intelligence Scale (WAIS).

In accord with the course of recovery observed in an earlier study by Thomsen (1975), acute global aphasia in this series of patients frequently evolved into a specific anomia. This pattern is illustrated by the serial findings in a 17-year-old student (see Figure 14.7A) who had a left temporal mass lesion and a diffuse injury of mild to moderate severity. She initially exhibited impairment of naming, word association, and alexia, whereas residual language deficit was confined to anomia. In contrast,

---

→

FIGURE 14.7. *(A) Baseline and follow-up language profiles of a 17-year-old student with residual anomia that was initially accompanied by a receptive impairment after surgical evacuation of a left temporal intracerebral hematoma. (B) Baseline and follow-up findings in a 19-year-old student which show persistent impairment of expressive and receptive language associated with cognitive deficit and progressive ventricular enlargement. He sustained a severe diffuse injury (coma = 21 days) complicated by bifrontal subdural hematomas. VN, Visual Naming; TNR, Tactile Naming, Right Hand; TNL, Tactile Naming, Left Hand; SR, Sentence Repetition; COWA, Controlled Word Association; WD, Writing to Dictation; WC, Writing–Copying; TOKENS, Token Test; ACWP, Auditory Comprehension of Words and Phrases; RC, Reading Comprehension. From Levin, Grossman, Sarwar, and Meyers (1981). Reproduced with permission by the publisher.*

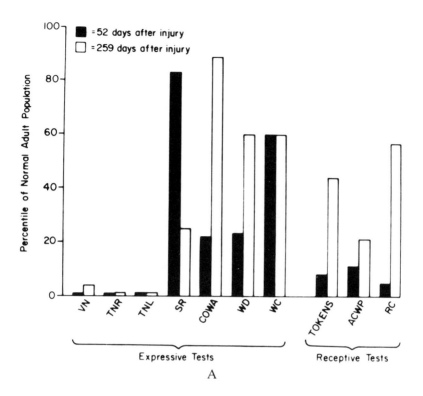

A

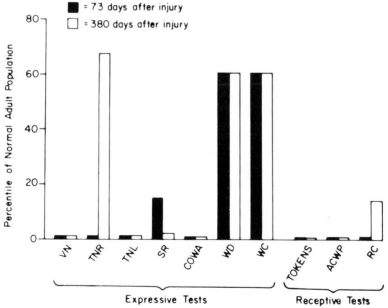

B

Figure 14.7B depicts persistent, generalized language defects in an 18-year-old patient who sustained a severe CHI (coma = 21 days) complicated by bilateral frontoparietal subdural hematomas. He evidenced a concomitant decline in cognitive ability, as reflected by a disparity between follow-up results on the WAIS and his high school test scores.

To summarize, the studies of long-term recovery of language after CHI show an overall trend of improvement that may eventuate in restoration of language or specific defects ("subclinical" language disorder) in naming or word finding in about two-thirds of the patients who are acutely aphasic. Generalized language deficit, which is associated with global cognitive impairment, persists in patients who sustain severe CHI.

Assessment of Aphasia After Closed Head Injury

Clinical Evaluation of Conversational Speech

SPEECH DURING THE PERIOD OF
POSTTRAUMATIC AMNESIA

As mentioned above in the review of mechanisms of injury, the early postcomatose stage of recovery from CHI is typically characterized by an amnesic condition during which the patient is confused. Reduplicative paramnesia (Benson, Gardner, & Meadows, 1976)—that is, the mistaken identification of a person, place, or event for one previously experienced, confabulation, and profound impairment of memory—may be misinterpreted as signs of language disorder. The distinction may be particularly difficult in a patient whose fluent speech is disconnected and perseverative. Confused, nonaphasic speech after CHI was evident in a patient studied in Galveston.

A 24-year-old right-handed woman was transferred from a community hospital to the University of Texas Medical Branch 3 hr after she sustained a CHI in a motor vehicle accident on 28 January 1978. The GCS score was 8 when she was initially examined. The cerebral ventricles and cisterns were poorly visualized on CT, suggesting the presence of diffuse cerebral swelling. Although she obeyed commands after 4 days, her disorientation persisted until 5 March. Spontaneous speech during the confusional period was continuous, rambling, and disorganized in this fearful, agitated woman. When queried on 27 February regarding the reason for her hospitalization, she responded, "Something that came up natural being born somewhere in here." Later in the day the patient elaborated that she was in the hospital "to have a baby" and that the year was 1952 (she was born in 1953). Reminiscent of the patients described by Weinstein and Kahn (1955), during examination the following day, she commented that she was hospitalized because of "being stabbed." This statement was interpreted as a reference to her intravenous tubes. Assessment of language on 19 April, however, disclosed completely normal findings on the MAE.

Analysis of this patient's utterances provided little evidence of consistent paraphasic errors, particularly when she was asked structured questions that focused on specific objects rather than expository material. Repeated questioning within the limits of her short attention span disclosed no evidence of receptive impairment similar to that found in patients with Wernicke's aphasia. Administration of tests of naming and word finding to this patient during posttraumatic amnesia (PTA) would likely have yielded defective scores. Weinstein and Kahn (1955) described patients with brain damage of diverse etiologies, including diffuse cerebral disturbance, who exhibited misnaming that was qualitatively atypical for aphasia. Anomic errors were frequently associated with objects that bore a relation to the patient's illness and frequently occurred during a period of disorientation, confabulation, and denial of illness. The authors observed that, in contrast to patients with classical anomic aphasia, patients exhibiting nonaphasic misnaming frequently showed no evidence of groping for words in their spontaneous speech nor did their naming necessarily improve when correction was offered.

Conversely, the presence of paraphasic errors in conversational speech after CHI may be misinterpreted as evidence for disorientation and confusion. This condition is likely to be found in CHI patients with mass lesion or depressed skull fracture involving the left hemisphere. In such cases, a multiple-choice format of testing orientation may be useful, as well as relatively nonverbal tests during the early stages of recovery.

POSTCONFUSIONAL STAGE OF RECOVERY

Few studies of aphasia during the early stages of recovery from CHI have concurrently assessed orientation. Consequently, there is a possibility that PTA had not completely resolved at the time language was evaluated.

Clinical examination of language in consecutive CHI admissions at the Boston City Hospital was found by Heilman et al. (1971) to yield 13 cases of aphasia, including 9 patients with anomic aphasia and 4 cases of Wernicke's aphasia. Aphasics accounted for 2% of the Boston series, a base rate very close to that obtained in a previous study of consecutive CHI admissions (Arseni, Constantinovici, Iliescu, Dobrota, & Gagea, 1970). In the Boston study, the authors defined anomic aphasia as a fluent aphasia in which the patient demonstrates verbal paraphasia for all kinds of material especially to confrontation. Wernicke's aphasia was defined as a fluent aphasia with paraphasia, impaired comprehension for spoken and written language, and poor repetition. Broca's aphasia was defined as nonfluent aphasia with relatively intact comprehension. No patient had a Broca's aphasia or exhibited total disruption of language. Heilman et al. (1971) excluded patients with intracranial surgery (other than evacuation of subdural hematoma). This strategy of patient selection, combined with the relatively high proportion of falls relative to motor vehicle accidents, may have restricted patients with mass lesions, thereby resulting in fewer aphasic cases compared with those of other neurotrauma centers.

Heilman et al. (1971) distinguished the anomia in their CHI patients from nonaphasic misnaming (Weinstein & Kahn, 1955). In contrast to the narrow range of anomic errors (e.g., related to illness) in cases of nonaphasic misnaming, the anomic CHI patients described by Heilman et al. exhibited diverse naming defects in spontaneous speech and writing. We have also been able to distinguish anomic aphasia from nonaphasic misnaming by delaying evaluation of language until the injured patient recovers to a normal level of orientation. This strategy revealed initial findings characteristic of Wernicke's aphasia in a patient who later evidenced anomic aphasia.

On 17 October 1975, a 17-year-old student was transferred to the University of Texas Medical Branch 3 hr after a motor vehicle accident in which she received a CHI. The GCS score on admission was 8. Although the patient obeyed commands on the day of admission, delayed neurological deterioration was reflected by the development of a right hemiparesis and progressive aphasia. Three days postinjury a partial left temporal lobectomy was performed with evacuation of an intracerebral hematoma. The patient remained confused for a month after injury but exhibited gradual improvement of receptive language. Administration of the MAE 2 months after injury disclosed findings consistent with an anomic aphasia. There were frequent errors of circumlocution (e.g., she described an island as "a place where you fish"), semantic approximation (e.g., she described the trunk of an elephant as a "nose"), and a tendency to substitute names of concrete objects for geometric designs (e.g., she described a triangle as "the thing you use when you play pool"). As shown in Figure 14.7A, the patient's long-term recovery of language was complete, except for a subtle residual anomic disturbance that was evident only under testing conditions.

Anomic aphasia may also persist after resolution of PTA in patients with severe diffuse CHI who evidence no other focal neurologic signs. In a study of 26 CHI patients without mass lesions who had been in coma for at least 24 hr, Thomsen (1975) found that aphasic symptoms were present during the first 2 or 3 weeks after injury in 12 cases. Verbal paraphasia (i.e., substitution of inappropriate words) and anomia were the most common defects; receptive impairment and dysgraphia were also frequently observed, whereas paragrammatism and other symptoms suggestive of Broca's aphasia were rarely seen. We have observed a patient who bears a close resemblance to the series of diffuse head injuries described by Thomsen.

A 20-year-old right-handed man was admitted to the University of Texas Medical Branch with a severe CHI (GCS score = 5) but no focal motor deficit. The CT scan suggested generalized brain swelling without a mass lesion. Baseline assessment 4 months after injury disclosed anomic errors that deteriorated into jargon (e.g., the handle of a fork was described as a "forkline" and the posterior aspect of the leg was described as a "negline"). Circumlocution was evidenced by his response when the examiner pointed to the pedals of a piano: "If you want a different sound, push them down." Word finding was defective on a test of letter–word association.

Clinical examination of language has disclosed a broad range of language defects in CHI patients. Thomsen (1976) characterized the findings in a series of patients with left-hemisphere mass lesions as "multisymptomatic aphasia." She used this term to describe patients who exhibited anomia, agraphia, and impaired comprehension; one-third of the patients in her series had global or receptive aphasia. Anomic aphasia was less common, and there were no cases of Broca's aphasia. Posttraumatic dyslexia and dysgraphia have also been reported by other authors (de Morsier, 1973).

NONAPHASIC DISORDERS OF SPEECH

Posttraumatic speech disorders that may occur without aphasia include mutism, stuttering, echolalia, palilalia, and dysarthria.

Mutism. Total abolition of speech may occur after termination of coma in patients capable of following commands during the transition between spontaneous eye opening and recovery of orientation. As previously described, transient mutism is characteristic of aphasia after head injury in children.

Prolonged if not permanent speechlessness is observed in adults who are persistently vegetative or exhibit akinetic mutism (Cairns, 1952; Plum & Posner, 1980). The akinetic type is a form of subacute or persistent mutism with little or no vocalization. Behaviorally this condition is distinguished from the vegetative state by its immobility. The features common to both conditions include apparent wakefulness with restoration of the sleep–wake cycle and inability to demonstrate cognitive function through interaction with the environment. When akinetic mutism is a sequel to CHI, diffuse cerebral injury is to be suspected.

Geschwind (1974) distinguished between nonaphasic and aphasic mutism. The aphasic type, which was thought to occur rarely in adults with CHI (cf. de Morsier, 1973), is accompanied by linguistic errors in writing. Nonaphasic mutism is associated with acute onset of right hemiplegia; writing is normal and there are no signs of aphasia when speech is restored. Following Bastian (1898), Geschwind referred to this condition as aphemia rather than aphasia. In such cases mutism may arise from focal lesions, often involving the basal ganglia. We have studied a case of subcortical mutism, which is described below.

In a prospective study of patients admitted to neurosurgery services in Houston and Galveston, posttraumatic mutism was present in nine patients (nearly 3% of the series) despite recovery of consciousness and communication through a nonspeech channel (Levin et al., 1983). CT scans revealed subcortical lesions situated primarily in the putamen and internal capsule of four patients, whereas four of the five without subcortical lesions had left-hemisphere cortical injury. The patients without subcortical injury visualized by CT exhibited a longer duration of impaired consciousness consistent with diffuse brain injury and showed more long-term linguistic deficits. The four patients with basal ganglia lesions included two children and an adolescent, a finding consistent with other evidence that basal ganglia lesions in CHI may be more common in the pediatric age range.

Stuttering.   Published studies suggest that stuttering is a more common sequel of penetrating missile wound than of CHI (Peacher, 1945). De Morsier (1973), however, noted a fluency disorder in more than half of his series of CHI patients, including four cases with posttraumatic stuttering. Helm, Butler, and Benson (1978) implicated bilateral injury in patients with acquired stuttering after CHI.

Echolalia and Palilalia.   Echolalia is the repetition of words spoken by others, whereas palilalia is the automatic repetition of one's own words. Echolalia may follow a period of mutism in cases with diffuse cerebral dysfunction (CHI) or may occur in patients with transcortical motor aphasia, that is, disturbed expressive and receptive language with preserved repetition. Apart from generalized cerebral disturbance, these disorders have been associated with large frontal lesions. According to Geschwind (1974), echolalia and Palilalia are uncommon in patients with lesions primarily involving the perisylvian region of the dominant hemisphere.

Stengel (1947) distinguished between the automatic and mitigated forms of echolalia. The former is parrotlike with no elaboration of the input. Mitigated echolalia is the questioning repetition of words spoken by others, often with a change of the personal pronoun. Stengel postulated that mitigated echolalia may facilitate comprehension in patients with receptive language disturbance. Accordingly, the transition from automatic to mitigated echolalia may be a sign of clinical improvement that parallels the developmental sequence in children. Stengel also observed that the mitigated type may be confined to social conversation and less evident when the patient is directly questioned by an unfamiliar speaker.

Thomsen (1976) reported 3 cases of echolalia in a series of 50 patients with severe CHI. Of the 2 echolalic patients with left-hemisphere mass lesions, 1 initially had a global aphasia and the other had minimal spontaneous speech. The third patient, who sustained a severe diffuse CHI with residual hydrocephalus, evidenced echolalia and palilalia. In contrast to the general association of echolalia with impoverished spontaneous speech (see Geschwind, 1974), Thomsen commented that the patient with diffuse CHI "talked almost constantly without any inhibition" (p. 220). We have studied a patient who developed a similar echolalia after CHI.

An 18-year-old right-handed student was brought to the emergency room of the University of Texas Medical Branch shortly after an automobile accident on 11 May 1980. Initial examination disclosed a GCS score of 6, fixed and dilated pupils, and a right hemiparesis. A CT scan on the day of injury was normal. She slowly improved and eventually followed commands on 9 June. After transfer to the Del Oro Rehabilitation Hospital in Houston on 16 June she remained confused and disoriented until 26 June. During this period, the patient's spontaneous speech changed from an overall impoverishment to a greater than normal flow in which automatic echolalia was prominent. Observations by Mary Ellen Hayden and Ron Levy during the course of rehabilitation showed a transition to mitigated echolalia which resolved by the middle of July. Repetition was most evident in the presence of persons familiar to the patient. Aphasia examination on 16 July disclosed intact spontaneous speech and relatively normal naming. Echolalia had resolved, but repetition of sentences and verbal associative fluency were markedly impaired. Comprehension of complex commands on the Token Test was also defective, whereas the patient could read and comprehend single words and phrases. Further progress in rehabilitation was complicated by her disinhibited behavior, a finding in agreement with Stengel's (1947) interpretation of echolalia as a failure of inhibitory control.

In summary, echolalia and palilalia are infrequent sequelae of CHI that are found in cases with severe diffuse CHI or large mass lesions in the dominant hemisphere. The absence of any reference to echolalia and palilalia in several studies supports the contention that they rarely occur after CHI (Levin et al., 1976; Najenson et al., 1978; Sarno, 1980).

Dysarthria. Sarno (1980) defined dysarthria as a speech disorder arising from pathology in the motor speech system that is evident in defects of the acoustic aspects of the speech stream (i.e., articulation, resonance, stress, and intonation). The severity of dysarthria varies from articulatory imprecision to completely unintelligible speech. Dysarthria may be due to a lesion of either the central or the peripheral nervous system. Peacher (1945) reviewed the cases of dysarthria recorded by U.S. Army hospitals during World War II. Of the injuries producing dysarthria, which were primarily missile wounds, 69% involved a lesion of the peripheral nerves. Trauma to the facial nerve was the most common site of lesion, although Peacher did not distinguish between central and peripheral facial nerve injuries.

Investigators of speech disorder after CHI have frequently reported dysarthria in patients with focal mass lesion of the left hemisphere (Alajouanine, Castaigne, Lhermitte, Escourolle, & De Ribaucourt, 1957; de Morsier, 1973; Thomsen, 1975) and in cases of diffuse cerebral injury (Sarno, 1980, 1984; Sarno et al., 1986; Thomsen, 1976). Dysarthric patients are frequently hemiparetic or may be quadraplegic. Serial assessment of language after severe CHI has suggested that dysarthia often accompanies aphasia during the early stage of recovery from CHI, and may persist after restoration of language. This dissociation is illustrated in a patient admitted to the University of Texas Medical Branch.

A 33-year-old right-handed carpenter sustained a severe CHI in a motorcycle accident on 17 December 1977. Evaluation in the emergency room shortly after injury disclosed a GCS score of 4. A CT scan showed a large left parietotemporal epidural hematoma, which was evacuated on the day of admission. Although he progressively improved and followed commands on 20 December, a left facial palsy and right hemiparesis remained. The combined aphasia and severe dysarthria rendered his speech unintelligible. By the first week in January, the patient's language and speech disorder partially resolved, although he continued to evidence anomia and impaired comprehension. A CT scan 10 months postinjury disclosed a large hypodense area at the site of the operated hematoma and a small hypodense area in the genu of the left internal capsule which was interpreted as a small lacunar infarct. He was transferred to a rehabilitation center prior to neuropsychological evaluation but returned a year later for testing. Despite frequent articulatory defects, expressive and receptive language skills had uniformly recovered, as reflected by normal scores on all subtests of the MAE.

In contrast to this patient's findings, Sarno (1980, 1984) and Sarno et al. (1986) reported that subclinical language deficit (e.g., decreased word fluency) was present in all dysarthric patients in a series of CHI cases. The findings in the Galveston patients suggest that the correspondence between language skills and motor speech varies depending upon the interval between injury and assessment.

We may conclude from these studies that assessment of communicative disorder after CHI should include evaluation of dysarthria. The tests for articulatory agility and rating speech characteristics that are included in the Boston Diagnostic Aphasia Battery (Goodglass & Kaplan, 1983) are brief and useful for this purpose.

Quantitative Findings on Aphasia Examination

The administration of standardized examinations for aphasia has yielded a characteristic profile of language disturbance after CHI. This strategy has disclosed that "subclinical" aphasic disorder—that is, evidence of language processing deficit on testing in the absence of clinical manifestations of classical aphasia (Sarno, 1980, 1984; Sarno et al., 1986)—is a frequent sequel of CHI. Moreover, quantitative assessment has facilitated the study of long-term recovery (cf. Levin et al., 1981).

Profiles of language disorder after CHI have been developed using the MAE (Benton, 1967; Benton & Hamsher, 1978) and the NCCEA (Spreen and Benton, 1969). The MAE evaluates expressive language on subtests of naming pictures of objects (Visual Naming), Sentence Repetition, Digit Repetition, and retrieving words beginning with a designated letter (Controlled Word Association). Benton and Hamsher (1978) included a spelling test in their 1978 revision of the MAE. Comprehension of oral language is evaluated by the Token Test and a receptive test in which the patient points to the picture corresponding to a word or phrase presented orally (Aural Comprehension of Words and Phrases). Reading comprehension is tested using a similar format. The NCCEA

(Spreen & Benton, 1969) includes similar tests, in addition to tests of naming objects presented tactually (Tactile Naming), construction of sentences (Sentence Construction), identification of objects by name, oral reading, writing names, writing to dictation and copying, and articulation. Both examinations yield a percentile score based on normative data for each subtest; the manual for the NCCEA also provides percentile scores based on performance of aphasics. Gaddes and Crockett (1973) published normative data for children on the NCCEA. The Boston Diagnostic Aphasia Test (Goodglass & Kaplan, 1983) also provides a profile of language abilities. It incorporates tests for articulation, repetition of automatized sequences, and rating of spontaneous speech.

We administered portions of the MAE and NCCEA to a consecutive series of patients with CHIs of varying severity (Levin et al., 1976). In this study, injury that produced no neurological deficit or loss of consciousness longer than a few minutes was designated as Grade I; Grade II referred to an injury producing coma not longer than 24 hr, and Grade III designated an injury that resulted in a period of coma exceeding 24 hr. A language subtest score that fell below the second percentile of the normative population was considered defective. Whereas clinical examination of spontaneous speech disclosed evidence of aphasia in only eight patients (16% of the series), nearly one-half of the patients were impaired in naming objects (Figure 14.8). Word finding difficulty (Controlled Word Association) and impaired writing to dictation were also common expressive defects in this series. In contrast, Figure 14.8 shows that repetition of sentences was well preserved. Nearly one-third of the patients had difficulty in comprehending complex oral commands on the Token Test. The results provided strong support for the presence of subclinical language deficit in apparently nonaphasic CHI patients, including cases with injuries of moderate severity.

Sarno et al. (1986) elucidated the characteristics of subclinical aphasia and speech disorder after CHI in a study of 125 CHI patients who were rendered comatose for periods ranging from 15 min to 6 months and who were referred to the Rusk Institute for Rehabilitation Medicine in New York. On the basis of clinical evaluation and administration of subtests of the NCCEA (median injury–test interval of 45 weeks), the authors classified the patients into categories of grossly obvious aphasia, dysarthria with language deficit reflected by test scores ("subclinical" aphasia), and language deficit without dysarthria. The author found that the proportion of patients with each category of language disturbance was approximately equal. The aphasic group ($n = 37$) consisted of 19 patients (51%) with fluent aphasia, 13 (35%) with nonfluent aphasia, and 5 (14%) with global aphasia. As depicted in Figure 14.6, aphasic

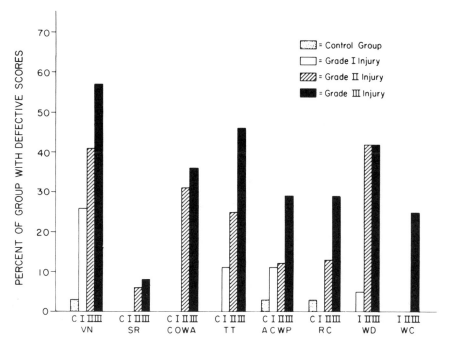

FIGURE 14.8. *Percentage of head-injured and control patients with defective scores in the Multi-lingual Aphasia Examination. VN, Visual Naming; SR, Sentence Repetition; COWA, Controlled Word Association, TT, Token Test; ACWP, Auditory Comprehension of Words and Phrases; RC, Reading Comprehension; WD, Writing to Dictation; WC, Writing–Copying. From Levin, Grossman, and Kelly (1976). Reproduced with permission of the publisher.*

patients had linguistic test scores that fell below the other groups. Most aphasics had defective scores on all four language subtests that were administered, whereas 56% of the subclinical patients failed at least two of the four tests. The patients with dysarthria had word fluency and sentence repetition scores that fell below the pure subclinical group. No CHI patients in this series, however, obtained completely normal scores.

Figure 14.6 shows the test results of the CHI patients in Sarno et al.'s (1986) study transformed into percentile scores for an aphasic population. Accordingly, any score below the ninetieth percentile is impaired in relation to normal subjects. The mean scores indicate reduced word fluency in the subclinical groups, although visual naming is also compromised. Consistent with the results of the Galveston study, Sarno's subclinical patients without dysarthria had adequate sentence repetition, whereas the dysarthric patients exhibited difficulty on this task. Impaired comprehension of complex oral commands was also found in patients without obvious aphasia. In a discussion of the results obtained in the Galveston study and her own investigation of language disturbance after CHI, Sarno concluded, "The use of sophisticated, neurolinguistic measures with this population is needed to detect subtle deficit which can permit enlightened clinical judgment".

Analysis of Discourse in Head-Injured Patients

DISPARITY BETWEEN DISCOURSE AND RESULTS
ON STRUCTURED TESTS

Recent studies have shown that head injury and other etiologies of acquired brain damage can produce a residual impairment of discourse ability despite recovery of performance on quantified, albeit structured, language tests as described in the previous section. Consistent with descriptions of residual speech following severe head injury as tangential, if not confabulatory, several studies have reported diminished efficiency of communication in the discourse of CHI patients (Ehrlich, 1988; Mentis & Prutting, 1987; Novoa & Ardila, 1987; Penn & Cleary, 1988; Ulatowska, Freedman-Stern, Doyel, & Macaluso-Haynes, 1983; Wyckoff, 1984). The studies by Erlich (1988), Mentis and Prutting (1987), and Wyckoff (1984) were confined to CHI patients, whereas the other investigations included other etiologies. Techniques employed in studies of discourse include asking patients to generate stories in response to a standard series of pictures depicting an interpersonal situation (e.g., comic strip), retelling a story, and generating a procedural narrative such as how to buy groceries (Wyckoff, 1984). An important methodological aspect of this work is recording the narrative and evaluating the interrater reliability for scoring the variables of interest.

In a study that analyzed the discourse for two narratives (in response to a comic strip and retelling a story) and explaining how to buy groceries, Wyckoff (1984) compared the findings obtained in 11 survivors of severe CHI (including 5 patients who were considered to be aphasic according to a standardized battery of language tests) with a group of normal subjects. The discourse of the head-injured patients was characterized by slow speech, in which a greater percentage of syllabic utterances were dysfluencies, and generally diminished productivity. The head-injured patients produced about one-half to two-thirds of the amount of accurate content relative to the discourse of normal speakers. Moreover, the discourse of head-injured patients contained fewer cohesive ties between utterances, a feature exemplified by failure to provide a referent. Wyckoff concluded that discourse analysis could potentially identify difficulty in functional communication, which would otherwise be overlooked by traditional, standardized language tests. At the same time, she suggested that further study utilizing spontaneous conversation with another speaker could potentially identify additional deficits, such as difficulty in topic maintenance.

In a study of 10 nonaphasic CHI patients who returned for linguistic examination at least 6 months posttrauma, Ehrlich (1988) analyzed the stories that they recited in response to the "Cookie Theft" picture from the Boston Diagnostic Aphasia Examination (Goodglass & Kaplan, 1983). The only difference that emerged in the comparison of narratives by these patients with those of normal adults was a reduction in the amount of information per unit of time. This pattern reflected the tendency of CHI patients to utter lengthier, slower spoken language.

METHODS OF DISCOURSE ANALYSIS

More detailed analysis of discourse in CHI adults has involved assessment of cohesion using the technique developed by Halliday and Hasan (1976). Accordingly, two items are cohesively related (i.e., a cohesive tie) if the interpretation of one of the elements in a text depends on reference to another (based on grammar and vocabulary). This methodology has shown that head-injured survivors frequently fail to provide the speaker with a referent. Wyckoff (1984) recorded fewer cohesive ties per communication in the discourse of 11 survivors of severe CHI compared with that of normal subjects. Mentis and Prutting (1987) studied cohesion in the discourse of three patients who had sustained a severe CHI at least 1 year earlier. In common with the patients studied by Ehrlich (1988), these CHI survivors were nonaphasic according to clinical examination and their scores on a conventional aphasia test battery. A conversation and narrative language sample (e.g., description of the patient's work) with a familiar partner were videotaped. Although the number of cohesive ties was similar in the conversation of the two groups, the normal subjects had a greater number of cohesive ties in their narratives compared with the CHI patients, who exhibited no variation under the two conditions. The investigators postulated that word retrieval problems contributed to the reduced number of cohesive ties in the narratives of the head-injured patients.

A somewhat different method of discourse analysis was employed by Ulatowska et al. (1983), who asked 15 moderately aphasic patients to generate an account of a memorable experience, retell a short fable, develop a story based on a sequence of drawings, and derive morals for a story. Stories by the patients reflected a reduction in the quantity and complexity of language (e.g., smaller number of episodes in the story, simplification of plots) and fewer words per clause in describing a memorable experience. The aphasics were particularly impaired in producing morals of stories that reflected abstract thinking.

RELATIONSHIP OF IMPAIRED DISCOURSE
TO FRONTAL LOBE LESIONS

Of the few published studies of discourse analysis in brain-damaged patients, only sparse data have been reported on localization of lesion. This issue is relevant to linguistic deficit in head-injured patients because the frontal region is the most common site of focal lesions. To this end, Novoa and Ardila (1987) tested 21 patients with prefrontal lesions resulting from several etiologies, including head trauma. Administration of various linguistic tasks and open-ended questions disclosed that patients with left frontal lesions had diminished verbal output and exhibited a tendency toward perseveration, confabulation, and disorganized ideas. The investigators also noted that patients with prefrontal injuries had difficulty in responding with interpretative statements, a finding similar to the problem in abstraction that was reported by Ulatowska et al. (1983).

The relationship of localization of lesion within the frontal region to discourse was studied by Kaczmarek (1984) using tasks similar to the procedures used by Ulatowska et al. (1983). The patients were asked to repeat by themselves stories that had been told by the examiner, describe a situation depicted by pictures, and generate stories about specific topics, both familiar to the patient and more abstract. Although Kaczmarek studied brain tumor patients, the study is described here because of its relevance to head-injured patients. The most prominent finding in the patients' discourse was their inability to organize information, as reflected by their excessive perseverations, digressions, confabulations, and use of stereotyped phrases. The perseverations, which were especially frequent in the patients with left dorsolateral frontal lesions, typically occurred when the patients were initiating their narratives, and they often failed to continue.

IMPLICATIONS OF DISCOURSE STUDIES

The recent trend toward quantitative analysis of discourse extends the concept of subclinical language disorder in patients who are not obviously aphasic by clinical examination. Although longitudinal studies are needed to characterize the recovery of deficient discourse, this capacity clearly merits further investigation. As pointed out earlier in this chapter, the communication problems of CHI patients often reflect the combined effects of impaired cognition and language. Moreover, the tangential, perseverative, and slow discourse of many survivors of severe CHI contributes to their disability and social isolation. Future studies could utilize neuroimaging to analyze the relationship of lesions in specific frontal lobe sites to various abnormalities in discourse. Inclusion of appropriate comparison groups, such as CHI patients with extrafrontal lesions, and assessment of cognitive functions (e.g., planning, flexibility in reasoning) purportedly subserved by the frontal lobes would be informative. In this connection, it remains to be seen whether patients with frontal lesions exhibit deficits analogous to inefficient discourse on nonverbal tasks that involve organization of patterns or designs.

Aphasia in Children After Closed Head Injury

CEREBRAL PLASTICITY AND RECOVERY OF FUNCTION

Investigations of early insult to the human brain have suggested that it possesses considerable plasticity for language development. Lenneberg (1967) proposed that recovery from aphasia parallels the degree to which specialization for language has become lateralized, that is, the commitment of the left hemisphere. From observations of aphasia in children, he postulated that cerebral dominance is established from 2 to 10 years of age. Young children would thus be able to displace language to the right hemisphere after injury to the left hemisphere. This postulation is also consistent with the observation that a right-hemisphere lesion more frequently produces aphasia in young children than in older patients. In contrast to evidence that the development of hemispheric dominance may be a gradual process beginning at age 2 (Woods & Carey, 1979), more recent research has documented that left-hemisphere lesions in the postnatal period result in subtle persisting deficits in object naming and auditory language comprehension (Vargha-Khadem, O'Gorman, & Watters, 1985). In addition to interhemispheric plasticity, Hécaen (1976) suggested that intrahemispheric reorganization may subserve the rapid recovery from expressive aphasia in children. Studies of infantile hemiplegia have shown no evidence of residual aphasia and only transient or mild aphasia when hemispherectomy is performed on young children with hemiplegia who have acquired language prior to surgery (Basser, 1962; Teuber, 1978). The integrity of language after early brain injury may be achieved, however, at the expense of functions primarily subserved by the right hemisphere (Teuber, 1978). For a more detailed discussion of the relationship between brain maturation and recovery from aphasia, the reader is referred to Aram's chapter 13.

The impression of greater capacity for recovery from CHI in children

has received support from a study at the Children's Hospital in Philadelphia which showed a mortality of only 6% in cases with a severe
injury defined by an initial GCS score of 8 or less (Bruce et al., 1979).
Whereas Bruce et al. reported that 90% of the children achieved a good
recovery or were only moderately disabled, more detailed studies employing psychological assessment have documented permanent cognitive deficit in more than one-third of children who sustain severe head
injuries (Brink, Garrett, Hale, Woo-Sam, & Nickel, 1970). In summary, it
may be anticipated that cognitive impairment contributes to the clinical
picture in children who are referred for assessment of aphasia after
severe CHI.

DESCRIPTION AND CLINICAL COURSE OF APHASIA
AFTER HEAD INJURY IN CHILDREN

Guttmann (1942) published one of the earliest systematic studies of
aphasia in children. In his review of previous descriptions, he commented that childhood aphasia was historically viewed as a congenital
disorder, whereas acquired aphasia was less well known. The author
attributed the prevailing concept of acquired aphasia as a rare disorder
in children to a lack of familiarity with its distinctive features. In a series
of 30 children (2–14 years of age) that included 9 cases of head injury,
Guttmann pointed out that his patients generally did not exhibit obvious
paraphasic errors and were less likely than adults to complain of difficulty in speech. Consequently, Guttmann suggested that acquired aphasia in children may be overlooked or misinterpreted as an unwillingness
to speak. Fourteen of the 16 children with left-hemisphere lesions, 1 of
the 13 with right-hemisphere lesions, and 1 child with bilateral injury
were aphasic. The author characterized the children's initial language
disturbance as an absence of spontaneous speech, followed by a poverty
of expression, hesitancy, and dysarthria when speech returned. In view
of incomplete follow-up data and technical limitations, Guttmann re-
frained from definitive statements regarding prognosis or localization of
lesion.

Alajouanine and Lhermitte (1965) studied 32 aphasic children with
left-hemisphere lesions, including 13 patients with head injury who
ranged in age from 6 to 15 years of age. Consistent with Guttmann's
(1942) earlier observations, the most striking feature of the aphasic disorder was poverty of expression, including oral and written language and
gestures. Dysarthria, which was present in two-thirds of the children,
was associated with hemiplegia. The authors found that, in contrast to
aphasia in adults, fluent paraphasic speech was rare and perseveration
was absent even in children with temporal lesions. The 7 children with

paraphasic errors were older than 10 years of age. In agreement with Guttmann's findings, only one-third of the children had a receptive deficit for oral speech, although nearly two-thirds were alexic. Comparison of the aphasic children who were under 10 years of age with those from 10 to 15 years of age disclosed that the younger patients had a more profound reduction of verbal expression and a more consistent disruption of articulation. Follow-up examinations at 6 and 12 months after the appearance of aphasia disclosed normal or nearly normal language in 22 and 24 children, respectively. The authors observed subtle alterations of language in 14 children on tests of narration, construction of sentences, and definition of words.

Hécaen (1976) described 26 children ($3\frac{1}{2}$–15 years of age) with focal cortical lesions of whom 16 (7 left, 6 right, 3 bilateral) sustained a CHI. Nineteen children were aphasic, including 88% of those with left-hemisphere lesions and 33% of those with right-hemisphere lesions. Consistent with previous reports of acquired aphasia in children, Hécaen considered the two essential features of language disorder in his patients to be the loss of initiation of speech (if not mutism) and the absence of paraphasia. Articulation disorder was also common. Impaired auditory verbal comprehension was found only in children with temporal lobe lesions. Alexia resolved rapidly, whereas disturbance of writing was the most common symptom during the acute period and the least likely to resolve. Acalculia was also frequently present in the aphasic children. Although Hécaen's findings lend support to the impression of more rapid resolution of aphasia in children, only one-third of his cases recovered fully. Although Hécaen's series confirmed the widely held view that aphasia in children is nonfluent, recent case reports have documented fluent aphasia when the focal lesion encroaches on Wernicke's area (van Dongen, Loonen, & van Dongen, 1985).

Insofar as Hécaen investigated acquired aphasia, he confined his study to children who had developed language prior to injury (the youngest aphasic in Hécaen's series was $3\frac{1}{2}$ years of age). We had the opportunity, however, to study serially the recovery of a $2\frac{1}{2}$-year-old girl in whom language development was advanced (e.g., she spoke in sentences, recited the alphabet, and wrote her name prior to injury) and a decided right-hand preference had been established. The child sustained a CHI in a motor vehicle accident on 20 March 1975. When examined in the emergency room shortly after injury, the GCS score was 6; she had a right hemiparesis and a third-nerve palsy. An angiogram showed no evidence of mass lesion. She followed commands after 10 days, but remained mute. The patient gradually vocalized and uttered the *b* sound on 9 April when shown the alphabet. She verbalized single words and brief phrases and joined in singing but failed to initiate speech. Clinic visits over the subsequent 5 years disclosed progressive improvement in language to a nearly normal level within 1 year after injury. During the 6 months following injury, the only residual noted in a speech evaluation was a slight hesitancy. The patient shifted her manual preference to the left hand and left foot, although strength on her right side was greatly improved.

Studies of pediatric head trauma have focused on quantitative assessment of language (Ewing-Cobbs, Levin, Eisenberg, & Fletcher, 1987; Levin & Eisenberg, 1979). Levin and Eisenberg administered the NCCEA to a consecutive series of children (6–12 years of age) and 42 adolescents (13–18 years of age) after they regained orientation. No child was mute or unresponsive at the time of testing. The series comprised 60% mild injuries (no coma) and 40% with more severe CHI (coma duration ranged from 1 hr to more than 3 weeks). The results showed that residual language defect was present in about one-third of the patients. Consistent with findings in adults with CHI, anomia was the most prominent deficit and verbal repetition was least affected. Comprehension of oral language was impaired in 11% of the children studied. More recently, Ewing-Cobbs et al. (1987) reported evidence for greater vulnerability of linguistic functions that were in a phase of rapid development at the time of injury. Findings obtained about 1 month postinjury disclosed that writing to dictation and copying were more impaired in children than in adolescents who had sustained CHI of comparable severity. In general, naming, other expressive functions, and writing were more sensitive to severity of injury than was receptive ability. Taken together, these results suggest that subclinical language disorder occurs after CHI in children with a frequency comparable to that found in adults.

Effects of Severity of Injury

Severity of Diffuse Injury

The duration of coma and persistence of PTA are widely viewed as indices of diffuse injury severity. The divergence in findings on the effects of duration of coma on language may reflect differences in the definition of coma and the interval between injury and assessment. Brooks, Aughton, Bond, Jones, and Rizvi (1980) defined duration of coma in reference to the GCS: no eye opening, failure to obey commands, and absence of comprehensible speech. In contrast, we employed the interval during which the patient was unable to follow commands (Levin et al., 1976).

Most investigators have reported no relationship between duration of coma and severity or persistence of language disturbance (Brooks et al., 1980; de Morsier, 1973; Groher, 1977; Sarno, 1980, 1984; Sarno et al., 1986). The data of patients with mass lesions, however, are typically merged with data of diffuse CHI cases. We reported significant correlations between duration of coma and test scores on visual naming, word fluency, comprehension of aural language, and reading comprehension. Review of individual scores on scatterplots disclosed cases with brief coma and a patient with a left-hemisphere mass lesion who evidenced language disturbance. The correlations were nonsignificant on other subtests of the MAE. In a follow-up study of long-term recovery (median interval of 1 year) of language, we confirmed that persistent impairment of both expressive and receptive abilities was related to a prolonged period of coma (Levin et al., 1981). Brooks et al. (1980) found that residual word fluency was correlated with the duration of PTA, which was estimated by retrospectively questioning the patient.

Severe diffuse CHI is frequently presumed in patients with a long period of coma in the face of a normal CT scan. Severity of generalized injury may also be reflected by an acute CT scan showing compression of the ventricles and cisterns by cerebral swelling. The possibility of differential recovery of language in patients with this CT pattern has not been studied. In summary, we may conclude that prolonged coma is neither a necessary nor a sufficient condition for residual aphasia.

Focal Brain Lesions

Localization of lesion in aphasia is reviewed by Damasio in chapter 3. This section provides a cursory summary of findings in patients with head injury. In acute CHI the presence of a focal mass lesion (i.e., hematoma or contusion) is visualized in most cases by a CT scan. Figure 14.2, a CT scan obtained on the day of injury, shows an area of increased density consistent with an intracerebral hematoma. Smaller lesions, such as hemorrhagic contusions, are also appreciated by CT. Although magnetic resonance imaging can detect intracranial lesions not seen on CT, it frequently requires a longer scanning interval and is more sensitive to artifact produced by the patient's movement. Moreover, bringing conventional life support equipment into a magnetic field can pose problems.

In general, the type of aphasia associated with a specific locus of lesion corresponds to the language disorder produced by nontraumatic vascular lesions in the same region (Alajouanine et al., 1957). This generalization has received support from studies of adults with left temporal intracerebral hematoma who exhibit fluent, paraphasic speech and impaired comprehension (Debray-Ritzen, Hirsch, Pierre-Kahn, Bursztejn, & Labbé, 1977; Stone et al., 1978). Injury to the dominant temporal lobe or extensive left-hemisphere damage accounted for most of the aphasic CHI patients with focal lesions described by Thomsen (1976). The presence of a focal lesion concomitant with diffuse injury may result in an apparent "crossed aphasia." From neurologic findings, CT results, and observations made during surgery, we recorded six patients with predominant right-hemisphere lesions who exhibited a linguistic defect on at least one subtest of the MAE (Levin et al., 1976). In contrast to aphasics with major involvement of the left hemisphere, contralateral hemiparesis was not present in these patients. We also observed that clinical evidence of injury to the rostral brain stem was more closely associated with linguistic disturbance than were signs of hemispheric injury, a finding consistent with Ommaya and Gennarelli's (1974) model of CHI discussed earlier in this chapter.

Subcortical Lesions

Evidence for the participation of subcortical structures in language is reviewed in chapter 3. We have been impressed by the long periods of mutism in three patients, including two adolescents and an adult, in whom CT disclosed a subcortical intracerebral hematoma. The findings in one patient are summarized (see Figure 14.2).

A 12-year-old left-handed girl (inconsistent familial sinistrality) was evaluated 20 min after sustaining a CHI on 22 June 1979 when she was struck by a car. Examination in the emergency room disclosed a GCS of 6. She began to obey commands on 30 June but had a right hemiplegia and uttered no words or sounds. The CT scan disclosed a hemorrhagic contusion of the left putamen and anterior limb of the internal capsule (Figure 14.2). She remained mute until 15 July. Throughout the mute period she was dysgraphic, her spelling was impaired, and she wrote in block letters. A repeat CT scan showed density changes that suggested resolution of the hemorrhagic lesion in the basal ganglia. Detailed assessment of language on 13 August when she was fully oriented disclosed an impoverished lexical stock with infrequent initiation of spontaneous speech. The MAE showed a decrement in verbal associative fluency and defective comprehension (Token Test). Spontaneous speech was grossly intact when she was examined a year later. The follow-up tests disclosed a residual impairment in word fluency and impaired comprehension of complex commands (Token Test), although there was a trend of improvement.

Concomitant Neuropsychological Deficits

Hemispheric Disconnection

In view of the shearing and stretching of axons and resultant injury to the corpus callosum, hemispheric disconnection syndrome would appear to be a likely consequence of severe CHI. The first description of a hemispheric disconnection after CHI was the case reported by Lhermitte, de Massary, and Huguenin (1929) of a jockey who developed alexia without agraphia after falling off a horse. He had a right homonymous hemianopsia and a left inferior quadrantopsia. The patient could not read words but was capable of reading single letters. The second case study of hemispheric disconnection after CHI was published 40 years later (Schott, Michel, Michel, & Dumas, 1969), but there was no anatomic confirmation of injury to the callosum. The authors described tactile anomia, ideomotor apraxia, and agraphia confined to the left hand. A case of posttraumatic disconnection syndrome with neuropathologic verification was found to evidence ideomotor apraxia and agraphia confined to the left hand (Rubens, Geschwind, Mahowald, & Mastri, 1977). Neuropathologic findings showed marked thinning of the corpus callosum with demyelination and loss of axons.

We tested interhemispheric transfer of information by comparing naming of objects placed in the left or the right hand in a study of long-term recovery from acute aphasia following CHI (Levin et al., 1981). There was disproportionate impairment of naming objects placed in the left hand, a finding consistent with callosal dysfunction. Two cases with residual expressive and receptive deficits also exhibited ideomotor apraxia, as they could not do better than approximating familiar gestures when requested orally to perform them. We postulated that ideomotor apraxia in these patients may have resulted from interruption of intrahemispheric connections.

The presence of hemispheric disconnection may be clinically investigated by detailed assessment of ideomotor apraxia, testing writing in both hands, and examining the patient's ability to name objects placed in either hand. It is necessary to exclude the possibility of a primary sensory defect by determining whether the patient can visually match objects that are incorrectly named.

To investigate posttraumatic hemisphere-disconnection effects, Levin et al. (1989) administered dichotic listening and intermanual tests to 69 patients who had sustained CHIs of varying severity. Manual tests included naming objects palpated in either hand, transfer of postures from one hand to the other, and writing. Consistent with a prediction of decreased efficiency of interhemispheric transfer of information, the degree of ear asymmetry in dichotic listening performance was directly related to the severity of head injury as reflected by impaired consciousness. Suppression of responses to left-ear input was the most characteristic abnormality in severely injured patients, despite preservation of hearing. Depth and localization of parenchymal lesions characterized by magnetic resonance imaging were also related to the degree of ear asymmetry. Lesions situated in sites that could potentially interfere with callosal auditory or geniculocortical pathways produced a greater disparity in response to left- versus right-ear input than did parenchymal lesions in areas such as the frontal lobes. Striking dissociation between marked asymmetry in dichotic listening performance and unilateral deficits on the intermanual tests was exhibited by individual patients. These results provide further evidence for the effects of multifocal brain lesions involving the white matter on tests that require intra- and/or interhemispheric integration.

Other Neuropsychological Deficits

Descriptive studies after CHI have emphasized the frequent finding of concomitant neuropsychological deficits. Associated verbal impairment, which may be viewed as an integral aspect of aphasia, includes alexia, agraphia, and acalculia (Heilman et al., 1971; de Morsier, 1973). Heilman et al. observed that anomic patients frequently exhibit right–left confusion, finger agnosia, and difficulties in calculation, writing, and reading. The authors also found reversible amnesic disorder in four of the nine anomic patients.

Thomsen (1977) compared verbal learning and memory for words, sentences, and numbers in CHI patients with persistent aphasic symptoms and in nonaphasic CHI cases who had comparable durations of PTA. This study, which tested patients more than 2 years postinjury, disclosed that both groups had impaired verbal memory for information beyond immediate span when their performance was compared with that of a control group. Residual impairment of immediate memory (e.g., digit span) was confined to the aphasic CHI patients, whose learning and retention of unrelated words were inferior to those of nonaphasic head-injured patients.

In a quantitative study of language defects after CHI, we considered related deficits on visuoperceptive and visuomotor tasks (Levin et al., 1976). Although we found a trend suggesting an association, it was not significant when these patients were compared with other CHI patients who were spared linguistic disturbance.

Historically, the relationship between aphasia, of any etiology, and intellectual function has been a controversial issue. We approached the issue by differentiating acutely aphasic CHI patients whose language fully recovered from patients with specific residual defects or chronic impairment of both expressive and receptive abilities (Levin et al., 1981). Patients with persistent aphasic disorder had marked cognitive deficit on both verbal and visuospatial subtests of the WAIS, whereas the other patients recovered to low normal or average intellectual level.

Behavioral Disturbances

The sequelae of CHI frequently include alterations in behavior (see Levin & Grossman, 1978). Severe head injury may result in thinking disturbances reflected by intrusion of irrelevant material into spontaneous speech. Patients disabled by CHI often lack insight into the severity of their deficits and the inappropriateness of their verbalizations. Motor retardation and withdrawal to isolated activities are also common in these patients. To a lesser degree, depression and anxiety may be present and affect the course of speech therapy, although these sequelae are not closely related to the severity of initial injury. Studies that have employed CT to localize focal brain lesions secondary to vascular disease or trauma have indicated that depression is more severe following left-hemisphere insult (Robinson & Szetela, 1981). The program of research by Robinson and his coworkers has included CHI and stroke patients. Analysis of the relationship between type of aphasia and affective change has shown that nonfluent aphasics are more depressed than fluent and global aphasics, according to self-report and ratings by clinicians (Robinson & Benson, 1981). Whether this vulnerability to depression in nonfluent aphasics is attributable to the closer proximity of their left-hemisphere brain lesions to the frontal pole, interruption of catecholaminergic pathways, or greater awareness of deficit in these patients awaits further study.

Special Aspects of Speech Therapy

The general topic of speech therapy for aphasia is discussed by M. T. Sarno in chapter 16. Although the techniques for remediation of aphasic symptoms after head injury may not differ fundamentally from the methods used for aphasics with cerebral vascular disease, the speech therapist should be particularly sensitive to related problems in young patients recovering from CHI. Providing feedback to assist the head-injured patient in monitoring linguistic errors and appropriateness of content may facilitate psychosocial functioning. This aspect of speech therapy assumes a prominent role when we consider that neuropsychological impairment and behavioral disorder far overshadow the contribution of focal motor deficit to chronic disability in head-injured patients. The intrusion of irrelevant and unrealistic statements into the conversational speech of brain-injured patients has been mentioned by various authors (see Levin & Grossman, 1978). Although no firm evidence shows that monitoring of speech content may respond favorably to therapeutic intervention, this potential role of the speech therapist warrants further study.

The application of techniques for memory training of head-injured patients may also broaden the role of the speech therapist. Instruction of the patient to evoke visual images to integrate and retrieve verbal material has been the most widely studied technique (Jones, 1974), although other methods have been proposed. The employment of visual imagery as a mnemonic aid would ostensibly be useful in patients with focal left-hemisphere injury. This possibility, however, awaits confirmation by definitive outcome studies.

Summary

The considerable heterogeneity in the mechanisms of brain injury produced by penetrating missile wounds and closed head injury is reflected by differences in aphasic symptoms. Nonfluent expressive aphasia is common in patients with left-hemisphere missile injury, but rarely found in adults with closed head injury. Anomic disturbance predominates in clinically obvious aphasia after closed head injury and may be demonstrated by appropriate testing in patients with relatively intact spontaneous speech. In contrast, acquired aphasia produced by closed head injury in children is characterized by a reduction in output with hesitancy, failure to initiate speech, and possibly mutism. Although the prognosis for recovery from aphasia is generally better in patients with closed head injury than in patients with cerebral vascular disease, residual defects in complex verbal skills are frequently present. Patients with closed head injuries who become aphasic frequently exhibit concomitant neuropsychological deficits, including hemispheric disconnection syndrome, verbal memory impairment, and acalculia.

Acknowledgments

Preparation of this manuscript and the author's research were supported by grant NS 21889. The author is indebted to A. L. Benton for providing valuable advice and reviewing the manuscript, and to Anita Padilla for assistance in manuscript preparation.

References

Adams, J. H., Mitchell, D. E., Graham, D. I., & Doyle, D. (1977). Diffuse brain damage of immediate impact type. *Brain, 100,* 489–502.

Alajouanine, T., Castaigne, P., Lhermitte, F., Escourolle, R., & De Ribaucourt, B. (1957). Étude de 43 cas d'aphasie posttraumatique. *Encéphale, 46,* 1–45.

Alajouanine, T., & Lhermitte, F. (1965). Acquired aphasia in children. *Brain, 88,* 653–662.

Annegers, J. F., Grabow, J. D., Kurland, L. T., & Laws, E. R. (1980). The incidence, causes, and secular trends of head trauma in Olmsted County, Minnesota. *Neurology, 30*(9), 912–919.

Arseni, C., Constantinovici, A., Iliescu, D., Dobrota, I., & Gagea, A. (1970). Considerations on posttraumatic aphasia in peace time. *Psychiatria, Neurologia, Neurochirurgia, 73,* 105–115.

Basser, L. S. (1962). Hemiplegia of early onset and the faculty of speech with special reference to the effects of hemispherectomy. *Brain, 85,* 427–460.

Bastian, H. C. (1898). *A treatise on aphasia and other speech defects.* London: H. K. Lewis.

Benson, D. F., Gardner, H., & Meadows, J. C. (1976). Reduplicative paramnesia. *Neurology, 26,* 147–151.

Benton, A. L. (1967). Problems of test construction in the field of aphasia. *Cortex, 3,* 32–58.

Benton, A. L., & Hamsher, K. (1978). *Manual for the multilingual aphasia examination.* Iowa City: University of Iowa.

Brink, J. D., Garrett, A. L., Hale, W. R., Woo-Sam, J., & Nickel, V. L. (1970). Recovery of motor and intellectual function in children sustaining severe head injuries. *Developmental Medicine and Child Neurology, 12,* 565–571.

Brooks, D. N., Aughton, M. E., Bond, M. R., Jones, P., & Rizvi, S. (1980). Cognitive sequelae in relationship to early indices of severity of brain damage after severe blunt head injury. *Journal of Neurology, Neurosurgery and Psychiatry, 43,* 529–534.

Bruce, D. A., Raphaely, R. C., Goldberg, A. I., Zimmerman, R. A., Bilaniuk, L. T., Schut, L., & Kuhl, D. E. (1979). Pathophysiology, treatment and outcome following severe head injury in children. *Child's Brain, 5,* 174–191.

Cairns, H. (1952). Disturbances of consciousness with lesions of the brain-stem and diencephalon. *Brain, 75,* 109–146.

Debray-Ritzen, P., Hirsch, J.-F., Pierre-Kahn, A., Bursztejn, C., & Labbé, J.-P. (1977). Atteinte transitoire du langage écrit en rapport avec un hématome du lobe temporal gauche chez une adolescente de quatorze ans. *Revue Neurologique, 133,* 207–210.

de Morsier, G. (1973). Sur 23 cas d'aphasie traumatique. *Psychiatria Clinica, 6,* 226–239.

Ehrlich, J. S. (1988). Selective characteristics of narrative discourse in head-injured and normal adults. *Journal of Communication Disorders, 21,* 1–9.

Ewing-Cobbs, L., Levin, H. S., Eisenberg, H. M., & Fletcher, J. M. (1987). Language functions following closed-head injury in children and adolescents. *Journal of Clinical and Experimental Neuropsychology, 9,* 5:575–592.

Gaddes, W. H., & Crockett, D. J. (1973). *The Spreen-Benton aphasia tests, normative data as a measure of normal language development* (Research Monograph, No. 25, pp. 1–76). Victoria, B.C.: University of Victoria, Neuropsychology Laboratory.

Geschwind, N. (1974). *Selected papers on language and the brain.* Dordrecht, Holland: Reidel.

Goodglass, H., & Kaplan, E. (1983). *The assessment of aphasia and related disorders* (2nd ed.). New York: Lea & Febiger.

Graham, D. I., & Adams, J. H. (1971). Ischaemic brain damage in fatal head injuries. *Lancet, 1,* 265–266.

Groher, M. (1977). Language and memory disorders following closed head trauma. *Journal of Speech and Hearing Research, 20,* 212–223.

Gurdjian, E. S., & Gurdjian, E. S. (1976). Cerebral contusions: Reevaluation of the mechanism of their development. *Journal of Trauma, 16,* 35–51.

Guttmann, E. (1942). Aphasia in children. *Brain, 65,* 205–219.

Halliday, M., & Hassan, R. (1976). *Cohesion in English.* London: Longman.

Hécaen, H. (1976). Acquired aphasia in children and the ontogenesis of hemispheric functional specialization. *Brain and Language, 3,* 114–134.

Heilman, K. M., Safran, A., & Geschwind, N. (1971). Closed head trauma and aphasia. *Journal of Neurology, Neurosurgery and Psychiatry, 34,* 265–269.

Helm, N. A., Butler, R. B., & Benson, D. F. (1978). Acquired stuttering. *Neurology, 28,* 1159–1165.

Jeannett, B., Teasdale, G., Galbraith, S., Pickard, J., Grant, H., Braakman, R., Avezaat, C., Maas, A., Minderhoud, J., Vecht, C. J., Heiden, J., Small, R., Caton, W., & Kurze, T. (1977). Severe head injuries in three countries. *Journal of Neurology, Neurosurgery and Psychiatry, 40,* 291–298.

Jones, M. K. (1974). Imagery as a mnemonic aid after left temporal lobectomy: Contrast between material-specific and generalized memory disorders. *Neuropsychologia, 12,* 21–30.

Kaczmarek, B. L. J. (1984). Neurolinguistic analysis of verbal utterances in patients with focal lesions of frontal lobes. *Brain and Language, 21,* 52–58.

Kraus, J. F., Black, M. A., Hessol, N., Ley, P., Rokaw, W., Sullivan, C., Bowers, S., Knowlton, S., & Marshall, L. (1984). The incidence of acute brain injury and serious impairment in a defined population. *American Journal of Epidemiology, 119,* 186–201.

Lenneberg, E. (1967). *Biological foundations of language.* New York: Wiley.

Levin, H. S., & Eisenberg, H. M. (1979). Neuropsychological impairment after closed head injury in children and adolescents. *Journal of Pediatric Psychology, 4,* 389–402.

Levin, H. S., Gary, H. E., Jr., & Eisenberg, H. M. (1989). Duration of impaired consciousness in relation to side of lesion after severe head injury. *Lancet, 5,* 1001–1003.

Levin, H. S., & Grossman, R. G. (1978). Behavioral sequelae of closed head injury: A quantitative study. *Archives of Neurology (Chicago), 35,* 720–727.

Levin, H. S., Grossman, R. G., & Kelly, P. J. (1976). Aphasic disorder in patients with closed head injury. *Journal of Neurology, Neurosurgery and Psychiatry, 39,* 1062–1070.

Levin, H. S., Grossman, R. G., Sarwar, M., & Meyers, C. A. (1981). Linguistic recovery after closed head injury. *Brain and Language, 12,* 360–374.

Levin, H. S., High, W. M., Jr., Williams, D. H., Eisenberg, H. M., Amparo, E. G., Guinto, F. C., & Ewert, J. (1989). Dichotic listening and manual performance in relation to magnetic resonance imaging after closed head injury. *Journal of Neurology, Neurosurgery and Psychiatry, 52,* 1162–1169.

Levin, H. S., Madison, C. F., Bailey, C. B., Meyers, C. A., Eisenberg, H. M., & Guinto, F. C. (1983). Mutism after closed head injury. *Archives of Neurology (Chicago), 40,* 601–606.

Levin, H. S., O'Donnell, V. M., & Grossman, R. G. (1979). The Galveston orientation and amnesia test: A practical scale to assess cognition after head injury. *Journal of Nervous and Mental Disease, 167,* 675–684.

Lhermitte, J., de Massary, J., & Huguenin, R. (1929). Syndrome occipital avec alexie pure d'origine traumatique, par. *Revue Neurologique, 2,* 703–707.

Ludlow, C. L., Rosenberg, J., Fair, C., Buck, D., Schesselman, S., & Salazar, A. (1986). Brain lesions associated with nonfluent aphasia fifteen years following penetrating head injury. *Brain, 109,* 55–80.

Mentis, M., & Prutting, C. A. (1987). Cohesion in the discourse of normal and head-injured adults. *Journal of Speech and Hearing Research, 30,* 88–98.

Mohr, J. P., Weiss, G., Caveness, W. F., Dillon, J. D., Kistler, J. P., Mierowsky, A. M., & Rish, B. L. (1980). Language and motor deficits following penetrating head injury in Vietnam. *Neurology, 30,* 1273–1279.

Najenson, T., Sazbon, L., Fiselzon, J., Becker, E., & Schechter, I. (1978). Recovery of communicative functions after prolonged traumatic coma. *Scandinavian Journal of Rehabilitation Medicine, 10,* 15–21.

Newcombe, F. (1969). *Missile wounds of the brain.* London: Oxford University Press.

Novoa, O. P., & Ardila, A. (1987). Linguistic abilities in patients with prefrontal damage. *Brain and Language, 30,* 206–225.

Ommaya, A. K., & Gennarelli, T. A. (1974). Cerebral concussion and traumatic unconsciousness: Correlation of experimental and clinical observations on blunt head injuries. *Brain, 97,* 633–654.

Peacher, W. G. (1945). Speech disorders in World War II. II. Further studies. *Journal of Nervous and Mental Disease, 102,* 165–171.

Penn, C., & Cleary, J. (1988). Compensatory strategies in the language of closed head injured patients. *Brain Injury, 2*(1), 3–17.

Plum, F., & Posner, J. B. (1980). *The diagnosis of stupor and coma.* Philadelphia, PA: Davis.

Robinson, R. G., & Benson, D. F. (1981). Depression in aphasic patients: Frequency, severity, and clinical-pathological correlations. *Brain and Language, 12,* 282–291.

Robinson, R. G., & Szetela, B. (1981). Mood change following left hemispheric brain injury. *Annals of Neurology, 9,* 447–453.

Rubens, A. B., Geschwind, N., Mahowald, M. W., & Mastri, A. (1977). Posttraumatic cerebral hemispheric disconnection syndrome. *Archives of Neurology (Chicago), 34,* 750–755.

Russell, W. R., & Espir, M. L. E. (1961). *Traumatic aphasia. A study of aphasia in war wounds of the brain.* London: Oxford University Press.

Russell, W. R., & Smith, A. (1961). Posttraumatic amnesia in closed head injury. *Archives of Neurology (Chicago), 5,* 4–17.

Sarno, M. T. (1980). The nature of verbal impairment after closed head injury. *Journal of Nervous and Mental Disease, 168*(11), 685–692.

Sarno, M. T. (1984). Verbal impairment after closed head injury: Report of a replication study. *Journal of Nervous and Mental Disease, 172*(8), 475–479.

Sarno, M. T., Buonaguro, A., & Levita, E. (1986). Characteristics of verbal impairment in closed head. *Archives of Physical Medicine and Rehabilitation, 67,* 400–405.

Schiller, F. (1947). Aphasia studied in patients with missile wounds. *Journal of Neurology, Neurosurgery and Psychiatry, 10,* 183–197.

Schott, B., Michel, F., Michel, D., & Dumas, R. (1969). Apraxie idéomotrice unilatérale gauche avec main gauche anomique: Syndrome de déconnexion calleuse? *Revue Neurologique, 120,* 359–365.

Spreen, O., & Benton, A. L. (1969). *Neurosensory center comprehensive examination for aphasia: Manual of directions.* Victoria, BC: Neuropsychology Laboratory.

Stengel, E. (1947). A clinical and psychological study of echo-reactions. *Journal of Mental Science, 93,* 598–612.

Stone, J. L., Lopes, J. R., & Moody, R. A. (1978). Fluent aphasia after closed head injury. *Surgical Neurology, 9,* 27–29.

Teasdale, G., & Jennett, B. (1974). Assessment of coma and impaired consciousness: A practical scale. *Lancet, 2,* 81–84.

Teuber, H.-L. (1978). The brain and human behavior. In R. Held, H. W. Leibowitz, & H.-L. Teuber (Eds.), *Perception.* Berlin: Springer Verlag.

Thomsen, I. V. (1975). Evaluation and outcome of aphasia in patients with severe closed head trauma. *Journal of Neurology, Neurosurgery and Psychiatry, 38,* 713–718.

Thomsen, I. V. (1976). Evaluation and outcome of traumatic aphasia in patients with severe verified focal lesions. *Folia Phoniatrica, 28,* 362–377.

Thomsen, I. V. (1977). Verbal learning in aphasic and non-aphasic patients with severe head injury. *Scandinavian Journal of Rehabilitation Medicine, 9,* 73–77.

Ulatowska, H. K., Freedman-Stern, R., Doyel, A. W., & Macaluso-Haynes, S. (1983). Production of narrative discourse in aphasia. *Brain and Language, 19,* 317–334.

van Dongen, H. R., Loonen, C. B., & van Dongen, K. J. (1985). Anatomical basis for acquired fluent aphasia in children. *Annals of Neurology, 17*(3), 306–309.

Vargha-Khadem, F., O'Gorman, A. M., & Watters, G. V. (1985). Aphasia and handedness in relation to hemispheric side, age at injury and severity of cerebral lesion during childhood. *Brain, 108,* 677–696.

Walker, A. E., & Jablon, S. (1961). A follow-up study of head wounds in World War II. *V. A. Medical Monograph.* Washington, D.C.: U.S. Government Printing Office.

Weinstein, E. A., & Kahn, R. L. (1955). *Denial of illness.* Springfield, IL: Charles C. Thomas.

Woods, B. T., & Carey, S. (1979). Language deficits after apparent clinical recovery from childhood aphasia. *Annals of Neurology, 6,* 405–409.

Wyckoff, L. H. (1984). Narrative and procedural discourse following closed head injury. Doctoral dissertation, University of Florida, Gainesville.

15

The Psychological and Social Sequelae of Aphasia

JOHN E. SARNO

The emotional dimensions of aphasia are important considerations for clinicians because the disorder has ramifications that extend far beyond the pathology in linguistic processing. The loss of normal communication strikes at the very roots of a person's sense of self. Identity is based primarily on relationships, which in turn depend largely on communication (M. T. Sarno, 1986). Aphasia, therefore, must affect all aspects of an individual's personal and social life.

Although it is growing, the literature on emotionality and personality disturbances specifically associated with aphasia is limited. Most studies deal with broader categories, such as the psychological and social sequelae of stroke and closed head injury. Some of these studies are reviewed here, however, so that we may extract from them whatever is relevant to this topic. Although some of the specific references to aphasia are anecdotal, they are reviewed nevertheless for the same reason.

Review of the Literature

Let us first consider some contributions of historical interest. Kurt Goldstein (1942) focused on what he identified as the CATASTROPHIC REACTION (CR), characteristic of many patients with aphasia, and argued that it resulted from a disturbance in the patient's ability to maintain "biologic homeostasis" rather than from a sense of inadequacy. Neglecting the concept of the unconscious, which had been well formulated by Freud and his followers by that time, Goldstein postulated that brain

499

ACQUIRED APHASIA, SECOND EDITION

damage produced a failure of the entire organism, a "biologic" rather than a psychic response, and that patients' reactions represented their attempts to maintain biologic homeostasis.

One could argue, however, that these same behaviors represent a desperate effort of the individual's psychic apparatus to maintain equilibrium (sanity, emotional stability) in the face of insults to the higher functions (language, cognition, perception) and that psychic stability is an integral aspect of biologic homeostasis rather than a thing apart. Whatever the merits of Goldstein's (1942) hypothesis, the description of the CR has been of great value to clinicians (Schuell, Jenkins, & Jiménez-Pabón, 1964).

Although Luria (1963) did not systematically study the impact of brain damage on emotionality, he acknowledged that premorbid personality played an important part in the process of recovery from aphasia.

A number of clinicians have called attention to the importance of the emotional concomitants of aphasia. Schuell et al. (1964), Wepman (1951), and Eisenson (1973) made frequent references to emotional phenomena and emphasized the necessity of considering them in therapeutic interaction with patients. Both Wepman and Eisenson stressed the occasional need for psychotherapy.

A Psychodynamically Oriented Report

In 1961 Friedman reported systematic observations of a group of aphasic patients in a group therapy setting over a period of 7½ months. He found that all of the patients expressed feelings of isolation, loneliness, sensitivity, and psychological impoverishment; almost all suffered feelings of lowered self-esteem that caused them to avoid and reject people, in fear of rejection. These feelings persisted even in the group therapeutic setting, from which they tended to withdraw. Behavior was generally regressive, as exemplified by the defensive use of dependency needs, projection, denial, and exaggeration of their deficits. The importance of language as a mechanism for exerting mastery over the environment was demonstrated in problems with reality testing experienced by these patients.

The Ullman Monograph

Ullman (1962) published the results of a systematic observation of behavioral changes in 300 patients admitted to a stroke study over a 3-year period. No attempt was made to categorize emotional responses on the basis of the site or the extent of the lesion. Some of his conclusions are relevant to the purposes of this chapter. In analyzing reactive responses to the stroke, leaving aside the patient with diffuse impairment of brain function, Ullman found that the severity and duration of "physical disability," in which category aphasia was included, were the most important determinants of the nature of the patient's response: Persistence of a deficit led to depression, hopelessness, and feelings of futility. Next in order of importance was the life situation to which the patient was returning. Premorbid personality was characterized as being "all important" but resisted classification that would predict whether a given patient would respond well.

Ullman described depression as reactive but differing from that seen in the usual psychiatric population. He found that the real problems confronting these patients often made it difficult to distinguish between (a) appropriate feelings of despair, loneliness, and so forth, and (b) depression attributable to the patient's premorbid personality. High on his list of reasons for psychiatric hospitalization of the stroke patient was depression secondary to aphasia. Other factors, not specifically related to aphasia, were antisocial behavior, inability to adapt to altered life circumstances, and latent psychosis precipitated by the stroke. Sexual sequelae, most particularly impotence, were found to be a reaction to psychological conflict, rather than the result of pathophysiological alterations.

Horenstein's Review

Horenstein (1970) reviewed the effects of cerebrovascular disease on personality and emotionality, drawing attention to a number of important clinical phenomena that accompany or are the result of stroke. Of these, he singled out depression as representing a grief reaction, its existence and severity relating to the type and severity of the neural deficits, as well as the patient's awareness of the illness, premorbid capacity for adaptation, intellectual level, and feelings of self-worth. Horenstein noted, however, that the reaction is not specific to stroke but occurs with any catastrophic illness. Other determinants of severity and duration of depression are the personal and social situation of the patient, for example, the loss of an accustomed role at home, in the community, or vocationally; the quality of family relationships; and the adequacy of plans for the posthospitalization period. Because of the importance of the severity and extent of neural deficits, Horenstein emphasized the therapeutic program as a practical means of combatting depression; to the same end, he stressed the need for careful and effective planning for the patient's future. The development of independence is paramount both for practical purposes and for its contribution to the patient's feelings of self-esteem. These observations are all particularly relevant to the patient with significant aphasia. In his review, Horenstein also considered denial of illness (or its manifestations) in a psychological context (distinct from the perceptual phenomenon). This reaction has been discussed by a number of authors (Baretz & Stephenson, 1976; Gainotti, 1972; Ullman, 1962; Weinstein & Kahn, 1955) and is often encountered in the patient with aphasia. Logically, it is related to the patient's prior personality; those who had difficulty facing reality in the past will surely react in the same way to problems posed by aphasia. Baretz and Stephenson (1976) considered it a necessary stage for many patients, serving the purpose of "buying time" as they struggle to adapt to their new reality, but probably only temporarily staving off the depression that must inevitably come. Baretz and Stephenson and Horenstein called attention to the effect of denial in its various forms on the professionals who work with patients. I shall return to this in a later section.

Most of those who have written on the subject of denial explicitly or implicitly suggest the need for psychiatric help for such patients, particularly when the degree of denial interferes with rehabilitation progress or is clearly leading to a deep depression.

Horenstein (1970) included in his review a discussion of the pseudobulbar state as possibly being confused with depression. In addition to inappropriate laughing and crying, other possible symptoms include a fixed facial expression, nonspastic articulatory and swallowing problems, partial mutism, and motor compulsions. All of these are rather dramatic manifestations of anatomicophysiological aberrations and much more than one commonly sees with the aphasic, who cries easily when exposed to emotionally laden material, either happy or sad in content. The emotional lability of the aphasic patient does not have the distinctly "organic" flavor of the pseudobulbar state described by Horenstein. Indeed, he stated that in almost all cases that have been documented the bilateral corticobulbar lesions are generally symmetrical and widespread. On the other hand, although the most frequent stroke lesion is unilateral, one does have the impression that there has been a loss of inhibition or control in the labile aphasic patient, suggesting a physiogenic process but reinforcing the concept that the left hemisphere plays a monitoring rather than a generative role in emotional expression (Lamendella, 1977).

Gainotti's Study

A report by Gainotti (1972), although primarily designed to explore the differences in emotional behavior associated with the hemispheric side of a lesion, did make specific reference to the emotional reactions of the patient with aphasia. He identified emotional reactions in four groups: a category of seven reactions under the heading CATASTROPHIC REACTIONS, five affective states characterized as DEPRESSIVE MOODS, four INDIFFERENCE REACTIONS, and a category of OTHER REACTIONS, which included confabulations, delusions, and hate for limbs. Patients with left-hemisphere lesions manifested catastrophic or anxiety–depression symptoms more frequently than did patients with lesions of the non-dominant hemisphere, whereas indifference reactions were more common among the latter group. When he subdivided the left-hemisphere patients according to the presence or absence of aphasia, Gainotti noted further differences. So-called Broca's aphasics had statistically more dramatic, sudden, and short-lived emotional outbursts than did other aphasics (Wernicke's aphasics did not weep at all), whereas the amnesic aphasics showed a different pattern of anxiety reaction that seemed to reflect greater awareness and control. Wernicke's aphasics were also quite different from nonaphasics and patients with right-brain damage in the frequent use of emotional language (swearing, cursing, religious imprecations), although in this they were almost matched by Broca's aphasics. The latter group showed the highest incidence of aggressive behavior (25% compared with about 10% for most of the other groups). Twenty-five percent of the fluent aphasics seemed unaware of their language problem, matching the proportion of right-hemisphere patients who were anosognosic, but the fluent aphasics did not manifest other characteristics of "belle indifference" as did the right-brain–damaged patients. In fact, Wernicke's aphasics expressed discouragement in greater numbers than did all other groups and matched others in drawing attention to their failures, clear evidence of some degree of awareness of and concern about their deficits.

The concept that the right hemisphere processes, that is, recognizes and expresses emotional phenomena, appears to be generally accepted. Judging by the observation of left-brain–damaged patients, the left hemisphere apparently functions to control emotions whose origins are elsewhere in the brain; however, the degree of control may depend on the patient's awareness of the aphasic deficit. Of aphasic patients, amnesic aphasic patients are most aware of their deficits and retain the greatest degree of control over their emotional reactions. Those with

Broca's aphasia appear to be quite aware, but their anxiety and/or depression, and quite possibly their anger, diminish their control. Fluent aphasic patients are the most complicated: Gainotti's (1972) data suggest that they, too, are anxious and depressed but present a confusing pattern of awareness and control. The inappropriateness of the behavior of some patients with Wernicke's aphasia is well known to clinicians, and the intimations of psychosis in a small number of patients is now a classical observation (Benson, 1980; Horenstein, 1970). The parapsychotic behavior of the occasional patient with Wernicke's aphasia may be the consequence of both affective and cognitive incompetence resulting primarily from the pathological lesion.

Smythies (1970) suggested that psychoses are the result of qualitative changes in brain physiology (as opposed to quantitative ones in the neuroses) that may be the result of biochemical aberrations. Such changes may be of significant enough magnitude in Wernicke's aphasia to mimic a classical psychosis. The frequent involvement of the temporal lobe in Wernicke's aphasia lends further credence to a special affective deficit because of the association of that area with emotional processes (Geschwind, 1977; Klüver & Bucy, 1939; Papez, 1937).

Further complicating the problem of fluent aphasia are the suggestions that deficits in auditory processing lead to paranoid ideas in the patient (Benson, 1980) and confusion in the mind of the examiner (Ziegler, 1952). Finally, the jargon of these patients may result in an occasional diagnosis of schizophrenia.

Benson's Review

In this excellent review of the psychiatric problems associated with aphasia, Benson (1980) discussed some common psychosocial sequelae: alterations in lifestyle, change in employment status (sometimes with consequent financial problems), loss of social position and change of roles within the family, simultaneous loss of physical capacity in cases of hemiparesis, real or imagined loss of sexual function, erosion of self-esteem, and reactions of grief and depression. Benson also discussed the changes in emotionality associated with the locus of the lesion: the depression and frustration of nonfluent patients sometimes leading to a catastrophic reaction with anger, hostility, loud crying, or withdrawal; refusal to eat or participate in treatment; and alteration in sleep patterns and personal hygiene. Because of the depth of depression, suicide is a possibility. Based on his experience, however, Benson thought the risk of suicide to be greater in patients with posterior lesions, the fluent aphasic patients. The only suicide in my experience was a nonfluent patient with a considerable right-sided motor deficit.

Change in emotional state is likely a highly individual matter, determined by the intensity of the person's intolerance for his or her altered state. In fact, a common observation among experienced aphasiologists is that little correlation exists between the severity or mildness of the aphasia and its impact on the patient. For instance, someone with a relatively mild aphasia may be devastated and inconsolable. The same lack of correlation has been noted between the type of aphasia and emotional impact. As Benson pointed out, the problems in fluent aphasia are different, stemming from the language comprehension deficit and the tendency to use jargon, both of which patients are often unaware and frequently unconcerned. Since these patients often are not understood and have trouble comprehending what is said to them, they may become paranoid, in much the same way as someone with acquired deafness. When this is combined with impulsiveness, these patients can be difficult to manage.

Benson also discussed other neurobehavioral disturbances, including confusional states, apathy, memory problems, and true dementia (as in someone with Alzheimer's disease). He also examined the difficult questions of how aphasia affects intelligence and how one establishes the legal competence of an aphasic person.

Language and the Limbic System

A review of the basic literature on communication and emotional behavior suggests that one is most likely to see a point of convergence by considering the function of the limbic system. Study of language has been limited almost entirely to neocortical systems, but more recent allusions have been made to the phylogenetically older and primarily subcortical limbic areas that are intriguing and attractive.

The term LIMBIC SYSTEM refers to a group of structures deep within the substance of the brain that have gradually come to be associated in humans with emotional behavior and attitudes and more recently with communication drives. It incorporates both cortical and subcortical structures which in lower animals primarily serve the sense of smell and which became converted to other functions as biologic imperatives changed with evolution. Papez (1937) is credited with having provided a theoretical base for the idea that the phylogenetically old rhinencephalon was the source of emotional and motivational behavior. Since then a great deal of research activity has corroborated this concept, including the work of Bard and Mountcastle (1947), Brodal (1947), Pribram and Kruger (1954), and MacLean (1952), who was the first to use the term limbic system.

Lamendella's Review

Motivated by the desire to draw attention to the role of the limbic system in human communication, Lamendella (1977) reviewed the subject in detail and presented some original concepts as a result of his study. Because they bear so closely on the subject matter of this chapter, some of his observations and conclusions are reported.

Lamendella's major thesis was that the limbic system plays an important role in human social and communicative behavior. In fact, he suggested that this system may be responsible for most human nonpropositional communication activity. He sees the limbic system as poised between and acting upon both vegetative (species-preserving) functions, through its connections with the hypothalamus, and the neocortex, which is involved with those higher level functions that define the human species: social and communicative behavior. Following a review of the anatomy, physiology, and phylogeny of the system as it is presently conceptualized, Lamendella presented evidence linking the limbic system to primate social and communication function and then identified five levels of forebrain activity that participate in human communication, three of which are included within the limbic system. The highest level, that of propositional communication, incorporates the dominant and nondominant hemispheres, the latter of which he suggested is closely related to nonpropositional processes that originate in the limbic system and are intertwined with affective subsystems. He suggested that the dominant left hemisphere, in addition to being the locus of propositional speech, appears to play an inhibitory role vis-à-vis affective function.

The emotional lability of patients with left-hemisphere lesions, many of whom are aphasic, is given as evidence of the loss of this inhibitory function. On the other hand, the indifference behavior of patients with right-hemisphere lesions would point to an impairment of the limbic–right-hemisphere system, which underlies affective function, according to his concepts.

What is most relevant to the subject of this chapter is the section of Lamendella's paper relating limbic structure and linguistic communication. He presented two ideas in this regard. First, AUTOMATIC speech is to be distinguished from PROPOSITIONAL speech, the latter being represented in the left hemisphere and, therefore, often disordered when there is damage to that area. He believes that automatic speech may be processed in multiple loci, including limbic, basal ganglia, thalamic, or midbrain structures and, therefore, may be relatively preserved in a patient with classical aphasia (Bay, 1964; Critchley, 1970; Head, 1926; Jackson, 1932; Luria, 1970). Second, Lamendella stated that one type of automatic speech has referential meaning: that which has emotional content. He believed that such speech (including obscenities and vulgarisms) actually originates in the limbic system because of its affective nature and that these utterances have the dual purpose of relieving affective pressures within the individual, as well as of evoking "limbic" responses in the person being spoken to. These affective pressures, in his view, include all of the primitive vegetative functions with which the limbic system is involved, colorfully identified by Pribram (1971) as the four Fs.

One additional reference surely suggests a powerful relationship between emotional and communication functions. This is the observation of B. W. Robinson (1976) concerning a patient who was severely aphasic and right hemiparetic and who subsequently developed a manic–depressive psychosis. During the manic phase, both his motor deficit and aphasia disappeared, only to return when the mania was controlled with medication. This remarkable pattern could be repeated by manipulating the medication; that is, when the medication was stopped and the patient became depressed again, aphasia and the motor deficit returned. Robinson interpreted this phenomenon to suggest the existence of two separate speech systems, but Lamendella hypothesized that strong emotional stimuli originating in the limbic system might possibly overcome or circumvent the loss of control over speech and motor systems normally exercised by the left hemisphere.

Summarizing his concept, Lamendella suggested that, although high-level neocortical systems may be largely responsible for communication now enjoyed by human beings, there is reason to believe that the complex systems for communication developed at lower brain levels down through phylogenetic strata continue to play a role in human communication. Most germane to our topic, this role is most relevant where emotions and speech conjoin.

Personal Reports

A fairly substantial literature comprising the personal reports of people who have experienced aphasia should be mentioned because it is appropriate to include material that may heighten one's awareness of the magnitude of the emotional devastation suffered by the person with aphasia.

Eric Hodgins (1964), a writer of great talent, was painfully successful in conveying his terror in the immediate poststroke period and the great frustration, panic, and despair that characterized his life in the months following his stroke. Guy Wint (1967), a journalist, historian, and excellent writer, succeeded in portraying a sense of utter desolation and isolation. One almost experiences his loss of the flavor of life, his fanatic need at first to find a cure for his illness somewhere in the world, and, failing this, his withdrawal into a gray, peopleless existence.

Wint and other writers have mentioned memory problems in their descriptions of their aphasia (Dahlberg, 1977; Moss, 1976; Segré, 1976). One has the sense that they were not talking about word-finding problems. Another recurrent report has been the loss of the ability to dream (Moss, 1976; Wint, 1967), which has not been explained, to the best of my knowledge.

Wint's (1967) writing is so captivating that it can lead to unjustified generalizations. It is likely that his emotional reactions, although not rare by any means, reflected his own personality. However, the loss of the ability to manipulate language in someone whose life was the written word, who was no doubt equally proud of his ability to discourse on subjects of great moment, must have been almost unbearable. An appropriate generalization is that language is so much a part of the personality of each of us that its loss goes far beyond the practical inconveniences of impaired communication, whether mild or severe. We are verbal animals, and our capacity for communication is very likely inextricably entwined with both emotional and intellectual function. Lenneberg (1967) made this point in part, suggesting that the biologic roots of language may reside in a person's emotional apparatus.

Wint appears to have possessed an unusual capacity for psychological insight and the ability to describe his feelings. His description of hallucinatory experiences (pp. 88, 89), including olfactory ones, gives one the impression that these are "organic" rather than psychodynamic in origin, that they are the result of sensory processes gone awry as a result of specific brain damage. This idea is in consonance with current thinking that attributes the psychoses to substantive changes in brain physiology (Smythies, 1970). The subject of hallucinosis and delusional phenomena has been well reviewed by Horenstein (1970); however, as with many other studies, the discussion does not pertain specifically to the aphasic patient. His review supports the impression gained from reading Wint (1967) that disordered sensory processes are probably responsible for hallucinations.

Returning to a review of personal accounts, two that refer specifically to aphasia (Moss, 1976; Segré, 1976) should be noted. Moss was 43 years of age at onset and indicates that his aphasia was global in the early stages and secondary to a "permanent blockage of the left internal carotid artery." Both he and Segré placed a great deal of emphasis on the loss of intellectual ability (memory loss, concreteness, loss of the ability to abstract). Moss described the inability to use words "internally" early in the course of his illness. Regarding emotional phenomena, he stressed the importance of premorbid personality; he apparently had struggled with feelings of inferiority prior to his stroke and found that he used the same compensatory behavior patterns after the stroke as he had before. He concluded that the basic personality does not change.

Segré (1976) did not provide a clear picture of the site of his lesion, although he mentioned an embolus of cardiac origin, and indeed it is not certain that he was aphasic, although he probably was. Nevertheless, he wrote an excellent review of his psychic and cognitive reactions early in the paper that includes many of the reactions that have been mentioned thus far. He drew attention to the importance of the attitude of the patient's family, that it be neither overprotective nor anxious, and stated that when the aphasic is encouraged by family and others with an overly optimistic prognosis, he or she may react with feelings of anxiety, depression, and the "complex of inferiority" when confronted with the reality of the situation.

One must be impressed with the aphasic's feelings of isolation and loneliness, of traversing a path unknown to the healthy, and of being unable to share the experience with anyone, primarily because of the impaired ability to communicate. Those of us who work with aphasic patients can probably serve them well by demonstrating our awareness of their emotional turmoil through verbalizing for them what they are experiencing. A clinical observation is that patients prefer commiseration to expressions of optimism. If, in addition, as suggested by Baretz and Stephenson (1976), we employ strategies designed to help the patient live through the dark days, we will have discharged our clinical responsibilities consonant with the best principles of the healing arts.

Studies on Depression

The years since the publication of the first edition of this book (J. E. Sarno, 1981) have produced some interesting and provocative work, most notably in the study of depression. R. G. Robinson and Benson (1981) stimulated great interest with the observation that a higher incidence of depression occurs in left-brain–damaged aphasic patients, particularly those with anterior lesions, than in right-brain–damaged patients. Acknowledging that their findings could be explained on the basis of psychological reactions to impairment, based on studies on rats, they hypothesized that disruption of catecholamine pathways might be responsible for the higher incidence of depression in nonfluent aphasia patients since the posterior frontal lobe is rich in such pathways. However, Egelko et al. (1989) found that the incidence of depression was higher in right-brain–damaged (nonaphasic) patients, whereas lesion laterality was found to be irrelevant in other studies (Gordon et al., in press; Sinyor et al., 1986).

Sinyor et al. (1986) presented a balanced assessment of the current state of knowledge on this subject: Although lesion location may play a role in poststroke depression, social, vocational, personality, and family factors also should be considered in the overall evaluation (Sinyor et al., 1986). Gordon et al. (in press) reviewed the subject of diagnosing depression in brain-damaged patients and concluded that the conflicting reports reflected "inadequate recognition of coexisting clinical syndromes and cognitive deficits that may alter the validity of assessment; the difficulty in applying evaluation tools developed for traditional psychiatric patients to brain damaged individuals; and methodological differences between the present study and prior research."

In the search for dependable diagnostic criteria in the study of depression, it was observed that certain patients reacted abnormally to ingested dexamethasone: Those with so-called endogenous depression failed to suppress serum cortisol levels when presented with a challenge dose of the drug. This test was called the dexamethasone suppression test (DST). When the DST was employed with populations of stroke patients, however, it did not consistently identify those who were depressed. In one study (Grober, Gordon, Hibbard, Aletta, & Sliwinski, 1990), where the diagnosis of depression was based on DSM III criteria, the DST failed to identify more than half the poststroke patients who were depressed and erroneously classified as depressed almost half the patients who were not. The authors concluded that the accurate diagnosis of depression in brain-damaged patients requires sensitive psychological tools, capable of accounting for the sometimes confusing array of neurological and cognitive sequelae of brain damage, of which aphasia is one of the more prominent.

As of this writing the subject must be considered unresolved. Lacking clear-cut evidence that lesion location and biochemical aberrations are the primary basis for depression, it is appropriate to retain the concept that the major factors in the depression of aphasia are the patient's overall reactions to the catastrophe and to specific aphasic deficits, as described above. Although it is enticing to hope that the chemistry laboratory will ultimately provide diagnostic and therapeutic answers to the profound problems that characterize the emotional sequelae of aphasia, in the immediate future, a continuing commitment to diagnostic evaluation, based on the knowledge of human behavior and psychopathology, is required. With the possible exception of the premorbidly mentally deficient or frankly psychotic patients, the onset of aphasia is a personal, familial, and social catastrophe, bringing with it profound changes in all of these spheres. The spectrum of possible reactions is broad, based on age, education, station in life, economic status, family composition and dynamics, premorbid personality, time since onset, previous history of illness, awareness of deficit, cognitive deficiencies, and other less obvious factors. Because of this bewildering array of variables, the issue of patients' reactions is exceedingly difficult to study.

Identification of Psychological and Social Sequelae

The last decade has seen a number of studies devoted to the psychological and social sequelae of aphasia. Christensen and Anderson (1989) confirmed the reports of earlier studies (Artes & Hoops, 1976; Kinsella & Duffy, 1978) that the spouses of stroke patients experienced a variety of negative reactions including shock, guilt, bitterness, depression, loneliness, and irritability. The spouses had to face role changes and altered social lives. Christensen and Anderson confirmed statistically that these negative sequelae were a greater problem for the spouses of patients with aphasia. Williams and Freer (1986) found that spouses of aphasia patients perceived a deterioration in lifestyles, emotional support, and sexual relationships. The authors suggested the need for both counseling and education about aphasia for the spouses of patients with both mild and severe aphasia. Documenting an impression held by many professionals who work with aphasic patients and their families, a survey conducted by the National Aphasia Association in 1987 revealed that 90% of 210 patients reported feeling isolated and 70% believed people avoided them because of their communication difficulties.

A very pertinent study was reported by Herrmann and Wallesch (1989). Close relatives of 20 patients with chronic, severe, nonfluent aphasia documented a variety of negative psychosocial changes in four categories: professional, social, familial, and psychological. Although the lists were not exhaustive, they included a large number of the changes observed by aphasia therapists, psychologists, and physicians who work intimately with these patients. Of particular importance, the authors noted that the patients and their families had received no psychotherapeutic aid or counseling, and the relatives had received neither care instructions nor prognostic information on discharge from the hospital so that they might develop realistic expectations.

Jaffe, one of the few psychiatrists with expertise in the diagnosis and treatment of emotional disorders in aphasic patients, wrote an excellent treatise on the subject (1981). He pointed out that patients with aphasia are subject to the full range of psychiatric disorders seen in the general population, but, because of the communication problem, the disorders may be difficult to detect and may not be recognized until the patients manifest such behavior as crying, psychomotor retardation, sleep or eating disturbance, significant weight change, manic hyperactivity, delusional behavior (e.g., paranoia), overt suicide attempts, physical destructiveness or assault, drug or alcohol abuse, panic attacks, or noncompliance with treatment regimens. Jaffe suggested that the extreme stress of having developed a "brain disease" may cause psychiatric illness to first appear, assuming that no such difficulty has appeared in the patient's past history. Jaffe questioned whether some of the "symptoms" of aphasia, such as the catastrophic reaction, are transformed versions of familiar psychiatric disorders, and argued that the so-called Type A personality may react more violently to the frustration of nonfluent aphasia than the more relaxed Type B person. Jaffe's description of the fears and outright phobias that aphasic persons may develop as a result of their linguistic incompetence is particularly pertinent. Patients are very apprehensive about making calculation mistakes (e.g., giving the wrong amount of money to a clerk), taking telephone messages inaccurately, forgetting names, and performing a host of other tasks encountered in daily life. Because of their perpetual concern, patients often withdraw rather than face the embarrassment of making mistakes.

Jaffe also commented that aphasia robs the patient of the solace usually available to people who have suffered a devastating loss by being able to talk about it to loved ones. He described this as "healing conversation" and characterized aphasia as being particularly cruel in that it interferes with a "major vehicle of its own treatment." Additionally, Jaffe described the exaggerations of premorbid personality traits that make patients almost unrecognizable to their intimates and that may create family problems if they are not properly diagnosed and managed. He also discussed the very difficult problem of determining mental competence in aphasia, which often creates great legal problems. Because of their impairment in expressing themselves verbally or in writing, aphasic patients are often thought to be mentally incompetent. If this is complicated by comprehension deficits, as in a person with global aphasia, it may be almost impossible to establish competence. Benson (1980) suggested that this is probably best judged by someone highly trained in aphasia who knows the patient intimately. Jaffe's paper makes it clear that a knowledge of psychodynamics may be very helpful in assessing the emotional reactions of the person with aphasia, although it may be difficult because of the communication disorder.

Hibbard, Grober, Gordon, Aletta, and Freeman (1990) have studied the treatment of poststroke depression and developed a set of cognitive therapeutic principles based upon detailed knowledge of patients' deficits, both physical and nonphysical. These include motor and sensory deficits, level of alertness and ability to concentrate, memory, capacity for abstract thinking, aphasia, visual–perceptual difficulties, and disturbances in the comprehension and/or expression of emotion. In developing the psychotherapeutic program, the following should be considered: the patients' awareness of these deficits and of the effect on their thinking and personality; the patients' premorbid personality, lifestyle, and interests; and whether the patients have adequately mourned their losses. Hibbard et al. also acknowledged the necessity of knowing what family members are thinking and doing; what distortions they may have about the patient's deficits, potential, and so forth; and whether they have mourned the losses and changes wrought by the stroke on the patient and themselves.

Although the literature remains sparse, interest in the evaluation of the psychological and social sequelae of stroke and aphasia has clearly increased. Let us now consider the subject of treatment.

Treatment

Almost anything one might do to meet the psychosocial needs of patients with aphasia would be welcome after their history of neglect. In general, patients and their families have had to fend for themselves, which undoubtedly has increased their anxiety and depression. Historically, physical concerns have always received priority in medicine, even in the field of rehabilitation medicine whose avowed philosophy is to concern itself with the whole spectrum of patients' needs. Most physicians training in this specialty are exposed to much more about the sensorimotor sequelae of brain damage than the cognitive, language, or affective disorders. It is perhaps inevitable, then, that the major thrust for remediation in this area would come from speech pathologists, psychologists, psychiatrists, social workers, rehabilitation counselors, and nurses.

Not all of the emotional needs of the aphasic patient (as well as other brain-damaged patients) have been neglected, however. Patients fortunate enough to have received speech therapy generally have found that their therapists have tried to minister to emotional needs in conjunction with their primary task of improving language skills. Many aphasia therapists have been unsung heroes. Some have sought specialized training in psychotherapy, and sometimes they enlist the aid of a psychologist for advice regarding their interaction with patients.

A successful collaboration between a speech–language pathologist and a psychologist is most poignantly illustrated in the following case history. (The case also points up other therapeutic principles applicable to this group of patients). The patient was a married woman in her late 40s who sustained a stroke as a result of a brain hemorrhage. She was severely aphasic, essentially global, and remained so throughout the period described. There was no sensorimotor deficit. At 6 months poststroke she was profoundly depressed and had disabling pain in both the right upper and lower limbs. As is usual, the pain was attributed to the thalamic syndrome, a poorly defined diagnosis that is inevitably made when a brain-damaged patient has pain. Accordingly, drugs were prescribed, both for the pain and depression; however, neither problem was relieved, and at one point she attempted suicide.

Her case then was reviewed by a rehabilitation team, which concluded that the pain was psychogenic in origin and that, in addition to medication, some form of psychotherapy must be attempted. Her suffering was attributed to psychogenic regional pain (Walters, 1961), no doubt induced by her rage at the persistent aphasia. The psychotherapist concluded that the depression resulted from at least three factors:

1. The patient was an exceedingly compulsive, perfectionistic person with a hypertrophied sense of responsibility.
2. In becoming aphasic she believed she had failed her mother, who had always doted on her, and with whom there was a kind of psychological symbiotic relationship.
3. She decided she had also failed her husband, a simple man who had leaned heavily on his wife emotionally. She was the strong, competent one in the family; his primary role was to provide for them financially.

Many painful, laborious months then ensued, during which the psychologist and speech pathologist tried hard to get the patient to understand the reasons for her pain and depression and to establish new perspectives. In the early days of the program, she attempted suicide once more. She was seen by each therapist at least three times weekly; the therapists met frequently to discuss strategies. As expected, the aphasia made psychotherapy difficult but not impossible. Fortunately, the patient's comprehension was better than her expression, and the therapists employed both talking and writing. Medications were continued under the supervision of a psychopharmacologist.

Perseverance was rewarded after many weeks, and the patient gradually emerged from the emotional depths. Although the aphasia remained global, first the pain disappeared, then her mood improved markedly. (As the patient's depression lifted, her mother's deepened.) The patient gradually came to accept the fact that, although aphasic, she was still a competent person, capable of resuming her role as wife, companion, and daughter. Eventually she became a volunteer at the hospital and began to take trips with her husband. Having no physical disability, she was fully capable of carrying on as a homemaker when she was no longer depressed and in pain. Although a few years have passed, she continues to visit the psychologist from time to time.

In addition to the obvious, the case emphasizes the need for a collaborative approach. In this case speech pathologist, psychologist, physician, and psychopharmacologist worked together. This case also suggests that anatomic–pathologic explanations for symptoms (e.g., pain and depression) may be dangerous, leading to a hopeless prognosis and reliance on drugs as the only therapy available. Furthermore, this patient's story contradicts the commonly held view that psychotherapy cannot be done with a severely aphasic person. A variety of techniques and methods likely can be effective. In addition, the therapeutic value of the sustained efforts of caring professionals is probably beyond measure.

Hibbard et al. (1990) have described a program for poststroke depression based on behavior therapy principles. The program is impressive in its detail and sensitivity to patient and family issues. It includes consideration of the particular problems associated with aphasia, as well as pointed reference to the importance of family therapy. The need for this type of program would seem self-evident.

Borenstein, Linell, and Wåhrborg (1987) described an intensive 5-day "course" for patients with aphasia and family members, conducted by a speech pathologist, a psychologist, and a neurologist. The aims were to educate about aphasia, improve language function through stimulation, and identify and attempt to ameliorate personal and interpersonal problems. Follow-up evaluation a year later revealed an improved capacity of patients and their families to deal with psychological problems despite little linguistic change. Borenstein et al. (1987) also reported experience with eight young people with chronic aphasia (mean time postonset of 3 years) enrolled in a "folk high school," a type of institution unique to Scandinavia and Finland, where the emphasis is on personal development and social integration rather than formal schooling. Although no formal speech therapy was available, the students showed improvement in linguistic proficiency and a tendency to lessened depression at the end of the 30-week course.

In his book, *A Survey of Adult Aphasia,* Davis (1983) reviewed many of the psychological consequences of aphasia and suggested how they may be managed by the speech–language pathologist. It is recommended reading for speech therapists working with adult aphasic patients.

In summary, I must reiterate that treatment of social and psychological problems consequent to the development of aphasia is generally not provided. Clearly, however, there is growing awareness of its importance to improve the quality of life of both patients and their families and possibly even to enhance linguistic ability. Despite the communication problems inherent in working with an aphasic person, the ideal to which we should strive is to provide some form of counseling or psychotherapy for all patients and their families. A variety of therapeutic approaches most likely can be used successfully. Group therapy for patients only, patients and their families, or family members only, can all be of great value for both education and psychotherapeutic purposes. Although the literature is not extensive, it uniformly supports the value of therapy.

There is little question that pharmacotherapy plays a role in the management of some patients with aphasia. Although it cannot yet function as a substitute for psychotherapy and education, it can be very valuable in lessening depression or anxiety, which then allows the patient to be more attentive to other therapeutic endeavors. On occasion, when a fruitful interaction between patient and therapist is not possible, pharmacotherapy may be the only effective therapeutic modality.

Experience suggests that an enlightened approach to the psychological and social problems of people with aphasia mandates the participation of a team of professionals. Unfortunately, they are not always available and, even when they are, economic realities may prevent their participation. One can only hope that social maturity will someday make it possible for aphasic patients and their families to have access to all the services necessary to alleviate their distressing condition.

Acknowledgments

The revision of this chapter was supported in part by grant RO 1 NS 25367-OIAI from the National Institute of Deafness and Other Communication Disorders (NIDCD), and by grant G0083000039 from the National Institute of Handicapped Research, U.S. Department of Education.

References

Artes, R., & Hoops, R. (1976). Problems of aphasic and nonaphasic stroke patients as identified and evaluated by patients' wives. In Y. Lebrun & R. Hoops (Eds.), *Recovery in aphasics*. Amsterdam: Swets & Zeitlinger, B.V.

Bard, P., & Mountcastle, V. B. (1947). Some forebrain mechanisms involved in expression of rage with special reference to the suppression of angry behavior. *Research Publications—Association for Research in Nervous and Mental Disease, 27*, 362–404.

Baretz, R. M., & Stephenson, G. R. (1976). Unrealistic patient. *New York State Journal of Medicine, 76*, 54–57.

Bay, E. (1964). Principles of classification and their influence on our concepts of aphasia. In A. V. S. de Rueck & M. O'Connor (Eds.), *Disorders of language*. Boston, MA: Little, Brown.

Benson, D. F. (1980). Psychiatric problems in aphasia. In M. T. Sarno & O. Höök (Eds.), *Aphasia: Assessment and treatment*. Stockholm: Almqvist Wiksell; New York: Masson.

Borenstein, P., Linell, S., & Wåhrborg, P. (1987). An innovative therapeutic program for aphasia patients and their relatives. *Scandinavian Journal of Rehabilitation Medicine, 19*, 51–56.

Borenstein, P., Wåhrborg, P., Linell, S., Hedberg, E., Asking, M., & Ahlsen, E. (1987). Education in "Folk High School" for younger aphasic people. *Aphasiology, 1*, 263–266.

Brodal, A. (1947). The hippocampus and the sense of smell: A review. *Brain, 70*, 179–222.

Christensen, J., & Anderson, J. (1989). Spouse adjustment to stroke: Aphasic versus non-aphasic partners. *Journal of Communication Disorders, 22*, 225–231.

Critchley, M. (1970). *Aphasiology and other aspects of language*. London: Arnold.

Dahlberg, C. C. (1977). Stroke. *Psychology Today, 2*, 121–128.

Davis, G. A. (1983). *A survey of adult aphasia* (pp. 290–308). Englewood Cliffs, NJ: Prentice-Hall.

Egelko, S., Simon, D., Riley, D., Gordon, W., Ruckdeschel-Hibbard, M., & Diller, L. (1989). First year after stroke: Tracking cognitive and affective deficits. *Archives of Physical Medicine and Rehabilitation, 70*, 297–302.

Eisenson, J. (1973). *Adult aphasia: Assessment and treatment*. Englewood Cliffs, NJ: Prentice-Hall.

Friedman, M. H. (1961). On the nature of regression in aphasia. *Archives of General Psychiatry, 5*, 60–64.

Gainotti, G. (1972). Emotional behavior and hemispheric side of the lesion. *Cortex, 8*, 41–55.

Geschwind, N. (1977). Behavioral changes in temporal lobe epilepsy. *Archives of Neurology (Chicago), 34*, 453.

Goldstein, K. (1942). *After effects of brain injuries in war*. New York: Grune & Stratton.

Gordon, W., Hibbard, M., Egelko, S., Riley, E., Simon, D., Diller, E., Ross, E., & Lieberman, A. (in press). Issues in the diagnosis of post-stroke depression.

Grober, S., Gordon, W., Hibbard, M., Aletta, E., & Sliwinski, M. (1990). The utility of the dexamethasone suppression test in the diagnosis of post-stroke depression. Personal communication.

Head, H. (1926). *Aphasia and kindred disorders of speech*. Cambridge: Cambridge University Press.

Herrmann, M., & Wallesch, C. (1989). Psychosocial changes and psychosocial adjustment with chronic and severe non-fluent aphasia. *Aphasiology*, 3, 513–526.

Hibbard, M., Grober, S., Gordon, W., Aletta, D., & Freeman, A. (in press). Cognitive therapy and the treatment of post-stroke depression. *Topics in Geriatric Rehabilitation, 5*, 43–55.

Hodgins, E. (1964). *Episode*. New York: Atheneum.

Horenstein, S. (1970). Effects of cerebrovascular disease on personality and emotionality. In A. L. Benton (Ed.), *Behavioral change in cerebrovascular disease*. New York: Harper.

Jackson, J. H. (1932). On the nature of duality of the brain. In J. Taylor (Ed.), *Selected writings of John Hughlings Jackson*. London: Hodder & Stroughton.

Jaffe, J. (1981). The psychiatrist's approach to managing the aphasic patient. In R. T. Wertz (Ed.), *Seminars in speech, language and hearing* (Vol. 2, No. 4). New York: Thieme-Stratton.

Kinsella, G., & Duffy, F. (1978). The spouse of the aphasic patient. In Y. Lebrun & R. Hoops (Eds.), *The management of aphasia*. Amsterdam: Swets & Zeitlenger, B.V.

Klüver, H., & Bucy, P. (1939). Preliminary analyses of functions of the temporal lobes in monkeys. *Archives of Neurology and Psychiatry*, 42, 979–1000.

Lamendella, J. T. (1977). The limbic system in human communication. In H. Whitaker & H. A. Whitaker (Eds.), *Studies in neurolinguistics* (Vol. 3). New York: Academic Press.

Lenneberg, E. H. (1967). *Biological foundation of language*. New York: Wiley.

Luria, A. R. (1963). *Restoration of function after brain injury*. New York: MacMillan.

Luria, A. R. (1970). *Traumatic aphasia*. The Hague: Mouton.

MacLean, P. D. (1952). Some psychiatric implications of physiologic studies on frontotemporal portion of limbic systems (visceral brain). *Electroencephalography and Clinical Neurophysiology, 4*, 407–418.

Moss, S. (1976). Notes from an aphasic psychologist, or different strokes for different folks. In Y. Lebrun & R. Hoops (Eds.), *Recovery in aphasics*. Amsterdam: Swets & Zeitlinger, B.V.

National Aphasia Association. (1987). *Questionnaire Survey*. New York: National Aphasia Association.

Papez, J. W. (1937). A proposed mechanism of emotion. *Archives of Neurology and Psychiatry,* 38, 725–743.

Pribram, K. M. (1971). *Languages of the brain: Experimental paradoxes and principles of neuropsychology*. Englewood Cliffs, NJ: Prentice-Hall.

Pribram, K. M., & Kruger, L. (1954). Functions of the "olfactory brain." *Annals of the New York Academy of Sciences*, 58, 109–138.

Robinson, B. W. (1976). Limbic influences on human speech. *Annals of the New York Academy of Sciences*, 280, 761–771.

Robinson, R. G., & Benson, D. F. (1981). Depression in aphasic patients: Frequency, severity, and clinical-pathological correlations. *Brain and Language*, 14, 282–291.

Sarno, J. E. (1981). Emotional aspects of aphasia. In M. T. Sarno (Ed.), *Acquired aphasia*. New York: Academic Press.

Sarno, M. T. (1986). *The Fifth Annual Hemphill Lecture.* Chicago, IL: Rehabilitation Institute of Chicago.

Schuell, H. M., Jenkins, J., & Jiménez-Pabón, E. (1964). *Aphasia in adults.* New York: Harper.

Segré, R. (1976). Autobiographical consideration on aphasic rehabilitation. *Folia Phoniatrica, 28,* 129–140.

Sinyor, D., Jacques, P., Kaloupek, D. G., Becker, R., Goldenberg, M., & Coopersmith, H. (1986). Poststroke depression and lesion location. An attempted replication. *Brain, 109,* 537–546.

Smythies, J. R. (1970). *Brain mechanisms and behavior.* New York: Academic Press.

Ullman, M. (1962). *Behavioral change in patients following strokes.* Springfield, IL: Thomas.

Walters, A. (1961). Psychogenic regional pain alias hysterical pain. *Brain, 84,* 1–18.

Weinstein, E., & Kahn, R. (1955). *Denial of illness.* Springfield, IL: Thomas.

Wepman, J. M. (1951). *Recovery from aphasia.* New York: Ronald Press.

Williams, S., & Freer, C. (1986). Aphasia: Its effect on marital relationships. *Archives of Physical Medicine and Rehabilitation, 67,* 250–252.

Wint, G. (1967). *The third killer.* New York: Abelard-Schuman.

Ziegler, D. W. (1952). Word deafness and Wernicke's aphasia. *Archives of Neurology and Psychiatry, 67,* 323–331.

16

Recovery and Rehabilitation in Aphasia

MARTHA TAYLOR SARNO

At the first Academy of Aphasia meeting in Chicago in 1963, Arthur Benton aptly stated that the history of aphasia "begins at the beginning," for as long as humans have enjoyed the gift of language they have been subject to language disturbances through injury or disease. Informal attempts to "retrain" individual aphasic patients have occurred throughout history, probably as a consequence of the seemingly natural inclination of humans to want to heal each other. Although language disturbances were of at least sufficient interest to physicians to be recorded as early as 3500 B.C. (Benton, 1964), Benton and Joynt (1960) cited that Nicolo Massa and Francisco Arceo in 1558 described some of the first patients who, via natural recovery and intervention, recovered language completely after surgical intervention following head trauma. Other authors have reported early "treatments"; however, they are not in any way similar to aphasia rehabilitation as it is known in the twentieth century. In Mettler's (1947) classic text, *History of Medicine*, for example, Avicenna is cited as recommending cashew (anacardium) "for virtually all psychiatric and neurological afflictions, especially aphasia" (p. 538). Undoubtedly, cautery, cupping, alchemy, and leeching were also tried before the seventeenth century.

In the seventeenth century, Johann Schmidt (1624–1690), reported on two apoplectic patients with language disturbances. One patient recovered letter recognition, and the other recovered reading skills with training (Benton & Joynt, 1960). In the well-known account of his own aphasia in 1783, Samuel Johnson attributed the beginning of his speech recovery to the fact that his doctor had pressed blisters into his back and from his ear to his throat (Critchley, 1970). Professor Lordat reeducated himself in speech and writing until he resumed his chair of medicine at Montpellier, thereby providing support for his preconceived ideas about the dissociation of speech from thought. Later his self-observations raised questions about whether he did, indeed, suffer from aphasia (Bay, 1969; Lordat, 1843). In the nineteenth century a professor of medicine at the Albany Medical College in New York, Thomas Hun (1847), broke new ground when he wrote about the rehabilitation of a 35-year-old poststroke aphasic patient. Hun recommended that systematic exercises in spelling, writing, and reading be carried out by the patient's wife, and he credited her with the patient's recovery. Harold Goodglass (1985) cited an 1879 paper that summarized a case conference and described a 49-year-old aphasic patient who was treated repeatedly by "applying a strong current to his skin with an electric brush." Regarding treatment, the professor wrote,

> Something may be accomplished by improving his nutrition. So let us give two drams of compound hypophosphates and half an ounce of cod liver oil thrice daily. Let's also use stimulation of the affected muscles, particularly the muscles of the tongue. We may in this manner stimulate what is the obscure connection with the nervous centers themselves. Numerous attempts have been made to stimulate the central nervous system by applications of continuous current over the seat of the disease in the brain. But the results thus far have never been as good as those obtained by stimulating locally the muscles of phonation. (pp. 308–309)

Paul Broca was one of the first to discuss the feasibility of retraining in aphasia. In his 1885 paper, "Du siège de la faculté du langage articule," Broca described some anecdotal experiences with retraining and theorized that aphasics could be taught language in the same way one teaches a child since the left hemisphere has been differentially developed for language and other intellectual processes.

Although Bateman had suggested in 1890 that there was "sufficient evidence that re-education is a valuable means to re-establish man's noblest prerogative—the faculty of articulate language" (p. 229), Charles K. Mills's (1904) paper was the first in English to address recovery and rehabilitation in aphasia. Mills, founder of the neurology service at Philadelphia General Hospital, reported the training of a poststroke aphasic patient whom he and Donald Broadbent saw in a London Hospital and described in 1879 (Broadbent, 1879) and 1880 (C. K. Mills, 1880/1904). The training methods employed were largely determined by the patient, who began by systematically repeating letters, words, and phrases. When the paper was published in 1904, only a small literature existed, in

German, concerning the rehabilitation of aphasia. Henry Head later commended Mills's work because it was not based on the more pedantic methods of training widely advocated at that time and it acknowledged that the aphasic, because of prior experience and already organized brain function, presented a different teaching problem than the child (Weisenburg & McBride, 1935, 1964). Mills described an experience with a 45-year-old physician whom he, Weisenburg, and the patient's secretary systematically retrained at the patient's home over a 2-year period. In this case the "physiological alphabet" designed by Wyllie (1894), essentially an articulatory–phonetic approach, was used as the basis for training.

Although Mills's work was done over a century ago, his observations and approach to aphasia rehabilitation are remarkably similar to much present-day practice and thought. Mills's paper is notable in that it discussed some of the methods used with aphasic patients at the turn of the century and showed concern with nonlinguistic aspects of the patients' rehabilitation management (i.e., emotional factors, premorbid intelligence, and education). He discussed the possible influence of semantic, lexical, and cognitive factors in recovery and suggested that different methods were appropriate for different patients and syndromes. He also noted that aphasia after trauma has a better outcome than after cerebrovascular accident (CVA) and that not all patients benefit from retraining to the same degree. He acknowledged that spontaneous recovery may influence the course and extent of recovery.

During World War I several hospitals were established for the treatment of the brain injured, particularly in Germany. This establishment occurred despite the fact that the treatment of aphasia was not accepted by neurologists, and securing their cooperation in establishing retraining programs was, therefore, difficult (Goldstein, 1942). In Vienna Emil Froeschels treated a large number of brain-injured patients between 1916 and 1925 (Schuell, Jenkins, & Jiménez-Pabón, 1964). Isserlin (1929) had a program in Munich, and Poppelreuter (1915) in Cologne. Henry Head's (1926, 1963) two-volume treatise on aphasia was based on his experience in England with 26 posttraumatic patients, primarily the victims of gunshot wounds during World War I. Nielsen (1936) reported residual language impairments in 16 of 200 head-injured patients who were treated at Hospital #1 at Cape May from 1918 to 1919. Frazier and Ingham (1920), Gopfert (1922), and Franz (1924) also reported experiences retraining aphasic patients during this period.

Goldstein's extensive and intensive experiences in Frankfurt during both world wars, especially at the Institut Zur Erforschung der Folgeerscheinungen von Hirnverletzungen, provided one of the most comprehensive descriptions of the systematic treatment of a large number of head-injured patients, of whom 90–100 were followed for a 10-year period (Goldstein, 1942). The Frankfurt facilities included a hospital, psychological laboratory, school, workshop, and research institute. Goldstein's work (1942, 1948) constituted some of the most detailed early observations of attempts to retrain large numbers of aphasic patients.

Except for Mills's (1904) report, knowledge of aphasia rehabilitation before World War II was based primarily on the literature that emerged from wartime experiences. Only occasional reports appeared describing the retraining of poststroke aphasic civilians. Notable among these was the detailed description by Mills (1904) and the case reported by Singer and Low (1933) of a 39-year-old woman who suffered an apparent vascular infarct after a full-term delivery and showed continuous language improvement with consistent training over a 10-year period. Two years after onset, the patient's only verbal response was the reiterative, "o dedar," and she could neither read nor write. After 10 years she reportedly used a vocabulary of 500 words freely and intelligibly with those she knew well. Autopsy findings 25 years later revealed complete absence of hinder parts of the second and third frontal convolutions.

Weisenburg and McBride's landmark 5-year study concerned the general topic of aphasia without special reference to recovery, but the authors did comment on the effectiveness of reeducation in a study of 60 patients of less than 60 years of age, a majority of whom had suffered strokes. They concluded that reeducation increased the rate of recovery, assisted in facilitating the use of compensatory means of communication, and improved morale (Weisenburg & McBride, 1935, 1964). Their work documented the psychotherapeutic benefits of treatment.

During World War II several army hospitals established special programs for aphasic brain-injured soldiers, which provided a basis for the literature that began to emerge concerning recovery and rehabilitation. Programs were established at Percy Jones General Hospital in Battle Creek, Michigan (Sheehan, 1946), Halloran General Hospital on Staten Island (Huber, 1946), the Aphasia Clinic at the University of Michigan (Backus, 1945; Backus, Henry, Clancy, & Dunn, 1947), and McGuire General Hospital in Richmond, Virginia (Peacher, 1945). Eisenson (1949) reported on aphasic patients he studied at Halloran General Hospital on Staten Island and Cushing General Hospital, Framingham, Massachusetts, in 1947. At the Thomas M. England General Hospital in Atlantic City, Louis Granich, following the retraining model set forth by Kurt Goldstein, published a book-length report detailing the retraining of eight aphasic patients (Granich, 1947).

In England, Butfield and Zangwill (1946) followed the recovery course of 66 aphasic patients, the majority of whom were posttrauma. After reeducation, speech was judged to be significantly improved, both in patients who began therapy less than 6 months after onset (one-half of the group) and in patients who began therapy more than 6 months after onset (one-third of the group). The authors also reported that the best outcome was obtained in those with aphasia due to trauma rather than other causes. Their published case studies, some of which monitored improvement only following the period of spontaneous recovery, provided evidence that speech and language could be improved by training.

Until World War II aphasia and its concomitant neurological deficits in the stroke patient were viewed as natural components of the aging process. In that era the civilian population did not consider treatment of aphasia as an option. It was believed that the aphasic patient, generally elderly, could count on an extended family to meet daily needs. Wepman (1951), however, drew attention to the large population of untreated civilians who, like the war veterans, could benefit from therapy.

One of the first comprehensive reports emerging from World War II was Joseph Wepman's (1951) book based on data obtained at the Aphasia Center of DeWitt General Hospital in Auburn, California. Wepman described the retraining of a population of 68 aphasic patients (mean age = 25.8 years) who began treatment 6 months posttrauma. He utilized training methods modeled after traditional language educational techniques. Aphasic patients made a gain of better than five school grades in language skills. Wepman's conviction was that premorbid personality had a profound influence on outcome, and he concluded that aphasia after brain trauma is amenable to improvement with training. Specifically, he found that individuals with expressive aphasia, followed by those with receptive and global aphasia, recovered the highest levels of language performance.

Luria (1948) reported the outcome of a large series of patients with traumatic aphasia treated at the Institute of Neurology, Academy of Medical Sciences. He concluded that systematic retraining based on a careful psycholinguistic analysis and aimed at developing compensatory function provides the foundation for the successful restoration of verbal skills.

Up to the period immediately following World War II, the word STROKE carried the highly charged connotation "stricken by God," which surely delayed its adoption into everyday usage. In the preface to Wepman's *Recovery from Aphasia* (1951), Wendell Johnson used PARALYTIC STROKE, and, in the text, Wepman used quotation marks around STROKE.

Several historical factors stand out as having had important influence in making the treatment of aphasia the common practice that it is today. These include the advent of speech pathology as a health profession, the emergence of rehabilitation medicine as a medical specialty, the mass media explosion, a larger and more affluent middle class, and increased public expectations of medicine in an age of technology. The latter has been particularly true in the industrialized areas of the world, where it is widely believed that treatment is possible for every human ill. Furthermore, whereas talk of chronic disease was once considered taboo, it is now openly and widely discussed.

In the past two decades the volume of clinical and research activity in aphasia rehabilitation has multiplied many times. Furthermore, the aphasia population is considerably larger now, given the overall increase in size of the general population, life span, and percentage of patients surviving stroke. An increase in the incidence of motor vehicle accidents and the increased rate of survival after head trauma have also added to the pool of individuals with aphasia. Concurrent with an increased aphasia population has been an increase in the number of facilities offering aphasia rehabilitation services.

While social and attitudinal changes were taking place, the field of speech pathology grew rapidly. Affiliates (members and certificate holders) in the American Speech–Language–Hearing Association (ASHA) increased from 1623 in 1950 to 35,000 in 1980. By January 1990, the number grew to 60,249. During the same period, the medical specialty of rehabilitation medicine burgeoned and is now an integral part of the health system.

In the United States, changing attitudes about chronic disease, the hope of modern medicine, and a more vocal lay press continued to sharpen interest in the subject of aphasia. The press reported on public figures who incurred strokes with aphasia, such as Sir Winston Churchill in 1953, President Dwight D. Eisenhower in 1957, and Ambassador Joseph Kennedy in 1962. In connection with President Eisenhower's stroke, Eugene J. Taylor, a medical writer long associated with Dr. Howard A. Rusk, wrote a series of articles that appeared on the front page of *The New York Times* describing stroke, particularly aphasia.

Several informational publications designed for use by the families and friends of patients with aphasia also appeared in the post–World War II period (American Heart Association, 1969; Backus et al., 1947; Boone, 1965; J. E. Sarno & Sarno, 1969b; Simonson, 1971; Taylor, 1958). One of these, "Understanding Aphasia" (Taylor, 1958), is still widely read and has been published in 11 languages.

Workbooks, manuals, and other treatment guides for home use, as well as personal accounts by individuals who acquired aphasia after stroke, attested to strong public interest in the problem of aphasia. The treatment materials included workbooks by Longerich and Bordeaux (1954), Taylor and Marks (1955, 1959), Keith (1972, 1977, 1984, 1987), Stryker (1975), Traendly (1977), Brubaker (1978, 1984), Kilpatrick (1980), Morganstein and Smith (1982), and M. C. Smith and Morganstein (1988). Most notable of the personal accounts were those of Ritchie (1961), Hodgins (1964), Wint (1967), Buck (1968), Moss (1972), Cameron (1973), Wulf (1973), Dahlberg and Jaffee (1977), and Lavin (1985).

After World War II the University of Michigan Aphasia Clinic, established during the war by Ollie Backus and Harlan Bloomer, the Speech Pathology Department of the Mayo Clinic under the late Josephine Simonson and Joe Brown, and the Speech Pathology Services of the Howard A. Rusk Institute of Rehabilitation Medicine, New York University Medical Center, under Martha Taylor Sarno, were among the few civilian programs where significant numbers of aphasic patients were treated. Many programs at Veterans Administration (VA) hospitals, originally organized to treat traumatic aphasia, continued to provide service to stroke patients in peacetime. The Aphasia Section of the Neurology Service at the Minneapolis VA Hospital under Hildred Schuell is a notable example of a VA program that made a major contribution to the aphasia rehabilitation literature. Schuell and her colleagues studied an aphasic population of 155 patients, 75 of whom were available for follow-up testing; these patients provided a rich data base for Schuell's major publication (Schuell et al., 1964). Two other active VA aphasic centers were those at Van Nuys, California, under Nielsen, and at Framingham, Massachusetts (later moved to Boston), under Edwin M. Cole (H. Goodglass, personal communication, 1990).

In the past two decades journals devoted to brain–language issues (e.g., *Aphasiology, Brain and Language,* and *Cortex*) have become indispensable information sources for aphasiologists. The Academy of Aphasia, a scholarly society established in 1962 and dedicated to the study of aphasia, meets annually and has among its members aphasiologists of international reputation (M. T. Sarno, 1986b). Following the example of several European national associations for aphasia, the National Aphasia Association (NAA) was founded in the United States in 1987. Its purposes include public education, patient recovery, and establishment of regional support groups called Aphasia Community Groups (ACGs), through a network of regional representatives and the support of research.

Critical Factors in the Evaluation of Recovery and Treatment

Before reviewing the literature on contemporary methods and the value of treatment, it is essential to consider some inherent limitations in investigating the treatment of aphasia. Chief among these is the question of what is meant by RECOVERY. No one disputes the idea that, at the very least, recovery refers to improvement in communication, but problems arise when one attempts to characterize recovery in qualitative and quantitative terms. If complete recovery is to occur, it usually happens within a matter of hours or days following onset. Once aphasia has persisted for weeks or months, a complete return to a premorbid state is usually the exception.

A discrepancy often exists among patients' perceptions of "recovery," their performances on aphasia tests, and the clinical manifestations of aphasia. Patients show a wide range of interpretations of recovery. Most do not consider themselves recovered unless they have fully returned to previous levels of language competence (Yarnell, Monroe, & Sobel, 1976). When unrecovered patients are content with their level of competence and consider themselves recovered, this is a psychological perception and should not be confused with an objective evaluation of communication abilities. In the final analysis, the true test of outcome in aphasia rehabilitation can be assessed only by patients' perceptions of the quality of their lives. A number of quality of life measures have been developed for this purpose (e.g., J. E. Sarno, Sarno, & Levita, 1973; Schwartz, 1983).

Following this line of thought, it is reasonable and probably desirable to distinguish between two separate recovery dimensions: one that is totally objective and attempts to identify, as far as it is possible, whether and to what extent the patient has regained previous language abilities, and a second, which in humanistic terms may be more important, that measures the degree of recovery of functional communication. Few investigators have considered this relevant dimension of patient recovery in their research.

The concept of a "functional" dimension of communication behavior emerged logically from the experience of treating patients with aphasia in the rehabilitation medicine setting (Holland, 1982; M. T. Sarno, 1983, 1984; Taylor, 1965). Rehabilitation medicine has traditionally acknowledged that the ability of patients to function in their daily lives, the so-called activities of daily living, does not necessarily correlate directly with the extent of physical disability. J. E. Sarno, Sarno, and Levita (1971) addressed functional communication recovery and demonstrated that improvement in quantitative measures of language performance did not necessarily represent improvement in functional communication.

If one wishes to do research on recovery and treatment, the problem becomes more complicated. Not only must one keep in mind the dichotomies noted above, but also the difficult problems revolving around how one classifies patients; establishes levels of severity; and accounts for previous language competence, age, education, socioeconomic status, intellectual level, personality, and, of critical importance, therapist competence. The virtual impossibility of finding homogeneous groups of patients on whom to try a variety of treatment methods limits the validity of all studies. To further complicate the situation, it is difficult, if not impossible, to obtain comparable control groups of patients since it is an ethical imperative that all patients have the opportunity to receive treatment. These comments are not intended to discourage potential investigators, but rather to emphasize the factors that need to be considered when designing research in this area. Students will do well to keep them in mind as they read the aphasia literature.

It is clear that recovery and treatment are important research topics. There are about 84,000 new aphasia patients in the United States each year, the majority of whom desire treatment (Brust, Shafer, Richter, & Bruun, 1976). The United States Census Bureau (1975, p. 25) predicts that by the year 2000, 31 million people will be over the age of 65. In the past two decades the 65 and older population has increased by 56% whereas the under-65 population has grown by only 19% (United States Department of Health and Human Services, 1988). The proportion of persons over 65 had increased from 4% in 1900 to 11% in 1980 and is projected to reach 21–22% of the total population by the year 2030 (Spencer, 1984). Together with this burgeoning population, rehabilitation service providers are faced with the constraints of tighter reimbursement policies, which result in shorter hospital stays and outpatient treatment duration. Hence, it has become increasingly important to establish valid treatment principles.

Studies on the Efficacy of Therapy in the Poststroke Aphasic Patient

In view of the limited literature on aphasia rehabilitation after stroke up to World War II, those who pioneered attempts to rehabilitate civilian aphasic patients after the war had to rely on knowledge obtained from experiences with wartime casualties. The aphasia literature based on posttraumatic aphasia suggested that (a) retraining is effective, (b) posttraumatic aphasia has a better outcome than aphasia resulting from stroke, (c) the early initiation of speech therapy enhances recovery, and (d) younger patients fare best (Butfield & Zangwill, 1946; Eisenson, 1949; Wepman, 1951). Eventually studies of the effectiveness of speech therapy with the post-CVA patient began to appear.

Despite the many important difficulties inherent in studying efficacy (Prins, Schooner, & Vermeulen, 1989; M. T. Sarno, 1976; Wertz et al., 1981, 1986), a number of investigators have addressed the general issue of treatment efficacy. One of the first studies in the postwar period presented an outcome analysis of 203 aphasic patients, primarily poststroke, who received speech therapy and comprehensive rehabilitation services in a rehabilitation setting (Marks, Taylor, & Rusk, 1957). Outcome was based primarily on clinical judgments of whether patients moved from lower to higher diagnostic or functional groups. Functional categories ranged from "institutional adequacy" to "vocational adequacy." The results indicated considerable functional benefit for aphasic patients exposed to language training in a rehabilitation medicine setting, especially those with a predominantly expressive language disorder.

An untreated control group was included in the retrospective study of 69 patients conducted by Vignolo (1964), who concluded that reeducation has a specific effect if it is administered for more than 6 months.

Sands, Sarno, and Shankweiler (1969) studied 30 treated poststroke aphasic patients in a rehabilitation medicine setting and reported a median gain for all patients of 10 percentage points in language function as measured by the Functional Communication Profile (FCP; M. T. Sarno, 1969; Taylor, 1965). Three patients did not improve.

In a prospective study (M. T. Sarno, Silverman, & Sands, 1970), 31 patients who were at least 3 months poststroke and classified as alert global aphasics were randomly assigned to three treatment conditions: programmed instruction, "traditional" speech therapy, and no treatment. Although the groups were equated for time since onset, the duration of symptoms in the sample ranged widely from 3 months to 10 years poststroke. Treatment ranged from 4 to 36 weeks, with a mean of 17.1 weeks. All patients showed small gains, but there were no significant differences in gains for any of the groups.

A. Smith (1971) and A. Smith, Champoux, Leri, London, and Muraski (1972) studied 80 relatively young (mean age = 51.3 years) treated aphasic patients. Sixty-seven patients had vascular etiology, and 13 patients were posttraumatic. Of the group, 55% showed improvement in speech, 67% in comprehension, 61% in reading, and 54% in writing.

Hagen (1973) studied the effects of treatment in 20 males with communication disorders after stroke (mean age = 52.6 years). Ten patients received therapy for 1 year, whereas the other 10 patients did not. Although both groups exhibited spontaneous improvement during the first 3 months, only those receiving treatment continued to improve beyond what is generally considered the spontaneous recovery period.

Basso, Faglioni, and Vignolo (1975) studied 185 subjects primarily poststroke (mean age = 48.1 years). Ninety-one treated patients were compared with 94 who were untreated. A positive effect of treatment in oral expression was reported even when undertaken 6 months after onset.

Kertesz and McCabe (1977) reported findings on 93 patients controlled for time since onset. Seventy-four had CVAs caused by occlusion, 12 had hemorrhaged, and 7 had suffered trauma. The degree of improvement was greatest in the period between 1.5 and 3 months poststroke. Patients with posttraumatic aphasia had a better outcome than those with aphasia secondary to vascular disease. Where comparisons were possible, no significant differences were found between treated and untreated patient groups.

Levita (1978) compared FCP results for 17 treated and 18 untreated aphasic patients. Treated patients received therapy during the period between 4 and 12 weeks postonset. No significant differences were found between the groups. The results suggested that patients who received traditional speech therapy could not be differentiated from untreated control patients at 3 months postonset.

In a major treatment study of 162 treated patients and 119 untreated controls conducted in Milan, Basso, Capitani, and Vignolo (1979) addressed the relationship of time since onset, type of aphasia, overall initial severity, and presence or absence of treatment and improvement. A significant positive effect on improvement in all language skills was found for the treated patients, which included some who began rehabilitation after the presumed spontaneous recovery period.

Shewan and Kertesz (1984) followed 100 post-CVA aphasic patients under four treatment conditions: language oriented treatment (LOT) and stimulation-facilitation provided by speech pathologists, supportive communication provided by nurses, and no treatment. Significant differences were evident between the groups treated by speech pathologists and the untreated group. The patients treated by speech pathologists made the greatest gains. The nurse-treated group did not differ significantly from the group that was untreated or those treated by the speech pathologists. The two groups treated by the speech pathologists did not differ significantly from each other.

Lincoln et al. (1984) randomly assigned 104 patients at 10 weeks poststroke to a treatment group and 87 to a no-treatment group for a 24-week period. Their results indicated "that speech therapy did not improve language abilities more than was achieved by spontaneous recovery". There was some evidence that "for the small number of patients who can cope with more intensive and prolonged treatment speech therapy is beneficial" (p. 1199).

Shewan (1988) analyzed samples of connected language with the Shewan Spontaneous Language Analysis system. In a treated group of 36 and an untreated group of 11 aphasic subjects, samples taken at 2–4 weeks postonset and again 3 months after the first sample indicated that only one variable, "time talked," differed significantly in favor of the treated group.

Prins, Schoonen, and Vermeulen (1989) studied 32 patients in a 5-month treatment program assigned to receive one of two different types of language treatment or no treatment. No significant differences were found among patients receiving systematic therapy, conventional stimulation therapy, and no therapy.

In a study of 76 treated patients and 92 untreated patients, Poeck, Huber, and Willmes (1989) found that treated patients improved significantly more than untreated patients. A similar rate of improvement was found for individuals with chronic aphasia beyond the period of spontaneous recovery.

Specific Treatment Variables

In the VA Cooperative Study (Wertz et al., 1981), 67 poststroke patients were randomly assigned to individual or group treatment for 8 hr per week for 11–44 weeks. Individual therapy was "traditional" stimulus–response type treatment of specific language deficits. Group therapy consisted of indirect "stimulation" through group interaction, and discussion with no direct treatment of specific language deficits. The investigators concluded that both types of therapy were effective.

Hartman and Landau (1987) compared a group of patients who received conventional speech therapy for a 6-month period by professional speech pathologists with a group attending emotional supportive counseling sessions with professional speech pathologists. Sixty patients who began treatment at 1 month postonset were randomly assigned to each of the two groups. No differences were found between the groups on Porch Index of Communicative Ability (PICA) results.

David, Enderby, and Bainton (1982) conducted a study of 96 patients in which they found no differences between randomly assigned patients who were treated for 15–20 weeks. One group was treated by professional speech pathologists, and the other by volunteers who provided general support and stimulation. Both groups had almost identical recovery courses.

In a follow-up to his 1981 study Wertz et al. (1986) studied 121 aphasic patients under three different treatment conditions: conventional treatment, home treatment, and deferred treatment. Conventional treatment was administered by a speech-language pathologist for 12 weeks. Home treatment was provided for 12 weeks by a family member or friend. Both conditions were followed by 12 weeks of no treatment. The deferred-treatment group received no treatment for 12 weeks, followed by 12 weeks of conventional treatment with a speech-language pathologist. Mean postonset time for all groups was between 6.5 and 8 weeks. The conventionally treated group improved significantly more than the deferred-treatment group. The outcome of the home-treated group did not differ significantly from that of either of the other groups. That group did, however, improve more on all measures than the untreated group and less on all measures than the conventionally treated group.

In a study conducted by the consortium of VA centers, R. C. Marshall et al. (1989) compared three treatment conditions for a 12-week period: home therapy administered by trained volunteers, conventional speech pathology treatment, and no treatment. Thirty-seven males were involved in the study. All of the patients improved in all treatment conditions, and the conventionally treated group did significantly better than the no-treatment group.

Other Variables

Some investigators have focused on specific variables as particularly relevant to recovery from aphasia. This section reviews some of the studies that have drawn conclusions regarding the influence of these variables on recovery course and outcome.

SPONTANEOUS RECOVERY

There is general agreement that some natural recovery takes place in the majority of patients with or without intervention, usually in the period immediately following onset. However, there is a lack of consensus about the duration of the spontaneous recovery period (Darley, 1970; Reinvang & Engvik, 1980; M. T. Sarno, 1980d).

Luria referred to a period of 6–7 months postonset as the time when spontaneous restitution takes place. Forty-three percent of his post-traumatic group showed residual signs requiring reeducation or psychotherapy after that period (Luria, 1963).

Culton (1969) found that both rapid spontaneous recovery of language function and spontaneous recovery in intellectual function occurred in the first month following the onset of aphasia in a group of 21 untreated poststroke aphasic patients. These increases were not evident in the second month postonset.

Vignolo (1964), Basso et al. (1975), Kertesz and McCabe (1977), and Demeurisse et al. (1980) all concluded that the greatest improvement occurs in the first 2–3 months postonset. Butfield and Zangwill (1946), Sands et al. (1969), and Vignolo (1964) found that the recovery rate dropped significantly after 6 months. Others believe that spontaneous recovery does not occur after 1 year (Culton, 1969; Kertesz & McCabe, 1977).

M. T. Sarno and Levita (1971) studied 28 untreated poststroke patients with severe aphasia in the first 6 months poststroke and found that greater change took place within a 3-month than a 6-month postonset period.

Brust et al. (1976) surveyed 850 acute stroke patients during the first month poststroke and found aphasia present in 177 patients (21% of the group) during the acute phase; 32% ($n = 57$) were classified as fluent and 68% ($n = 120$) as nonfluent. In the period 4–12 weeks poststroke, aphasia improved in 74% of the patients and cleared in 44%. At 3 months poststroke, 12% of the fluent group and 34% of the nonfluent group were still considered impaired. In this study, those with fluent aphasia in the first month poststroke presented the best prognosis for improving before the end of the spontaneous recovery period.

Lomas and Kertesz (1978) tested 31 aphasic stroke patients within 30 days (mean = 11.5 days) and at 3 months (mean = 97 days) poststroke. Eight language tests (i.e., yes–no responses, repetition and imitation, naming, Token Test, spontaneous speech in picture description and conversational questions, word fluency, sentence completion, and responsive speech) were administered. Improvement on these eight comprehension, repetition, and expression tasks were documented for all aphasics, confirming the observation that spontaneous recovery occurs in the first 3 months.

Holland et al. (1985) documented the spontaneous recovery of language in a global aphasic patient from the first to the fourteenth day postonset.

Fifty-two stroke patients with aphasia who did not receive speech therapy during the first 6 months postonset were studied by Lendrem and Lincoln (1985). PICA test (Porch, 1967, 1973) results and FCP ratings from 10 to 34 weeks after CVA supported the view that most recovery occurs in the first 3 months poststroke, particularly between weeks 4 and 10.

AGE AND RECOVERY

Healthy elderly individuals generally begin to experience language changes during the sixth decade. Aphasia is usually superimposed on the quantitative and qualitative changes present in the language behavior of the healthy elderly (Bayles & Kaszniak, 1987; Davis, 1984; Obler & Albert, 1981; Wertz, 1984). On naming tasks, for example, correctness scores decline significantly between the seventh and eighth decades (Obler, Nicholas, & Albert, 1985), and on comprehension tasks a performance decrement begins in the sixth decade and continues through the eighth decade (Obler et al., 1985). Discourse measures, by contrast, show increasing elaborateness with advancing age (Obler, 1980). Furthermore, the duration of speech tends to be 20—25% longer for elderly (66–75 years) than for younger (24–27 years) subjects (B. L. Smith, Wasowicz, & Preston, 1987). For a review of this topic, the reader is referred to chapter 12 by Au, Obler, and Albert.

Aphasiologists generally consider age an important variable in recovery outcome (Darley, 1972; Davis & Holland, 1981; Eisenson, 1949; Sands et al., 1969; Sarno, 1976; Schuell et al., 1964; Vignolo, 1964; Wepman & Jones, 1958); however, reports of the effects of age on recovery are not consistent (Basso et al., 1979; Sarno, 1976; Yarnell et al., 1976). Age is reported as both a decisive (Sands et al., 1969; Shewan & Kertesz, 1984; Vignolo, 1964) and weak variable (Basso et al., 1979; Culton, 1969, 1971; Kertesz & McCabe, 1977; M. T. Sarno & Levita, 1971; M. T. Sarno, Silverman, & Levita, 1970). For example, in a comparison of the 10 oldest (mean age = 82.4, range = 77–93) and 10 youngest (mean age = 38.1, range = 19–49) patients in a sample of 74 patients, Holland and Bartlett (1985) found that advanced age was a significant deterrent to recovery. Holland, Greenhouse, Fromm, & Swindell (1989) and Sasanuma (1988) also showed less improvement in the older aphasic patient. In contrast, Kertesz (1984) recently observed remarkably good recovery in elderly patients, whereas some young patients remained severely disabled. Wertz and Dronkers (1988) reviewed data from the VA cooperative study, and concluded that age was not a factor in recovery. In a study of untreated patients between 4 and 34 weeks poststroke, Lendrem and Lincoln (1985) found spontaneous recovery to be independent of age. Pickersgill and Lincoln (1983) found language recovery to be relatively independent of age in moderate and severe patients.

Reports of recovery outcome in groups of posttraumatic aphasics in wartime have concluded that younger patients do better than older patients (Eisenson, 1949; Wepman, 1951). The largest number of patients with aphasia in peacetime, however, are those secondary to stroke, usually in older group (M. T. Sarno, 1968, 1975; Schuell et al., 1964). Some studies limited subjects to younger aphasic patients. In the now classic study of Weisenburg and McBride (1935), for example, patients over the age of 60 were excluded "to prevent a picture complicated by senile changes" (p. 119).

The wide discrepancy in the literature with respect to the influence of age on recovery from aphasia is probably related to a great degree to differences in methodology.

One of the first studies to address the influence of chronological age on recovery in the adult, poststroke aphasic patient followed 66 treated aphasic patients ranging from 51 to 77 years of age (mean = 61.4 years) from 4 to 52 weeks poststroke (M. T. Sarno, 1980b). When the extremes of the group were compared, the 10 oldest and youngest, and the 10 least and most improved, age did not emerge as a significant variable in recovery.

GENDER AND RECOVERY

It has been suggested that language in males is more discretely lateralized than in females (McGlone, 1980) and, as a result, that left-hemisphere strokes result in aphasia more often in men than in women (McGlone, 1977). One of the few studies that found gender a significant factor in recovery from aphasia was that of Basso, Capitani, and Moraschini (1982) which studied 264 males and 121 females in Milan. In this study females recovered significantly more in oral expression than males, but did not show significant differences in recovery of auditory verbal comprehension ability. Pizzamiglio, Mammurcari, and Razzaro (1985) studied 48 males and 41 females with aphasia before and after a 3-month language therapy treatment period. There was significantly greater improvement in auditory comprehension in the 15 females than in the 19 males in the global aphasia group.

Other studies, however, have concluded that sex is not a significant factor in recovery from aphasia (Gloning et al., 1976; Kertesz & McCabe, 1977; C. Rose, Boby, & Capildeo, 1976; M. T. Sarno, Buonaguro, & Levita, 1985; Shewan & Kertesz, 1984; Wade, Hewer, & Wood, 1984b).

TYPE AND SEVERITY OF APHASIA AND RECOVERY

Some investigations have concluded that patients with different aphasia syndromes recover differently. For example, researchers have observed that conduction and anomic aphasics have a good prognosis for recovery (Benson, 1970; Kertesz, 1979a, 1979b). In Kertesz and McCabe's (1977) study, Broca's aphasics had the highest rate of recovery. The lowest rate of recovery occurred in the untreated global aphasic and anomic groups. There was a high correlation among different types of aphasia during the first 3 months poststroke. Vignolo (1964) concluded that expressive disorders were resistant to recovery. In contrast, Marks et al. (1957) found that expressive-type aphasics benefited most from speech therapy. Basso et al. (1975) reported no significant differences in rate of recovery between Broca's and Wernicke's aphasics. Benson (1979b) and Kertesz and McCabe (1977) found that patients with mixed transcortical aphasia showed little if any recovery.

Prins, Snow, and Wagenaar (1978) found no qualitative or quantitative differences between groups (fluent, mixed, nonfluent, severely nonfluent), despite differences in severity. Using fluency alone as the basis for classification, there was no differentiation among types of a- phasia. Even though fluency had a high correlation with degree of sever- ity, the pattern of change over the course of a year, that is, the relatively greater improvement in comprehension than in spontaneous speech, was the same for all types of aphasia.

Schuell et al. (1964) reported the best recovery in patients that they classified as having simple aphasia (decrements in all language modalities) and the poorest outcome in those with irreversible aphasic syndrome.

In M. T. Sarno and Levita's (1979) study, data were systematically obtained on 34 patients from 8 to 52 weeks poststroke. Fluent aphasics reached the highest level of functional communication and made the greatest gain (36 FCP overall percentage points), whereas nonfluent and global aphasic patients made smaller gains (24 and 25 FCP overall per- centage points, respectively). Prins et al. (1978) reported that some global aphasic patients recovered sufficiently to be reclassified as nonfluent.

Kertesz (1984) charted the evolution of aphasic syndromes based on his studies (Kertesz, 1981; Kertesz & McCabe, 1977) and reported that (a) global aphasia evolved toward severe Broca's aphasia with significantly improved comprehension, (b) Broca's aphasia improved in fluency and grammar evolving toward anomic aphasia, and (c) Wernicke's aphasia evolved toward anomic or conduction aphasia.

Pashek and Holland (1988) found anomic aphasia to be a common end point for both fluent and nonfluent patients at 1 year postonset. The incidence of evolution was greatest in patients with Wernicke's aphasia.

In general, most investigators report that the patients with severe aphasia do not recover as well as those with mild aphasia (Kertesz &

McCabe, 1977; Sands et al., 1969; Schuell et al., 1964; Selnes, Niccum, Knopman, & Rubens, 1984). Differential recovery has also been confirmed in studies where outcome in untreated global aphasics was compared with outcome in a treated group (M. T. Sarno, Silverman, & Sands, 1970).

In contrast to previous studies in which patients with the greatest severity level improved least, Shewan (1988) found more improvement in the severe group than in either the mild or the moderate group at 6 months postonset.

ETIOLOGY AND RECOVERY

Researchers generally agree that those patients with posttraumatic aphasia show greater recovery than patients with aphasia after vascular lesions (Butfield & Zangwill, 1946; Vignolo, 1964). In fact, some cases of aphasia after closed head injury have been reported to recover completely (Kertesz, 1979a; Kertesz & McCabe, 1977). Kertesz (1979b) also noted that global aphasics secondary to closed head injury may improve to a mild anomic state. A similar evolution is not generally observed in patients with vascular lesions who have a similar degree of initial impairment.

In Schuell et al.'s (1964) series, the least recovered patients were those in the most seriously impaired patient group, which also had the highest incidence of complete thrombosis of the internal carotid and middle cerebral arteries or the middle cerebral artery alone.

In another study by Kertesz and McCabe (1977), patients with aphasia subsequent to subarachnoid hemorrhage showed varying recovery rates, apparently related to the extent of the bleed and the presence of infarcts or tissue destruction. Some of the most severe instances of jargon and global aphasia in the Kertesz series (1979a) occurred in patients with ruptured middle cerebral aneurysms.

In a study of recovery from acute aphasia in 21 young adults at least 6 months after closed head injury, Levin, Grossman, Sarwar, and Meyers (1981) reported that the 9 who recovered normal levels of language performance had mild diffuse brain injury. Six with global cognitive deficit, including language impairment, had suffered more severe diffuse damage. The remaining 6 patients whose only residual was anomia were split in etiology: Half had mild diffuse brain injury, whereas the others had focal left-hemisphere damage.

Dell, Batson, Kasden, and Paterson (1983) described four cases of posttraumatic aphasia associated with subdural hematoma. The onset of aphasia was delayed from a few hours to weeks after injury with rapid deterioration of language behavior. Timely surgical intervention led to rapid resolution of the aphasia through decompression.

Thirty-nine patients who sustained penetrating head injuries resulting in nonfluent aphasia were studied by Ludlow et al. (1986). CAT scans of the 13 patients with persistent syntax processing deficits, as long as 15 years postinjury, showed left-hemisphere lesions of greater extent, number, and deep posterior extension than those in the 26 patients in the recovered group.

NEURORADIOLOGIC CORRELATES OF RECOVERY

Yarnell et al. (1976) systematically analyzed CAT scans of 14 aphasic patients up to 8 months poststroke and concluded that the size, location, and number of lesions documented by the scans showed a high degree of correlation with recovery from aphasia. Those patients with significant dominant-hemisphere lesions, either one large or many small ones, fared poorly, whereas those with lesser lesions did better. Bilateral lesions, at times unrecognized clinically, helped to account for significant aphasia residuals. Bilateral, in part temporal, or single large dominant-hemisphere lesions correlated with acute severe global aphasic states. Fluent aphasics showed predominantly left posterioparietal lesions.

Kertesz (1979a) found similar CAT scan correlations for global aphasia. He reported that the computerized tomography (CT) scans of patients reclassified as Broca's from global aphasia at 3–6 months showed the greatest amount of temporoparietal damage (Kertesz, 1979a). Yarnell et al. (1976) reported little prognostic value in angiographic and radioscintigraphic findings. CT scans did not help in predicting who might profit from language retraining in Reinvang's study (1980).

Pieniadz, Naeser, Koff, and Levine (1983) studied the relationship between CT scan hemispheric asymmetries and recovery from stroke in 14 right-handed global aphasic patients more than 7 months poststroke. Increased recovery in auditory comprehension was significantly correlated with atypical increased right occipital widths. The degree of right occipital width, more frequently observed in left handers in the LeMay (1977) control population, correlated $-.63$ ($p < .02$) with Token Test scores. The degree of combined atypical right occipital and atypical left frontal width asymmetries correlated $-.53$ ($p < .05$) with naming ability on the Boston Diagnostic Aphasia Examination (BDAE; Goodglass & Kaplan, 1972, 1983).

A number of neuroradiologic correlates of the linguistic components of recovery were identified in the aphasia study conducted at the Hennepin County Medical Center. The study found that in 39 patients at 5 months poststroke CAT scan correlates of the recovery of auditory comprehension, as measured by the Token Test, implicated the role of two specific sites of lesion: the left posterior superior temporal and left infrasylvan supramarginal regions (Selnes, Knopman, Niccum, Rubens, & Larsen, 1983).

In a second report based on the same study, recovery of single-word comprehension, as assessed by the Word Discrimination subtest of the BDAE, correlated with CT scans. Lesions in Wernicke's area did not necessarily imply a persistent impairment of single-word comprehension, but at the sentence level there was a strong relationship between recovery of comprehension and sparing of Wernicke's area (Selnes et al., 1984).

In a third report, Knopman et al. (1983) found CT scan correlates for persistent nonfluency as well. In that study, scans obtained at 5 months postonset revealed that persistent nonfluency in 17 patients was associated with lesions in the rolandic cortical region and underlying white matter. Thirty patients who were fluent by 1 month postonset lacked extensive rolandic lesions. The 6 patients who became fluent by the sixth month had less extensive lesions than those with persistent dysfluency.

Knopman, Rubens, Selnes, Klassen, and Meyer (1984) also correlated the recovery of auditory comprehension by combining scores from the Word Discrimination subtest of the BDAE, the Token Test, and a measure of comprehension of syntactically complex sentences, with cerebral blood flow findings. Evidence was found for the participation of the right hemisphere in language comprehension during the first 3 months of recovery, with return of function to left-hemisphere regions at 5–12 months poststroke.

Knopman, Selnes, Niccum, and Rubens (1984) also found a relationship between oral naming and CT findings. Of 54 left-hemisphere stroke patients, all of whom had moderate to severe naming deficits at initial testing, one-third, with lesions smaller than 60 cm in volume, achieved normal scores after 6 months on a shortened version of the Boston Naming Test (Kaplan, Goodglass, & Weintraub, 1983). Those with similar lesions who showed persistently deficient naming had two discrete sites of lesion: the superior temporal–inferior parietal (semantic paraphasias) and insula–putamen (phonologic paraphasias). Several patients were exceptions, showing recovery of naming despite lesions at these sites.

Naeser and Helm-Estabrooks (1985) looked at CT scan correlations with respect to Melodic Intonation Therapy (MIT) as measured by pre- and posttreatment scores on the BDAE. Data obtained on eight patients, half showing good and half poor response, showed that those who responded positively to MIT had lesions involving Broca's area and/or white matter deep to it. They did not show large lesions in Wernicke's area, the temporal isthmus, or the right hemisphere.

RECOVERY OF LINGUISTIC RULES

Ludlow (1977) administered taped measures of free speech and selected language tasks to 10 treated aphasics, 5 untreated aphasics, and 5 normal controls nine times during the first 3 months post-CVA. Analyses included a measure of sentence length, an index of grammaticality, an index of sentence production, and a tabulation of transformations. In this study, the aphasic patients did not develop a new and simplified language system in connected speech, but tended to recover the same structures used premorbidly. The relative frequency of the use of grammatical structures was similar to that of normal speakers. A common pattern of syntactic sequence was observed in the course of recovery for both treated and untreated patients. Ludlow noted no changes in language competence and concluded that recovery can be interpreted as an increase in the proficiency of language use (language performance). Furthermore, there was no difference in the sequence of recovery with respect to type of aphasia (fluent vs. nonfluent).

Reinvang (1976) investigated sentence recovery in two aphasics: a 44-year-old patient with Broca's aphasia secondary to stroke and a 73-year-old head-injured patient with Wernicke's aphasia. An analysis of spontaneous speech and tasks of sentence repetition and sentence judgment comprised the bases for his findings. Reinvang reported that syntactically normal utterances were produced with regularity in the patients' speech samples and that an increase in utterance length was a dominant feature in recovery. The main form of deviant utterances was incomplete sentences.

RECOVERY PATTERNS

The hypothesis that comprehension improves more than expression has been supported by a number of studies (Kenin & Swisher, 1972; Lebrun, 1976; Prins et al., 1978; Vignolo, 1964).

Prins et al. (1978) obtained a tape-recorded speech corpus based on a linguistic paradigm, Token Test scores, and a sentence comprehension test from 54 aphasic patients (fluent, mixed, nonfluent, severely nonfluent) at three specified time intervals (6-month intervals) in the first poststroke year. No overall clinical improvement in spontaneous speech occurred in any group. Sentence comprehension improved significantly in all four groups.

Kenin and Swisher (1972) concluded that the greatest improvement occurs on imitative tasks and that auditory comprehension improves more than expressive language in nonfluent aphasics.

A. Smith (1971) and A. Smith et al. (1972) studied 80 relatively young treated aphasic patients (mean age = 51.3 years). Sixty-seven patients had vascular etiology, and 13 patients were posttraumatic. Fifty-five percent of the group showed improvement in speech, 67% in comprehension, 61% in reading, and 54% in writing.

Lomas and Kertesz (1978) analyzed recovery patterns in 31 aphasic patients and found equal improvement on all language tasks for patients with good comprehension, and more selective improvement largely in comprehension and imitative tasks for patients with severely impaired auditory comprehension.

Reinvang and Engvik (1980) concluded that the profile of linguistic impairment tended to be maintained during the 2–6 month period. Half of the patients showed a global impairment, and half a pattern of specific impairment. The most significant improvement was noted on oral language and a clinical rating of communication ability. Patients improved only moderately in writing, showed improvement in the ability to follow commands, but showed no improvement in agnosic or conceptual skills.

In a small group of treated patients classified as global aphasics at 3 months poststroke, the greatest improvement was noted in auditory comprehension and the least in propositional speech (M. T. Sarno & Levita, 1981).

Basso, Capitani, and Zonobio (1982) reported that the recovery of comprehension and expression, both oral and written, always turned out to be linked in treated patients. In untreated patients improvement was often noted in comprehension without a corresponding improvement in oral or written expression.

In a study assessing the recovery of connected language across a 1-year period in 47 aphasic (CVA) subjects, Shewan (1988) found that verbal output increased significantly for a majority of the classical types and severities of aphasia. Global and Broca's aphasics showed significant improvement in melody and articulation (articulatory–prosodic variables), whereas the fluent groups changed mainly on content variables. In general, patients made the greatest changes on those variables on which they were initially most impaired.

TIME SINCE ONSET AND RECOVERY

Time since onset is often cited as an important variable with respect to improvement (Marshall & Phillips, 1983; Sarno & Levita, 1979). The general consensus has been that language changes take place earlier rather than later.

In a retrospective study of the evolution of aphasia, Vignolo (1964) reported that as the time interval from onset increased before treatment was initiated, the number of patients improving decreased. Patients who received training for more than 6 months were compared with those who received training for less than 6 months, and the findings showed that the long-term group improved to a greater degree. Time since onset emerged as an important prognostic factor: 2 and 6 months from onset seemed to be important milestones.

Sands et al. (1969) reported greater improvement in a group of patients who began treatment up to 2 months poststroke than in a group that started treatment after 4 months. In the VA cooperative study the deferment of treatment for 12 weeks did not influence outcome (Wertz et al., 1986). The influence of early treatment on gains in language function was also demonstrated in A. Smith et al.'s (1972) study. Basso et al. (1975) found the least recovery in patients with the longest duration of symptoms.

Reinvang and Engvik (1980) reported a significant degree of improvement in the period 2–6 months postonset. Prins et al. (1978) noted significant time changes in spontaneous speech variables in the first year poststroke. Changes after the first year poststroke were noted by Marks et al. (1957) and Sands et al. (1969). On the other hand, Kertesz and McCabe (1977) reported little or no change after the first year.

In the M.T. Sarno and Levita study (1979), 34 treated aphasic patients were systematically examined during the first year poststroke. Patients were evenly distributed across fluent, nonfluent, and global diagnostic categories. Scores on the Neurosensory Center Comprehensive Examination for Aphasia (NCCEA; Spreen & Benton, 1969, 1977) and clinical ratings on the FCP (M. T. Sarno, 1969; Taylor, 1965) provided the data base. In the 4- to 8-week period, little change was observed on any of the measures administered. However, in the 12- to 26-week period, all diagnostic groups, particularly those designated as fluent, made gains on all measures.

Figure 16.1 shows patients' changes over time on NCCEA subtests. Each graph shows the pattern of subtest performance at given time intervals. As shown in Figure 16.2, fluent and nonfluent groups were similar in their performance and essentially equidistant from normal performance levels on the FCP at 12 weeks poststroke. Figure 16.2 shows that for the whole group performances generally improved during the 6- to 12-month period. The greatest changes on the NCCEA subtests from 6 to 12 months were made by the global group, and the smallest gains by the fluent group, which was the reverse of the findings in the 3- to 6-month period. The most remarkable finding for this period was the magnitude of improvement on the Token Test achieved by the

NCCEA

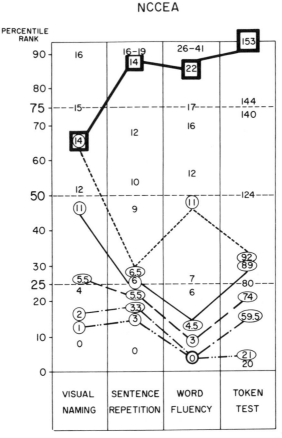

FIGURE 16.1. *Median raw scores for total group, Neurosensory Center Comprehensive Examination for Aphasia.* ·······= 4 weeks poststroke; ·····= 8 weeks poststroke; --- = 12 weeks poststroke; ——— = 26 weeks poststroke; —— = 8th percentile rank normal. [From Sarno & Levita, 1979. Reproduced by permission of the American Heart Association, Inc.]

global group. In the all-inclusive period from 1 month to 1 year, the general trend indicated improvement in all areas. The primary finding of the study was the continuation of improvement in all patients up to 1 year poststroke, which agrees with the reports of other investigators and personal accounts of aphasic patients (Dahlberg & Jaffee, 1977; Moss, 1972; Sands et al., 1969; A. Smith, 1971; Vignolo, 1964).

Despite the fact that global aphasic patients showed the greatest improvement in the latter part of the first poststroke year, they failed to evolve to another type of aphasia. As shown in Figure 16.2, no member

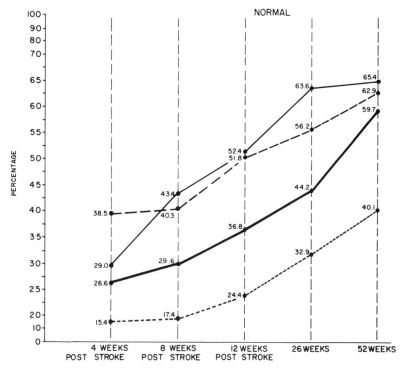

FIGURE 16.2. *Overall scores over time poststroke, based on median scores by group, Functional Communication Profile.* ····=global; ——— = fluent; —— = nonfluent; —— = total group. *[From Sarno & Levita, 1979. Reproduced by permission of the American Heart Association, Inc.]*

of the global aphasic group exceeded a 40% overall FCP score. In contrast to the findings of Lomas and Kertesz (1978) and Kertesz and Mc-Cabe (1977), the nonfluent group showed the least change from 3 months to 1 year poststroke. The discrepancy between changes observed on structured language tasks (NCEEA) and functional ratings was striking and is probably at least in part accounted for by extra-linguistic compensatory mechanisms, rather than by specific changes in linguistic processing. In this study, time since onset emerged as a potent variable in recovery (M. T. Sarno & Levita, 1979).

PSYCHOSOCIAL AND RELATED FACTORS

A. Smith (1971) and M. T. Sarno, Silverman, and Levita (1970) found no relationship between educational level, occupational status before illness, and recovery. In a retrospective study, Keenan and Brassell (1974) reported that health and employment had little if any prognostic value. C. Rose et al. (1976) found that sex, length of stay in a hospital, speech diagnosis, and presence of hemiplegia were not significant prognostic factors. In another study (M. T. Sarno & Levita, 1971), individuals who were employed at the time of stroke recovered more than those who were unemployed.

Several aphasiologists have cited the presence of certain psychological symptoms, such as depression, anxiety, and paranoia, as factors that have a negative effect on outcome (Benson, 1979a, 1979b, 1980; Lebrun, 1980; Dunkle, K. E. and Hooper, C. R., 1983). Other studies have emphasized the patient's psychological state and premorbid personality as important prognostic factors (Eisenson, 1973; Wepman, 1951). The influence of fatigue (R. Marshall & King, 1973; R. Marshall & Watts, 1976), discouraging instructions, and nonverbal negative messages on task performance (Chester & Egolf, 1974) have also been studied (Stoicheff, 1960). Eisenson (1949, 1964, 1973) felt that patients with outgoing personalities had a better prognosis than those with introverted, dependent, rigid personalities.

SUMMARY

Until the early 1950s, aphasia rehabilitation was essentially limited to patients with aphasia secondary to trauma as the result of missile wounds. Since then, poststroke aphasic patients, who are generally older than posttraumatic patients, have been seeking and receiving therapy. Reports of the efficacy of aphasia rehabilitation are generally positive; however, the limits of spontaneous recovery and the relative influence of many variables on outcome remain inconclusive.

Approaches to the Treatment of Aphasia

The preceding section reviewed certain aspects of recovery and the social and medical currents that led directly to the demand for aphasia remediation. This demand has grown steadily over the years, and with it there has been a proliferation of treatment methods. As noted earlier large numbers of aphasic patients have been treated, especially since World War II, in hospitals, rehabilitation medicine centers, and other facilities where speech therapy services are generally provided by speech–language pathologists. As with aphasia classification and testing, therapeutic approaches have been based on theoretical concepts of the nature of language and the pathology of aphasia. The following outlines some of the main currents in treatment.

Literally hundreds of specific techniques are cited in the literature.

Aphasia therapy is rarely the same in any two treatment settings. The lack of therapeutic uniformity has undoubtedly impeded carefully controlled studies on the effects of language retraining (Taylor, 1964a). Most methods derive essentially from traditional pedagogic practices, relying heavily on repetition (Darley, 1975; M. T. Sarno, 1974, 1975, 1980a). For a detailed elaboration of therapeutic techniques, the reader will want to consult Chapey's (1986) volume.

Approaches to aphasia therapy have generally followed one of two models: a SUBSTITUTE SKILL MODEL or a DIRECT TREATMENT MODEL, both of which are based on the assumption that the processes that subserve normal performance need to be understood if rehabilitation is to succeed (Goodglass, 1987).

In general, treatment methods can be categorized as those that are largely indirect-stimulation–facilitation and those that are essentially direct-structured–pedagogic (Benson, 1979b; Burns & Halper, 1988; Darley, 1975; Kertesz, 1979a; M. T. Sarno, 1980a; Taylor, 1964a).

The two principles that underlie most treatment methods reflect contrasting views of aphasia as either impaired access to language or a "loss" of language. The stimulation methods generally follow an impaired access theory, and pedagogic approaches are based on a theory of aphasia as a language loss.

In practice, however, much of aphasia therapy addresses the "performance" aspect of language in which repeated practice and "teaching" strategies are assumed to help restore impaired skills through a "task-oriented" approach (i.e., naming practice). One of the commonly used techniques involves self-cuing and repetition exercises that manipulate components of grammar and vocabulary. Another approach involves "stimulating" the patient to use residual language by encouraging conversation in a permissive setting where a patient's responses are unconditionally accepted and topics are of personal interest (M. T. Sarno, 1990).

Following a behavioral model, Luria (1963, 1966) put forth the view that aphasia treatment promotes the reorganization of the brain. He considered that both premorbid personality and differences in lesions might have an effect on this process and identified three types of restoration: (a) deinhibition of temporarily depressed functions, (b) substitution of the opposite hemisphere in language mediation, and (c) radical reorganization of functional systems.

Both Goldstein (1948) and Lenneberg (1967) felt that the aphasia therapist would be most effective by helping patients to compensate for impaired function. In fact, they suggested that compensatory adjustments were intrinsic to the homeostatic tendencies of the organism.

In an experiment that focused on stimulating a patient's access to a lexicon rather than on the lexicon itself, Seron, Deloche, Bastard, Chassin, and Hermand (1979) found it more efficient to restore the access process than to restore specific lexical items, as in the traditional method. These findings were consonant with those of Holland (1970) and Wiegel-Crump and Koenigsknecht (1973).

Stimulation—Facilitation Approaches

Wepman (1951, 1953) believed that the primary role of the aphasia therapist was to "stimulate" language in order to facilitate language performance. He suggested that the manner of stimuli presentation was of paramount importance and that it was not the role of the therapist to "teach" vocabulary or syntax. One technique he suggested was the presentation of filmstrips selected for individual patients according to their levels of interest and competence (Wepman & Morency, 1963).

Schuell et al. (1964) also felt that the speech clinician's role was not as teacher, and they, too, developed stimulation techniques, especially in the auditory mode. The aphasia therapist was viewed as someone who tries to stimulate disrupted processes to function maximally and called language stimulation the "backbone of aphasia therapy." Basic to Schuell et al.'s approach was the belief that sensory stimulation is the only method available for making complex events happen in the brain.

Schuell et al.'s (1964) approach to aphasia rehabilitation was based on the premise that auditory processing impairments underlie aphasia. She stressed adequate stimulation, carefully controlled for length, rate, and loudness. She saw individual therapy as more effective than group therapy because of the individual differences among patients. Within this framework, one language modality is used to stimulate another in a program carefully graded for complexity. Schuell stressed the importance of repetition and overt responses from patients, with a minimum of correcting or explaining on the part of the therapist. She also considered the treatment atmosphere as important in its influence on a patient's self-esteem and believed that establishing rapport with the patient is an important treatment variable. The details of Schuell's rationale and approach to aphasia therapy are elaborated in her book (Schuell et al., 1964).

Wepman (1972, 1976) held to the view that no specific formula was to be followed in administering treatment for aphasia and that the efforts should be stimulating, indirect, and general. He believed that therapeutic intervention should consider using topics known to be of interest to the patient in his premorbid life and should be elaborated largely through an increased focus on visualization. Wepman viewed stimulation as the core of therapy and objected to attempts to have the patient produce specific words or syntactic forms. Whatever the patient produced should be accepted as "his best possible response at the moment."

Wepman (1976) proposed that language is inextricably related to thought but not identical with it, that it is the product of thought and the servant of the highest human mental processing. He saw the process of stimulation in speech therapy as an "embellishment of thought," removing the implied criticism of corrective therapy and never asking for or trying in any way to elicit verbal expression.

Wepman (1951) rejected the notion of aphasia as a specific speech or language disorder and interpreted the disturbance as a "disorder affecting the patient's total reaction pattern due to a disturbance of the integrating capacity of the cortex" (p. 85). His "indirect" stimulation approach was the natural result of his views on the nature of the disorder. He saw direct psycholinguistic attacks on the aphasic manifestation as most likely to become rigid language approaches and, therefore, placed a premium on innovation, ingenuity, and individual creativity in aphasia therapy.

In the case of patients with phonetic impairment, Wepman (1976) and many others (Dabul & Bollier, 1976; Millikan & Darley, 1967; Rosenbek, Kent, & LaPointe, 1984; J. E. Sarno & Sarno, 1969a, 1969b, 1979; Schuell et al., 1964) have recommended direct methods of articulation therapy along traditional lines in which the basis is primarily imitative practice with visual and kinesthetic cues.

The possibility that linguistic principles might apply to reeducation in aphasia has been raised by a number of authors (Jakobson, 1955; Morley, 1960; Pincas, 1965; Scargill, 1964; Taylor, 1964b) who have presented a theoretical orientation toward language reacquisition in aphasia on the basis of what is known about neurological, linguistic, and psycholinguistic aspects of natural language development. Ludlow (1977) reported a common order of recovery of syntactic structures in the aphasics she studied, which was unrelated to type of aphasia or whether patients were treated. She suggested that this sequence of syntactic recovery might provide a logical basis for a treatment regimen.

Using a programmed instruction approach, Naeser (1975) succeeded in showing an average 10% improvement in the production of three basic declarative sentence types in four male aphasic patients. Naeser also reported a carryover of 36% improvement in sentences of the same type but with which the patients had not been trained.

Wiegel-Crump (1976) studied two treatment approaches, programmed and nonstructured, with the goal of increasing syntax retrieval. After 4 weeks of highly structured therapy, improvement in syntax generation did not generalize from specific items drilled in therapy to additional nondrilled items. The level of improvement on nondrilled items did not differ significantly from the level of improvement on drilled items.

Behavior Modification

The application of behavior modification principles to aphasia therapy is a good example of method following theoretical concept. It was perhaps inevitable that an attempt would be made to apply the work of B. F. Skinner to aphasia therapy. Skinner's theory of operant conditioning rests on the assumption that the desired behavior, or a behavior similar to it, exists in the patient's behavioral inventory and can be manipulated so that it will occur in a targeted manner in response to a specific stimulus. Although this assumption is supported by several studies, Lenneberg (1967) thought that aphasia was a retrieval rather than a learning impairment and that conditioning procedures would, therefore, not be effective in restoring language to a patient with a well-established aphasia.

Tikofsky and Reynolds (1963) found that conditioning occurred in aphasic subjects more slowly than in normal subjects. Goodkin (1968) reported that verbal perseveration and inappropriateness were altered in two aphasic subjects using a conditioning protocol. H. Lane and Moore (1962) successfully conditioned aphasics who could not discriminate between the phonemes /t/ and /d/.

M. Smith (1974) applied operant conditioning in a 32-year-old aphasic patient 6 months poststroke and a 65-year-old patient 11 months poststroke. Using an informal operant conditioning technique, the two patients were trained to choose prepositions that correctly identified spatial relationships among objects. They learned a sequencing strategy that enabled them to arrange three word cards to describe an object display that they could not describe spontaneously. The experimental results suggested that conditioning techniques might enable non-language mechanisms to solve, or help solve, language problems.

Holland (1969) discussed the nature of reinforcers and the need for careful attention either to gradually changing the topography of the behavior in question or to systematically altering the stimulus conditions in which the desired behavior is supposed to occur—the process of successive approximation in clinical application. A programmed instruction approach views language rehabilitation as an educative process and rigorously applies operant conditioning methods drawn from learning theory and principles drawn from psycholinguistic analysis to guide the content and order of presentation of the linguistic elements taught (Boone, 1967; Holland, 1969, 1970; Taylor, 1964b). It is based on the belief that learning involves several distinguishable stages, including recognition, imitation, repetition of the model based on memory needed for echoed performance, and finally spontaneous selection of a response from a repertoire of learned responses.

The results of several experiments requiring aphasics to perform a variety of tasks on automated devices have suggested that even severely impaired aphasics can learn to match visual configurations, perform visual oddity tasks, and write their names. Rosenberg (1965) used automated training procedures in an experiment designed to assess and train aphasics to make perceptual discriminations basic to reading. The programs were effective in teaching certain discriminations, as well as in increasing the rate of response and retention of the material. Edwards (1965) investigated differential responses to tasks involving the matching of visual stimuli by more than 100 severely impaired aphasics and found that all but 4 of the patients successfully completed the program. In still another study, Filby and Edwards (1963) taught form discrimination to 12 severely impaired aphasics and 10 normal subjects. In the optimal learning conditions of the experiment, the aphasic group did not differ significantly from the controls and also did not exhibit catastrophic reactions or other forms of disruptive responses.

Holland and Levy (1971) expressed the view that aphasics learn by having consequences applied to their behavior and that the clinician's primary concern should be to screen subject matter and control reinforcement through programmed instruction. Based on the premise that aphasic patients need to have tasks reduced to small steps with more than an average number of repetitions, and a more systematically structured teaching procedure, the technology of programmed instruction lends itself to experimentation (Taylor, 1964a; Taylor & Marks, 1959; Taylor & Sands, 1966).

Holland and Sonderman (1974) attempted to teach 24 aphasic patients tasks from the Token Test in a programmed approach. Patients had a mean age of 54.45 years and a mean time since onset of 5.6 years. All except 2 head trauma patients had aphasia secondary to CVA. Patients were rated on a severity scale and divided into low and high groups according to Token test scores. The mild and mild–moderate patients demonstrated significant improvement as a result of training, whereas the moderate and severe patients did not. Training was more effective for those who initially did well; however, no patient was error free. In general, the patients did not easily transfer the language skills acquired in the program to similar untrained tasks.

Weigl (1961) developed an approach to therapy called DEBLOCKING, which is based on the factor of context. It is essentially a systematic use of a patient's intact modalities. For example, if a patient is having difficulty with auditory recognition, he or she may be helped in recognizing a given spoken word by stimulation with the written word through the visual channel. Deblocking seems to be naturally in tune with clinical approaches that build new responses upon a patient's most intact language skill or those that rely on multisensory stimulation. Ulatowska and Richardson (1974) provided a detailed description of the use of a deblocking technique to reintegrate the mechanisms for correlating sound and meaning in a longitudinal single-case report of an aphasic patient with a severe impairment of auditory comprehension. The visual mode of presentation of linguistic material was used to provide a stable representation of speech units and to allow reinforcement of auditory representations. The patient was given tasks of repetition, reading aloud, and sequencing, using progressively more complex material.

Treatment of the Patient with Speech Dyspraxia

The disorder of articulation referred to as speech dyspraxia seldom, if ever, is manifest in the absence of a coexisting Broca's aphasia, however mild. The speech dyspraxia component of this multifaceted communication disorder appears to be especially amenable to direct therapeutic intervention using approaches adapted primarily from traditional articulation therapy techniques, including stress and intonation drills. These approaches, designed to improve phonetic placement accuracy, typically depend on imitation, stress, and progressive approximation, which are drilled using kinesthetic, visual, and auditory cues. Generally, the stimuli used as the bases for these exercises are selected in a presumed order of difficulty, beginning with nonoral imitation, followed by sounds, words, phrases, and finally utterances.

Treatment techniques for speech dyspraxia have been described by many clinicians (Deal & Florance, 1978; Halpern, 1981; Rosenbek, 1978; Rosenbek, Lemme, Ahern, Harris, & Wertz, 1973; Rubow, Rosenbek, Collins, & Longstreth, 1982; Wertz, 1984; Wertz, LaPointe, & Rosenbek, 1984; Wiedel, 1976). Dworkin, Abharion, and Johns (1988) reported an effective treatment regimen in a study of a single subject. Various rhythmic techniques in which the patient generates the rhythm also have been reported as facilitory methods to increase articulation accuracy (Rosenbek, Hansen, Baughman, & Lemme, 1974; Schuell et al., 1964). In contrast, Shane and Darley (1978) found that articulation precision tended to deteriorate under externally imposed rhythmic stimulation. As discussed later, melodic intonation therapy also has been employed as a facilitory technique in the treatment of the patient with speech dyspraxia.

In Sands, Freeman, and Harris's (1978) study, the phonemic errors made by a Broca's aphasia patient with speech dyspraxia who received speech therapy for 10 years were analyzed and compared. The errors that prevailed in the first poststroke year were compared with his performance 10 years later. The features of place and manner of production had improved and omission errors were virtually eliminated, although voicing and addition errors persisted.

Some Innovative Treatment Methods

Beyn and Shokhor-Trotskaya (1966) reported on the effect of a specific plan of therapy with 25 poststroke patients. They attempted to "prevent the appearance of some of the speech defects of aphasic patients which, up to now, seemed to be inevitable" (p. 98), specifically the "telegraphic style" of responses. They avoided teaching nominative words, teaching at first only simple words that could function as a whole sentence, such as "no," "there," "here," "give," "tomorrow," and "thanks." Only when words appeared spontaneously in a patient's speech were nouns introduced into therapy. They wrote, "The results of the rehabilitation of active speech varied; but the most important fact is that telegraphic style, which is inevitable with other methods of rehabilitation, did not emerge in any of our patients" (p. 104).

Graphic representations have also been used in treatment. Luria (1966) used a "card index plan" to train a posttraumatic, mildly impaired aphasic who had difficulty producing fluent narrative speech. The patient was trained to write down fragments of the theme he was to relate on separate cards and to speak from them. Luria's idea was that the function of a defective internal system can be replaced by an external aid; in this instance writing was used to facilitate speech.

Hatfield and Zangwill (1974) employed a picture story method in which they explored the capacity of aphasic patients to communicate a sequence of events by drawing. The underlying notion was that ideational processes in aphasia may be substantially intact despite severe defects in speaking and writing.

Weniger, Huber, Stachowiak, and Poeck (1980) reported on a

therapeutic regimen based on linguistic principles, which they concluded is superior to conventional methods. (See Chapter 7 for a review of studies in the treatment of sentence processing.)

Visual Communication Therapy

Visual communication therapy (VIC; Gardner, Zurif, Berry, & Baker, 1976) is an experimental technique designed for the global aphasic. It follows earlier work done by Premack (1971), who reported an experiment in which a chimpanzee was taught a simple communication system, and Velletri-Glass, Gazzaniga, and Premack (1973), who trained global aphasic patients to use cutout paper symbols as an artificial language system. VIC employs an index card system of arbitrary symbols representing syntactic and lexical components. Patients learn to recognize the symbols and manipulate them so as to (a) respond to a command and (b) express needs, wishes, or other emotions. The system attempts to circumvent the use of natural oral language, which is severely impaired and often unavailable to the global aphasic patient. Gardner et al. concluded that the evidence supports the view that some severely aphasic patients can master the basics of an artificial language. Moreover, several indexes suggested that the communication effectiveness of the system was appreciated and that some of the cognitive operations entailed in natural language are preserved despite severe aphasia. The experimenters expressed the idea that the method may have greater relevance as a means of exploring residual mental function in global aphasics than as a system of therapy (Gardner et al., personal communication, 1979).

An adaptation and application of the VIC system called the computer-aided visual communication (C-VIC) system was developed by Steele and his coworkers (Steele, Weinrich, Kleczewska, Carlson, & Wertz, 1987; Steele, Weinrich, Wertz, Kleczewska, & Carlson, 1989a; Weinrich, Steele, & Illes, 1985).

Visual Action Therapy

Visual action therapy (VAT), developed at the Boston Veterans Administration Medical Center by Helm-Estabrooks and her associates, is designed to train global aphasic patients to use symbolic gestures representing visually absent objects (Helm & Benson, 1978; Helm-Estabrooks, Fitzpatrick, & Barresi, 1982). The tasks leading to this goal include associating pictured forms with specific objects, manipulating real objects appropriately, and finally producing symbolic gestures that represent the objects used (e.g., cup, hammer, razor).

Melodic Intonation Therapy

Sparks, Helm, and Albert (1974) elaborated a programmed therapeutic regimen called melodic intonation therapy (MIT), based on the observation that language that may not be available in spontaneous speech can sometimes be produced in association with an intoned melody. The system presumes an intact right hemisphere, thought to be the locus of melodic production, and also presumed that functional language can be retrieved if it is associated with rhythm and melody. In a series of carefully graded steps, therapists slowly introduce melody, rhythm, and verbal content, gradually including the patients' participation in the process and diminishing their own, eventually leaving the patient as the sole "performer." The MIT program uses a number of relevant and high-probability phrases and sentences that are intoned/chanted, which, if successful, leads ultimately to speech. Candidates for this technique includes patients who have good auditory comprehension, facility for self-correction, markedly limited verbal output, reasonably good attention span, and emotional stability (Helm, 1976; Helm-Estabrooks, 1983; N. Marshall & Holtzapple, 1976).

Amerind and Other Gesture Systems

In an attempt to utilize systematized gestural language to facilitate oral production, American Indian sign language has been modified in a method that combines common gestural sign with oral speech production (Amerind) (Skelly, 1979). The technique was systematically studied in six patients with long-standing severe speech dyspraxia (cortical dysarthria). Three of the six patients progressed to two-word sentences and another to single-word usage (Skelly, Schinsky, Smith, & Fust, 1974). Subsequent reports have supported the use of Amerind as an effective technique in selected cases (Rao et al., 1980; Rao & Horner, 1978).

Moody (1982) detailed the successful training of a man with global aphasia in a method called "total communication," which combines a modification of Australasian sign language (ANSL) and speech. Kirshner and Webb (1981) succeeded in training a 39-year-old aphasic woman more than 100 signs in a combined Amerind and Ameslan sign language.

Coelho and Duffy (1987) trained 12 chronically severe aphasic subjects in the use of a manual sign vocabulary and reported a clear and significant relationship between severity of aphasia and success in acquiring and generalizing manual signs. The authors concluded that there may be a threshold of aphasia severity above which acquisition is negligible.

Functional Communication Pragmatic Therapy

In the functional communication treatment (FCT) method developed by Aten, Caliguri, and Holland (1982), emphasis is placed on restoration of communication in the broadest sense. Language is considered to be only one, but admittedly an important, aspect of communication. Therapy is designed to improve patients' information processing in the activities necessary to conduct activities of daily living, social interactions, and self-expression of both physical and psychological needs. FCT is "a refocusing of traditional treatment goals and methods rather than a novel approach requiring radically different activities" (Aten, 1986).

Promoting Aphasics' Communicative Effectiveness (PACE; Davis & Wilcox, 1985), a technique intended to reshape structured interaction between clinicians and patients into more natural communicative exchanges, includes several pragmatic components common to natural conversation. These include taking turn as both senders and receivers of messages, and making use of multiple modes of communication. The therapist, therefore, provides feedback intrinsically, as a party to the conversation and as a partner might in a natural communicative situation (Davis & Wilcox, 1985).

Narrative discourse has begun to be explored as a basis for language therapy (Ulatowska & Chapman, 1989).

Alternative/Augmentative Communication Systems and Devices

The early work of Velletri-Glass et al. (1973) and Gardner et al. (1976) demonstrated that global aphasic patients could be trained to use an artificial language. This work, as well as the reported success in training patients to use a combination of symbolic gestures and speech production (Rao et al., 1980), suggested that systems and/or devices might have application in aphasia rehabilitation. New technology, especially synthetic speech and microcomputers, might serve as either a compensatory means of communication or a facilitory technique to enhance treatment (Katz 1984, 1987). A review of this topic can be found in Kratt (1990).

The technology has varied widely. Microcomputers were the basis for an approach that Seron, Deloche, Monlard, and Rousselle (1980) found effective in treating aphasic patients with writing disorders. Beukelman, Yorkston, and Dowden (1985), Colby, Christinaz, and Graham (1978), and Colby, Christinaz, Parkinson, Graham, and Karpf (1981) explored the facilitation of word-retrieval in an anomic patient using an intelligent speech prosthesis. Johannsen-Horbach, Cegla, Mager, and Schempp

(1985) reported success in training severely impaired aphasics to use alternative systems. V. W. Lane and Samples (1981) and Bailey (1983) trained aphasics in the use of Blissymbolics. Katz and Nagy (1983) improved accuracy and recognition time in reading commonly used words. R. H. Mills (1982) reported improvement in auditory comprehension in an aphasic patient who, when followed at a later date, showed additional gains with continued exposure to training (R. H. Mills & Hoffer, 1985). Bruce and Howard (1987) demonstrated that computer-generated phonemic cues were effective in improving naming in five Broca's aphasic patients. Garrett, Beukelman, and Low-Morrow (1989) developed an augmentative system for a Broca's patient. Hunnicutt (1989) developed a word retrieval facilitation program for aphasics. Steele et al. (in press) and Weinrich, Steele, Carlson, and Kleczweska (1989) replicated and extended the findings of Gardner et al. (1976) and Baker et al. (1975) by training aphasic patients to use a computerized version of the VIC system.

Summary

The foregoing review is far from complete and intended only to give some idea of the scope of aphasia rehabilitation experience and literature that has been reported, especially since World War II. Clearly, the approaches are usually based on theoretical concepts of the nature of aphasia and its remediation. Until the definitive neurophysiology of communication has been described, there is no recourse but to continue the process of experimentation, with clinicians adopting those strategies and systems that they find the most effective and best suited to the individual patient.

Few studies have compared treatment methods, which is understandable in view of the seemingly insurmountable methodological problems associated with such research and our present state of knowledge. Although we cannot be absolutely certain of the rationale for therapy, large numbers of patients nevertheless seek treatment and require management. The following section represents an approach to this and related ethical questions and dilemmas.

Toward a Comprehensive Approach to Aphasia Rehabilitation

A critical factor in aphasia rehabilitation is that once the condition is stabilized, very few patients recover normal communication function, with or without speech therapy. This unfortunate reality requires that aphasia rehabilitation be viewed as a process of patient management in the broadest sense of the word. The task then becomes primarily one of helping the patient and his or her intimates adjust to the alterations and limitations imposed by the disability. Many experienced clinicians have addressed this problem, citing a variety of factors contributing to its complexity: type and severity of the language deficit, physical disability, premorbid personality patterns, cognitive status, time since onset, cultural and educational background, associated neuropsychological deficits, and general physical condition (Benson, 1979b, Darley, 1970, 1972, 1975; Eisenson, 1973; Reinvang, 1980; M. T. Sarno, 1980a; Schuell et al., 1964; Wepman, 1951). The multiplicity of factors suggests that effective rehabilitation management requires the participation of a variety of disciplines, including medicine, psychology, physical and occupational therapy, social work, vocational counseling, and, most critically, aphasia therapy. In this regard the advent of the medical specialty of rehabilitation medicine has been fortuitous, for it provides a well-organized setting in which all of these services can be mobilized for the benefit of the patient with aphasia. The greatest responsibility in this process falls to the aphasia therapist. I return later to a description of how the speech–language pathologist works with an aphasic. Let us first look at the patient and catalog some of the important clinical–behavioral features of the disorder.

The Patient with Aphasia

Ullman (1962) observed that the variability of patients' psychological reactions is rarely determined by the type or location of their lesions, but is an expression of the whole life experience of the person who has had a stroke. Regarding this Ullman wrote,

> [We] need to focus not on an abstract appraisal of psychopathological patterns but on understanding the current life situation and consequent meaning of the stroke to the patient at this particular moment in his life. Repeatedly one gets the feeling in talking with these patients that had the stroke occurred a year or two earlier, or a year or two later, their reactions would have been quite different. At times it climaxes a process of resignation and surrender set in motion years before; at other times it initiates such a process. In some patients it touches off a last-ditch stand dedicated to the pursuit of unattained life goals and ambitions. Occasionally it opens up new vistas for the elaboration of secondary gain from illness. Unrealistic strivings for independence and unrealistic dependency are perhaps the two main channels into which irrational modes of adaptation flow. (pp. 60–61)

In a study of aphasic patients participating in a group psychotherapy program, Friedman (1961) investigated the nature of psychological regression in aphasia. Beyond the communication difficulties posed by aphasia, Friedman observed that each patient remained psychologically isolated, an individual island. Patients did not maintain a consistent level of group participation and expressed intense feelings that they were very different from other people. Both withdrawal and projection were apparent as each patient acted in isolation and yet complained of this characteristic in others. Friedman's study suggested that aphasia can result in regressive behavior with impaired reality testing. Patients became overly dependent, as shown by their recurring demands that they be given more help by their therapists and preferably in smaller groups in which individualized attention would be provided (Friedman, 1961).

The work of Ullman (1962) and Friedman (1961) provided insight into the magnitude and complexity of the psychological and social ramifications of aphasia. (For a review of these aspects, see chapter 15). Often individual psychotherapy (Aronson, Shatin, & Cook, 1956; Blackman, 1950) and family counseling (Linell & Steg, 1980; Malone, 1969; J. E. Sarno & Sarno, 1979) have been provided, even though traditionally psychological therapies rely heavily on the use of language.

An effective management tool is the selective and discriminating use of speech therapy to stimulate and support the patient through the various stages of recovery (Brumfitt & Clarke, 1980; M. T. Sarno, 1980a; Tanner, 1980).

Experienced therapists recognize that while working on a specific communication deficit, they are simultaneously dealing psychotherapeutically with a readjusting personality (Wepman, 1951). Speech therapy, therefore, serves different purposes at different points along the way. Sometimes it allows patients to "borrow time," as Baretz and Stephenson (1976) aptly stated. At other times it helps them to a realistic assessment of language capacity, which they need at that moment. In a study by Shewan and Cameron (1984), the spouses of patients who received speech therapy became more aware of the patients' problems than did the partners of untreated patients. Occasionally depression lifts after speech therapy has been initiated, reflecting the supportive and nurturing nature of the therapeutic relationship rather than an objective improvement in recovery of speech and language (Ullman, 1962).

Viewed in this way, aphasia rehabilitation can be understood as a dynamic process consisting of a series of stages similar to the stages of mourning, through which the majority of patients evolve. In her classic characterization of the stages of adjustment to death and dying, Kubler-Ross (1969) provided a model that can be applied to the reactions of loss manifested by the aphasic patient. She specified five stages: denial and isolation, anger, bargaining, depression, and acceptance. Both real and symbolic losses can be experienced by aphasic patients. Loss of the ability to communicate has real meaning because speech is such a vital human function. But aphasics may experience symbolic loss as well, because of altered perceptions of their familial, social, and vocational roles. Some patients, of course, never emerge from a state of severe depression (Espmark, 1973).

The perception of loss leads to grief, which is not a single reaction but a complex process involving many emotions and attempts to adjust to and cope with loss. A number of authors have suggested a sequence of phases in grieving. Engle (1964) listed shock and disbelief, awareness, and restitution–recovery. Schneider (1974) suggested that the stages proposed by Kubler-Ross and other authors could be characterized as attempts to overcome the sense of loss, which include denial, rage, and bargaining; awareness of the loss; and acceptance of the loss. The stages of grief are universal, but vary with respect to their order and duration.

Based on these theories, one may postulate three stages through which the aphasic patient passes: depression–denial, anger, and adaptation. In the first stage patients usually withdraw from friends and social situations. Some patients experience a vague, dreamlike state, with a lack of interest in surroundings and no apparent concern over what has happened. They may be lethargic, complaining of chronic fatigue and manifesting universal signs of helplessness. They often make unrealistic plans based on complete recovery, set deadline dates for recovery, or otherwise stall for time while the depression resolves. Health professionals are generally unaccepting of these behaviors and tend to express anger at a patient's "unrealistic attitude," reflecting their own biases and needs for success. As a consequence of these dynamics, therapists are not generally kindly disposed to patients who are preoccupied, self-involved, or seclusive, or who express hopeless attitudes.

Speech therapy can serve an important purpose during this stage. By directly addressing the patient's linguistic deficits and channeling attention and energies toward constructive ends, speech therapy may produce a noticeable reduction in depression. Therapy tasks in this instance act as an equivalent for work, which has long been recognized as an antidote for depression. The title of a chapter written in a personal account of a stroke patient (Wulf, 1973), "My Lifeline to Sanity, The Marvels of Speech Therapy," is a testimony to the positive psychological impact of speech therapy.

In his *Autobiographical Considerations on Aphasia Rehabilitation*, Renato Segré (1976) suggested that there is value in allowing the aphasic patient to delay speaking and to economize on the length and complexity of utterances. He wrote,

> It is important not to interrupt these resting periods because they represent a defense and compensation measure . . . some aphasics enjoy their verbal silence. It is a kind of spiritual rest, of quiet criticism of other people's opinions; a kind of personal formula to reach a better optimism. (p. 136)

In the second stage, the expression of anger that the severely impaired patient originally internalized, in particular, the expression of anger by nonverbal means, may be difficult to interpret. Some patients act out physically or precipitate confrontations with family or staff members. During this stage the patient is particularly difficult to manage. By understanding this phase as a natural and necessary part of the recovery course, those around the patient can continue to provide a supportive environment.

The third and last stage is a period of acceptance and adaptation that continues for the remainder of the patient's life. In this period patients mobilize and bring to bear all of their resources and begin to compensate for deficits. In a one-year poststroke patient, the pattern of linguistic impairment is generally stabilized, and, although some improvement may continue indefinitely beyond this period, full recovery is rare if not achieved by then.

There is a great tendency to overestimate the capacity of an aphasic to return to work, particularly if the verbal deficits are mild. If the patient's work depends upon cognitive and verbal skills, even at fairly low levels, great caution should be exercised since it is impossible to accurately evaluate a patient's performance except on the job. Premature attempts to return to work may be psychologically devastating. Generally, it is advisable to postpone such plans for as long as possible.

The process of finding acceptable vocational alternatives is very difficult, time-consuming, and often unsuccessful. Vocational counseling can also be effective in helping the patient adjust to the reality of his or her problem. Professional rehabilitation counselors are best equipped to explore and evaluate a patient's vocational potential and carry out the long and arduous process of evaluating work performance and job requirements.

Many experienced aphasia clinicians have stressed the importance of the patient's family in the rehabilitation process (Boone, 1967; Brocklehurst, Morris, Andrews, Richards & Laycock, 1981; Godfrey & Douglass, 1959; Malone, 1969; Schuell et al., 1964; Wepman, 1951; Williams & Freer, 1986). Some of the potentially negative reactions of the family include overprotectiveness, hostility, anger, unrealistic expectations, overzealousness, lack of knowledge of the dimensions of the disorder, and inability to cope with practical difficulties. Also, the apparently natural tendency of family members to minimize the patient's communication impairment, particularly in the early stages of recovery, requires understanding and tactful management (Buxbaum, 1967; Helmick, Watamori, & Palmer, 1976; M. T. Sarno, 1971). Some consideration has been given to varieties of family therapy as a means of reducing some of these reactions (Kinsella & Duffy, 1978; Norlin, 1986; Rollin, 1984; Währborg & Borenstein, 1989; Worral, 1989) and to precrisis intervention (Shadden, 1987).

In general, the quality of premorbid relationships tends to be intensified in the aftermath of a catastrophic event; those that were problematic may deteriorate further, whereas the bond between a loving couple may become stronger. The reversal of roles, changes in levels of dependency, and a changed economic situation, so often a consequence of chronic disability, can have a critical negative impact on the patient and the family. One must utilize all available resources in such cataclysmic situations to minimize deleterious effects on the patient. Formal programs designed to educate and counsel report the need for such programs as an integral part of the services provided by agencies that treat aphasic patients (Boone, 1967; Crewe, 1969; Derman & Manaster, 1967; Newhoff & Davis, 1978; Rolnick, 1969; Strauss, Burrucker, Cicero, & Edwards, 1967; Turnblom & Meyers, 1952; Watzlawick & Coyne, 1980).

In a positive family milieu, patients are encouraged to develop regular daily routines as close to premorbid patterns as possible and are treated as contributing members of the family. They are allowed to progress at their own speed, and the family facilitates their participation in avocational activities that suit their interests and abilities. A great deal of patience, understanding, and information are essential to achieve these difficult goals.

Experience suggests additional guidelines. Patients need to be allowed some sense of control. Respecting their rights to participate in some of their own rehabilitation planning helps to restore feelings of self-worth. In this regard, the emphasis on function rather than complete recovery, pointing up success rather than performance failure, adds to the patients' sense of themselves as viable persons (Baretz & Stephenson, 1976; M. T. Sarno, 1986a; Tanner, 1980). It is essential to listen to patients, particularly to their expression of loss. Commiserations is often more comforting than optimistic prognostic statements.

Group speech therapy, stroke clubs, and other social groups are frequently used resources that can be effective tools in the management of some patients with chronic aphasia. They generally serve best after the acute, spontaneous recovery period, when patients are more aware of their deficits and less preoccupied with symptoms. By this time the patient may be more interested in and capable of interacting with others and can gain support by sharing feelings with those who have gone through the same experience. The National Aphasia Association (NAA) was founded in the United States in 1987, following the lead of existing organizations established in Finland in 1971, Germany in 1978, the United Kingdom in 1980, Sweden in 1981, and Montreal, Quebec, in 1988. Knowledge that one is not alone often helps to reduce depression and loneliness (Benson, 1979a; M. T. Sarno, 1980a).

Group therapy with peers also provides a permissive atmosphere in which patients can meet new friends and ventilate feelings. Not all aphasic patients can benefit from group therapy. A positive effect seems related to level of comprehension, time since onset, and personality factors. Although group therapy generally plays an important role in aphasia rehabilitation, much of its effectiveness depends on the skill of the group leader. Since group dynamics can be volatile and emotionally loaded, the inexperienced, untutored aphasia therapist would do best to avoid this therapy format. It is also difficult in small programs to have a sufficiently large pool of patients to create reasonably homogeneous groups.

The foregoing briefly describes a philosophy of rehabilitation that takes into account the broad spectrum of problems and residuals presented by aphasic patients. It is based primarily on experiences with the poststroke patient; however, the principles apply as well to the closed-head–injured aphasic patient, with some adjustments regarding the recovery timetable. The picture is also somewhat more complicated in that closed-head–injured patients usually present a greater number of behavioral, cognitive, and perceptual deficits. They are also generally younger, posing a great many social problems that are less apt to be present in the middle-aged and older person with aphasia (M. T. Sarno, 1980c; M. T. Sarno, Buonaguro, & Levita, 1987).

The late Hildred Schuell (Schuell et al., 1964) had great concern for the humanitarian aspects of aphasia rehabilitation. Some of her thoughts provide an apt conclusion for this section:

> There has always been a good deal of discussion about the art and the science of professions that include clinical practice as well as laboratory research. If by art one means appreciation of the fact that one is dealing with human life, and by science one means precise information, both are necessary and must go hand in hand. In a sense they have always done so. This is to say that asking questions and making observations is not the exclusive domain of

either art or science, or the clinic or the laboratory. The dichotomy seems to reflect the either-orishness that Aristotelian language habits have tended to impose on our thinking.

What the clinician cannot get along without, and what great artists and scientists alike have always had, is a kind of reverence for human life. . . . The great literature of all times and places has had something to say about the human condition as searching and as probing as the questions scientists have asked about the nature of the universe and the nature of man. Scientists have learned that one cannot leave the observer out of the operation, and clinicians know one cannot leave the laboratory out of the clinic. (p. 347)

The Aphasia Therapist

The aphasia therapist may be the most critical variable in the patient's rehabilitation. No approach or treatment technique can be effective unless it is implemented by an experienced, sophisticated, mature therapist.

To the experienced clinician, it is clear that no single technique is adequate to produce normal communication function and that the ideal overall approach, given our present state of knowledge, remains eclectic and specifically tailored to the individual patient. Fundamental to this therapeutic philosophy is the acknowledgment and appreciation of the uniqueness of the individual. This statement is not included here simply to pay lip service to the humanistic idea that we are all as individual as our fingerprints, but to underline in the most practical sense that no two aphasic persons are exactly alike in pathology, personality, linguistic deficits, reactions to catastrophic illness, life experience, spiritual values, and a host of other factors; that the influence of these factors carries different weight and strength at different stages of recovery; and that they are all inextricably related to recovery outcome.

A number of principles underlie daily practice. The first of these was stated by Brumfitt and Clarke (1980): Speech therapy is a "special case of the general art of psychotherapy" (p. 2). Basic to each therapeutic technique is the concept that it must contribute to the patient's psychological comfort and, conversely, should never feed into depression, frustration, anger, feelings of low self-esteem, or other negative emotions. This is uppermost in the mind of the experienced, enlightened therapist and dictates the selection of therapeutic activities. At the outset the therapist chooses those techniques or exercises that allow the patient to use preserved skills, thereby increasing the chances for successful performance. As therapists come to know patients better, they learn which activities facilitate the most successful performance and employ these as often as possible. These early therapeutic sessions should foster the growth of a trusting relationship between patient and therapist and lead to the therapist's image as a forgiving, accepting, and approving ally. A strictly pedagogic approach based upon preconceived notions of what is to be taught (except perhaps in the patient with mild aphasia or speech dyspraxia) must lead to failure, for what the therapist must attempt to do at this point is to help patients toward an acceptance of themselves as they are. This task is difficult and requires much time and patience, for aphasic patients see themselves as inferior and altered in the profoundest sense. A strong ego is required if the aphasic can continue to feel important and worthy of respect. Unfortunately, aphasia assaults even the strongest ego. Therapists, therefore, must become the patients' advocates while at the same time learning in greater detail what the patients can and cannot do.

Experience has revealed that the choice of remedial techniques is far less important than how they are applied. Any language-rehabilitation method may be used in aphasia therapy providing, of course, it is adapted to the individual patient. One must be careful to keep material at a level commensurate with the patient's ability to perform successfully. The choice of vocabulary, length of phrase or sentence, and grammatical or semantic complexity must often be restricted, although material should never be presented in anything other than an adult context. The effective therapist never pursues treatment activities that the patient perceives as meaningless. It is also essential that the therapist construct a program that makes use of cues that appear to enhance the possibility of evoking correct responses. For example, if a patient seems to be capable of completing words if the first letter is provided, this could be the basis for a sequence of drills; or if a patient is able to produce a word verbally if he or she writes it first, then this is a perfectly legitimate therapeutic strategy. As in all rehabilitation efforts, repetition and reinforcement are important.

Kindness and good intentions are insufficient for effective aphasia therapy. The competent therapist must also have a thorough knowledge of aphasia so as to be able to explain to patients and their families the causes of symptoms, reactions, and other behaviors. Sometimes these explanations require endless repetition before they can be comprehended and incorporated by the patient.

The subject of motivation always arises in the treatment of disabling neurological disorders. Experience suggests that, except for severely depressed individuals, who are unable to put forth much effort, patients generally produce everything they are capable of producing. Therapists must not allow their expectations to contaminate the therapeutic interaction; this is not uncommon and is usually motivated by laudatory aspirations—therapists want to see their patients improve—but is nonetheless counterproductive. Patients with involvement of subcortical areas may have low levels of activation, a purely physiological process independent of psychological motivation. The distinction between these two processes must be understood.

A clinical observation with particular relevance to aphasia therapy is the fact that anxiety invariably deteriorates performance. Although this is true regardless of whether an individual is suffering from a neurological disorder, it has special significance in the brain-damaged patient. The therapeutic setting and the quality of interaction between patient and therapist should be relaxed, quiet, and comfortable in order to elicit the patient's best performance. Families sometimes report that the patient performs better at home than in therapeutic sessions. This observation is probably related to the familiarity of the home setting.

One task requiring great skill is managing the process of treatment termination. For some patients speech–language rehabilitation need not go beyond a 2- or 3-week period of participation in selected language exercises and becoming informed about their condition. Others may require some form of speech rehabilitation (group and/or individual sessions) indefinitely. The criteria for termination cannot be reduced to a simple formula, for it depends upon multiple factors, including the patient's level of linguistic ability, psychological state (including adjustment to disability, level of anxiety or depression, dependency needs, ego strength, and self-esteem), family situation, opportunity for social contact, and vocational status. The aphasia therapist should strive to involve the patient in the termination process over a period of time, avoiding an abrupt discontinuation. The treatment termination process requires expert clinical judgment in evaluating and balancing a patient's linguistic skills, expectations, adequacy of support systems, and other relevant factors. Effective interaction with the patient in the treatment termination process demands tact, understanding, knowledge, and experience.

Experienced aphasia therapists evoke much respect and admiration for they engage in work that is always difficult and frequently underestimated considering the skill, wisdom, patience, and understanding that are required. Through knowledge of aphasic deficits, specific treatment techniques, and the needs of the patient, they make ever-changing judgments and decisions about patients' requirements from moment to moment, often balancing patients' needs for nurturance with the reality of their limitations.

Many ethical moral dilemmas face those who manage the rehabilitation of aphasic patients. One principal issue is a result of the necessity to select those individuals who will receive treatment. Rehabilitation medicine services are not only scarce in many situations, but they are also not a right or entitlement. Services are usually provided on a selective basis to those individuals believed to have the potential to "benefit." This process assumes that we know who can benefit (Caplan & Haas, 1987; Haas & Caplan, 1988; M. T. Sarno, 1986a, 1988). Many who are experienced in aphasia rehabilitation management believe that all aphasic persons should be given a trial treatment period to determine their candidacy for further treatment and that trials should be provided at different points in the recovery course. Goal setting, the patient's right to self-determination, and the criteria appropriate in determining the termination of therapy are also important ethical issues (M. T. Sarno, 1986a, 1990).

Conclusion

Historical realities suggest that the realm of recovery and rehabilitation in aphasia does not yet enjoy a firm basis in objective data. Until now a great deal of what is known and practiced depends upon clinical experience and the slow development of maturity and skill in those who undertake this difficult work. Systematic investigation to date has not sufficiently clarified the physiology and pathophysiology of communication or provided therapeutic blueprints for persistent disorders such as aphasia. To a large extent, successful treatment is compensatory in nature and the effective therapist is one who has learned from experience how to maximize the process of adjustment.

Despite the reality of anatomical and physiological pathology in aphasia, those who engage in this work have not been deterred. New knowledge and research have opened promising areas for exploring and developing more sophisticated rehabilitation techniques. Contemporary studies on language processing, new applications of microcomputer technology, the development of alternative communication systems, and research in the management of depression offer hope for improving treatment management. The study of human brain mechanisms is one of the last frontiers of biology, and as such will continue to be an irresistible challenge.

Acknowledgments

The preparation of the revised chapter was supported in part by the National Institute of Deafness and Other Communication Disorders (NIDCD) grant R01NS25367-01A1, on which the author is principal investigator, and the National Institute of Disability and Rehabilitation Research (NIDRR) grant G008300000. I am grateful to Antonia Buonaguro,

Sandra Beckman, and John Sarno for their assistance and support in the revision of this chapter and Laureen VanOudenrode for preparing the final manuscript.

References

American Heart Association. (1969). *Aphasia and the family* (Publication EM 359). Dallas: American Heart Association.

Aronson, M., Shatin, L., & Cook, J. (1956). Socio-psychotherapeutic approach to the treatment of aphasic patients. *Journal of Speech and Hearing Disorders, 21,* 352–364.

Aten, J. L. (1986). Function communication treatment. In R. Chapey (Ed.), *Language intervention strategies in adult aphasia* (2nd ed.). Baltimore, MD: Williams & Wilkins.

Aten, J. L., Caligiuri, M. P., & Holland, A. L. (1982). The efficacy of functional communication therapy for chronic aphasic patients. *Journal of Speech and Hearing Disorders, 47*(1), 93–96.

Backus, O. (1945). Rehabilitation of aphasic veterans. *Journal of Speech Disorders, 10,* 149–153.

Backus, O., Henry, L., Clancy, J., & Dunn, H. (1947). *Aphasia in adults.* Ann Arbor: University of Michigan Press.

Bailey, S. (1983). Blissymbolics and aphasia therapy: A case study. In C. Code & D. Muller (Eds.), *Aphasia therapy.* London: Arnold.

Baker, E., Berry, T., Gardner, H., Zurif, E., Davis, L., & Veroff, A. (1975). Can linguistic competence be dissociated from natural language functions? *Nature (London), 254,* 609–619.

Baretz, R., & Stephenson, G. (1976). Unrealistic patient. *New York State Journal of Medicine, 76*(Pt. 1), 54–57.

Basso, A., Capitani, E., & Moraschini, S. (1982). Sex differences in recovery from aphasia. *Cortex, 18,* 469–475.

Basso, A., Capitani, E., & Vignolo, L. (1979). Influence of rehabilitation on language skills in aphasic patients: A controlled study. *Archives of Neurology (Chicago), 36,* 190–196.

Basso, A., Capitani, E., & Zonobio, M. E. (1982). Pattern of recovery in oral and written expression and comprehension in aphasic patients. *Behavioural Brain Research, 6*(2), 115–128.

Basso, A., Faglioni, P., & Vignolo, L. (1975). Etude controlée de la réeducation du language dans l'aphasie: Comparaison entre aphasiques traites et non-traites. *Revue Neurologique, 131,* 607–614.

Bateman, F. (1890). *On aphasia and the localization of the faculty of speech* (2nd ed.). London: Churchill.

Bay, E. (1969). The Lordat case and its import on the theory of aphasia. *Cortex, 5,* 302–308.

Bayles, K. A., & Kaszniak, A. W. (1987). *Communication and cognition in normal aging and dementia.* Boston, MA: Little, Brown.

Benson, D. F. (1970). Language rehabilitation: Presentation 10. In A. Benton (Ed.), *Behavioral change in cerebrovascular disease.* New York: Harper.

Benson, D. F. (1979a). Aphasia. In K. M. Heilman & E. Valenstein (Eds.), *Clinical neuropsychology.* New York: Oxford University Press.

Benson, D. F. (1979b). *Aphasia, alexia, and agraphia.* New York: Churchill-Livingstone.

Benson, D. F. (1980). Psychiatric problems in aphasia. In M. T. Sarno & O. Hook (Eds.), *Aphasia: Assessment and treatment.* Stockholm: Almqvist & Wiksell; New York: Masson.

Benton, A. L. (1964). Contributions to aphasia before Broca. *Cortex, 1,* 314–327.

Benton, A. L., & Joynt, R. J. (1960). Early descriptions of aphasia. *Archives of Neurology (Chicago), 3,* 109–126.

Beukelman, D., Yorkston, K., & Dowden, P. (1985). Communication Augmentation: A Casebook of Clinical Management. San Diego: College Hill Press.

Beyn, E., & Shokhor-Trotskaya, M. (1966). The preventive method of speech rehabilitation in aphasia. *Cortex, 2,* 96–108.

Blackman, N. (1950). Group psychotherapy with aphasics. *Journal of Nervous and Mental Disease, 111,* 154–163.

Boone, D. (1965). *An adult has aphasia.* Danville, IL: Interstate.

Boone, D. (1967). A plan for rehabilitation of aphasic patients. *Archives of Physical Medicine and Rehabilitation, 48,* 410–414.

Borenstein, R., & Brown, G. (1990). *Neurobehavioral aspects of cerebrovascular disease.* New York: Oxford University Press.

Broadbent, D. (1879). A case of peculiar affection of speech, with commentary. *Brain, 1,* 484–503.

Broca, P. (1885). Du siège de la faculté du langage articule. *Bulletin de la Societe d'Anthropologie (Paris), 6,* 377–399.

Brubaker, S. H. (1978). *Workbook for aphasia: Exercises for the re-development of higher level language.* Detroit, MI: Wayne State University Press.

Brubaker, S. H. (1984). *Workbook for language skills.* Detroit, MI: Wayne State University Press.

Bruce, C., & Howard, D. (1987). Computer-generated phonemic cues: An effective aid for naming in aphasia. *British Journal of Disorders of Communication, 22,* 191–201.

Brumfitt, S., & Clarke, P. (1980, July). *An application of psychotherapeutic techniques to the management of aphasia.* Paper presented at the Summer Conference of Aphasia Therapy, Cardiff, England.

Brust, J., Shafer, S., Richter, R., & Bruun, B. (1976). Aphasia in acute stroke. *Stroke, 7,* 167–174.

Buck, M. (1968). *Dysphasia: Professional guidance for family and patient.* Englewood Cliffs, NJ: Prentice-Hall.

Burns, M. S., & Halper, A. S. (1988). Speech/language treatment of the aphasias. Rockville, MD: Aspen Publishers.

Butfield, E., & Zangwill, O. (1946). Re-education in aphasia: A review of 70 cases. *Journal of Neurology, Neurosurgery and Psychiatry, 9,* 75–79.

Buxbaum, J. (1967). Effect of nurturance on wives' appraisals of their marital satisfaction and the degree of their husband's aphasia. *Journal of Counseling Psychology, 31,* 240–243.

Cameron, C. (1973). *A different drum.* Englewood Cliffs, NJ: Prentice-Hall.

Caplan, A., & Haas, J. (1987, August). *Ethical and policy issues in rehabilitation medicine* (Hastings Center Report, Spec. Suppl. pp. 1–20). Briarcliff Manor, NY: Hastings Center.

Chapey, R. (1986). *Language intervention strategies in adult aphasia* (2nd ed.). Baltimore, MD: Williams & Wilkins.

Chester, S., & Egolf, D. (1974). Nonverbal communication and aphasia therapy. *Rehabilitation Literature, 35,* 231–233.

Coelho, C. A., & Duffy, R. J. (1987). The relationship of the acquisition of manual signs to severity of aphasia: A training study. *Brain and Language, 31*(2), 328–45.

Colby, K. M., Christinaz, D., & Graham, S. (1978). A computer-driven, personal, portable and intelligent speech prosthesis. *Computers and Biomedical Research, 11,* 337–343.

Colby, K. M., Christinaz, D., Parkinson, R. C., Graham, S., & Karpf, C. (1981). A word finding computer program with a dynamic lexical-semantic memory for patients with anomia using an intelligent speech prosthesis. *Brain and Language, 14,* 272–281.

Crewe, M. (1969, January-February). Training course: Stroke in your family. *Rehabilitation Record*, pp. 32–34.

Critchley, M. (1970). *Aphasiology and other aspects of language*. London: Arnold.

Culton, G. (1969). Spontaneous recovery from aphasia. *Journal of Speech and Hearing Research, 12*, 825–832.

Culton, G. (1971). Reaction to age as a factor in chronic aphasia in stroke patients. *Journal of Speech and Hearing Disorders, 36*, 563–564.

Dabul, B., & Bollier, B. (1976). Therapeutic approaches to apraxia. *Journal of Speech and Hearing Disorders, 41*, 268–276.

Dahlberg, C., & Jaffee, J. (1977). *Stroke: A physician's personal account*. New York: Norton.

Darley, F. (1970). Language rehabilitation: Presentation 8. In A. Benton (Ed.), *Behavioral change in cerebrovascular disease*. New York: Harper.

Darley, F. (1972). The efficacy of language rehabilitation in aphasia. *Journal of Speech and Hearing Disorders, 37*, 3–21.

Darley, F. (1975). Treatment of acquired aphasia. In W. J. Friedlander (ed.), *Advances in Neurology, 7*. New York: Raven Press. 111–145.

David, R., Enderby, P., & Bainton, D. (1982). Treatment of acquired aphasia—speech therapists and volunteers compared. *Journal of Neurology, Neurosurgery and Psychiatry, 45*, 957–961.

Davis, G. A. (1984). Effects of aging on normal language. In A. L. Holland (Ed.), *Language in adults: Recent advances*. San Diego, CA: College Hill Press.

Davis, G. A., & Holland, A. L. (1981). Age in understanding and treating aphasia. In D. S. Beasley & G. A. Davis (Eds.), *Aging communication processes and disorders*. New York: Grune & Stratton.

Davis, G. A., & Wilcox, M. J. (1985). *Adult aphasia rehabilitation: Applied pragmatics*. San Diego, CA: College Hill Press.

Deal, J., & Florance, C. (1978). Modification of the eight-step continuum for treatment of apraxia of speech in adults. *Journal of Speech and Hearing Disorders, 43*, 89–95.

Dean, E. C., Skinner, C. M., & Edmonstone, A. (1987). An efficacy study of functional communication therapy: preliminary findings. In E. Scherzer, R. Simon, & J. Stark (Eds.), *Proceedings of the First European Conference on Aphasiology*. Vienna: Austrian Workers Compensation Board.

Dell, S. O., Batson, R., Kasden, D. L., & Paterson, T. (1983). Aphasia in subdural hematoma. *Archives of Neurology (Chicago), 40*(3), 177–179.

Demeurisse, G., Verhos, M., & Capon, A. (1984). Resting CBF sequential study during recovery from aphasia due to ischemic stroke. *Neuropsychologia, 22*, 241–246.

Derman, S., & Manaster, A. (1967). Family counseling with relatives of aphasic patients at Schwab Rehabilitation Hospital. *Journal of the American Speech and Hearing Association, 9*, 175–177.

Dunkle, K. E., & Hooper, C. R. (1983). Using language to help depressed elderly aphasic persons. *Social Casework, 64*(9), 539–545.

Dworkin, J. P., Abharion, G. G., & Johns, D. F. (1988). Dyspraxia of speech: The effectiveness of a treatment regimen. *Journal of Speech and Hearing Disorders, 53*(3), 289–94.

Edwards, A. (1965). Automated training for a "matching-to-sample" task in aphasia. *Journal of Speech and Hearing Research, 8*, 39–42.

Eisenson, J. (1949). Prognostic factors related to language rehabilitation in aphasic patients. *Journal of Speech and Hearing Disorders, 14*, 262–264.

Eisenson, J. (1964). Aphasia: A point of view as to the nature of the disorder and factors that determine prognosis for recovery. *International Journal of Neurology, 4*, 287–295.

Eisenson, J. (1973). *Adult aphasia: Assessment and treatment*. Englewood Cliffs, NJ: Prentice-Hall.

Engle, G. (1964). Grief and grieving. *American Journal of Nursing, 64*, 93.

Espmark, S. (1973). Stroke before 50: A follow-up study of vocational and psychological adjustment. *Scandinavian Journal of Rehabilitation, Supplement*, No. 2.

Filby, Y., & Edwards, A. (1963). An application of automated-teaching methods to test and teach form discrimination to aphasics. *Journal of Programmed Instruction, 2*, 25–33.

Franz, S. (1924). Studies in re-education: The aphasics. *Journal of Comparative Psychology, 4*, 349–429.

Frazier, C., & Ingham, S. (1920). A review of the effects of gunshot wounds of the head. *Archives of Neurology and Psychiatry, 3*, 17–40.

Friedman, M. (1961). On the nature of regression. *Archives of General Psychiatry, 5*, 60–64.

Gardner, H., Zurif, E., Berry, T., & Baker, E. (1976). Visual communication in aphasia. *Neuropsychologia, 14*, 275–292.

Garrett, K., Beukelman, D., & Low-Morrow, D. (1989). A comprehensive augmentative communication system for an adult with Broca's Aphasia. *Augmentative and Alternative Communication, 5*, 55–61.

Gloning, K., Trappl, R., Heiss, W., & Quatember, R. (1976). Prognosis and speech therapy in aphasia. In Y. Lebrun & R. Hoops (Eds.), *Recovery in aphasics*. Amsterdam: Swets & Zeitlinger, B.V.

Godfrey, C., & Douglass, E. (1959). Recovery in aphasia. *Canadian Medical Association Journal, 80*, 618–624.

Goldstein, K. (1942). *After-effects of brain injuries in war: Their evaluation and treatment*. New York: Grune & Stratton.

Goldstein, K. (1948). *Language and language disturbances*. New York: Grune & Stratton.

Goodglass, H. (1985). Aphasiology in the United States. *International Journal of Neuroscience, 25*, 307–311.

Goodglass, H. (1987). Neurolinguistic principles and aphasia therapy. In M. Meier, A. Benton, & L. Diller (Eds.), *Neuropsychological rehabilitation*. New York and London: Guilford Press.

Goodglass, H., & Kaplan, E. (1972). *The assessment of aphasia and related disorders* (1st ed.). Philadelphia, PA: Lea & Febiger.

Goodglass, H., & Kaplan, E. (1983). *The assessment of aphasia and related disorders* (2nd ed.). Philadelphia, PA: Lea & Febiger.

Goodkin, R. (1968). Use of concurrent response categories in evaluating talking behavior in aphasic patients. *Perceptual Motor Skills, 26*, 1035–1040.

Gopfert, H. (1922). Beitrage zur Frage der Restitution nach Hirnverletzung. *Zeitschrift für die Gesamte Neurologie und Psychiatrie, 75*, 411–459.

Granich, L. (1947). *Aphasia: A guide to retraining*. New York: Grune & Stratton.

Haas, J. & Caplan A. (1988a). *Archives of Physical Medicine and Rehabilitation: Special Issue on Ethics, 69*, 5.

Haas, J., & Caplan, A. (1988b). *Case studies in ethics and rehabilitation*. Briarcliff Manor, NY: Hastings Center.

Hagen, C. (1973). Communication abilities in hemiplegia: Effect of speech therapy. *Archives of Physical Medicine and Rehabilitation, 54*, 454–463.

Halpern, H. (1981). Therapy for agnosia, apraxia, and dysarthria. In R. Chapey (Ed.), *Language intervention strategies in adult aphasia*. Baltimore, MD: Williams & Wilkins.

Hartman, J., & Landau, W. (1987). Comparison of formal language therapy with supportive counseling for aphasia due to acute vascular accident. *Archives of Neurology (Chicago), 44*, 646–649.

Hatfield, F., & Zangwill, O. (1974). Ideation in aphasia: The picture story method. *Neuropsychologia, 12,* 389–393.

Head, H. (1926). *Aphasia and kindred disorders of speech* (Vols. 1 & 2). London: Cambridge University Press.

Head, H. (1963). *Aphasia and kindred disorders of speech* (2nd ed.). New York: Hafner.

Helm, N. (1976). *Assessing candidacy for melodic intonation therapy.* Paper presented at American Speech and Hearing Association Convention, Houston, Texas.

Helm, N., & Benson, D. F. (1978). *Visual action therapy for global aphasia.* Presentation at the 16th annual meeting of the Academy of Aphasia, Chicago, IL.

Helm-Estabrooks, N. (1983). Exploiting the right hemisphere for language rehabilitation. Melodic intonation therapy. In E. Perecman (Ed.), *Cognitive processing in the right hemisphere.* New York: Academic Press.

Helm-Estabrooks, N., Fitzpatrick, P. M., & Barresi, B. (1982). Visual action therapy for aphasia. *Journal of Speech and Hearing Disorders, 47,* 385–389.

Helmick, J., Watamori, T., & Palmer, J. (1976). Spouses understanding of the communication disabilities of aphasic patients. *Journal of Speech and Hearing Disorders, 41,* 238–243.

Hodgins, E. (1964). *Episode.* New York: Atheneum.

Holland, A. L. (1969). Some current trends in aphasia rehabilitation. *Journal of the American Speech and Hearing Association, 11,* 3–7.

Holland, A. L. (1970). Case studies in aphasia rehabilitation using programmed instruction. *Journal of Speech and Hearing Research, 35,* 377–390.

Holland, A. L. (1982). Observing functional communication of aphasic adults. *Journal of Speech and Hearing Disorders, 47*(1), 50–56.

Holland, A. L., & Bartlett, C. S. (1985). Some differential effects of age on stroke-produced aphasia. In H. K. Ulatowska (Ed.), *The aging brain: Communication in the elderly.* San Diego, CA: College Hill Press.

Holland, A. L., Greenhouse, J. B., Fromm, D., & Swindell, C. S. (1989). Predictors of language restriction following stroke: A multivariate analyses. *Journal of Speech and Hearing Research, 32,* 232–238.

Holland, A. L., & Levy, C. (1971). Syntactic generalization in aphasics as a function of relearning an active sentence. *Acta Symbolica, 2,* 34–41.

Holland, A. L., Miller, J., Reinmuth, O., Bartlett, C., Fromm, D., Pashek, G., Stein, D., & Swindell, C. (1985). Rapid recovery from aphasia: A detailed language analysis. *Brain and Language, 24*(1), 156–173.

Holland, A. L., & Sonderman, J. (1974). Effects of a program based on the Token Test for teaching comprehension skills to aphasics. *Journal of Speech and Hearing Research, 17,* 589–598.

Huber, M. (1946). Linguistic problems of brain-injured servicemen. *Journal of Speech and Hearing Disorders, 11,* 143–147.

Hun, T. (1847). A case of amnesia. *American Journal of Insanity, 7,* 358.

Hunnicutt, S. (1989). Access: A lexical access program. *Proceedings of RESNA 12th Annual Conference* (pp. 284–235). New Orleans, LA.

Isserlin, M. (1929). Die pathologische physiologie der sprache. *Ergebnisse der Physiologie, Biologischen Chemie und Experimentellen Pharmakologie, 29,* 129.

Jakobson, R. (1955). Aphasia as a linguistic problem. In H. Werner (Ed.), *On expressive language.* Worcester, MA: Clark University Press.

Johannsen-Horbach, H., Cegla, B., Mager, U., & Schempp, B. (1985). Treatment of chronic global aphasia with a non-verbal communication system. *Brain and Language, 24,* 74–82.

Kaplan, E., Goodglass, H., & Weintraub, S. (1983). *Boston naming test* (2nd ed.). Philadelphia, PA: Lea & Febiger.

Katz, R. C. (1984). Using microcomputers in the diagnosis and treatment of chronic aphasic adults. *Seminars in Speech-Language-Hearing, 5,* 11–22.
Katz, R. C. (1987). Efficacy of aphasia treatment using microcomputers. *Aphasiology, 1,* 141–175.
Katz, R. C., & Nagy, V. (1983). A computerized approach for improving word recognition in chronic aphasic patients. In R. H. Brookshire (Ed.), *Clinical aphasiology: Conference proceedings.* Minneapolis, MN: BRK Publishers.
Keenan, J., & Brassell, E. (1974). A study of factors related to prognosis for individual aphasic patients. *Journal of Speech and Hearing Disorders, 39,* 257–269.
Keith, R. (1972). *Speech and language rehabilitation: A workbook for the neurologically impaired* (Vol. 1). Danville, IL: Interstate.
Keith, R. (1977). *Speech and language rehabilitation: A workbook for the neurologically impaired* (Vol. 2). Danville, IL: Interstate.
Keith, R. (1984). *Speech and language rehabilitation* (2nd ed., Vol. 2). Austin, TX: Pro-Ed.
Keith, R. (1987). *Speech and language rehabilitation* (3rd ed., Vol. 1). Austin, TX: Pro-Ed.
Kenin, M., & Swisher, L. (1972). A study of pattern of recovery in aphasia. *Cortex, 8,* 56–68.
Kertesz, A. (1979a). *Aphasia and associated disorders: Taxonomy, localization and recovery.* New York: Grune & Stratton.
Kertesz, A. (1979b). Recovery and treatment. In K. M. Heilman & E. Valenstein (Eds.), *Clinical neuropsychology.* New York: Oxford University Press.
Kertesz, A. (1981). Evolution of aphasic syndromes. *Topics in Language Disorders, 1*(4), 15–27.
Kertesz, A. (1984). Recovery from aphasia. In F. C. Kese (Ed.), *Advances in Neurology, 42,* New York: Raven Press.
Kertesz, A., & McCabe, P. (1977). Recovery patterns and prognosis in aphasia. *Brain and Language, 100,* 1–18.
Kilpatrick, K. (1980). *Working with words.* Akron, OH: Visiting Nurse Service.
Kinsella, G. J., & Duffy, F. (1978). The spouse of the aphasic patient. In Y. Lebrun & R. Hoops (Eds.), *The management of aphasia.* Amsterdam: Swets & Zeitlinger, B.V.
Kirshner, H. S., & Webb, N. G. (1981). Selective involvement of the auditory-visual modality in an acquired communication disorder: Benefit from sign language therapy. *Brain and Language, 13,* 161–170.
Knopman, D. S., Rubens, A. B., Selnes, O. A., Klassen, H. C., & Meyer, M. W. (1984). Mechanisms of recovery from aphasia: Evidence from serial XE-133 cerebral blood flow studies. *Annals of Neurology, 15*(6), 530–535.
Knopman, D. S., Selnes, O. A., Niccum, N., & Rubens, A. B. (1984). Recovery of naming in aphasia-relationship to fluency, comprehension and CT findings. *Neurology, 34*(11), 1461–1470.
Knopman, D. S., Selnes, O. A., Niccum, N., Rubens, A. B., Yoch, D., & Larsen, D. (1983). A longitudinal study of speech fluency in aphasia-CT correlates of recovery and persistent nonfluency. *Neurology, 33*(9), 1170–1178.
Kratt, A. W. (1990). Augmentative and alternative communication (AAC): Does it have a future in aphasia rehabilitation? *Aphasiology,* (4), 321–338.
Kubler-Ross, E. (1969). *On death and dying.* New York: Macmillan.
Lane, H., & Moore, D. (1962). Reconditioning a consonant discrimination in an aphasic: An experimental case history. *Journal of Speech and Hearing Disorders, 27,* 232–241.
Lane, V. W., & Samples, J. M. (1981). Facilitating communication skills in adult aphasics: Application of blissymbolics in a group setting. *Journal of Communication Disorders, 14,* 157–167.
Lavin, J. H. (1985). *Stroke: From crises to victory.* New York: Franklin Watts.

Lebrun, Y. (1976). Recovery in polyglot aphasics. In Y. Lebrun & R. Hoops (Eds.), *Recovery in aphasics*. Amsterdam: Swets & Zeitlinger, B.V.

Lebrun, Y. (1980). The aphasic condition. In M. T. Sarno & O. Hooks (Eds.), *Aphasia: Assessment and treatment*. Stockholm: Almqvist & Wiksell; New York: Masson.

LeMay, M. (1977). Asymmetries of the skull and handedness. *Journal of Neurological Sciences, 32,* 243–253.

Lendrem, W., & Lincoln, N. B. (1985). Spontaneous recovery of language abilities in stroke patients between 4 and 34 weeks post-stroke. *Journal of Neurology, Neurosurgery and Psychiatry, 48,* 743–748.

Lenneberg, E. (1967). *Biological foundations of language*. New York: Wiley.

Levin, H. S., Grossman, R. G., Sarwar, W., & Meyers, C. A. (1981). Linguistic recovery after closed head-injury. *Brain and Language, 12*(2), 360–74.

Levita, E. (1978). Effects of speech therapy on aphasics' responses to the Functional Communication Profile. *Perceptual and Motor Skills, 47,* 151–154.

Lincoln, N. B., Mulley, G. P., Jones, A. C., McGuirk, E., Lendrew, W., & Mitchell, J. R. (1984). Effectiveness of speech therapy for aphasic stroke patients—a randomized control trial. *Lancet, 1,* 1197–1200.

Linell, S., & Steg, G. (1980). Family treatment in aphasia-experience from a patient association. In M. T. Sarno & O. Hook (Eds.), *Aphasia: Assessment and treatment*. Stockholm: Almqvist & Wiksell; New York: Masson.

Lomas, A., & Kertesz, A. (1978). Patterns of spontaneous recovery in aphasic groups: A study of adult stroke patients. *Brain and Language, 5,* 388–401.

Longerich, M., & Bordeaux, J. (1954). *Aphasia therapeutics*. New York: Macmillan.

Lordat, J. (1843). Analyse de la parole pour servir à la théorie de divers cas d'alalie et de puralie (de mutisme et d'imperfection du parler) que les nosologistes ont mal connus. (Leçons tirées du cours de physiologie de l'ancée scolaire, 1842–1843). *Journal de la Societe de Medecine Pratique de Montpelier, 7,* 333, 417; *8,* 1.

Ludlow, C. L. (1977). Recovery from aphasia: A foundation for treatment. In M. Sullivan & M. Krommers (Eds.), *Rationale for adult aphasia therapy*. Omaha: University of Nebraska Medical Center.

Ludlow, C. L., Rosenberg, J., Dair, C., Buck, D., Schesselman, S., & Salazar, A. (1986). Brain lesions associated with nonfluent aphasia fifteen years following penetrating head injury. *Brain, 109,* 55–80.

Luria, A. R. (1948). *Rehabilitation of brain functioning after war traumas*. Moscow: Academy of Sciences Press.

Luria, A. R. (1963). *Restoration of function after brain injury*. New York: Macmillan.

Luria, A. R. (1966). *Human brain and psychological processes*. New York: Harper.

Malone, R. (1969). Expressed attitudes of families of aphasics. *Journal of Speech and Hearing Disorders, 34,* 146–151.

Marks, M., Taylor, M. L., & Rusk, H. (1957). Rehabilitation of the aphasic patient: A survey of three years experience in a rehabilitation setting. *Neurology, 7,* 837–843.

Marshall, N., & Holtzapple, P. (1976). Melodic intonation therapy: Variations on a theme. In R. Brookshire (Ed.), *Clinical aphasiology: Conference proceedings*. Minneapolis, MN: BRK Publications.

Marshall, R., & King, P. (1973). Effects of fatigue produced by isokinetic exercise on the communication ability of aphasic adults. *Journal of Speech and Hearing Research, 16,* 222–230.

Marshall, R., & Watts, M. (1976). Relaxation training: Effects on the communicative ability of aphasic adults. *Archives of Physical Medicine and Rehabilitation, 57,* 464–467.

Marshall, R. C. & Golper, L. A. (1983). Letter on treatment of acquired aphasia. *Journal of Neurology, Neurosurgery and Psychiatry, 46,* 689.

Marshall, R. C., & Philipps, D. S. (1983). Prognosis for improved verbal communication in aphasic stroke patients. *Archives of Physical Medicine & Rehabilitation. 64*, 597–600.

Marshall, R. C., Wertz, R. T., Weiss, D. G., & Aten, J. L. (1989). Home treatment for aphasic patients by trained professionals. *Journal of Speech and Hearing Disorders, 54*, 462–470.

McGlone, J. (1977). Sex differences in the cerebral organization of verbal functions in patients with unilateral brain lesions. *Brain, 100*, 775–793.

McGlone, J. (1980). Sex differences in human brain asymmetry: A critical survey. *Behavioural Brain Sciences, 3*, 215–263.

Mettler, C. C. (1947). *History of medicine.* Philadelphia, PA: Blakiston.

Millikan, C., & Darley, F. L. (1967). *Brain mechanisms underling speech and language.* New York: Grune & Stratton.

Mills, C. K. (1880, May). *Medical Bulletin* (cited in C. K. Mills, 1904).

Mills, C. K. (1904). Treatment of aphasia by training. *JAMA, Journal of the American Medical Association, 43*, 1940–1949.

Mills, R. H. (1982). Microcomputerized auditory comprehension training. In R. H. Brookshire (Ed.), *Clinical aphasiology: Conference proceedings.* Minneapolis, MN: BRK Publishers.

Mills, R. H., & Hoffer, P. (1985). Computers and caring: An integrative approach to the treatment of aphasia and head injury. In R. C. Marshall (Ed.), *Case studies in aphasia rehabilitation.* Baltimore, MD: University Park Press.

Moody, E. J. (1982). Sign-language acquisition by a global aphasic. *Journal of Nervous and Mental Disease, 170*, 113–116.

Morganstein, S., & Smith, M. C. (1982). *Thematic language stimulation.* Tucson, AZ: Communication Skill Builders.

Morley, H. (1960). Applying linguistics to speech and language therapy for aphasics. *Language and Learning, 10*, 135–149.

Moss, C. (1972). *Recovery with aphasia: The aftermath of my stroke.* Urbana: University of Illinois Press.

Naeser, M. A. (1975). A structured approach teaching aphasics basic sentence types. *British Journal of Disorders of Communication, 10*, 70–76.

Naeser, M. A., & Helm-Estabrooks, N. (1985). CT scan lesion evaluation and response to MIT with nonfluent aphasia cases. *Cortex, 21*(2), 203–225.

Newhoff, M., & Davis, G. (1978). A spouse intervention program: Planning, implementation, and problems of evaluation. In R. H. Brookshire (Ed.), *Clinical aphasiology: Conference proceedings.* Minneapolis, MN: BRK Publishers.

Nielson, J. (1936). *Agnosia, apraxia, aphasia: Their value in cerebral localization.* (Copyright 1936 by J. M. Nielsen, Los Angeles, California and 1946 by Hoeber, New York).

Norlin, P. F. (1986). Familiar faces, sudden strangers: Helping families cope with the crises of aphasia. In R. Chapey (Ed.), *Language intervention strategies in adult aphasia* (2nd ed.). Baltimore, MD: Williams & Wilkins.

Obler, L. K. (1980). Narrative discourse style in the elderly. In L. K. Obler & M. L. Albert (Eds.), *Language and communication in the elderly.* Lexington, MA: D. C. Heath.

Obler, L. K., & Albert, M. L. (1981). Language in the elderly aphasic and in the dementing patient. In M. T. Sarno (Ed.), *Acquired aphasia.* New York: Academic Press.

Obler, L. K., Nicholas, M., & Albert, M. L. (1985). On comprehension across the adult life span. *Cortex, 21*, 273–280.

Pashek, G. V., & Holland, A. L. (1988). Evolution of aphasia in the first year post-onset. *Cortex, 24*(3), 411–423.

Peacher, W. G. (1945). Speech disorders in World War II. *Journal of Speech Disorders, 10*, 155–161, 287–291.

Pieniadz, J. M., Naeser, M. A., Koff, E., & Levine, H. L. (1983). CT scan cerebral hemisphere asymmetries-measurements in stroke patients with global aphasia: Atypical asymmetries. *Cortex, 19*(3), 371–91.

Pickersgill, M. J. and Lincoln, N. B. (1983). Prognosis indicators and the pattern of recovery of communication in aphasic stroke patients. *Journal of Neurology, Neurosurgery and Psychiatry, 46,* 130–139.

Pincas, A. (1965). Linguistics and aphasia. *Australian Journal of the College of Speech Therapists, 15,* 20–28.

Pizzamiglio, L., Mammurcari, A., & Razzaro, C. (1985). Evidence for sex differences in brain organization in recovery in aphasia. *Brain and Language, 25*(2), 213–223.

Poeck, K., Huber, W., & Willmes, K. (1989). Outcome of intensive language treatment in aphasia. *Journal of Speech and Hearing Disorders, 54,* 471–479.

Poppelreuter, W. (1915). Ueber psychische ausfall sercheinungen nach hirveretzungen. *Muenchener Medizinische Wochenschrift, 62,* 489–491.

Porch, B. E. (1967). *Porch Index of Communicative Ability: Therapy and development* (Vol. 1). Palo Alto, CA: Psychologists Press.

Porch, B. E. (1973). *Porch Index of Communicative Ability: Administration, scoring, and interpretation* (Vol. 2). Palo Alto, CA: Consulting Psychologists Press.

Premack, D. (1971). Language in chimpanzee? *Science, 172,* 808–822.

Prins, R. S., Schoonen, R., & Vermeulen, J. (1989). Efficacy of two different types of speech therapy for aphasic stroke patients. *Applied Psycholinguistics, 10,* 85–123.

Prins, R. S., Snow, C., & Wagenaar, E. (1978). Recovery from aphasia: Spontaneous speech versus language comprehension. *Brain and Language, 6,* 192–211.

Rao, P., Basil, A. G., Koller, J. M., Fullerton, B., Diener, S., & Burton, P. (1980). The use of American-Indian Code by severe aphasics adults. In M. Burns & J. Andrews (Eds.), *Neuropathologies of speech and language diagnosis and treatment: Selected papers.* Evanston, IL: Institute for Continuing Education.

Rao, P., & Horner, J. (1978). Gesture as a deblocking modality in a severe aphasic patient. In R. Brookshire (Ed.), *Clinical aphasiology: Conference proceedings.* Minneapolis, MN: BRK Publications.

Reinvang, I. (1976). Sentence production in recovery from aphasia. In Y. Lebrun & R. Hoops (Eds.), *Recovery in aphasics.* Amsterdam: Swets & Zeitlinger, B.V.

Reinvang, I. (1980). A plan for rehabilitation of aphasics. *Scandinavian Journal of Rehabilitation Medicine, Supplement,* No. 7, 120–129. (In A. R. Fugl-Meyer [Ed.], *Stroke with hemiplegia,*Proceedings of a Symposium in Umea, Sweden, May 5–7, 1978.)

Reinvang, I., & Engvik, E. (1980). Language recovery in aphasia from 3–6 months after stroke. In M. T. Sarno & O. Hook (Eds.), *Aphasia: Assessment and treatment.* Stockholm: Almqvist & Wiksell; New York: Masson.

Ritchie, D. (1961). *Stroke: A study of recovery.* New York: Doubleday.

Rollin, W. J. (1984). Family therapy and the aphasic adult. In J. Eisenson (Ed.), *Adult aphasics.* Englewood Cliffs, NJ: Prentice-Hall.

Rolnick, I. (1969). Speech pathology services in a home health agency: The visiting nurse association of Detroit. *Journal of the American Speech and Hearing Association, 11,* 462–463.

Rose, C., Boby, V., & Capildeo, R. (1976). A retrospective survey of speech disorders following stroke, with particular reference to the value of speech therapy. In Y. Lebrun & R. Hoops (Eds.), *Recovery in aphasics.* Amsterdam: Swets & Zeitlinger, B.V.

Rosenbek, J. C. (1978). Treating apraxia of speech. In D. F. Johns (Ed.), *Clinical management of neurogenic communication disorders.* Boston, MA: Little, Brown.

Rosenbek, J. C. (1984). Advances in the evaluation and treatment of speech apraxia. *Advances in Neurology, 42,* 327–335.

Rosenbek, J. C., Hansen, R., Baughman, C., & Lemme, M. (1974). Treatment of developmental apraxia of speech: A case study. *Language, Speech and Hearing Services in the Schools, 5,* 13–22.

Rosenbek, J. C., Kent, R. D., & LaPointe, L. L. (1984). Apraxia of speech: An overview and some prospectives. In J. C. Rosenbek, M. McNeil, & A. Aronson (Eds.), *Apraxia of speech: Physiology and acoustics—linguistic management.* San Diego, CA: College Hill Press.

Rosenbek, J. C., Lemme, M., Ahern, M., Harris, E., & Wertz, R. (1973). A treatment for apraxia of speech in adults. *Journal of Speech and Hearing Disorders, 38,* 462–472.

Rosenberg, B. (1965). The performance of aphasics on automated visuo-perceptual discrimination, training, and transfer tasks. *Journal of Speech and Hearing Research, 8,* 165–181.

Rubow, R., Rosenbek, J. C., Collins, M. J., & Longstreth, D. (1982). Vibrotactile stimulation for intersystemic reorganization in the treatment of apaxia of speech. *Archives of Physical Medicine and Rehabilitation, 63,* 150–153.

Sands, E., Freeman, F., & Harris, K. (1978). Progressive changes in articulatory patterns in verbal apraxia: A longitudinal case study. *Brain and Language, 6,* 97–105.

Sands, E., Sarno, M. T., & Shankweiler, D. (1969). Long-term assessment of language function in aphasia due to stroke. *Archives of Physical Medicine and Rehabilitation, 50,* 203–207.

Sarno, J. E., & Sarno, M. T. (1969a). The diagnosis of speech disorders in brain damaged adults. *Medical Clinics of North America, 53,* 561–573.

Sarno, J. E., & Sarno, M. T. (1969b). *Stroke: The condition and the patient.* New York: McGraw-Hill.

Sarno, J. E., & Sarno, M. T. (1979). *Stroke: A guide for patients and their families.* (rev. ed.). New York: McGraw-Hill.

Sarno, J. E., Sarno, M. T., & Levita, E. (1971). Evaluating language improvement after completed stroke. *Archives of Physical Medicine and Rehabilitation, 52,* 73–78.

Sarno, J. E., Sarno, M. T., & Levita, E. (1973). The Functional Life Scale. *Archives of Physical Medicine and Rehabilitation, 54,* 214–220.

Sarno, M. T. (1968). Method for multivariant analysis of aphasia based on studies of 235 patients in a rehabilitation setting. *Archives of Physical Medicine and Rehabilitation, 49,* 210–216.

Sarno, M. T. (1969). *The Functional Communication Profile: Manual of directions.* New York: Howard A. Rusk Institute of Rehabilitation Medicine, New York University Medical Center.

Sarno, M. T. (1971). The role of the family in aphasia. In T. D. Hanley (Ed.), *The family as supportive personnel in speech and hearing remediation* (Proceedings of a Post-Gradute Course). Santa Barbara: University of California.

Sarno, M. T. (1974). Aphasia rehabilitation. In S. Dickson (Ed.), *Communication disorders: Remedial principles and practices.* Glenview, IL: Scott, Foresman.

Sarno, M. T. (1975). Disorders of communication in stroke. In S. Licht (Ed.), *Stroke and its rehabilitation.* Baltimore, MD: Williams & Wilkins.

Sarno, M. T. (1976). The status of research in recovery from aphasia. In Y. Lebrun & R. Hoops (Eds.), *Recovery in aphasics.* Amsterdam: Swets & Zeitlinger, B.V.

Sarno, M. T. (1980a). Aphasia rehabilitation. In M. T. Sarno & O. Hook (Eds.), *Aphasia: Assessment and treatment.* Stockholm: Almqvist & Wiksell; New York: Masson.

Sarno, M. T. (1980b). Language rehabilitation outcome in the elderly aphasic patient. In L. K. Obler & M. L. Albert (Eds.), *Language and communication in the elderly: Clinical, therapeutic, and experimental issues.* Lexington, MA: D. C. Heath.

Sarno, M. T. (1980c). The nature of verbal impairment after closed head injury. *Journal of Nervous and Mental Disease, 168*, 685–692.

Sarno, M. T. (1980d). Review of research in aphasia: Recovery and rehabilitation. In M. T. Sarno & O. Hook (Eds.), *Aphasia: Assessment and treatment.* Stockholm: Almqvist & Wiksell; New York: Masson.

Sarno, M. T. (1981). Recovery and rehabilitation in aphasia. In M. T. Sarno (Ed.), *Acquired aphasia.* New York: Academic Press.

Sarno, M. T. (1983). The functional assessment of verbal impairment. In G. Grimby (Ed.), *Recent advances in rehabilitation medicine.* Stockholm: Almqvist & Wiksell, International.

Sarno, M. T. (1984). Functional measurement in verbal impairment secondary to brain damage. In C. V. Granger & G. E. Gresham (Eds.), *Functional assessment in rehabilitation medicine.* Baltimore, MD: Williams & Wilkins.

Sarno, M. T. (1986a). *The silent minority: The patient with aphasia* (Hemphill Lecture). Chicago, IL: Rehabilitation Institute of Chicago.

Sarno, M. T. (1986b). *The academy of aphasia: A twenty-five year history 1960–1985.* New York Academy of Aphasia.

Sarno, M. T. (1988). The case of Mr. M.: The selection and treatment of aphasic patients. In J. Haas, A. L. Caplan, & D. Callahan (Eds.), *Case studies in Ethics and Medical Rehabilitation.* Briarcliff Manor, NY: Hastings Center.

Sarno, M. T. (1990). The Management of Aphasia. In R. A. Borenstein & G. G. Brown (Eds.). *Neurobehavioral aspects of cerebrovascular disease.* New York: Oxford University Press.

Sarno, M. T., Buonaguro, A., & Levita, E. (1985). Gender and recovery from aphasia after stroke. *Journal of Nervous and Mental Disease, 173*(10), 605–609.

Sarno, M. T., Buonaguro, A., & Levita, E. (1987). Aphasia in closed head injury and stroke. *Aphasiology, 1*(4), 513–516.

Sarno, M. T., & Levita, E. (1971). Natural course of recovery in severe aphasia. *Archives of Physical Medicine and Rehabilitation, 52*, 75–179.

Sarno, M. T., & Levita, E. (1979). Recovery in treated aphasia during the first year post-stroke. *Stroke, 10*, 663–670.

Sarno, M. T., & Levita, E. (1981). Some observations on the nature of recovery in global aphasia. *Brain and Language, 13*, 1–12.

Sarno, M. T., Silverman, M., & Levita, E. (1970). Psychosocial factors and recovery in geriatric patients with severe aphasia. *Journal of the American Geriatric Society, 18*, 405–409.

Sarno, M. T., Silverman, M., & Sands, E. (1970). Speech therapy and language recovery in severe aphasia. *Journal of Speech and Hearing Research, 13*, 607–623.

Sasanuma, S. (1988). Studies of dementia: In search of the linguistic/cognitive interaction underlying communication. *Aphasiology, 2*, 191–193.

Scargill, M. (1964). Modern linguistics and recovery from aphasia. *Journal of Speech and Hearing Disorders, 19*, 507–513.

Schneider, J. (1974). *The stresses of living: Loss.* Paper presented at Michigan State University (cited in Tanner, 1980).

Schuell, H., Jenkins, J., & Jiménez-Pabón, E. (1964). *Aphasia in adults.* New York: Harper.

Schwartz, G. E. (1983). Geriatric Evaluation by Relative's Rating Instrument (GERRI). *Psychopharmacology Bulletin, 24*(4), 713–716.

Segré, R. (1976). Autobiographical considerations on aphasic rehabilitation. *Folia Phoniatrica, 28*, 129–140.

Selnes, O. A., Knopman, D. S., Niccum, N., Rubens, A. B., & Larsen, D. (1983). Computed tomographic scan correlates of auditory comprehension deficits in aphasia. A prospective recovery study. *Annals of Neurology, 13*(5), 558–566.

Selnes, O. A., Niccum, N., Knopman, D. S., & Rubens, A. B. (1984). Recovery of single-word comprehension-CT scan correlates. *Brain and Language, 21*(1), 72–84.

Seron, X., Deloche, G., Bastard, V., Chassin, G., & Hermand, N. (1979). Word-finding difficulties and learning transfer in aphasic patients. *Cortex, 15,* 149–155.

Seron, X., Deloche, G., Monlard, G., & Rousselle, M. (1980). A computer-based therapy for the treatment of aphasic subjects with writing disorders. *Journal of Speech and Hearing Disorders, 45,* 45–58.

Shadden, B. B. (1987). Precrisis intervention: A tool for meeting the needs of significant others involved with aphasic older adults. *Topics in Language Disorders, 7*(3), 64–76.

Shane, H., & Darley, F. L. (1978). The effect of auditory rhythmic stimulation on articulatory accuracy in apraxia of speech. *Cortex, 14,* 444–450.

Sheehan, V. (1946). Rehabilitation of aphasics in an army hospital. *Journal of Speech and Hearing Disorders, 11,* 149–157.

Shewan, C. M. (1988). Expressive language recovery in aphasia using the Shewan Spontaneous Language Analysis (SSLA) System. *Journal of Communication Disorders, 21,* 155–169.

Shewan, C. M., & Cameron, H. (1984). Communication and related problems as perceived by aphasic individuals and their spouses. *Journal of Communication Disorders, 17*(3), 175–87.

Shewan, C. M., & Kertesz, A. (1984). Effects of speech and language treatment on recovery from aphasia. *Brain and Language, 23,* 272–299.

Simonson, J. (1971). *According to the aphasic adult.* Dallas, Texas: University of Texas Southwestern Medical School.

Singer, H., & Low, A. (1933). The brain in a case of motor aphasia in which improvement occurred with training. *Archives of Neurology and Psychiatry, 29,* 162–165.

Skelly, M. (1979). *Amer-Ind Gestural Code based on Universal American Indian Hand Talk.* New York: American Elsevier.

Skelly, M., Schinsky, L., Smith, R., & Fust, R. (1974). American Indian sign (AMERIND) as a facilitator of verbalization for the oral verbal apraxic. *Journal of Speech and Hearing Disorders, 39,* 445–456.

Smith, A. (1971). Objective indices of severity of chronic aphasia in stroke patients. *Journal of Speech and Hearing Disorders, 26,* 167–207.

Smith, A., Champoux, R., Leri, J., London, R., & Muraski, A. (1972). *Diagnosis, intelligence and rehabilitation of chronic aphasics* (Final Report). Ann Arbor: University of Michigan, Department of Physical Medicine and Rehabilitation.

Smith, B. L., Wasowicz, J., & Preston, J. (1987). Temporal characteristics of the speech of normal elderly adults. *Journal of Speech and Hearing Research, 30,* 522–529.

Smith, M. (1974). Operant conditioning of syntax in aphasia. *Neuropsychologia, 12,* 403–405.

Smith, M. C., & Morganstein, S. (1988). *Thematic picture stimulation.* Tucson, AZ: Communication Skill Builders.

Sparks, R., Helm, N., & Albert, M. (1974). Aphasia rehabilitation resulting from melodic intonation therapy. *Cortex, 10,* 303–316.

Spencer, G. (1984). U.S. Bureau of the Census. "Projects of the population of the United States, by age, sex, and race: 1983 to 2080." *Current Population Reports,* Series P-25, No. 952.

Spreen, O., & Benton, A. (1969). *Neurosensory Center Comprehensive Examination for Aphasia* (1st ed.). Victoria, BC: University of Victoria, Department of Psychology.

Spreen, O., & Benton, A. (1977). *Neurosensory Center Comprehensive Examination for Aphasia* (2nd ed). Victoria, BC: University of Victoria, Department of Psychology.

Steele, R. D., Weinrich, M., Kleczewska, M. K., Carlson, G. S., & Wertz, R. T. (1987). Evaluating performance of severely aphasic patients on a computer-aided visual communication system. In R. H. Brookshire (Ed.), *Clinical aphasiology: Conference proceedings.* Minneapolis, MN: BRK Publishers.

Steele, R. D., Weinrich, M., Wertz, R. T., Kleczewska, M., & Carlson, G. (1989). Computer-based visual communication in aphasia. *Neuropsychologia, 27,* 409–426.

Stoicheff, M. (1960). Motivating instructions and language performance of dysphasic subjects. *Journal of Speech and Hearing Research, 3,* 755–85.

Strauss, A., Burrucker, J., Cicero, J., & Edwards, R. (1967, November-December). Group-work with stroke patients. *Rehabilitation Record,* pp. 30–32.

Stryker, S. (1975). *Speech after stroke: A manual for the speech pathologist and the family member.* Springfield, IL: Thomas.

Tanner, D. (1980). Loss and grief: Implications for the speech-language pathologist and audiologist. *Journal of the American Speech and Hearing Association, 22,* 916–926.

Taylor, M. L. (1958). *Understanding aphasia: A guide for family and friends.* New York: Howard A. Rusk Institute of Rehabilitation Medicine, New York University Medical Center.

Taylor, M. L. (1964a). Language therapy. In H. Burr (Ed.), *The aphasic adult: Evaluation and rehabilitation.* Charlottesville, VA: Wayside Press.

Taylor, M. L. (1964b). Linguistic considerations of the verbal behavior of brain damaged adults. *Linguistic Reporter, 6,* 1–2.

Taylor, M. L. (1965). A measurement of functional communication in aphasia. *Archives of Physical Medicine and Rehabilitation, 46,* 101–107.

Taylor, M. L., & Marks, M. (1955). *The basic 100 words: Aphasia rehabilitation manual and workbook.* New York: McGraw-Hill.

Taylor, M. L., & Marks, M. (1959). *Aphasia rehabilitation manual and therapy kit.* New York: Howard A. Rusk Institute of Rehabilitation Medicine, New York University Medical Center.

Taylor, M. L., & Sands, E. (1966). Application of programmed instruction techniques to the language rehabilitation of severely impaired aphasic patients. *Journal of the National Society of Programmed Instruction, 5,* 10–11.

Tikofsky, R., & Reynolds, G. (1963). Further studies of non-verbal learning and aphasia. *Journal of Speech and Hearing Research, 6,* 133–143.

Traendly, C. A. (1977). *Aphasia rehabilitation.* Tigard, OR: C. C. Publications.

Turnblom, M., & Meyers, J. (1952). A group discussion program with the families of aphasic patients. *Journal of Speech and Hearing Disorders, 17,* 393–396.

Ulatowska, H. K., & Chapman, S. B. (1989). Discourse consideration for aphasia management. *Seminars in Speech and Language, 10*(4), 298–31.

Ulatowska, H. K., & Richardson, S. (1974). A longitudinal study of an adult with aphasia: Considerations for research and therapy. *Brain and Language, 1,* 151–166.

Ullman, M. (1962). *Behavioral changes in patients following strokes.* Springfield, IL: Thomas.

United States Census Bureau. (1975, February). *Current population report* (Publication No. 541). Washington, DC: U.S. Government Printing Office.

United States Department of Health and Human Services. (1988). *Aging America: Trends and projections, 1987–1988* ed. Washington, DC: U.S. Government Printing Office.

Velletri-Glass, A., Gazzaniga, M., & Premack, D. (1973). Artificial language training in global aphasics. *Neuropsychologia, 11,* 95–103.

Vignolo, L. (1964). Evolution of aphasia and language rehabilitation: A retrospective exploratory study. *Cortex, 1,* 344–367.

Wade, D. T., Hewer, R. L., & Wood, V. A. (1984a). Stroke: Influence of age on outcome. *Age Ageing, 13,* 357–362.

Wade, D. T., Hewer, R. L., & Wood, V. A. (1984b). Stroke: Influence of patients' sex and side of weakness on outcome. *Archives of Physical Medicine and Rehabilitation, 65,* 513–516.

Währborg, P., & Borenstein, P. (1989). Family therapy in families with an aphasic member. *Aphasiology, 3*(1), 93–98.

Watzlawick, P., & Coyne, J. (1980). Depression following stroke: Brief, problem-focused family treatment. *Family Process, 19*, 13–18.

Weigl, E. (1961). The phenomenon of temporary deblocking in aphasia. *Zeitschrift fuer Phonetik, Sprachwissenschaft und Kommunikationsforschung, 14*(Pt. 4), 337–364.

Weinrich, M., Steele, R. D., Carlson, G. S., & Kleczweska, M. (1989a). Processing of visual syntax in a globally aphasic patient. *Brain and Language, 36*, 391–405.

Weinrich, M., Steele, R. D., Kleczweska, M., Carlson, G. S., Baker, E. & Wertz, R. T. (1989b). Representations of verbs in a computerized visual communication system. *Aphasiology, 3*, 501–512.

Weinrich, M., Steele, R. D., & Illes, J. (1985). Implementation of a visual communicative system for aphasic patients on a microcomputer. *Annals of Neurology, 18*, 148.

Weisenburg, T., & McBride, K. (1935). *Aphasia: A clinical and psychological study*. New York: Commonwealth Fund.

Weisenburg, T., & McBride, K. (1964). *Aphasia: A clinical and psychological study* (2nd ed.), New York: Hafner.

Weniger, D., Huber, W., Stachowiak, F. J., & Poeck, K. (1980). Treatment of aphasia on a linguistic basis. In M. T. Sarno & O. Hook (Eds.), *Aphasia: Assessment and treatment*. Stockholm: Almqvist & Wiksell; New York: Masson.

Wepman, J. (1951). *Recovery from aphasia*. New York: Ronald Press.

Wepman, J. (1953). A conceptual model for the processes involved in recovery from aphasia. *Journal of Speech and Hearing Disorders, 18*, 4–13.

Wepman, J. (1972). Aphasia therapy: A new look. *Journal of Speech and Hearing Disorders, 37*, 201–214.

Wepman, J. (1976). Aphasia: Language without thought or thought without language? *Journal of the American Speech and Hearing Association, 18*, 131–136.

Wepman, J., & Jones, L. (1958). *The development of the Language Modalities Test for Aphasia* (Final Summary Report). Washington, DC: U.S. Department of Health, Education & Welfare.

Wepman, J., & Morency, A. (1963). Filmstrips as an adjunct to language therapy for aphasia. *Journal of Speech and Hearing Disorders, 28*, 191–194.

Wertz, R. T. (1984). Language disorders in adults: State of the clinical art. In A. L. Holland (Ed.), *Language disorders in adults*. San Diego, CA: College Hill Press.

Wertz, R. T., Collins, M. J., Weiss, D., Kurtzke, J. F., Friden, T., Brookshire, R. H., Pierce, J., Holtzapple, P., Hubbard, D. J., Porch, B. E., West, J. A., Davis, L., Matovitch, V., Morley, G. K., & Resureccion, E. (1981). VA cooperative study on aphasia: A comparison of individual and group treatment. *Journal of Speech and Hearing Disorders, 24*, 580–594.

Wertz, R. T., & Dronkers, N. (1988, September) *Effects of age on aphasia*. Paper presented at the American Speech-Language-Hearing Association Research Symposium on Communication Sciences and Disorders and Aging, Washington, DC.

Wertz, R. T., LaPointe, L. L., & Rosenbek, J. C. (1984). *Apraxia of speech: The disorder and its management*. New York: Grune & Stratton.

Wertz, R. T., Weiss, D. G., Aten, L. J., Brookshire, R. H., Garcia-Buñuel L., Holland, A. L., Kurtzke, J. F., Greenbaum, H., Marshall, R., Vogel, D., Carter, J., Barnes, N., & Goodman, R. (1986). Comparison of clinic, home and deferred language treatment for aphasia: A VA cooperative study. *Archives of Neurology (Chicago), 43*, 653–658.

Wiedel, I. M. H. (1976). The basic foundation approach for decreasing aphasia and verbal apraxia in adults (BFA). In R. H. Brookshire (Ed.), *Clinical aphasiology: Conference proceedings*. Minneapolis, MN: BRK Publishers.

Wiegel-Crump, C. (1976). Agrammatism and aphasia. In Y. Lebrun & R. Hoops (Eds.), *Recovery in aphasics*. Amsterdam: Swets & Zeitlinger, B.V.

Wiegel-Crump, C., & Koenigsknecht, R. (1973). Tapping the lexical store of the adult aphasic: Analysis of the improvement made in word retrieval skills. *Cortex, 9,* 410–417.

Williams, S. E., & Freer, C. A. (1986). Aphasia: Its effect on marital relationships. *Archives of Physical Medicine and Rehabilitation, 67,* 250–252.

Wint, G. (1967). *The third killer: Meditations on a stroke*. New York: Abelard.

Worral, L. S. (1989). Aphasia and family therapy: Innovative, but untested. *Aphasiology, 13* (5), 483–485.

Wulf, H. (1973). *Aphasia: My world alone*. Detroit, MI: Wayne State University Press.

Wyllie, J. (1894). *The disorders of speech*. Edinburgh: Oliver & Boyd.

Yarnell, P., Monroe, P., & Sobel, L. (1976). Aphasia outcome in stroke: A clinical neuroradiological correlation. *Stroke, 7,* 514–522.

Subject Index